T0198043

MEDICAL

SECRETS

MEDICAL

SECRETS

Sixth Edition

MARY P. HARWARD, MD, FACP
Internal Medicine and Geriatrics
Orange, California

ELSEVIER

ELSEVIER

1600 John F. Kennedy Blvd.
Ste 1800
Philadelphia, PA 19103-2899

MEDICAL SECRETS, SIXTH EDITION

ISBN: 978-0-323-47872-4

Notices

Knowledge and best practice in this field are constantly changing. As new research and experience broaden our understanding, changes in research methods, professional practices, or medical treatment may become necessary.

Practitioners and researchers must always rely on their own experience and knowledge in evaluating and using any information, methods, compounds, or experiments described herein. In using such information or methods they should be mindful of their own safety and the safety of others, including parties for whom they have a professional responsibility.

With respect to any drug or pharmaceutical products identified, readers are advised to check the most current information provided (i) on procedures featured or (ii) by the manufacturer of each product to be administered, to verify the recommended dose or formula, the method and duration of administration, and contraindications. It is the responsibility of practitioners, relying on their own experience and knowledge of their patients, to make diagnoses, to determine dosages and the best treatment for each individual patient, and to take all appropriate safety precautions.

To the fullest extent of the law, neither the Publisher nor the authors, contributors, or editors, assume any liability for any injury and/or damage to persons or property as a matter of products liability, negligence or otherwise, or from any use or operation of any methods, products, instructions, or ideas contained in the material herein.

Previous editions copyrighted in 2012, 2005, 2001, 1996, 1991.

Library of Congress Cataloging-in-Publication Data

Names: Harward, Mary P., editor.
Title: Medical secrets / [edited by] Mary P. Harward.
Description: Sixth edition. | Philadelphia, PA : Elsevier Inc., [2019] |
    Includes bibliographical references and index.
Identifiers: LCCN 2017058627 | ISBN 9780323478724 (pbk. : alk. paper)
Subjects: | MESH: Internal Medicine | Examination Questions
Classification: LCC RC58 | NLM WB 18.2 | DDC 616.0076--dc23 LC record available at
https://lccn.loc.gov/2017058627

Executive Content Strategist: James Merritt
Content Development Manager: Louise Cook
Publishing Services Manager: Catherine Jackson
Senior Project Manager: Sharon Corell
Book Designer: Bridget Hoette

Printed in the United States.

Last digit is the print number: 9   8   7   6   5   4   3   2

To our patients who have shared with us the secrets of their health and illness.

CONTRIBUTORS

William L. Allen, M. Div, JD
Associate Professor
Department of Community Health and Family Medicine
Program in Bioethics, Law, and Medical
Professionalism
University of Florida College of Medicine
Gainesville, Florida

Katherine Vogel Anderson, PharmD, BCACP
Associate Professor
University of Florida College of Pharmacy and Medicine
Gainesville, Florida

Rhonda A. Cole, MD, FACG
Associate Section Chief
Department of Gastroenterology
Associate Professor
Department of Internal Medicine
Baylor College of Medicine
Houston, Texas

Kathryn H. Dao, MD, FACP, FACR
Associate Director of Clinical Rheumatology
Baylor Research Institute
Dallas, Texas

Nathan A. Gray, MD
Assistant Professor of Medicine
Division of General Internal Medicine
Duke University School of Medicine
Durham, North Carolina

Gabriel Habib, Sr., MS, MD, FACC, FCCP, FAHA
Professor of Medicine and Cardiology
Baylor College of Medicine
Director of Education and Associate Chief
Section of Cardiology
Michael E. DeBakey VA Medical Center
Houston, Texas

Eloise M. Harman, MD
Staff Physician and MICU Director
Malcom Randall VA Medical Center
Professor Emeritus of Medicine
University of Florida College of Medicine
Gainesville, Florida

Mary P. Harward, MD, FACP
Internal Medicine and Geriatrics
Orange, California

Timothy R.S. Harward, MD, FACS
Vascular and Interventional Specialists of Orange
County
Orange, California

Teresa G. Hayes, MD, PhD
Associate Professor
Department of Internal Medicine
Hematology-Oncology Section
Baylor College of Medicine
Chief
Hematology-Oncology Section
Michael E. DeBakey VA Medical Center
Houston, Texas

Nisreen Husain, MD
Director
GI Motility
Department of Gastroenterology
Baylor College of Medicine
Houston, Texas

Ankita Kadakia, MD
Assistant Professor of Clinical Medicine
Division of Infectious Diseases
University of California San Diego Medical
Center – Owen Clinic
San Diego, California

Henrique Elias Kallas, MD, CMD
Assistant Professor
Departments of Medicine and Aging
University of Florida College of Medicine
Gainesville, Florida

Alexander S. Kim, MD
Assistant Professor of Medicine
Associate Program Director
Allergy/Immunology Fellowship Program
University of California, San Diego
San Diego, California

Roger Kornu, MD, FACR
Affiliated Physician
University of California, Irvine
Irvine, California

R. Anjali Kumbla, MD
Department of Hematology/Oncology
The Southeast Permanente Medical Group
Athens, Georgia

Daniel Lee, MD
Clinical Professor of Medicine
Division of Infectious Diseases
University of California San Diego Medical
Center—Owen Clinic
San Diego, California

Harrinarine Madhosingh, MD, FACP, FIDSA
Attending Physician
Infectious Disease
Central Florida Infectious Disease Specialists
Assistant Professor
Department of Medicine
University of Central Florida
Orlando, Florida

Ara Metjian, MD
Assistant Professor
Division of Hematology
Department of Medicine
Duke University School of Medicine
Durham, North Carolina

John Meuleman, MD
Geriatric Research, Education, and Clinical
    Center
University of Florida College of Medicine
Gainesville, Florida

Jeffrey M. Miller, MD
Chief
Division of Hematology/Oncology
Program Director
Hematology/Oncology Fellowship
Olive View—UCLA Medical Center
Cedars Sinai Medical Center
Kaiser Sunset
Associate Clinical Professor of Medicine
David Geffen School of Medicine at UCLA
Olive View UCLA Medical Center
Los Angeles, California

Yamini Natarajan, MD
Assistant Professor
Department of Gastroenterology
Baylor College of Medicine
Michael E. DeBakey VA Medical Center
Houston, Texas

Catalina Orozco, MD
Rheumatology Associates
Dallas Texas

Rahul K. Patel, MD, FACP, FACR
Medical Director
PRA Health Sciences
Dallas, Texas

Sharma S. Prabhakar, MD, MBA, FACP, FASN
Professor and Chief
Division of Nephrology
Vice-Chair
Department of Medicine
Texas Tech University Health Sciences Center
Lubbock, Texas

Nila S. Radhakrishnan, MD
Assistant Professor and Chief
Division of Hospital Medicine
Department of Medicine
University of Florida College of Medicine
Gainesville, Florida

Eric I. Rosenberg, MD, MSPH, FACP
Associate Professor and Chief
Division of General Internal Medicine
Department of Medicine
University of Florida College of Medicine
Associate Chief Medical Officer
University of Florida Health Shands Hospitals
Gainesville, Florida

Abbas Shahmohammadi, MD
Assistant Professor
Division of Pulmonary and Critical Care Medicine
Department of Medicine
University of Florida College of Medicine
Gainesville, Florida

Damian Silbermins, MD
Huntington Internal Medicine Group
Huntington, West Virginia

Amy M. Sitapati, MD
Clinical Professor of Medicine
Chief Medical Information Officer of Population Health
University of California San Diego Health
San Diego, California

David B. Sommer, MD, MPH
Neurology, Movement Disorders
Reliant Medical Group
Worcester, Massachusetts

Susan E. Spratt, MD
Associate Professor
Division of Endocrinology
Department of Medicine
Duke University School of Medicine
Durham, North Carolina

Adriano R. Tonelli, MD
Assistant Professor
Division of Pulmonary, Allergy, and
    Critical Care Medicine
Case Western Reserve University School of Medicine
Cleveland, Ohio

Whitney W. Woodmansee, MD
Endocrinology
Mayo Clinic—Jacksonville
Jacksonville, Florida

Jason A. Webb, MD, FAPA
Director of Education
Duke Center for Palliative Care
Assistant Professor
Department of Medicine
Department of Psychiatry and Behavioral Sciences
Duke University School of Medicine
Durham, North Carolina

PREFACE

Most of my post-training professional life has been concurrent with the six editions of this book, and I have seen astounding scientific and therapeutic changes with each new update of *Medical Secrets*. The chapters in the sixth edition reflect the many major changes in medical science, prevention, and therapy that have occurred since the book was first published in 1991. For instance, in the first edition the mortality rate from Acquired Immunodeficiency Syndrome (AIDS) was cited as 75% at 3 years, and treatment of AIDS as a chronic disease was not discussed. The sixth edition now notes the 36.9 million people *living* with Human Immunodeficiency Virus (HIV) and AIDS and includes questions on preventive treatments. Elsewhere, the Gastroenterology chapter contrasts the lack of even screening tests for hepatitis C in 1991 with questions on contemporary effective methods for hepatitis C treatment in 2018. Similar contrasts can be found in all the chapters. Also noteworthy are the chapters added to later editions on Medical Ethics and Palliative Medicine, acknowledging the increased presence of these disciplines in everyday medical practice.

The contributor list has also significantly changed since the first edition with new contributors to this edition adding their fresh perspectives. In addition, Drs. Cole, Habib, and Prabhaker deserve special recognition for faithfully updating their chapters from the first through the sixth editions.

I hope the students using this book will appreciate and acknowledge the perspectives in the previous editions, yet sense how quickly medicine adapts to new discoveries. Many of the quotes at the beginning of the chapters reflect the historical context of the disciplines and hopefully may prompt the reader to investigate the original sources. Perhaps some of the students reading the text today will be future contributors and remember how medicine was practiced "back during the time of the sixth edition."

Mary P. Harward, MD, FACP
Orange, California

CONTENTS

TOP 100 SECRETS

These secrets are 100 of the top board alerts. They summarize the most important concepts, principles, and salient details of internal medicine.

1. Informed consent is not merely a signature on a form but a process by which the patient and physician discuss and deliberate the indications, risks, and benefits of a test, therapy, or procedure and the patient's outcome goals.
2. Patients should participate in informed consent, even if they have impaired memory or communication skills, whenever they have sufficient decision-making capacity.
3. Decision-making capacity is determined by assessing the patient's ability to (1) comprehend the indications, risks, and benefits of the intervention; (2) understand the significance of the underlying medical condition; (3) deliberate the provided information; and (4) communicate a decision.
4. Many states now have specific physician-signed order forms to indicate a patient's end-of-life preferences for resuscitation and intensity of care.
5. All adults need one dose of tetanus, diphtheria, pertussis (Tdap) vaccine in place of one booster dose of tetanus-diphtheria (Td) vaccine to improve adult immunity to pertussis (whooping cough).
6. Zoster vaccine is indicated for adults ≥ 60 years old even if they have had an episode of herpes zoster infection.
7. Adolescent girls and boys should begin human papillomavirus (HPV) vaccine at age 11–12 to prevent HPV infection and reduce cervical cancer risk. Those who start at a later age can "catch up" through age 21 (men) or age 26 (women).
8. High-risk patients and those 65 years and older should receive two types of pneumococcal vaccine: pneumococcal conjugate vaccine (PCV13) and pneumococcal polysaccharide vaccine (PCV23) at least 12 months apart.
9. Antibiotic prophylaxis before dental procedures is recommended only for patients with (1) significant congenital heart disease; (2) previous history of endocarditis; (3) cardiac transplantation; and (4) prosthetic valve.
10. "Routine" preoperative testing is not helpful to reduce surgical risk. Laboratory and procedural tests should be ordered to address the acuity or stability of a medical problem or to investigate an abnormal symptom or physical sign identified during the consultation.
11. Preoperative consultation should include identification of risk factors for postoperative venous thromboembolism and appropriate treatment.
12. Patients undergoing major surgery who are at risk of adrenal suppression may need glucocorticoid therapy in the perioperative period. Some patients, though, may just need close monitoring postoperatively for signs of adrenal insufficiency.
13. "Tight" control of diabetes with target blood sugar of 80–110 mg/dL may not be beneficial postoperatively.
14. Metformin should be held and renal function closely monitored for patients undergoing surgery or imaging procedures involving contrast agents.
15. Asking the patient about personal and family history of bleeding episodes associated with minor procedures or injury is as effective in identifying bleeding diatheses as measuring coagulation studies.
16. Noninvasive stress testing has the best predictive value for detecting coronary artery disease (CAD) in patients with an intermediate (30–80%) pretest likelihood of CAD and is of limited value in patients with very low (<30%) or very high (>80%) likelihood of CAD.
17. Routine use of daily low-dose aspirin (81–325 mg) can reduce the likelihood of cardiovascular disease in high-risk patients with known CAD, diabetes, stroke, or peripheral or carotid vascular disease.
18. Routine daily low-dose aspirin use is associated with an increased risk of gastrointestinal bleeding, which can be reduced through the use of proton pump inhibitors.
19. Right ventricular infarction should also be considered in any patient with signs and symptoms of inferior wall myocardial infarction.

1

20. Diabetes is considered an equivalent of known CAD, and treatment and prevention guidelines for diabetic patients are similar to those for patients with CAD.
21. Patients with congestive heart failure (CHF) and left ventricular ejection fraction (LVEF) < 35% with class II or III New York Heart Association (NYHA) symptoms should be considered for implantable cardiac defibrillator.
22. Consider aortic dissection in the differential diagnosis of all patients presenting with acute chest or upper back pain.
23. Increasing size of an abdominal aortic aneurysm (AAA) increases the risk of rupture. Patients with AAA greater than 5 cm or aneurysmal symptoms should have endovascular or surgical repair. Smaller aneurysms should be followed closely every 6 to 12 months by computed tomography (CT) scan.
24. Patients presenting with pulselessness, pallor, pain, paralysis, and paresthesia of a limb likely have acute limb ischemia due to an embolus and require emergent evaluation for thrombolytic therapy or revascularization.
25. Patients with symptoms of transient ischemic attack are at high risk of stroke and require urgent evaluation for carotid artery disease and treatment that may include antiplatelet agents, carotid endarterectomy, statin drugs, antihypertensive agents, and anticoagulation.
26. All patients with peripheral arterial disease and cerebrovascular disease should stop smoking.
27. Asthma, chronic obstructive pulmonary disease (COPD), CHF, vocal cord dysfunction, and upper airway cough syndrome (UACS) can all cause wheezing.
28. Inhaled corticosteroid therapy should be considered for asthmatic patients with symptoms that occur with more than intermittent frequency.
29. Pulmonary embolism cannot be diagnosed by history, physical examination, and chest radiograph alone. Additional testing such as D-dimer level, spiral chest CT scan, angiography, or a combination of these tests will be needed to effectively rule in or rule out the disease.
30. Sarcoidosis is a multisystem disorder that frequently presents with pulmonary findings of abnormal chest radiograph, cough, dyspnea, or chest pain.
31. Hepatitis C virus infection can lead to cirrhosis, hepatocellular carcinoma, and severe liver disease requiring liver transplantation. Routine screening for infection is helpful for certain high-risk groups including those born in the United States between 1945 and 1965.
32. Travelers to areas with endemic hepatitis A infection should receive hepatitis A vaccine.
33. Celiac sprue should be considered in patients with unexplained iron-deficiency anemia or osteoporosis.
34. In the United States, gallstones are common among American Indians and Mexican Americans.
35. Esophageal manometry may be needed to complete the evaluation of patients with noncardiac chest pain that may be due to esophageal motility disorders.
36. The estimated glomerular filtration rate (eGFR) is now routinely reported when chemistry panels are ordered and can provide a useful estimate of renal function.
37. Angiotensin-converting enzyme (ACE) inhibitor or angiotensin receptor blocker (ARB) use should be evaluated for all diabetics, even those with normotension, for their renoprotective effects.
38. Diabetes is the most common cause of chronic kidney disease (CKD) in the United States, followed by hypertension.
39. When erythrocyte-stimulating agents are used for the treatment of anemia associated with CKD and end-stage renal disease, the hemoglobin level should *not* be normalized but maintained at 11–12 g/dL.
40. Almost 80% of patients with nephrolithiasis have calcium-containing stones.
41. Hyponatremia can commonly occur after transurethral resection of the prostate.
42. Thrombocytosis, leukocytosis, and specimen hemolysis can falsely elevate serum potassium levels.
43. Intravenous calcium should be given immediately for patients with acute hyperkalemia and electrocardiographic changes.
44. Hypoalbuminemia lowers the serum total calcium level but does not affect the ionized calcium.
45. Hypokalemia, hypophosphatemia, and hypomagnesemia are common findings in alcoholics who require hospitalization.
46. Lupus mortality rate is bimodal in distribution. It peaks in patients who die early from the disease or infection and again in patients who die later in life from cardiovascular diseases.
47. Inflammatory arthritis is characterized by morning stiffness, improvement with exercise, and involvement of small joints (although large joints may also be involved).

48. Patients with autoimmune disorders who smoke should be counseled to quit because tobacco has recently been linked to precipitation of symptoms and poorer prognosis.
49. Most rheumatologic diseases are diagnosed via clinical criteria based on thorough history, physical examination, and selective laboratory testing and imaging.
50. Early diagnosis of an inflammatory arthritis leads to intervention and improved clinical outcomes because there are many disease-modifying therapies available.
51. The most common immunoglobulin (Ig) deficiency is IgA deficiency, which can cause a false-positive pregnancy test.
52. Intranasal steroids are the single most effective drug for treatment of allergic rhinitis. Decongestion with topical adrenergic agents may be needed initially to allow corticosteroids access to the deeper nasal mucosa.
53. ACE inhibitors can cause dry cough and angioedema.
54. Beta blockers should be avoided whenever possible in patients with asthma because they may accentuate the severity of anaphylaxis, prolong its cardiovascular and pulmonary manifestations, and greatly decrease the effectiveness of epinephrine and albuterol in reversing the life-threatening manifestations of anaphylaxis.
55. Patients with persistent fever of unknown origin should first be evaluated for infections, malignancies, and autoimmune diseases.
56. Viruses are the most common causes of acute sinusitis; therefore, antibiotics are ineffective, unless symptoms are persistent (>10 days) or relapse after improvement.
57. Rocky Mountain spotted fever (RMSF) occurs through North and Central America with concentration in the southeastern and south central U.S. states with increasing incidence in Arizona (on Indian reservations). Empiric therapy for RMSF should be considered within 5 days of symptom onset for patients with febrile illnesses and a history of a tick bite who have been in these regions in the spring or summer (May to September).
58. Asplenic patients (either anatomic or functional) are susceptible to infections with encapsulated organisms (*Streptococcus pneumoniae, Haemophilus influenzae,* and *Neisseria meningitidis*) and should receive appropriate vaccinations for these organisms in addition to up-to-date childhood vaccinations. Needed vaccinations should be administered 14 days before elective splenectomy, if possible.
59. Allergic bronchopulmonary aspergillosis (ABPA) occurs in asthmatics and is evident by recurrent wheezing, eosinophilia, transient infiltrates on chest radiograph, and positive serum antibodies to *Aspergillus.*
60. Chagas disease, caused by *Trypanosoma cruzi,* can cause cardiomyopathy, cardiac arrhythmias, and thromboembolism.
61. Human immunodeficiency virus (HIV) infection is preventable and treatable but not curable.
62. Routine HIV testing should be considered for all patients aged 13–65 years.
63. A fourth-generation Ag/Ab combination enzyme immunoassay (EIA) is needed for diagnosis of acute primary HIV infection.
64. HIV-infected patients with undetectable viral loads can still transmit HIV.
65. HIV-infected patients with tuberculosis are more likely to have atypical symptoms and present with extrapulmonary disease.
66. All patients with HIV infection should be tested for syphilis, and all patients diagnosed with syphilis (and any other sexually transmitted disease) should be tested for HIV.
67. The presence of thrush (oropharyngeal candidiasis) indicates significant immunosuppression in an HIV-infected patient.
68. Transferrin saturation and ferritin are effective screening tests for hemochromatosis.
69. Methylmalonic acid can be helpful in the diagnosis of vitamin B_{12} deficiency in patients with low normal vitamin B_{12} levels.
70. Patients with chronic hemolysis should receive folate replacement (1 mg/day).
71. Chronic lymphocytic leukemia is the most common leukemia in adults and is often found in those older than 70 years.
72. Patients with antiphospholipid syndrome have an antiphospholipid antibody and the clinical occurrence of arterial or venous thromboses or both, recurrent pregnancy losses, or thrombocytopenia.
73. Solid tumor staging often uses American Joint Commission on Cancer (AJCC) TNM staging (T = tumor size and areas of invasion; N = regional nodal status; and M = distant metastases).
74. Each type of cancer is driven by different mutations and abnormal checkpoints for which many new, targeted immunotherapeutics have been developed.

75. Differential diagnosis when evaluating possible malignancy should always ensure an accurate treatment plan and may require multiple biopsies and other procedures prior to diagnosis.
76. Tobacco and alcohol use are significant risk factors for head and neck cancers.
77. The treatment plan for a malignancy is often chemotherapy but may include surgical oncology, radiation oncology, and palliative medicine.
78. The best initial screening test for evaluation of thyroid status in most patients is the thyroid-stimulating hormone (TSH). The exceptions are patients with pituitary and hypothalamic dysfunction.
79. Patients with type 1 and type 2 diabetes mellitus (DM) should be screened at regular intervals for the microvascular complications of retinopathy, neuropathy, and nephropathy.
80. Closely examine the feet of diabetic patients regularly, looking for ulcerations, significant callous formation, injury, and joint deformities that could lead to ulceration. Check dorsalis pedis and posterior tibial pulses to detect reduced blood flow and sensation with a monofilament.
81. Erectile dysfunction and decreased libido in men and amenorrhea and infertility in women are the most common symptoms of hypogonadism.
82. Hyperparathyroidism is the most common cause of hypercalcemia.
83. Ataxia can be localized to the cerebellum.
84. Gait dysfunction, urinary dysfunction, and memory impairment are symptoms of normal-pressure hydrocephalus.
85. In the appropriate setting, thrombolysis can markedly improve the outcome of stroke. Prompt initiation of thrombolytic therapy is essential.
86. The sudden onset of a severe headache may indicate an intracranial hemorrhage.
87. Optic neuritis can be an early sign of multiple sclerosis.
88. Cognitive behavioral therapy for insomnia (CBT-I) is the recommended treatment for insomnia, particularly for older adults.
89. Older adults are particularly susceptible to the anticholinergic effects of multiple medications, including over-the-counter antihistamines.
90. Anemia is not a normal part of aging, and hemoglobin abnormalities should be investigated.
91. Decisions regarding screening for malignancies in the elderly should be based not on the age alone but on the patient's life expectancy, functional status, and personal goals.
92. Systolic murmurs in the elderly may be due to aortic stenosis or aortic sclerosis.
93. Delirium in hospitalized patients is associated with an increased mortality risk.
94. When delirium occurs, the underlying cause should be thoroughly evaluated and treated.
95. Pneumonia is the most common infectious cause of death in the elderly.
96. Patients with life-limiting or serious illness can be referred for palliative care at any point in their illness process, regardless of prognosis.
97. A stimulant laxative should always be prescribed whenever opiates are prescribed for chronic pain management to manage opiate-induced constipation.
98. Patients can discontinue hospice care if their symptoms improve or their end-of-life goals change.
99. Opiates are the first line treatment for severe dyspnea at the end of life.
100. Opioid analgesics are available in many forms including tablets to swallow or for buccal application, oral solutions, lozenges for transmucosal absorption, transdermal patches, rectal suppositories, and subcutaneous, intravenous, or intramuscular injection administration.

MEDICAL ETHICS

William L. Allen, M Div, JD

I will use treatment to help the sick according to my ability and judgment, but I will never use it to injure or wrong them.

Attributed to Hippocrates
4th-Century Greek Physician

ETHICAL PRINCIPLES AND CONCEPTS

1. Define the following terms in relation to the patient and physician-patient relationship: *beneficence, nonmaleficence, autonomy*, and *justice*.
   - **Beneficence:** The concept that the physician will contribute to the welfare of the patient through the recommended medical interventions
   - **Nonmaleficence:** An obligation for the physician not to inflict harm upon the patient
   - **Autonomy:** The obligation of the physician to honor the patient's right to accept or refuse a recommended treatment, based on respect for persons
   - **Justice:** The obligation of the physician to avoid treating patients differently by providing better care or privileges to favored patients or by discriminating against less favored patients, especially on grounds of race, ethnicity, sex, sexual orientation, religion, creed, socioeconomic status, or disability

2. What is fiduciary duty?
   An obligation of trust imposed upon physicians requiring them to place their patients' best interests ahead of their own interests and, as the patient's advocate, to protect patients from exploitation or neglect of others in the health care system.

3. What is conflict of interest?
   A situation in which one or more of a professional's duties to a client or patient potentially conflicts with the professional's self-interests or when a professional's roles or duties to more than one patient or organization are in tension or conflict.

4. How should conflicts of interest be addressed?
   - Avoided, if possible
   - Disclosed to institutional officials or to patients affected
   - Managed by disinterested parties outside the conflicted roles or relationships

5. What is conscientious objection?
   Refusal to participate in or perform a procedure, prescription, or test grounded on a person's sincere and deeply held belief that it is morally wrong.

6. What is a conscience clause?
   A provision in law or policy that allows providers with conscientious objections to decline participation in activities to which they have moral objections, under certain conditions and limitations. The scope of the allowance should only protect the provider's conscience, not deny a patient legitimate care.

7. Describe futility.
   The doctrine that physicians are not required to provide treatment if there will be no medical benefit from it. It has become a very controversial term in recent times, in part because of inconsistency in definition and usage. In the narrowest definition, "futility" may refer to physiologic futility or the inability of a treatment or intervention to support bodily functions such as circulation or respiration or reverse the ultimate decline and cessation of these functions. More often, though, futility refers to the very low likelihood of an intervention succeeding in restoring physiologic function or health.

Patients and physicians may disagree about the level of probability that could be considered futile, though. Most health care institutions will establish policies for guidance in resolving such disagreements.

INFORMED CONSENT

8. **How should one request "consent" from a patient?**
   Consent is not a transitive verb. Sometimes a medical student or resident is instructed to "go consent the patient," implying that consent is an act that a health professional performs upon a passive recipient who has no role in the action other than passive acceptance. A health professional seeking consent from a patient should be asking the patient for either an affirmative endorsement of an offered intervention or a decision to decline the proposed intervention.

9. **What is consent or mere consent?**
   Consent alone, without a sufficiently robust level of information to justify the adjective "informed." Although "mere consent" may avoid a finding of battery (which is defined as harmful or offensive physical contact with a person without that person's consent), it is usually insufficient permission for the physician to proceed with a procedure or treatment.

10. **What is informed consent?**
    Consent from a patient that is preceded by and based on the patient's understanding of the proposed intervention at a level that enables the patient to make a meaningful decision about endorsement or refusal of the proposed intervention.

11. **What are the necessary conditions for valid informed consent?**
    - Disclosure of relevant medical information by health care providers
    - Comprehension of relevant medical information by patient (or authorized representative)
    - Voluntariness (absence of coercion by medical personnel or institutional pressure)

12. **What topics should always be addressed in the discussion regarding informed consent (or informed refusal)?**
    - Risks and benefits of the recommended intervention (examination, test, or treatment)
    - Reasonable alternatives to the proposed intervention and the risks and benefits of such alternatives
    - The option of no intervention and the risks and benefits of no intervention

KEY POINTS: INFORMED CONSENT

1. Informed consent involves more than a signature on a document.
2. Before beginning the informed consent process, the physician should assess the patient's capacity to understand the information provided.
3. The physician should make the effort to present the information in a way the patient can comprehend and not just assume the patient is "incompetent" because of difficulty in understanding a complex medical issue.
4. The patient's goals and values are also considered in the informed consent process.

13. **What are the different standards for the scope of disclosure in informed consent?**
    - **Full disclosure:** Disclosure of everything the physician knows. This standard is impractical, if not impossible, and is not legally or ethically required.
    - **Reasonable person** (sometimes called "prudent person standard"): Patient-centered standard of disclosure of the information necessary for a reasonable person to make a meaningful decision about whether to accept or to refuse medical testing or treatment. This standard is the legal minimum in some states.
    - **Professional practice** (also called "customary practice"): Physician-centered standard of disclosure of the information typically practiced by other practitioners in similar contexts. Sometimes the professional practice standard is the legal minimum in states that do not acknowledge the reasonable person standard.
    - **Subjective standard:** Disclosure of information a particular patient may want or need beyond what a reasonable person may want to know. This is not a legally required minimum but is ethically desirable if the physician can determine what additional information the particular patient might find important.

14. **What are the exceptions to the obligation of informed consent?**
    - **Implied consent:** For routine aspects of medical examinations, such as blood pressure, temperature, or stethoscopic examinations, explicit informed consent is not generally required, because presentation for care plausibly implies that the patient expects these measures and consent may be reasonably inferred by the physician. Implied consent does not extend to invasive examinations or physical examination of private or sensitive areas without explicit oral permission and explanation of purpose.
    - **Presumed consent:** Presentation in the emergency room does not necessarily mean that emergency interventions are routine or that the patient's consent is implied. The justification for some exception to informed consent is that most persons would agree to necessary emergency interventions; therefore, consent may be presumed, even though this presumption may turn out to be incorrect in some instances for some patients. Such treatment is limited to stabilizing the patient and deferring other decisions until the patient regains capacity or an authorized decision maker has been contacted.

15. **What should you do when a patient requests the physician to make the decision without providing informed consent?**
    When a patient seems to be saying in one way or another, "Doctor, just do what you think is best," it is appropriate to make a professional recommendation based on what the physician believes to be in the patient's best medical interests. This does not mean, however, that the patient does not need to understand the risks, benefits, and expected outcomes of the recommended intervention. This type of request is sometimes referred to as requested paternalism or waiver of informed consent. The physician should explain, in terms of risks and benefits of a recommended intervention, the reasons he or she recommends the intervention and why it would seem to be in the patient's best medical interest and then ask the patient to endorse it or to decline it.

16. **What is a physician's obligation to veracity (truthful disclosure) to patients?**
    In order for patients to have an accurate picture of their medical situation and what clinical alternatives may best meet their goals in choosing among various medical tests or treatments or to decline medical intervention, patients must have a truthful description of their medical condition. Such truthful disclosure is also essential for maintaining patient trust in the physician-patient relationship. Truthful disclosure, especially of "bad news," however, does not mean that the bearer of bad news must be brutal or insensitive in the timing and manner of disclosure.

17. **Define *therapeutic privilege*.**
    A traditional exception to the obligation of truthful disclosure to the patient, in which disclosures that were thought to be harmful to the patient were withheld for the benefit of the patient. In recent decades, this exception has narrowed almost to the vanishing point from the recognition that most patients want to know the truth and make decisions accordingly, even if the truth entails bad news. Nevertheless, some disclosures may justifiably be withheld temporarily, such as when a patient is acutely depressed and at risk of suicide. Ultimately, however, with appropriate medical and social support, the patient whose decisional capacity can be restored should be told the information that had been temporarily withheld for her or his benefit.

CONFIDENTIALITY

18. **What is medical confidentiality?**
    The private maintenance of information relating to a patient's medical and personal data without unauthorized disclosure to others. Maintaining the confidential status of patient medical information is crucial not only to trust in the physician-patient relationship but also to the physician's ability to elicit sensitive information from patients that is crucial to adequate medical management and treatment. The Health Information Portability and Accountability Act (HIPAA, a federal statute) as well as most state statutes provide legal protections for patients' personally identifiable health information (PHI), but the professional ethical obligation of confidentiality may exceed these minimal protections or apply in situations not clearly addressed by HIPAA or state statutes.

19. **What are recognized exceptions to patient medical confidentiality?**
    - Duty to warn (Tarasoff duty): A basis for justifying a limited exception to the rule of patient confidentiality when a patient of a psychiatrist makes an explicit, serious threat of grave bodily harm to an identifiable person(s) in the imminent future. The scope of this warning is limited to the potential victim(s) or appropriate law enforcement agency, and the health care provider may divulge only enough information to convey the threat of harm.

- Reporting of communicable disease to public health authorities (but not others).
- Reporting of injuries from violence to law enforcement.
- Reporting of child or elder abuse to protective social service authorities.

20. What is the obligation to veracity to nonpatients?
Physicians are not obligated to lie to persons who inquire about a patient's confidential information, but they may be required simply to decline to address such requests from persons to whom the patient has not granted access.

DECISION-MAKING CAPACITY

21. How do physicians assess decision-making capacity in patients?
Whereas most adult patients should be presumed to have intact decisional capacity, some patients may be totally incapacitated for making their own medical decisions. Totally incapacitated patients will generally be obvious cases, such as unconscious or sedated patients. But decisional capacity is not an all-or-nothing category, so it is not uncommon for patients to have variable capacity depending on the status of their condition and the complexity of the particular decision at hand. Thus, one crucial aspect of assessing decisional capacity is to determine whether the patient can comprehend the elements required for valid informed consent to the particular decision that needs to be made. Patients with mood disorders, such as acute depression, however, may be incapacitated by their mood, even if they comprehend the information.

22. What are common pitfalls in assessing patient decisional capacity or competence?
If one uses the **outcome approach,** the patient's capacity is determined based on the outcome of the patient's acceptance of the physician's recommendation. The physician may incorrectly assume that the refusal of a recommended treatment indicates incapacity. Refusal of a recommended treatment is not adequate grounds to conclude patient incapacity. Nor is patient acceptance of the physician's recommendation an adequate means of assessing patient capacity. An incapacitated patient may acquiesce to recommended treatment, whereas a capacitated patient may refuse the physician's best medical advice. If one uses the **status approach,** patients with a history of a mental illness or memory impairment may be considered incapacitated. Psychiatric conditions or other medical conditions that can result in incapacity may have resolved or may be under control with appropriate therapy that mitigates the condition's impact on patient capacity for decision making. Patients with memory impairment or dementia may also be able to express wishes regarding treatment. Patients who can express a clear preference should have that expression seriously regarded as assent or dissent, even if an authorized decision maker makes the legally sufficient informed consent or refusal.

23. What is the best approach to assessing patient capacity?
The **functional approach,** which determines the patient's ability to function in a particular context to make decisions that are authentic expressions of the patient's own values and goals. Determining whether a patient is capacitated for a particular medical decision entails assessing whether the patient is able to:
- Comprehend the risks and benefits of the recommended intervention, risks and benefits of reasonable alternative intervention, and the risks and benefits of no intervention.
- Manifest appreciation of the significance of his or her medical condition.
- Reason about the consequences of available treatment options (including no treatment).
- Communicate a stable choice in light of his or her personal values.
Appelbaum PS. Clinical practice. Assessment of patients' competence to consent to treatment. *N Engl J Med.* 2007;357:1834–1840.

24. What is involuntary commitment?
Assignment of a person to an inpatient psychiatric facility without patient consent when the appropriate criteria are met. These patients must be unable to provide informed consent owing to a mental illness *and,* owing to the same mental illness, pose a danger to themselves or to others. Similarly, patients who are seriously impaired by substance abuse may be involuntarily admitted to detoxification units or to longer term rehabilitation facilities.

25. What are assent and dissent?
Assent is the obligation prospectively to explain medical interventions in language and concepts the patient can comprehend even if the patient is deemed to be not capable of full informed consent, such as children or mentally impaired adults. The patient's agreement is elicited, even though the final decision requires parental, guardian, or other legally authorized decision maker's permission.

Conversely, dissent is the obligation to take seriously the refusal of children or mentally impaired adults when they are opposed to medical interventions or placements, unless the recommendations are so crucial to the patient's well-being that their dissent must be overridden to avert serious deterioration or harm to their interests.

ADVANCE DIRECTIVES

26. What is an advance directive?

A generic term for any of several types of patient instructions, oral or written, for providing guidance and direction in advance of a person's potential incapacity. The instructions and authorization in an advance directive do not take effect until the person loses decisional capacity and the advance directive ceases to be in effect if or when the patient regains capacity.

27. What are the types of advance directives?

Designation by a capacitated patient of the person the patient chooses to make medical decisions during any period when the patient is incapacitated, whether during surgery, temporary unconsciousness, or mental condition, as well as irreversible condition of lost decisional capacity. The decisions the designated person can make include withholding or withdrawal of treatment in life-limiting circumstances. This type may variously be called a "durable power of attorney for health care," a "surrogate health care decision maker," or a "proxy health care decision maker."

A **living will** is a formal expression of a patient's choices about end-of-life care and specifications or limitations of treatment, either with or without the naming of a person to reinforce, interpret, or apply what is expressed to the patient's current circumstances.

28. Who are statutorily authorized next-of-kin decision makers?

If a patient has not made a living will or designated a person to make decisions during periods of patient incapacity, state statutes determine the order of priority for persons related to or close to the patient to assume the role of making medical decisions on the patient's behalf. These are typically called "surrogates" or "proxies," but they differ from decision makers designated by the patient in the way they are selected, and, in many cases, they bear a greater burden of demonstrating that they know what the patient would want.

29. What are the standards of decision making for those chosen either by the patient or by statute to make decisions for the incapacitated patient?
   - **Substituted judgment:** The decision the patient would have made if she or he had not been incapacitated. In some cases, this will not be the same as what others may think is in the patient's best interest.
   - **Best interest:** Choosing what is considered most appropriate for the patient. If there is substantial uncertainty about what the patient would have chosen for herself or himself, then the traditional best interest standard is the appropriate basis for decision making.

END-OF-LIFE ISSUES

30. What are end-of-life care physician orders?

Orders that give direction regarding interventions at the time of death or cardiopulmonary arrest. Patient-directed measures such as advance directives or statutory next-of-kin decisions should be the basis for underlying medical decisions that entail informed consent or refusal issues at the end of life.

KEY POINTS: END-OF-LIFE ISSUES

1. Patients should be encouraged to discuss their wishes for end-of-life care with family members or close friends and physicians while still able to clearly express these wishes.
2. Forms such as Preferences of Life-Sustaining Treatment can designate the patient's specific requests to accept or decline therapies at the end of life.
3. Patients are frequently unaware of the numerous, complex therapies related to end-of-life care and may not be able to write down what is wanted. Designation of a surrogate decision maker with whom the patient discusses her or his values and goals related to end-of-life care can also ensure the patient's choices will be respected.

31. How are end-of-life care orders written?

- **Do not resuscitate (DNR) or do not attempt resuscitation (DNAR):** An order written by the attending physician to prevent emergency cardiopulmonary resuscitation (CPR) for a patient who has refused CPR as a form of unwanted treatment. The decision of an incapacitated patient's authorized decision maker may also be a basis for a written DNR order by the physician.
- **Physician Orders for Life-Sustaining Treatment (POLST):** Similar to the concept of DNR, but broadened to include all aspects of end-of-life care based on the choices of the patient or authorized decision maker, including withholding or withdrawal of care and palliative measures. Many states now have statutory acknowledgment that a properly executed POLST form, signed by a physician, should be followed by all health care providers for the patient. Available at www.polst.org. Accessed October 27, 2016.

32. What is brain death?

The term used to replace the traditional definition of death by cessation of heartbeat and respiration. In the legally operative definition of this term, it refers to whole brain death, cessation not only of higher cortical function but of brainstem function as well.

33. What is physician aid-in-dying?

The provision of a lethal amount of a medication that the patient voluntarily takes to end his or her life. Oregon, Washington, California, New Mexico, and Vermont have established legislation to allow these prescriptions, and other states are considering the issue. Montana, based on court ruling, also allows physician aid-in-dying.

BIBLIOGRAPHY

1. Beauchamp TL, Childress JF. *Principles of Biomedical Ethics.* 7th ed. Oxford: Oxford University Press; 2012.
2. Jonsen A, Siegler M, Winslade W. *Clinical Ethics: A Practical Approach to Ethical Decisions in Clinical Medicine.* 8th ed. New York: McGraw-Hill Education; 2015.
3. Lo B. *Resolving Ethical Dilemmas. A Guide for Clinicians.* 5th ed. Philadelphia: Lippincott Williams & Wilkins; 2013.

CHAPTER 2

GENERAL MEDICINE AND AMBULATORY CARE

Mary P. Harward, MD, FACP

When I see a new patient, I find it valuable, at the first meeting, consciously to look at the hands. Clues to diseases in the nervous system, heart, lung, liver, and other organs can be found there.... In medicine, a hand is never merely a hand; symbolically it is much more. That is why the "laying on of hands" is so important for the physician and patient.

John Stone (1936–2008)
"Telltale Hands" from
In the Country of Hearts: Journeys in the Art of Medicine, 1990

It's the humdrum, day-in, day-out everyday work that is the real satisfaction of the practice of medicine; ... the actual calling on people, at all times and under all conditions, the coming to grips with the intimate conditions of their lives, when they were being born, when they were dying, watching them die, watching them get well when they were ill, has always absorbed me.

William Carlos Williams (1883–1963)
"The Practice" from
The Autobiography of William Carlos Williams, 1951

LISTENING TO THE PATIENT

1. **What interviewing skills can help the physician identify all the significant issues for the patient?**
Remaining open-ended and encouraging the patient to "go on" until all the pertinent issues have been expressed by the patient. Other facilitative techniques to keep the patient talking include a simple head nod or saying, "and" or "what else?" Continue these facilitative techniques until the patient says, "nothing else." During the opening of the interview, the physician can listen to the patient's "list" of the concerns for that visit, without focusing on specific signs and symptoms at that time. Physicians too often interrupt the patient and direct the remaining interview, only focusing on what the physician deems important. A patient may have other, significant issues that are not immediately expressed, and the physician may miss this "hidden agenda" if the patient is interrupted. Once the patient has listed the concerns, the patient and physician can then decide which ones will be addressed at that visit and which ones can be deferred to future visits.

2. **How can the physician understand more clearly what the patient is trying to describe?**
By rephrasing the patient's response in the physician's words or simply restating what the patient said. Sometimes the physician simply needs to ask, "Can you find other words to describe your pain?" Emotional responses and pain are particularly difficult to put into words.

3. **What questions help characterize a symptom?**
   - **Where** does the symptom occur?
   - **What** does it feel like?
   - **When** does the symptom occur?
   - **How** is it affected by other things you do?
   - **Why** does the symptom occur (what brings the symptom on)?
   - **What** makes the symptom better?

EVALUATING THE TESTS

4. Define *sensitivity* and *specificity* of tests.
   - **Sensitivity:** The percentage of patients who have the disease that is being tested and have a positive test result
   - **Specificity:** The percentage of patients who do not have the disease and have a negative test result

5. What are the positive and negative predictive values of tests?
   - **Positive predictive value:** The percentage of patients who have a positive test result and have the disease that is being tested
   - **Negative predictive value:** The percentage of patients who have a negative test result and do not have the disease

6. How are these values calculated?
   See Fig. 2.1.

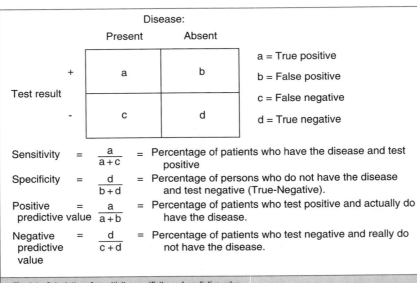

Fig. 2.1. Calculation of sensitivity, specificity, and predictive value.

7. What is the NNT?
   The number needed to treat that quantifies the number of patients who will require treatment with a therapy (with possibly no benefit to an individual patient) in order to ensure that at least one patient benefits from the therapy, usually defined as no occurrence of the adverse event or events that the therapy should prevent. Most publications now include this number. There is no absolute NNT that is appropriate for all therapeutic decisions, but it will depend on the risks of the therapy, the benefits of treatment, and the patient's goals for treatment. In general, the higher the NNT, the less effective the therapy.

SCREENING FOR MALIGNANCIES

8. What are the recommendations for colon cancer screening?
   The U.S. Preventive Services Task Force (USPSTF) recommends performing at least one of multiple screening procedures beginning at age 50 years and continuing through age 75 years. For patients of *average risk* who are *asymptomatic,* the physician may consider:

- gFOBT (guiac-based fecal occult blood test): Every year
- FIT (fecal immunochemical test): Every year
- FIT-DNA (multitargeted stool DNA test): Every 1–3 years
- Colonoscopy: Every 10 years (if no polyps on previous colonoscopy)
- CT (computed tomography) colonography: Every 5 years
- Flexible sigmoidoscopy: Every 5 years
- Flexible sigmoidoscopy with FIT: Flexible sigmoidoscopy every 10 years + FIT every year

Screening is not recommended after age 86 years. For patients aged 76–84 years, individual health, risk factors, and previous findings at screening should be considered before recommending screening procedure. Other organizations such as the National Comprehensive Cancer Care Network and American Gastroenterology Association have different recommendations.

Burt RW, Cannon JA, David DS, et al. Colorectal cancer screening. *J Natl Compr Conc Netw.* 2013;11:1538–1575.

Rex DK, Johnson DA, Anderson JC, et al. American College of Gastroenterology guidelines for colorectal cancer screening 2009. *Am J Gastroenterol.* 2009;104:739–750.

U.S. Preventive Services Task Force, Bibbins-Domingo K, Grossman DC, Curry SJ, et al. Screening for colorectal cancer: U.S. Preventive Services Task Force recommendation statement. *JAMA.* 2016;315:2564–2575.

9. **What are the guidelines for breast cancer screening?**
The most recent guidelines (2016) from the USPSTF for screening asymptomatic women with conventional mammography are summarized as:

Age	Recommendation
40–49 years (y)	Individual decision made by the woman based on her preferences
50–74 y	Every 2 years
≥75 y	No recommendation because of insufficient evidence

The USPSTF based these recommendations after review of the available evidence that mammograms reduce mortality and morbidity risks. The recommendations also considered the potential harms from screening including false-positive results and unnecessary biopsies. These guidelines are regularly updated. The American Cancer Society (ACS) recommends beginning annual screening at age 45 and continuing until age 55. Biennial screening should begin at age 55.

Oeffinger KC, Fontham ET, Etzioni R, et al. Breast cancer screening for women at average risk: 2015 guideline update from the American Cancer Society. *JAMA.* 2015;314:1599–1614.

U.S. Preventive Services Task Force. Screening for breast cancer: U.S. Preventive Services Task Force Recommendation Statement. *Ann Intern Med.* 2016;164:279–297.

10. **How should childhood cancer survivors be screened for breast cancer?**
For this group who received chest radiation, mammography should begin at age 25 years or 8 years after chest radiation exposure, whichever is earlier. Mammograms should be continued annually.

Oeffinger KC, Ford JS, Mokowitz CS, et al. Breast cancer surveillance practices among women previously treated with chest radiation for a childhood cancer. *JAMA.* 2009;301:404–414.

11. **What are the controversies related to prostate cancer screening?**
The prostate-specific antigen (PSA) currently used for prostate cancer screening does not have sufficient evidence to support its routine use in men of *average risk* for prostate cancer. False-positive and false-negative PSA tests occur. The evidence is also unclear as to whether treatment of prostate cancer, when discovered, prolongs life. Prostate cancer screening decisions should be made on an individual basis. As with mammograms, not all expert groups concur with the USPSTF recommendations. Currently trials are under way to try to more clearly identify appropriate prostate cancer screening tests.

U.S. Preventive Services Task Force. Screening for prostate cancer: U.S. Preventive Servicess Task Force Recommendation Statement. *Ann Intern Med.* 2012;157:120–135.

Wolf AM, Wender RC, Etzioni RB, et al. American Cancer Society guideline for the early detection of prostate cancer: update 2010. *CA Cancer J Clin.* 2010;60:70–98.

12. **When should screening begin for cervical cancer?**
At age 21 years. A Papanicolaou (Pap) smear every 3 years is the appropriate screening test. If women aged 30 to 65 years wish to undergo screening less frequently, the interval can be extended to every 5 years with the use of a Pap smear and human papillomavirus (HPV) tests. The USPSTF recommends ending screening in women after age 65 years if they have had appropriate routine screening.
    U.S. Preventive Services Task Force, Moyer VA. Screening for cervical cancer: U.S. Preventive Services Task Force Recommendation Statement. *Ann Intern Med.* 2012;156:880–891.

13. **Do women who have had a total hysterectomy (with cervix removal) for nonmalignant reasons need Pap smears?**
No. The yield of finding significant disease in this population is low.

14. **Is there an effective screening test for ovarian cancer?**
No, not at this time, although this is an area of active research. Although the pelvic examination, transvaginal ultrasound, and the tumor marker CA-125 have all been used as screening tests, none has been shown to reduce death from the disease.

15. **What is the role of chest x-rays and computed tomography scans in lung cancer screening?**
Although chest x-rays are not effective for lung cancer screening, the National Lung Screening Trial (NLST) showed that annual low-dose chest CT (LDCT) scans showed a reduction in lung cancer and all-cause mortality rate for patients who are:
    - Age 55–79 years
    - Current smoker OR former smoker who quit within the past 15 years
    - Smoker for at least 30 pack-years (currently or former)
    - Asymptomatic
    The USPTF recommends continuing screening until age 80 and discontinuing screening when a significant life-limiting illness develops or the patient has not smoked for 15 years. Centers for Medicaid and Medicare Services (CMS) covers LDCT for those meeting the above criteria and are 55–77 years old.
    National Lung Screening Trial Research Team, Aberle DR, Adams AM, et al. Reduced lung-cancer mortality with low-dose computed tomographic screening. *N Engl J Med.* 2011;365:395–409.
    U.S. Preventive Services Task Force: Lung cancer screening. Available at: https://www.uspreventiveservicestaskforce.org/Page/Document/UpdateSummaryFinal/lung-cancer-screening; December, 2013. [accessed 22.01.17].

CARDIOLOGY

16. **What is the first step to evaluate a patient with an initial blood pressure (BP) reading of 150/90 mm Hg?**
Confirm that the BP was measured under the right conditions including:
    - Comfortable seating in a chair
    - Uncrossed legs, feet resting on the floor
    - Support of patient's back and arm for BP measurement
    - No clothing covering the area of the cuff placement
    - Middle of the cuff placed on the upper arm across from the midpoint of the sternum
    - Waiting 5 minutes after the patient is seated comfortably (and remaining quiet) before measuring the BP
    - Adequate cuff size for the patient's arm (cuff bladder length is 80% and width is 40% of the patient's arm circumference)
    - Recording at least two measurements 30 seconds apart
    - Measurement of the BP in both arms at initial visit
    Multiple measurements at different times of the day (and possibily different settings) should be done to confirm the elevated BP. Home and work site measurements and ambulatory BP recordings are also helpful for hypertension confirmation.
    LeBlond RF, Brown DD, Suneja M, et al. *DeGowin's Diagnostic Examination.* 10th ed. New York: McGraw-Hill; 2015.

17. **What can cause a difference in BP between the right and the left arm?**
Arterial occlusion in the arm with the lower BP (subclavian artery stenosis), thoracic outlet syndrome, or aortic dissection. "Normal" BP difference should be <10 mm Hg. The arm with the higher reading should be used for future measurements. Sometimes no cause is found.

18. **Should systolic BP between 120 and 139 mm Hg and/or diastolic BP between 80 and 89 mm Hg be treated?**
Yes, with lifestyle modification. BP readings such as these are called "prehypertension" and are associated with increased risk of cardiovascular events. Pharmacologic therapy should be initiated if the BP increases to the hypertensive range (systolic ≥140 mm Hg or diastolic ≥90 mm Hg).
Chobanian AV, Bakris GL, Black HR, et al. The Seventh Report of the Joint National Committee on Prevention, Detection, Evaluation, and Treatment of High Blood Pressure: The JNC 7 Report. *JAMA.* 2003;289:2560.
James PA, Oparil S, Carter BL, et al. 2014 evidence-based guideline for the management of high blood pressure in adults: report from the panel members appointed to the Eighth Joint National Committee (JNC 8). *JAMA.* 2014;311(5):507–520.

19. **What lifestyle modifications are helpful for reducing BP?**
- Weight loss (to body mass index [BMI] of 18.5–24.9)
- Salt restriction (<6 g sodium chloride or <2.5 g sodium)
- Limited alcohol use (12 oz of beer, 5 oz of wine, 1.5 oz of 80-proof spirits daily)
- Stress management
- Smoking cessation
- Regular aerobic exercise
- Low–saturated fat diet rich in fruits and vegetables
U.S. Department of Health and Human Services. National Heart, Lung, and Blood Institute. NIH Publication: How is high blood pressure treated? Available at: https://www.nhlbi.nih.gov/health-topics/high-blood-pressure#Treatment.

20. **What are the risks of prehypertension?**
Coronary artery disease, myocardial infarction, and death from a cardiovascular event.

21. **What is the initial laboratory evaluation of newly diagnosed hypertension (HTN)?**
- Fasting blood glucose
- Complete blood count
- Total and HDL (high-density lipoprotein) cholesterol
- Potassium
- Creatinine, blood urea nitrogen (BUN)
- Calcium, albumin
- Urinalysis
- Electrocardiogram

22. **How can the patient's history identify secondary HTN due to medications and other substance use?**
Ask the patient about use of:
- **Over-the-counter medications:** Decongestants, stimulants (methylphenidate), appetite suppressants, nonsteroidal anti-inflammatory drugs (NSAIDs), and caffeine
- **Prescription medications:** NSAIDs, corticosteroids, antidepressants (venlafaxine, desvenlafaxine, bupropion), cyclosporine, oral contraceptive pills (OCPs), estrogen and progesterone preparations, erythropoietin, vascular growth factor antagonists
- **Illicit drugs (acute and chronic):** Cocaine, amphetamines, stimulants, MDMA (3,4-methylene-dioxymethamphetamine, or ecstasy), PCP (phencyclidine), cannabis (marijuana), and herbal designer drugs
- **Alcohol:** Alcohol history, CAGE questionnaire (see Question 156), family history of alcoholism

23. **How can the patient's history identify secondary HTN due to an endocrine disorder?**
Ask the patient about:
- **Cushing syndrome:** weight gain, central obesity, easy bruising, "moon" facies, abdominal striae
- **Hyperthyrodism:** weight loss, tachycardia, nervousness
- **Hypothyroidism:** weight gain, fatigue, constipation, dry skin
- **Pheochromocytoma:** labile HTN, sweating, headache, palpitations
- **Hyperaldosteronism:** fatigue, muscle weakness due to low potassium

24. **List two elements in the history that may suggest secondary HTN due to sleep apnea.**
Snoring and daytime sleepiness. (See also Chapter 6, Pulmonary Medicine, and Chapter 17, Neurology.)

> **KEY POINTS: RISK FACTORS FOR CORONARY ARTERY DISEASE IN PATIENTS WITH HYPERLIPIDEMIA**
>
> 1. Cigarette smoking (current)
> 2. Hypertension (>140/90 mm Hg)
> 3. Low HDL (<40 mg/dL)
> 4. Family history of premature CAD (father or brother <55 yr; mother or sister <65 yr)
> 5. Diabetes mellitus
> 6. Men age ≥45 yr
> 7. Women age ≥55 yr or premature menopause without estrogen replacement
>
> CAD, coronary artery disease; HDL, high-density lipoprotein.

25. **What findings suggest renal artery stenosis?**
    - Presence of peripheral vascular disease
    - Periumbilical bruit
    - HTN resistant to multiple drug therapy
    - Worsening hypertension control in patient taking prescribed medications
    - Worsening of renal function after initiation of angiotensin-converting enzyme (ACE) inhibitor or angiotensin receptor blocker (ARB)
    - Initial diagnosis of HTN in patient <35 years of age or >65 years of age
    - Cigarette smoking (current or former)
    - Known atherosclerotic disease in another organ
    - Elevated cholesterol
    - Elevated creatinine
    - "Flash" pulmonary edema

26. **Which patients should be screened for primary aldosteronism?**
    Those with:
    - HTN associated with unexplained hypokalemia or hypokalemia associated with low-dose diuretic therapy
    - HTN resistant to multidrug (three-drug) therapy
    - HTN associated with adrenal incidentaloma (adrenal lesion noted on imaging study done for another reason)
      Funder JW, Carey RM, Fardella C, et al. Case detection, diagnosis, and treatment of patients with primary aldosteronism: an Endocrine Society clinical practice guideline. *J Clin Endocrinol Metab.* 2008;93:3266–3281.

27. **What are the signs and symptoms of pheochromocytoma?**
    - Paroxysmal HTN
    - Excessive sweating
    - Palpitations
    - Anxiety
    - Nervousness
    - Tremulousness
    - Heat intolerance
    - Resistant HTN

28. **What causes of secondary HTN can be detected by physical examination?**
    - **Aortic insufficiency:** high-pitched blowing decrescendo diastolic murmur
    - **Aortic coarctation:** diminished femoral pulses and murmur best heard over the back (interscapular area)
    - **Renovascular disease:** periumbilical bruit
    - **Subclavian stenosis (or other peripheral arterial disease):** BP difference > 10 mm Hg between right and left arms
    - **Cushing syndrome:** abdominal striae, "buffalo hump," "moon" facies, acne, peripheral edema, supraclavicular fat pads
    - **Hyperthyroidism:** thyroid nodularity or tenderness, muscle weakness, tremor, lid lag

- **Sleep apnea:** obesity, particularly of neck
- **Alcoholism:** spider angiomata, hepatomegaly, gynecomastia

29. Can licorice ingestion elevate the BP?

Yes, although glycyrrhizic acid is found only in confectioner's black licorice. Most commercially sold licorice in the United States does not contain significant amounts, although glycyrrhizic acid may be found in chewing tobacco.

30. What is the target BP for HTN treatment?

In general, <140/90 mm Hg. Lower target levels may be indicated for patients with significant risk factors for cardiovascular complications such as diabetes, chronic kidney disease, peripheral arterial disease, or known coronary artery disease. The target goal for BP measured by automated oscillometric blood pressure (AOBP) is slightly lower. (See also Chapter 4, Cardiology.)

31. What are PCSK9 inhibitors?

Lipid-lowering drugs that target the enzyme proprotein convertase subtilisin kexin 9, which degrades low-density lipoprotein (LDL) receptors in the liver, leading to increased LDL cholesterol levels. These monoclonal antibodies may reduce the LDL cholesterol as much as 70% and are given as injections.

32. Which lipids can be measured without fasting?

Total cholesterol and HDL cholesterol. LDL cholesterol is calculated from the fasting triglyceride level, and total and HDL cholesterol levels are calculated by the following formula:

LDL cholesterol = Total cholesterol − (HDL cholesterol + Triglycerides/5)

33. What are the guidelines for treating cholesterol?

Treatment initiation values and treatment goals are based on the patient's underlying risk factors (age, tobacco use, HTN, family history, and low HDL) and coronary artery disease (CAD) risk equivalents. (CAD risk equivalents are symptomatic heart disease, known atherosclerotic disease in other vessels, and diabetes mellitus [DM].) See Table 2.1.

Table 2.1. Treatment Guidelines and Goals for Elevated Cholesterol

NO. OF RISK FACTORS* OR CAD RISK EQUIVALENTS†	LDL GOAL (mg/dL)	LDL LEVEL FOR INITIATION OF DRUG THERAPY (mg/dL)
Known CAD or CAD risk equivalent	<100	≥130 (100–129: drug optional)
2+	<130	≥130 if 10-yr risk 10–20% ≥160 if 10-yr risk < 10%
0–1	<160	≥190 (160–189: drug optional)

*Tobacco use, hypertension, low HDL cholesterol, family history of premature CAD, and age ≥ 45 yr (men) and ≥ 55 yr (women).
†Diabetes mellitus, symptomatic heart disease, known atherosclerotic disease, and abdominal aortic aneurysm.
CAD, coronary artery disease; HDL, high-density lipoprotein; LDL, low-density lipoprotein.
From Grundy SM, Cleeman JI, Bairey Merz CN. Implications of recent clinical trials for the National Cholesterol Education Program Adult Treatment Panel III Guidelines. *Circulation.* 2004;110:227–239.

34. List the lipid-lowering agents.

See Table 2.2.

KEY POINTS: ATHEROSCLEROTIC DISEASES ASSOCIATED WITH HIGH RISK OF CORONARY ARTERY DISEASE

1. Symptomatic carotid artery disease
2. Peripheral arterial disease
3. Abdominal aortic aneurysm

Table 2.2. Lipid-Lowering Agents

CLASS	DRUGS	MECHANISM	TG	LDL	HDL	SIDE EFFECTS
HMG-CoA reductase inhibitors or "statins" (drugs of choice for lowering LDL)	Fluvastatin Pravastatin Lovastatin Simvastatin Atorvastatin Rosuvastatin (in order of ↑ potency)	Inhibits HMG-CoA reductase (rate-limiting enzyme in cholesterol synthesis) ↑LDL receptor activity	↓, ↓↓ (dose-related)	↓↓↓	↑	Overall well tolerated ↑LFTs Rhabdomyolysis Myositis Drug interactions
Cholesterol absorption inhibitor	Ezetamibe	Inhibits cholesterol absorption from gut	↕	↓↓	↕	↑LFTs (w/statins) GI upset/bloating
Bile acid resins	Colestipol Cholestyramine Colesevelam	Bind bile acids ↑ Hepatic LDL receptor activity	↕, ↑	↓↓	↑	Constipation Steatorrhea Bloating Bind other drugs
Fibrates (drugs of choice for lowering TG)	Clofibrate Gemfibrozil Fenofibrate	↓VLDL synthesis ↑VLDL clearance	↓↓↓	↕, ↓*	↑	Overall well tolerated Gallstones Myopathy Drug interactions
Bile acid resins	Colestipol Cholestyramine Colesevelam	Bind bile acids ↑ Hepatic LDL receptor activity	↕, ↑	↓↓	↑	Constipation Steatorrhea Bloating Bind other drugs
Nicotinic acid (drug of choice for raising HDL)	Crystalline niacin Niaspan (long-acting niacin)	↓VLDL secretion ↓Adipose lipolysis	↓↓	↓	↑↑	Flushing with short-acting form ↑LFTs Glucose intolerance Hyperuricemia Rash
Omega 3 fatty acids	Fish oils	↓VLDL synthesis and secretion	↓↓	?	?	Glucose intolerance Smell like fish

*Fenofibrate has more LDL-lowering effect than gemfibrozil.

GI, gastrointestinal; HDL, high-density lipoprotein; HMG-CoA, 3-hydroxy-3-methylglutaryl coenzyme A; LDL, low-density lipoprotein; LFTs, liver function tests; TG, triglyceride;

35. How is the risk of a cardiac event calculated?

One risk assessment tool from the Framingham Heart Study can be calculated online and includes assessment based on sex, age, total cholesterol, tobacco use, HDL cholesterol level, and systolic BP (treated or untreated). Other tools include the Reynolds Risk Score and Pooled Cohort Equations.

Available at: http://www.framinghamheartstudy.org/risk-functions/index.php. Accessed January 14, 2017.

Available at: http://www.reynoldsriskscore.org/. Accessed January 29, 2017.

Available at: http://tools.acc.org/ASCVD-Risk-Estimator/.

36. What is the New York Heart Association (NYHA) classification of congestive heart failure (CHF)?

The NYHA classifies patients with known cardiac disease into four classes based on functional capacity and objective assessment (Table 2.3).

Table 2.3. New York Heart Association Classification of Congestive Heart Failure

CLASS	FUNCTIONAL CAPACITY (LIMITATION OF PHYSICAL ACTIVITY)	OBJECTIVE ASSESSMENT (EVIDENCE OF CARDIOVASCULAR DISEASE)
I	None	None
II	Slight	Minimal
III	Marked	Moderately severe
IV	Inability to carry on any activity without symptoms	Severe

37. What is the role of an angiotensin receptor–neprilysin inhibitor in the treatment of CHF?

To reduce mortality risk in patients with NYHA II–IV CHF classification. Such combination medications (e.g., sacubitril-valsartan) can be used in place of an ACE inhibitor or ARB in these patients.

McMurray JJ, Packer M, Desai AS, et al. Angiotensin-neprilysin inhibition versus enalapril in heart failure. *N Engl J Med.* 2014;371:993–1002.

38. What is Takotsubo cardiomyopathy?

Acute, reversible left ventricular dysfunction occurring in postmenopausal women after sudden and unexpected emotional or physical stress. The syndrome is also called *apical ballooning* or *stress cardiomyopathy.* The syndrome likely results from high levels of catecholamines related to the acute stress.

Akashi YJ, Goldstein DS, Barbaro G, et al. Takotsubo cardiomyopathy. A new form of acute, reversible heart failure. *Circulation.* 2008;118:2754–2762.

39. What are the characteristics of an innocent heart murmur? Mitral valve prolapse (MVP) murmur?

See Table 2.4.

Table 2.4. Innocent Heart Murmur Versus Murmur Due to Mitral Valve Prolapse (MVP)

CHARACTERISTIC	INNOCENT MURMUR	MVP MURMUR
Location	Base	Apex
Intensity	<3/6	>2/6
Timing in cardiac cycle	Early systole	Mid-to-late systole
Response to standing	Decreased	Begins earlier in systole
Response to Valsalva maneuver	Decreases	May increase
Associated findings	None	Midsystolic click

40. **List the cardiac conditions that require prophylactic antibiotics when a patient has certain dental procedures.**
    - Prosthetic cardiac valve or presence of prosthetic material used for cardiac valve repair
    - Previous infectious endocarditis (IE)
    - Congenital heart disease (CHD)
    - Cardiac transplantation with cardiac valvulopathy

41. **What other procedures require antibiotic prophylaxis for high-risk patients?**
    - Upper respiratory procedures that require incision or biopsy (tonsillectomy and adenoidectomy)
    - Procedures on infected skin and musculoskeletal tissue

42. **Is antibiotic prophylaxis indicated for procedures such as cystoscopy, prostate surgery, intestinal surgery, and colonoscopy in high-risk patients?**
    No.
    Chambers HF, Eliopoulos GM, Gilbert DN, et al, editors. The Sanford Guide to Antimicrobial Therapy. Sperryville VA: Antimicrobial Therapy, Inc.; 2016.
    Wilson W, Taubert KA, Gewitz M, et al. Prevention of infective endocarditis: Guidelines from the American Heart Association: From the American Heart Association Rheumatic Fever, Endocarditis, and Kawasaki Disease Committee, Council on Cardiovascular Disease in the Young, and the Council on Clinical Cardiology, Council on Cardiovascular Surgery and Anesthesia, and the Quality of Care and Outcomes Research Interdisciplinary Working Group, *Circulation*. 2007;116:1736–1754.

43. **Which dental procedures require endocarditis prophylaxis?**
    Those that involve manipulation of gingival tissues or periapical region of the teeth or any perforation of the oral mucosa.

44. **What antibiotics are used for prophylaxis for endocarditis?**
    See Table 2.5.

Table 2.5. Antimicrobial Prophylaxis for the Prevention of Bacterial Endocarditis in Patients With Underlying High-Risk Cardiac Conditions Undergoing Dental Procedures

ABLE TO TAKE ORAL MEDICATIONS?	ALLERGIC TO PENICILLIN OR AMPICILLIN?	ANTIBIOTIC	DOSAGE*
Yes	No	Amoxicillin	2 g
No	No	Ampicillin	2 g IM or IV
		Cefazoline or ceftriaxone	2 g
Yes	Yes	Cephalexin[†‡] or Clindamycin or Azithromycin or clarithromycin	2 g 600 mg 500 mg
No	Yes	Cefazolin or ceftriaxone[†] Clindamycin	1 g IM or IV 600 mg IM or IV

*Given as single dose 30–60 min before procedure.
[†]Or another first- or second-generation oral cephalosporin.
[‡]Do not use a cephalosporin in a patient with a history of anaphylactic-, urticarial-, or angioedema-type reaction to penicillin.
IM, intramuscular; IV, intravenous.
From Wilson W, Taubert KA, Gewitz M, et al. Prevention of infective endocarditis: guidelines from the American Heart Association: from the American Heart Association Rheumatic Fever, Endocarditis, and Kawasaki Disease Committee, Council on Cardiovascular Disease in the Young, and the Council on Clinical Cardiology, Council on Cardiovascular Surgery and Anesthesia, and the Quality of Care and Outcomes Research Interdisciplinary Working Group. *Circulation*. 2007;116:1736–1754.

45. **What are the common causes of atrial fibrillation?**
    Alcohol use (especially binge drinking), thyrotoxicosis, congestive heart failure, myocardial ischemia or infarction, pulmonary embolism, illicit or over-the-counter stimulant use, mitral valve disease, sinus node dysfunction (tachycardia-bradycardia or sick sinus syndrome), Wolff-Parkinson-White (WPW) syndrome, hypertensive cardiomyopathy, digoxin toxicity, cardiac surgery, sleep apnea.

46. What range of the international normalized ratio (INR) is the target treatment for most patients receiving anticoagulation for atrial fibrillation?
2.0–3.0.

47. If medications are taken with grapefruit juice, the absorption and blood level of the medication may be increased, resulting in toxicity. Which medications show this effect?

Alprazolam
Amiodarone
Benzodiazepines
Buspirone
Carbamazepine
Cyclosporine
Dextromethorphan
Diltiazem
Dihydropyridine calcium channel blockers
Erythromycin
Estrogens

Fexofenadine
Fluoxetine
3-Hydroxy-3-methylglutaryl coenzyme A
(HMG-CoA) reductase inhibitors
Itraconazole
Methylprednisone
Sertraline
Saquinavir
Sildenafil
Verapamil
Warfarin

48. How much grapefruit juice can be consumed by patients on these medications?
One cup of juice or one-half grapefruit is probably safe if taken at a different time from the medication. Drug interactions with grapefruit juice. *Med Lett.* 2004;46:2–3.

49. Which is a greater risk factor for cardiovascular disease: cigarette smoking or obesity?
Cigarette smoking.

DERMATOLOGY

50. List your treatment recommendations to an adolescent with mild, mixed noninflammatory acne (primarily comedones or "blackheads" and inflammatory acne [pustules and papules]).
- Avoid oily cosmetics.
- Do not rub the face.
- Use sunscreen.
- Use mild cleansing soap.
- Apply topical retinoic acid cream (or gel).
- Apply topical antimicrobials.
- Consider topical benzoyl peroxide with topical antimicrobial to limit antibiotic resistance.
- Can use salicylic acid as alternative to topical retinoid.

51. What oral contraceptive pills (OCPs) are approved for acne treatment?
- Norgestimate and ethinyl estradiol (Ortho Tri-Cyclen)
- Ethinyl estradiol 20 µg/drospirenone 3 mg (Yaz)
- Ethinyl estradiol and norethindrone (Estrostep)

52. Define *hidradenitis suppurativa* and *erythrasma*.
- **Hidradenitis suppurativa:** An apocrine sweat gland infection of the axilla, groin, breasts, or buttocks that can cause inflammation and scarring
- **Erythrasma:** A skin infection caused by *Corynebacterium minutissimum* that occurs in the axilla or groin or sometimes between the toes

53. How do you recognize tinea versicolor (pityriasis)?
As macular lesions of various colors such as red, pink, or brown. Slight scale may be present. Involved areas do not tan and are hypopigmented.

54. How do you treat pityriasis?
With topical corticosteroids and antihistamines for severe itching. Usually no treatment is needed, but acyclovir may be helpful for severe itching or cosmetic reasons, as may phototherapy.
Drago F, Veechio F, Rebora A. Use of high-dose acyclovir in pityriasis rosea. *J Am Acad Dermatol.* 2006;54:82–85.

55. **What is the ABCDE rule for melanoma?**
Skin lesions are likely melanoma if these characteristics are present:
- **A**symmetry
- **B**order irregularity
- **C**olor variation (usually purple or black)
- **D**iameter > 6 mm
- **E**nlargement of volution of color change, shape, or symptoms
  Friedman RJ, Rigel DS, Kopf AE. Early detection of malignant melanoma: the role of physician examination and self-examination of the skin. *CA Cancer J Clin.* 1984;35:130–151.

ENDOCRINOLOGY

56. **Describe the typical follow-up examination for a patient with non–insulin-dependent DM.**
History:
- Ask about the frequency, cause, and severity of hypoglycemic or hyperglycemic episodes.
- Update medication list.
- Review home glucose monitoring records, if used.
- Ask about any recent illnesses.
- Review diet, eating patterns, sleep behaviors, life stressors, and behavioral supports.
- Ask about dental symptoms and history.
- Inquire about use of tobacco, alcohol, and other substances.
- Review potential complications including known history or symptoms of retinopathy, nephropathy, and neuropathy.
- Review previous BP readings and lipid results.
- Review contraception choices for women of child-bearing potential.

Screening:
- Use screening tools to identify depression, anxiety, or eating disorders.
- Identify psychosocial problems and potential barriers to diabetes self-management.
- Assess for diabetes distress (coping difficulties with demands of diabetes care and monitoring).

Physical examination:
- Record height, height, and body mass index (BMI).
- Measure BP with orthostatic measurement if indicated by symptoms or medication use.
- Perform funduscopic examination.
- Palpate thyroid.
- Inspect skin.
- Examine feet (including inspection for lesions and calluses, assessment of sensation, and palpation of pedal pulses [dorsalis pedis, posterior tibial]).
- Assess reflexes (patellar, Achilles).
- Check sensation (proprioception, vibration, monofilament).
- Confirm annual ophthalmologic examination.
- Confirm annual dental examination.

57. **What laboratory testing should be ordered during follow-up visits?**
- Glycohemoglobin (HbA$_{1c}$) quarterly
- Fasting lipids, including triglycerides, total cholesterol, HDL cholesterol, LDL cholesterol
- Liver function tests
- Spot urinary albumin-to-creatinine ratio
- Serum creatinine, estimated glomerular filtration rate (eGFR)
- Thyroid-stimulating hormone (TSH) (if type 1 diabetes)
  American Diabetes Association. Standards of medical care in diabetes—2017. 3. Comprehensive medical evaluation and assessment of comorbidities. *Diabetes Care.* 2017;40:S25–32.

58. **What immunizations do diabetics need?**
- Completed childhood vaccine series (including MMR [measles-mumps-rubella], HPV [human papillomavirus], and varicella [chickenpox])
- Pneumococcal polysaccharide vaccine (PPSV23) with repeat dose after age 65 if initial dose received before age 65
- Pneumococcal conjugate vaccine (PCV13) if ≥ 65 years

- Influenza vaccine annually
- Tetanus-diphtheria booster every 10 years with at least one dose of tetanus-diphtheria with acellular pertussis (Tdap)
- Hepatitis B vaccine (if not received as a child) if < 60 years old with strong consideration for administration if ≥ 60 years
- Shingles vaccine if ≥ 60 years

Use of hepatitis B vaccination for adults with diabetes mellitus: recommendations of the Advisory Committee on Immunization Practices (ACIP). *Morbid Mortal Rep (MMWR)*. 2011;60:1709–1711.

KEY POINTS: COUNSELING TOPICS FOR PATIENTS WITH DIABETES

1. Exercise
2. Diet
3. Foot care
4. Medication adjustment when ill
5. Regular ophthalmologic follow-up
6. Regular dental follow-up
7. Up-to-date immunizations
8. Smoking cessation
9. Management of hypoglycemic and hyperglycemic episodes
10. Psychosocial support
11. Signs of diabetic distress

59. **What test is most useful for monitoring thyroid replacement therapy?**
Thyroid-stimulating hormone (TSH).

60. **List the skin findings of hyperthyroidism.**
- Warm, moist, "velvety" texture of skin
- Increased palmar or dorsal sweating
- Facial flushing
- Palmar erythema
- Vitiligo
- Altered hair texture
- Alopecia
- Pretibial myxedema

61. **What are the skin findings in hypothyroidism?**
- Decreased sweating
- Color changes to skin
- Coarse hair or hair loss
- Brittle nails
- Pretibial myxedema (due to hypothyroidism resulting from treatment of Graves disease)
- Generalized nonpitting edema (myxedema)
- Periorbital edema

62. **When should thyroid antibodies be ordered?**
To distinguish Hashimoto thyroiditis (and likely permanent hypothyroidism) from subclinical hypothyroidism, painless thyroiditis, or postpartum thyroiditis.

63. **What thyroid antibody test is ordered?**
Thyroid peroxidase antibody.

64. **What are the thyroid effects of lithium?**
- Goiter
- Hypothyroidism
- Chronic autoimmune thyroiditis
- Hyperthyroidism (uncommon)

65. **How is hypothyroidism due to lithium detected?**
By an elevated TSH. Hypothyroidism is most likely to occur in the first 2 years of therapy and is more common in women > 45 years of age.

66. **What are the risk factors for osteoporosis?**
Women ≥ 65 years old, men ≥ 70 years old, postmenopausal state, medication use (glucocorticoids, chronic heparin, vitamin A, cyclosporine, methotrexate, anticonvulsants, thyroid replacement, thiazolidinediones, proton pump inhibitors [possible], and anxiolytics), chronic illnesses (systemic lupus erythematosus; rheumatoid arthritis; psoriatic arthritis; cancer treatment; cystic fibrosis; inflammatory bowel disease; celiac disease; hyperthyroidism; hyperparathyroidism; hypercalciuria; vitamin D deficiency; osteogenesis imperfecta; human immunodeficiency virus [HIV]; alcoholism; diabetes; hypogonadotropic hypogonadism caused by low weight, eating disorders, excessive exercise, hyperprolactinemia, or hypopituitarism; and chronic liver disease), positive family history, cigarette smoking, excessive caffeine intake, low body weight, above average height, sustained amenorrhea, and lack of exercise.

67. **What is the role of estrogen-progesterone therapy in prevention and treatment of osteoporosis?**
Although estrogen-progesterone therapy has been shown to reduce fracture risk in postmenopausal women, recent data from the Women's Health Initiative (WHI) suggest that the risks of cardiac events, breast cancer, and stroke are increased in treated women and outweigh potential benefit.
    Rossouw JE, Anderson GL, Prentice RL, et al. Risks and benefits of estrogen plus progestin in healthy postmenopausal women: principal results From the Women's Health Initiative randomized controlled trial. *JAMA*. 2002;288:321–333.

68. **How should you instruct patients to take a bisphosphonate?**
    - Use weekly or monthly preparation.
    - Take the pill first thing in the morning with a full glass of water.
    - Do not take with other pills or food.
    - Do not eat, drink, or swallow any other pills for 30 minutes.
    - Maintain upright posture (either sitting or standing) for 30 minutes.

69. **What are some of the side effects of bisphosphonate therapy?**
    - Esophageal ulceration, gastritis, gastroesophageal reflux disease, possibly esophageal cancer
    - Joint and muscle pain
    - Long bone fracture (midshaft)
    - Osteonecrosis of the jaw
    - Flu-like illness after intravenous administration

70. **Which patients should not receive bisphosphonate therapy?**
Those with:
    - Chronic kidney disease (eGFR < 30 mL/min)
    - Chronic esophageal disease (achalasia, strictures, Barrett esophagus, varices)
    - Inability to maintain upright posture for 30–60 minutes after ingesting oral preparation

71. **What is the BMI?**
Body mass index. The BMI gives an estimate of risk of complications of obesity because it relates weight to height. Calculations can be obtained from tables or nomograms. Ideal BMI is < 25.
    Available at: https://www.nhlbi.nih.gov/health/educational/lose_wt/BMI/bmicalc.htm. Accessed January 22, 2017.

72. **List the complications of morbid obesity.**
    - HTN
    - Coronary artery disease
    - Impaired glucose tolerance (metabolic syndrome)
    - DM
    - Increased mortality risk from all causes, including cancer
    - Sleep apnea
    - Osteoarthritis
    - Depression
    - Recurrent skin infections (particularly intertriginous areas)
    - Cancers (breast, colon, uterine)

73. **What initial tests should be done to evaluate involuntary weight loss?**
    - Thorough interview to identify underlying depression or eating disorder
    - Complete blood count (CBC)
    - Electrolytes, glucose, calcium, liver function tests, blood urea nitrogen (BUN), and creatinine
    - TSH
    - Human immunodeficiency virus (HIV)
    - Erythrocyte sedimentation rate (ESR) or C-reactive protein (CRP)
    - Chest x-ray

    Additional testing will be guided by the results of additional history, physical examination, and these tests.

GASTROENTEROLOGY

74. **What medications can cause chronic constipation?**
    - Calcium channel blockers
    - Antihistamines
    - Opiates
    - Iron
    - Tricyclic antidepressants
    - Anticholinergics
    - Aluminum- and calcium-based antacids
    - Calcium supplements
    - Sucralfate
    - Disopyramide
    - Laxatives (if abused)
    - Antipsychotics
    - Antiparkinson drugs
    - Aluminum- and calcium-containing antacids
    - Antidiarrheal drugs
    - Diuretics
    - Beta-blockers

75. **What is the treatment of chronic constipation?**
    - Regular exercise.
    - Establishment of regular bowel schedules. The gastrocolic reflex and urge to have a bowel movement are greatest about 30 minutes after breakfast.
    - Adjustment of dose or discontinuance of medications that contribute to constipation, if possible.
    - Bulk-forming agents (psyllium, methylcellulose, and polycarbophil) that should be taken with adequate fluids.
    - Hyperosmolar agents (lactulose, sorbitol, and polyethylene glycol).
    - Stimulant laxatives (senna and bisacodyl) as needed.

    Lubiprostone is an approved medicine for the treatment of women with irritable bowel syndrome who have constipation as the main symptom and can also be used for chronic constipation. Lubiprostone improves the frequency of bowel movements and reduces straining and bloating. Side effects include nausea, headache, abdominal pain, and diarrhea. Methylnaltrexone is also available for use in opioid-induced constipation.

    Available at: https://www.uptodate.com/contents/methylnaltrexone-drug-information?source=see_link.

76. **Define *proctalgia fugax*.**
    A fleeting, deep pain in the rectum, possibly caused by muscle spasm. Tenderness is found on digital rectal examination.

77. **What NSAIDs have the greatest risk of gastrointestinal (GI) symptoms?**
    Piroxicam, indomethacin, and ketorolac. Ibuprofen has a low risk of GI bleeding, and cyclooxygenase-2 (COX-2) inhibitors have the lowest risk.

    Gonzalez EM, Patrignani P, Tacconelli S, et al. Variability among nonsteroidal antiinflammatory drugs in risk of upper gastrointestinal bleeding. *Arthritis Rheum.* 2010;62:1592–1601.

78. **How can the risk of gastric and duodenal ulcers with the use of NSAIDs be decreased?**
    By testing for and treating *Helicobacter pylori* infection in patients with history of peptic ulcer disease and use of proton pump inhibitors.
    Bhatt DL, Scheiman J, Abraham NS, et al. ACCF/ACG/AHA 2008 Expert Consensus Document on Reducing the Gastrointestinal Risks of Antiplatelet Therapy and NSAID Use. *Am J Gastroenterol.* 2008;103:1–18.

79. **What is the effect of omeprazole on clopidogrel?**
    Concurrent use of omeprazole and clopidogrel may result in decreased effectiveness of clopidogrel in reducing thrombotic events.

80. **What is fecal transplant?**
    Rectal deposition (through colonoscopy, naso/jejunal tube, or retention enema) of purified donor stool sample into a recipient who has had recurrent *Clostridium difficile* infections unresponsive to antibiotic therapy.

81. **What is the irritable bowel syndrome?**
    One of the most commonly diagnosed gastrointestinal disorders characterized with chronic abdominal pain and altered bowel habits (constipation, diarrhea, or both). (See Chapter 7, Gastroenterology.)

GYNECOLOGY

82. **What topics should you cover in the history of a 20-year-old, sexually active woman with the complaint of acute dysuria?**
    Ask about hematuria; vaginal discharge; flank pain; fever; chills; last menses; previous medical history including DM, gynecologic surgeries, urologic procedures, pregnancy, and recent antibiotic use; current sexual activity; use of barrier contraception; use of OCPs; illness or symptoms in sexual partner; recent new sexual partner; previous sexually transmitted diseases (STDs); and HIV test results, if done.

83. **What should the physical examination include in the same patient?**
    Temperature, pulse, BP, abdominal examination, evaluation for flank tenderness, and bimanual examination if cervicitis or vaginitis or both are likely by history.

84. **What laboratory tests should you order for this patient?**
    Urinalysis (dipstick) to examine for leukocyte esterase and hematuria; wet mount of vaginal discharge including addition of 10% potassium hydroxide (KOH), with pH measurement and smell test; and nucleic acid amplification test (NAAT) of vaginal fluid for *Chlamydia* spp. and *Neisseria gonorrhoeae* if cervical or adnexal tenderness is present. If the history and examination suggest acute cystitis without complications, empirical treatment can be started with trimethaprim-sulfamethoxazole (TMP-SMX [3 days]), nitrofurantoin monohydrate [5 days], or fosfamycin trometamol (single dose). Fluoroquinolones are considered second-line agents owing to concerns of antibiotic resistance. Pyridium is helpful for symptom relief. If there are risk factors for STDs, doxycycline for 7 days or single-dose azithromycin is the appropriate choice. Urine culture is not necessary for young healthy women without history of recent antibiotic use or recurrent urinary tract infections (UTIs), but should be done in areas of high antibiotic resistance. Older women with underlying medical problems are at greater risk of complications and should have urine culture and antibiotic treatment for 7 days' duration.

85. **List the common causes of abnormal vaginal bleeding in premenopausal women.**
    - Threatened or complete abortion
    - Ectopic pregnancy
    - Hypothyroidism
    - Hypercortisolism
    - Polycystic ovary syndrome
    - Thrombocytopenia
    - Bleeding diathesis
    - Vulvar infection, laceration, or tumor

- Vaginal laceration, tumor, or foreign body
- Cervical infection, erosion, polyp, or carcinoma
- Uterine infection, polyp, fibroids, or carcinoma
- Ovarian infection
- Intrauterine device
- Idiopathic

86. **How do you manage a woman with postmenopausal vaginal bleeding?**
With referral to a gynecologist for consideration of diagnostic studies to detect endometrial carcinoma.

87. **What is the interpretation of ASC-US result on Pap smear?**
Atypical squamous cells of uncertain insignificance. Women > 25 years should have testing for human papillomavirus (HPV) and referral for colposcopy and treatment if positive for HPV. Women aged 21–24 years may be managed with repeat Pap smear in 1 year.

88. **What is the interpretation of ASC-H result on Pap smear?**
Atypical squamous cells in which a high-grade squamous intraepithelial lesion (HSIL) cannot be excluded. These women should be referred for colposcopy and treatment.
   Massad LS, Einstein MH, Huh WK, et al. 2012 updated consensus guidelines for the management of abnormal cervical cancer screening tests and cancer precursors. *J Low Genit Tract Dis.* 2013;17:S1–27.

89. **List the characteristic vaginal discharges caused by *Candida albicans*, *N. gonorrhoeae*, bacterial vaginosis, and *Trichomonas vaginalis*.**
See Table 2.6.

Table 2.6. Characteristic Vaginal Diseases of Common Infections

ORGANISM	DISCHARGE CHARACTERISTICS
Candida albicans	Thick, white, curdlike, adherent to vaginal wall with satellite lesions and erythema on perineum
Neisseria gonorrhoeae	Mucopurulent with cervicitis
Gardnerella vaginalis (and other organisms)	Foul-smelling ("fishy" with KOH), thin, scanty, white, frothy, and adherent to vaginal wall pH >3.5 and <4.5
Trichomonas vaginalis	Copious, yellow-green, frothy

KOH, potassium hydroxide.

90. **What are clue cells?**
Epithelial cells covered with coccobacilli or curved rods. Clue cells are found in the vaginal discharge of patients with bacterial vaginosis.

91. **What is atrophic vaginitis?**
Symptoms of vaginal burning, pruritus, discharge, bleeding, and dyspareunia in postmenopausal women due to estrogen loss. Topical intravaginal estrogen can help with symptoms.

92. **What are the absolute contraindications to the use of OCPs?**
- Pregnancy or lactation
- Thrombophlebitis or known thrombophilia
- History of stroke
- History of thromboembolic event
- History of estrogen-dependent tumor (breast and endometrium)
- Active liver disease (cirrhosis, hepatocellular adenoma, or malignant hepatoma)
- Uterine bleeding of unknown cause
- Hypertriglyceridemia

- Heavy smoking (>15 cigarettes/day) in women > 35 years
- Systemic lupus erythematosus
- Migraine headaches with aura

93. **What are the preventive measures for cervical carcinoma?**
Safer sex practices and immunization with HPV vaccine. HPV vaccination should begin for boys and girls at age 11–12 years, preferably before sexual activity and HPV exposure. Teens can "catch up" with subsequent vaccine dose for young women through age 26, and young men through age 21. HPV vaccine is also recommended for those who did not get vaccinated previously and are:
    - young men who have sex with men, including young men who identify as gay or bisexual or who intend to have sex with men through age 26;
    - young adults who are transgender through age 26; and
    - young adults with certain immunocompromising conditions (including HIV) through age 26.
    Centers for Diseases Control and Prevention (CDC), Petrosky E, Bocchini JA Jr, Hariri S, et al. Use of 9-Valent human papillomavirus (HPV) vaccine: updated HPV vaccination recommendations of the Advisory Committee on Immunization Practices. *MMWR Morb Mortal Wkly Rep.* 2015;64:300–304.

94. **Describe the evaluation of a new breast nodule discovered in a 50-year-old woman during routine examination.**
    - **History:** Personal history of breast disorders and biopsies; family history of breast, ovarian, or colon cancer; use of hormone replacement therapy; and use of OCPs
    - **Physical examination:** Location, size, mobility, and consistency of nodule; presence or absence of nipple discharge; presence or absence of axillary adenopathy; and complete examination of contralateral breast and axilla
    - **X-ray:** Mammogram with appropriate needle aspiration or biopsy of suspicious lesions
    Most importantly, a new solitary nodule should always be biopsied even if a mammogram is normal.

95. **What is the role of genetic testing in the risk assessment for breast cancer?**
The gene mutations associated with an increased risk of breast and ovarian cancer (*BRAC1* and *BRAC2*) have been identified and can be commercially tested. The results may be difficult to interpret and women may be unduly concerned or relieved about their breast cancer risk if improperly interpreted. If a woman requests genetic testing because of a perceived increased family risk, she should be referred to a genetic counseling center or specialists where a thorough family history can be obtained and appropriate counseling and testing provided. Patients considered for referral include those with:
    - Two first-degree relatives with breast cancer, one of whom was diagnosed before age 50
    - Three or more first- or second-degree relatives with breast cancer
    - Both breast and ovarian cancer in first- and second-degree relatives in any combination
    - Bilateral breast cancer in first-degree relative
    - Male relative with breast cancer
    - First- or second-degree relative with breast and ovarian cancer
    Women of Askhenazi Jewish heritage should be referred if any first-degree or two second-degree relatives on the same family side have breast cancer.

96. **What is premenstrual syndrome (PMS)?**
A group of physical and psychological symptoms that occur approximately 5 days prior to menses consistently during a woman's menstrual cycle and lead to significant social and occupational dysfunction. Physical symptoms include abdominal bloating, fatigue, breast tenderness, and headaches. Emotional symptoms include depression, irritability, confusion, and feelings of isolation.

97. **What are the treatments for PMS?**
Selective serotonin reuptake inhibitors (SSRIs) such as fluoxetine, sertraline, paroxetine, and citalopram have the most clinical efficacy and may be given daily or begin on day 14 of the menstrual cycle or with symptom onset. Oral contraceptives are also an option. Gonadotropin-releasing hormone agonists are helpful, too, but may have significant side effects.

98. **What is PMDD?**
Premenstrual dysphoric disorder with symptoms of PMS in addition to at least one affective symptom such as anger, irritability, or emotional tension.

HEMATOLOGY

99. Which medications and supplements affect the effects of warfarin?
See Table 2.7.

Table 2.7. Effects of Medications and Supplements on Anticoagulation Effects of Warfarin

Anticoagulant Effect	
INCREASED (INCREASED INR)	**DECREASED (DECREASED INR)**
Acetaminophen	Antithyroid agents
Allopurinol	Barbiturates
Amiodarone	Bile acid sequestrants
Clopidogrel	Carbamazepine
Cranberry (including juice)	Coenzyme Q_{10}
5-FU	Dicloxacillin
Fenofibrate	Ginseng
Fluconazole	Nafcillin
Fluoroquinolones	Oral contraceptives
Fluvoxamine	St. John's wort
Gingko biloba	Sucralfate
Green tea	
H_2 receptor blockers	
HMG-CoA reductase inhibitors (except atorvastatin)	
Ketoconazole	
Metronidazole	
NSAIDs (COX-2 inhibitors)	
NSAIDs (nonselective)	
Omega-3 fatty acids	
Orlistat	
Phenytoin	
Proton pump inhibitors	
SSRIs	
Trimethoprim-sulfamethoxazole	
Tetracyclines	
Tricyclic antidepressant	
Venlafaxine	
Vitamin A	
Vitamin E	

COX-2, cyclooxygenase-2; 5-FU, fluorouracil; HMG-CoA, 3-hydroxy-3-methylglutaryl coenzyme A; INR, international normalized ratio; NSAIDs, nonsteroidal anti-inflammatory drugs; SSRIs, selective serotonin reuptake inhibitors.

INFECTIOUS DISEASES AND IMMUNIZATION

100. List the high-risk factors that indicate the need for the pneumococcal polysaccharide vaccine (PPSV23).
- Age ≥ 65 years
- Chronic cardiovascular disease such as congestive heart failure and cardiomyopathies
- Chronic pulmonary disease (including asthma, emphysema, and chronic obstructive pulmonary disease [COPD])
- DM
- Alcoholism
- Chronic liver disease, including cirrhosis
- Cerebrospinal fluid (CSF) leaks
- Asplenia, either functional (sickle cell disease/hemoglobinopathy) or anatomic
- Immunosuppression including leukemia, lymphoma, Hodgkin disease, other malignancy, multiple myeloma, chronic renal failure, nephrotic syndrome, solid organ transplants, chronic corticosteroid use, and HIV infection

- Cochlear implant
- Cigarette smoking

101. Who should receive pneumococcal conjugate vaccine (PCV13)?
All of the above, EXCEPT PCV 13 is not recommended for patients with chronic heart, liver, or lung disease; diabetes; and cigarette smoking.

102. What is the schedule for PCV13 and PPSV23 administration?
Generally for adults who have not received a pneumococcal vaccine, PCV13 is given first, followed by PPSV23 1 year later. If PPSV23 was initially received before age 65, an additional dose should be give after age 65 but always separated by 1 year from a dose of PCV13.

103. What is a VIS?
Vaccine Information Sheet, which is available for each vaccine and published by and provided by the CDC. The VIS provides information for the patient on who should receive the designated vaccine and potential benefits and side effects. Every patient should receive a current VIS at the time of vaccination. The most up-to-date VIS can be obtained from the CDC.

Available at: www.cdc.gov/vaccines/hcp/vis/index.html. Accessed January 24, 2017.

Kim DK, Riley LE, Harriman KH, et al. Recommended immunization schedule for adults aged 19 years or older, United States, 2017. *Ann Intern Med.* 2017;166:209–218. (Updated annually)

KEY POINTS: VACCINES FOR ADULTS

1. All adults should receive IIV or RIV annually. Older adults (65 years or older) may receive high dose IIV.
2. Td is administered every 10 years, but at least one dose of Td should be replaced with Tdap.
3. Adults who have egg allergy manifested as hives can receive IIV or RIV.
4. Patients receiving anticoagulants may safely receive IIV or RIV.
5. PCV13 and PPSV23 are both administered to adults 65 years or older and those with additional medical conditions at least 1 year apart.
6. HZV can be given to all adults > 60 years who do not have contraindications to a live vaccine regardless of known episode of herpes zoster infection.
7. History should be reviewed for high-risk conditions that may indicate need for MMR, HPV, HepA, HepB, MenACWY or MPSV4, MenB, and Hib.

HepA, hepatitis A vaccine; HepB, hepatitis B vaccine; Hib, *Haemophilus influenzae* type B conjugate vaccine; HPV, human papillomavirus vaccine; HZV, herpes zoster vaccine; IIV, inactivated influenza vaccine; MenACWY, serogroups A, C ,W, and Y meningococcal conjugate vaccine; MenB, serogroup B meningococcal vaccine; MMR, measles, mumps, and rubella vaccine; MPSV4, serogroups A, C, W, and Y meningococcal polysaccharide vaccine; PCV13, 13-valent pneumococcal conjugate vaccine; PPSV23, 23-valent pneumococcal polysaccharide vaccine; RIV, recombinant influenza vaccine; Td, tetanus and diphtheria toxoids; Tdap, tetanus toxoid, reduced diphtheria toxoid, and acellular pertussis vaccine.

---

104. List the symptoms of influenza.
Sudden onset of high fever
Myalgia
Headache
Malaise
Coryza
Sore throat
Also, influenza infection may present with mild upper respiratory tract symptoms without fever.

105. What are the complications of influenza?
- Pneumonia (either primary influenza pneumonia or secondary bacterial pneumonia)
- Encephalitis and myelitis
- Hepatitis and pancreatitis
- Myositis and rhabdomyolysis
- Asthenia and prolonged fatigue
- Reye syndrome (in children and adolescents)

106. How do you diagnose influenza?

By clinical findings supported by community epidemiologic data and confirmed by laboratory testing. Influenza A or B is very likely when a patient presents with the symptoms described in Question 104 during the time when influenza is known to circulate in your community. The Centers for Disease Control and Prevention publishes influenza updates October through May on its website. Local health departments also publish data from the local community. The suspicion of influenza can be confirmed through rapid tests done in the office from nasal or throat swabs. Some rapid tests may only detect influenza A, detect influenza A and B but not distinguish between the two strains, or distinguish between influenza A and B.

Available at: https://www.cdc.gov/flu/weekly/fluactivitysurv.htm. Accessed January 22, 2017.

107. What are the treatments for influenza?

The symptoms may be relieved by cough suppressants and acetaminophen. Aspirin should not be used during influenza epidemics. Antiviral agents that reduce the duration and severity of influenza are also indicated for severe disease. Amantadine and rimantadine were the first agents available to treat influenza but are effective only against influenza A and have central nervous system (CNS) side effects, particularly in the elderly. Newer neuroaminadase inhibitors (zanamivir and oseltamivir) are effective against both influenza A and B. Zanamivir is given as an inhaled powder. All of these drugs should be given within the first 48 hours from the onset of symptoms and reduce the symptomatic phase by about 1 day. These treatments may not be effective in severe influenza. Some oseltamivir resistance was noted during the H1N1 pandemic. Peramivir is available as an intravenous preparation if the patient is unable to receive oral or inhalation drugs. The upper respiratory symptoms are treated with acetaminophen or NSAIDs. Patients should rest as needed and remain hydrated.

108. How do you prevent influenza?

By practicing infection prevention habits (washing hands frequently, avoiding close contact with those who are ill with upper respiratory symptoms, covering a sneeze or cough with a tissue or elbow/upper sleeve), and administering seasonal influenza virus vaccine, given annually in the fall in physicians' offices, at the time of hospital discharge, and in local health departments. Many community groups, churches, pharmacies, and grocery stores also sponsor opportunities to receive vaccine. The vaccine is reformulated each year and should be given annually to ensure protection against the current year's circulating virus. Amantadine, rimantadine, and zanamivir may also be used for prevention in those exposed to influenza before receiving the vaccine or those unable to receive the vaccine.

109. Who should receive influenza seasonal vaccine?

All people older than 6 months who do not have contraindications to the vaccine.

110. Who should not receive seasonal influenza virus vaccine?

- People with documented severe reaction to egg (i.e., anaphylaxis)
- People with a history of Guillain-Barré syndrome after previous influenza virus vaccination

The CDC provides guidelines for evaluating the risk of influenza vaccine in these patients.

Grohskopf LA, Sokolow LZ, Broder KR, et al. Prevention and control of seasonal influenza with vaccines. *MMWR Morb Mort Wkly Rep.* 2016;65:1–54. (Updated annually)

111. Who should receive high-dose influenza vaccine?

Those > 65 years.

112. Which patients with wounds should receive tetanus immune globulin (TIG) in addition to tetanus and diphtheria toxoids (Td)?

Patients who received < three previous doses of Td or whose Td doses are unknown AND have one of the following wound characteristics:

- Contaminated with dirt, feces, or saliva
- Caused by puncture, sharp object penetration, frostbite, or burns
- >6 hours old
- >1 cm depth
- Devitalized

113. When is tetanus, diphtheria, and pertussis (Tdap) vaccine indicated?

As a replacement dose for Td toxoid in adults who have not received a previous Tdap dose. After receiving one dose of Tdap, Td toxoid can be used every 10 years for subsequent booster doses.

114. **What vaccines should a pregnant woman receive?**
Influenza vaccine and Tdap. Specific groups of pregnant women may consider hepatitis A, hepatitis B, and meningococcal vaccines.

115. **What is considered acceptable evidence of immunity to measles, mumps, or rubella (MMR)?**
- Born before 1957
- Documentation of MMR vaccine receipt
- Serologic evidence of immunity

116. **Is MMR a live vaccine?**
Yes, and therefore should not be given to pregnant women and patients with HIV infection or other immunosuppression.

117. **What types of meningococcal vaccines are available?**
Meningococcal conjugate vaccine, quadrivalent (MenACWY), meningococcal polysaccharide vaccine (MPSV4), and serogroup B meningococcal vaccine. Up-to-date recommendations for use and schedule of these vaccines are available at: https://www.cdc.gov/vaccines/schedules/hcp/imz/adult.html. Accessed January 30, 2017.

118. **Who should receive meningococcal vaccine?**
- All healthy adolescents
- New entrants to institutions with residential living (e.g., dormitories, military barracks)
- Those with anatomic or functional asplenia
- HIV-infected individuals
- Those with complement pathway deficiencies
- Microbiologists exposed to *Neisseria meningitidis*

119. **Who should receive hepatitis A virus (HAV) vaccine?**
- Frequent travelers to Mexico, the Caribbean, Asia (excluding Japan), Eastern Europe, South America, and Africa
- Patients with chronic liver disease
- Anticipated close household or babysitting contact with an international adoptee from a country of high or intermediate endemicity
- Illegal drug users
- Men who have sex with men
- Adults who receive clotting factor replacement
- Research staff who work with HAV-infected primates or HAV in a laboratory

120. **Who should be screened for hepatitis C virus (HCV)?**
Those who:
- Were born between 1945 and 1965
- Currently or previously inject or injected drugs
- Received clotting factor concentrates produced before 1987
- Have ever received long-term hemodialysis
- Have persistently abnormal alanine aminotransferase (ALT) levels
- Have HIV infection
- Were prior recipients of transfusions or organ transplants, including those who:
  - Received blood from a donor who later tested positive for HCV infection
  - Received a transfusion of blood, blood components, or an organ transplant before July 1992

121. **What suggestions would you give to a patient traveling outside the United States?**
- Review any travel precautions and needed vaccinations at www.cdc.gov/travel/.
- Consider purchase of travel insurance including evacuation coverage. Additional insurance is particularly important for Medicare beneficiaries because Centers for Medicare and Medicaid Services (CMS) does not cover medical care in foreign countries.
- Register your travel plans with the U.S. State Department at https://step.state.gov/step/ to receive travel notifications.

122. Which immunizations should a person who has had a splenectomy or functional asplenia (i.e., sickle cell disease) receive?
    - Pneumococcal: Both PCV13 and PPS23
    - Meningococcal: Give two doses of or MCV4 2 months apart **and** MenB
    - *Haemophilus influenzae* type B (HiB)
    - Usual schedules based on age and other risk factors for influenza vaccine, Tdap, hepatitis A, hepatitis B, and shingles vaccine

123. What causes Lyme disease? How does it present?
    Borrelia burgdorferi, a tick-borne spirochete. A characteristic rash (erythema migrans), followed in weeks to months by involvement of other organ systems (including cardiovascular and neurologic systems and joints) often accompanies the initial infection.

124. Who should receive prophylactic treatment for latent tuberculosis (TB)?
    Anyone with recent conversion of purified protein derivative (PPD) skin test to positive classified on the size of the induration:
    - **≥5 mm:** If immunosuppression due to medications, HIV infection, and recent contacts of TB cases, fibrotic changes on chest x-ray suggesting old TB
    - **≥10 mm:** Residents or employees of high-risk settings (prisons, nursing homes, homeless shelters, hospitals, residential care facilities for AIDS patients), recent (<5 years) immigrants from high-prevalence countries, mycobacteriology laboratory personnel, and injection drug users
    - **≥15 mm:** All others without risk factors
    An increase in induration of > 10 mm within 2 years is also considered a positive tuberculin skin test.

125. What organisms commonly cause nongonococcal urethritis (NGU) in men?
    - *Chlamydia trachomatis*
    - *Mycoplasma genitalium*
    - *Trichomonas vaginalis*
    - *Ureaplasma urealyticum* (more recently questionable)
    - Herpes simplex virus
    - Adenovirus

126. What organisms commonly cause epididymitis?
    - *C. trachomatis*
    - *N. gonorrhoeae*
    - *U. urealyticum*
    - Gram-negative organisms (older men)
    - *Mycobacterium tuberculosis*
    - *Brucella* spp.

NEUROLOGY

127. What are the prodromal symptoms of herpes zoster (shingles)?
    Headache, malaise, pain, and paresthesias (in the involved dermatome).

128. What is meralgia paresthetica?
    The entrapment of the lateral femoral cutaneous nerve producing pain and numbness over the anterolateral thigh.

129. What are risk factors for meralgia paresthetica?
    - DM
    - Pregnancy
    - Obesity
    - Sudden weight loss
    - Girdles, guns, belts, and other tight-fitting accessories

130. List the typical symptoms of migraine, tension, and cluster headaches.
    See Table 2.8.

Table 2.8. Symptoms of Migraine, Tension, and Cluster Headaches

SYMPTOM FEATURE	MIGRAINE	TENSION	CLUSTER
Location	Hemicranial	Entire head or bitemporal	Unilateral
Pain quality	Throbbing	Aching	Burning
Duration	2–6 hr	Days	1–2 hr
Frequency	Episodic	Daily	Flurry of attacks for several weeks
Associated symptoms	Prodrome	Neck and shoulder aching	Ipsilateral sweating, flushing, lacrimation, and rhinorrhea

131. **What is a "thunderclap" headache?**
Sudden onset of severe head pain with rapid escalation described by the patient as "the worst headache I've ever had." These patients require emergent evaluation with head CT scan and possibly lumbar puncture. The most common cause is subarachnoid hemorrhage, but it may also be due to carotid or vertebral dissection or cerebral vein thrombosis.

132. **What is amaurosis fugax?**
Sudden loss of vision in one eye associated with transient ischemic attack (TIA). It may be described as a "shade" coming down over the eye.

133. **List the symptom triad of Ménière syndrome.**
Paroxysmal vertigo, hearing loss, and tinnitus.

134. **What are the frequent causes of acute loss or impairment of smell?**
Head trauma and viral infection.

135. **What is Phalen's maneuver?**
Forced flexion (hyperextension) of the wrist. If carpal tunnel syndrome is present, the symptoms of pain and paresthesia are reproduced.

136. **Compare the neurologic findings in a patient with the following nerve root compressions: L4, L5, and S1.**
See Table 2.9.

Table 2.9. Findings in Nerve Root Compressions at L4, L5, and S1

ROOT	DISC	MUSCLE WEAKNESS	SENSORY LOSS	ABSENT REFLEX
L4	L3–4	Leg extensors (quadriceps)	Anterolateral thigh, medial lower leg	Patellar
L5	L4–5	First toe dorsiflexion (extensor hallucis longus), heel walking (tibialis anterior)	Dorsum of foot	None
S1	L5–S1	Toe walking (gastrocnemius)	Lateral foot and fifth toe	Ankle

ORTHOPEDICS

137. **What are the common causes of knee pain?**
- Osteoarthritis
- Inflammatory arthritis (rheumatoid, reactive, and psoriatic arthritis and gout)
- Chondromalacia
- Chondrocalcinosis (pseudogout)
- Baker cyst
- Septic arthritis
- Trauma (ligamental and meniscal injuries)

- Bursitis
- Iliotibial band syndrome
- Patellofemoral syndrome

138. What is trochanteric bursitis?
A painful inflammation of the bursa superficial to the greater trochanter of the femur. Symptoms include lateral pain described as being in the "hip," although the hip joint itself is not involved. The most classic finding is point tenderness over the greater trochanter.

139. Can hip pads prevent hip fractures?
Yes. Commercially available, small, lightweight pads can be easily worn daily and prevent hip fractures after falls.

140. Which toe fracture should be referred to an orthopedist?
Fractures of the proximal phalanx of the first toe. A fracture that involves the distal phalanx and extends into the interphalangeal joint also should be referred.

141. How do you treat a coccygeal fracture?
Conservatively with analgesics and seating cushions. Inflatable "donut" cushions should not be used because they can lead to pressure ulcers. Coccygeal fractures usually result from a fall.

142. How do you manage a patient with acute low back pain?
If a patient has no signs of nerve root compression and mild to moderate pain, usual activity should be encouraged. Nonpharmacologic treatments such as heat, massage, acupuncture, and spinal manipulation can be tried first. If medications are needed for pain control, NSAIDs are preferred and tramadol or duloxetine should be considered second-line choices. Tai-chi, mindfulness-based stress reduction, relaxation therapy, and exercise may also be helpful.

> Qaseem A, Wilt TJ, McLean RM, et al. Noninvasive treatments for acute, subacute, and chronic low back pain: a clinical practice guideline from the American College of Physicians. Ann Intern Med 2017;166:514–530.

143. What should be done if the patient has severe pain or signs of nerve root compression?
Bed rest may be needed but should be limited to only 2 days. Once a patient can sit comfortably, increasing exercise levels is warranted. Patients with occupations that require prolonged sitting or standing, bending, or lifting will need evaluation and counseling to prevent future back injury. NSAIDs are the preferred initial medications, if needed, and need for opioid therapy must be closely assessed before prescribing.

144. What are the rotator cuff muscles?
- Supraspinatus
- Infraspinatus
- Teres minor
- Subscapularis

145. What syndromes are associated with rotator cuff injury or dysfunction?
Impingement syndrome and rotator cuff tendinitis. Impingement syndrome occurs when the supraspinatus tendon is injured through repetitive motions and is "caught." Pain worsens with overhead arm movement and internal rotation. Symptoms of tendinitis are usually acute.

146. What is Tietze syndrome?
Mild inflammation of the costochondral junction that produces localized warmth, swelling, erythema, and pain. The symptoms are reproduced by palpation of the involved area.

BEHAVIORAL MEDICINE

147. What are the diagnostic criteria for major depression?
At least five of these symptoms must have been present nearly every day for 2 consecutive weeks:
- Depressed mood most of the day
- Diminished interest or pleasure in nearly all activities (anhedonia)
- Weight loss or gain or decrease or increase in appetite
- Insomnia or hypersomnia

- Psychomotor agitation or retardation
- Feelings of worthlessness or inappropriate guilt
- Fatigue or low energy
- Decreased ability to think or concentrate
- Recurrent thoughts of death, suicidal ideation, or suicide attempt

American Psychiatric Association. *Diagnostic and Statistical Manual of Mental Disorders.* 5th ed. Primary Care Version (DSM-V). Washington, DC: American Psychiatric Association Press; 2013.

148. **Which medical illnesses can also present with symptoms of depression?**
- **Endocrine disorders:** hyperthyroidism, hypothyroidism, Cushing syndrome, Addison disease, hypercalcemia, hyperparathyroidism
- **Rheumatic disorders:** rheumatoid arthritis, systemic lupus erythematosus, fibromyalgia
- **Neurologic disorders:** temporal lobe epilepsy, chronic intracranial hematoma, cerebrovascular accident, multiple sclerosis, frontal lobe tumor, Alzheimer disease, vascular dementia
- **Infections:** hepatitis, infectious mononucleosis, Lyme disease, HIV infection, TB, syphilis, influenza, viral illnesses
- **Nutritional deficiency:** vitamin B_{12}

149. **List the risk factors for suicide.**
- Male sex
- Single or widowed status
- Unemployment
- Social isolation
- Urban residence
- Recent loss of health
- Recent surgery
- History of impulsive behaviors
- History of suicide attempts
- History of chronic illness such as chronic pain, depression, organic brain syndromes, or psychosis
- History of alcoholism or substance abuse
- Family history of suicide

150. **What is an anniversary reaction?**
Occurrence of symptoms of depressed mood or undefined somatic symptoms as the anniversary of the death of a spouse, relative, or close friend approaches. An anniversary reaction may also occur after any significant loss such as that of a job, limb, or health or divorce.

151. **What is agoraphobia?**
Fear of being in public places. People with agoraphobia may live a reclusive life. Women are most often affected, and symptoms may present in adolescence or the early 20s. If panic attacks accompany agoraphobia, the patient has at least four of these symptoms when in a public place:
- Dyspnea or smothering feeling
- Palpitations
- Chest discomfort
- Choking sensation
- Dizziness, faintness
- Feelings of unreality
- Paresthesias
- Hot and cold flashes
- Sweating
- Trembling
- Feeling of doom or fear of death
- Fear of losing control

152. **What is bipolar disorder, type II?**
The bipolar syndrome characterized by at least one episode of major depression and at least one hypomanic episode. The hypomania is characterized by an abnormally elevated mood (for that individual), but the mood change does not impair function or require hospitalization. Type II bipolar disorder also requires maintenance medication therapy.

153. Are antipsychotic drugs associated with an increased risk of sudden cardiac death?
Yes, particularly in patients with dementia in whom these medications are frequently used for behavior management.
Ray WA, Chung CP, Murray KT. Atypical antipsychotic drugs and the risk of sudden cardiac death. *N Engl J Med.* 2009;360:225–235.

154. What are some of the early signs and symptoms of anorexia nervosa?
- Amenorrhea
- Weight loss
- Distorted body image (feeling "fat" even though clearly emaciated)

155. What skin finding is associated with anorexia nervosa?
Lanugo (abnormal fine hair growth on the arms and legs).

156. What is the CAGE test?
A reliable screening test for alcoholism. A positive answer to at least two of the questions warrants further evaluation for possible alcoholism.

C = Have you ever felt the need to **c**ut down on drinking?
A = Have you ever felt **a**nnoyed by criticism of your drinking?
G = Have you ever felt **g**uilty about your drinking?
E = Have you ever taken a morning **e**ye-opener?

Johnson B, Clark W. Alcoholism: A challenging physician-patient encounter. *J Gen Intern Med.* 1989;4:445–452.

157. Describe the stages of alcohol withdrawal and how soon after the last drink they occur.
- **Minor withdrawal syndromes** (6–36 hours): tremulousness, diaphoresis, tachycardia without mental status changes
- **Seizures** (6–48 hours): grand mal
- **Alcoholic hallucinosis** (12–48 hours): tactile, auditory, or visual hallucinations or combination with normal orientation
- **Delirium tremens** (48–96 hours): delirium, agitation, HTN, fever, diaphoresis that can be fatal
Isbell H, Fraser HF, Wikler A, et al. An experimental study of the etiology of rum fits and delirium tremens. *Q J Stud Alcohol.* 1955;16:1–33.

PULMONARY MEDICINE

158. What is Kartagener syndrome?
The triad of:
- Recurrent sinus and respiratory infections
- Bronchiectasis
- Situs inversus (occasionally)
Male patients may also have immotile spermatozoa. Kartagener syndrome should be considered in patients with recurrent sinusitis and bronchitis that are resistant to treatment.

159. What causes Kartagener syndrome?
An autosomal recessive disorder that leads to dysfunction of airways cilia. The dysfunctional cilia are unable to effectively clear and move mucous secretions of the respiratory tract.
Eliasson R, Mossberg B, Camner P, et al. The immotile cilia syndrome. *N Engl J Med.* 1977;297:1–6.

MISCELLANEOUS

160. Compare the characteristics of bacterial, viral, and allergic conjunctivitis.
See Table 2.10.

Table 2.10. Characteristics of Bacterial, Viral, and Allergic Conjunctivitis

CHARACTERISTIC	BACTERIAL	VIRAL	ALLERGIC
Foreign body sensation	–	±	–
Itching	±	±	++
Tearing	+	++	+
Discharge	Mucopurulent	Mucoid	–
Preauricular adenopathy	–	+	–

Adapted from Goroll AH, Mulley HG. *Primary Care Medicine: Office Evaluation and Management of the Adult Patient.* 4th ed. Philadelphia: Lippincott Williams & Wilkins; 2000, p 1079.

161. **Define *complex regional pain syndrome* (CRPS).**
A syndrome of severe pain, edema, and vasomotor abnormalities with accompanying bone, muscle, and skin atrophy in the arms, hands, legs, or feet. The pain is usually out of proportion to the inciting event. CRPS was previously referred to as "reflex sympathetic dystrophy" and "Sudek's atrophy."

162. **What conditions are associated with Dupuytren contractures?**
- DM
- Chronic liver disease
- Epilepsy
- Plantar fasciitis
- Carpal tunnel syndrome
- Rheumatoid arthritis
- Hand trauma
- Pulmonary TB
- Alcoholism

163. **What are the guidelines for prescribing opioids?**
- Initially use nonpharmacologic and nonopioid pharmacologic therapy. If opioid therapy is indicated, continue these therapies.
- Establish treatment goals with patient, including pain relief and expected function.
- Assess risk and benefits of therapy with patient.
- Define patient's responsibilities for continued opioid use.
- Initially use immediate-release preparations at the lowest effective dosage.
- When treating acute pain, prescribe a limited amount for the expected duration of the acute pain.
- Reevaluate risks and benefits with 1–4 weeks of starting opioid therapy or if dose escalation is needed.
- Reevaluate the continued benefits every 3 months with goal to taper dose when appropriate.
- Review state prescription drug monitoring programs to review any other controlled substance prescriptions from other health care providers.
- Consider urine drug testing before starting therapy and annually thereafter.
- Avoid use of opioids and benzodiazepines when possible.
  Dowell D, Haegerich Tm, Chou R. CDC guidelines for prescribing opioids for chronic pain. *MMWR Morbid Mort Wkly Repl.* 2016;65:1–49.

WEBSITES

1. https://www.cdc.gov/
2. http://immunize.org/
3. www.UpToDate.com

BIBLIOGRAPHY

1. Barker LR, Fiebach NH, Kern DE, eds. *Principles of Ambulatory Medicine.* 7th ed. Philadelphia: Lippincott Williams & Wilkins; 2006.
2. Cassell EJ. *Talking with Patients.* Cambridge, MA: MIT Press; 1985.

3. Fletcher RH, Fletcher SW. *Clinical Epidemiology. The Essentials.* 5th ed. Philadelphia: Lippincott Williams & Wilkins; 2012.
4. Goroll AH, Mulley AG. *Primary Care Medicine. Office Evaluation and Management of the Adult Patient.* 7th ed. Philadelphia: Lippincott Williams & Wilkins; 2014.
5. Nabel EG, ed. *ACP Medicine.* Hamilton, Ontario, Canada: BC Decker; 2009.
6. Stone J. *In the Country of Hearts. Journeys in the Art of Medicine.* New York: Delacorte Press; 1990.
7. Wallach J. *Interpretation of Diagnostic Tests.* 9th ed. Philadelphia: Lippincott Williams & Wilkins; 2011.

CHAPTER 3

MEDICAL CONSULTATION

*Eric I. Rosenberg, MD, MSPH, FACP, Nila S. Radhakrishnan, MD, and
Katherine Vogel Anderson, PharmD, BCACP*

GENERAL ISSUES

1. **Why do physicians request medical consultation?**
   - For assistance in making a diagnosis in a patient with symptoms and signs suggestive of an unknown disease or syndrome
   - For collaborative assistance in daily management of a hospitalized patient with multiple comorbid conditions
   - To obtain advice on specific disease management (such as diabetes or hypertension)
   - To obtain a procedure usually performed by a subspecialist (e.g., coronary angiogram in a patient with persistent angina)
   - To evaluate a patient's ability to safely undergo surgical procedures

2. **What questions assess the effectiveness of medical consultation?**
   - Is the consultation question answered?
   - Does the patient benefit from disease improvement or promotion of better long-term health?
   - Are the consultant's recommendations actually implemented?

3. **What factors increase the likelihood that the consultant's recommendations will be accepted by the referring physician?**
   - Clear and concise communication between the requesting physician and the consultant (Poor communication occurs 12–24% of the time in some studies.)
   - Prompt response to consultation request
   - Addressing the requesting physician's key clinical question
   - Continued follow-up until the referring physician clearly understands the consultant will no longer follow the patient

4. **What are the 10 commandments for effective consultation?**
   A classic list of principles proposed by Goldman to improve the quality of medical consultation that stated:
   - Determine the specific issues and question(s) prompting the consult.
     - Confirm if the designated consultant is the appropriate physician to answer the requesting physician's questions.
     - Determine the requesting physician's expectations regarding the outcome of the consult.
   - Establish the urgency of the consultation request by confirming:
     - How quickly the consultant is expected to evaluate the patient
     - How recommended tests are to be initiated
     - How recommendations are to be communicated back to the requesting physician
   - "Look for yourself."
     - Give recommendations only after personally evaluating the patient and data.
   - "Be as brief as appropriate."
     - Record a concise, prioritized, and focused summary of the patient's illness with a specific impression that answers the requesting physician's initial questions.
     - Utilize follow-up visits to address less urgent yet possibly contributory issues.
   - "Be specific."
     - Specify who will order specific indicated tests or medications.
     - If medications are recommended, include specific dosages, necessary laboratory monitoring, and treatment durations.
   - "Provide contingency plans."
     - Include written suggestions for evaluation and initial treatment of likely complication.
     - Provide specific contact information for the consultant if new questions arise before the next hospital bedside visit.

- "Honor thy turf."
  - Keep the patient's primary physicians updated on new information.
  - Avoid providing detailed recommendations on patient issues outside the specific questions of the consultation.
- "Teach ... with tact."
  - Share expertise openly and in a nonjudgmental fashion.
- Talk is cheap ... and effective."
  - Directly talking to the requesting physicians increases the likelihood that your recommendations will be followed.
- "Follow up."
  - Return to evaluate the patient to confirm that recommendations are implemented, to demonstrate shared commitment to the patient's convalescence, and to document any new recommendations.

  Goldman L, Lee T, Rudd P. Ten commandments for effective consultation. *Arch Intern Med.* 1983;143:1753–1755.

5. **What is a curbside consult, and why should it be avoided?**
   The practice of giving an impression and recommendation to a physician without actually interviewing and examining the patient and reviewing the laboratory, radiographic, and medical records data. "Curbsides" are sometimes appropriately requested in order to determine if a full consultation is needed. Consultants should avoid giving specific recommendations without having seen a patient because the premise for the curbside may be faulty. For example, if a consultant is asked what dosage of warfarin a patient should receive when the international normalized ratio (INR) is 4.5, a review of the record might reveal that the patient has no medical indication to be on warfarin, and the proper recommendation is to discontinue the medication rather than to reduce the dosage.

6. **What are some examples of common and appropriate areas of consultation for the internist?**
   - Chest pain
   - Uncontrolled hypertension
   - Uncontrolled diabetes (hyper- or hypoglycemia)
   - Newly diagnosed thyroid disease
   - Electrolyte abnormalities (hypo-/hypernatremia; hypo-/hyperkalemia)
   - Unstable vital signs (fever, hypoxia, tachycardia, tachypnea)
   - Edema
   - Delirium
   - Management of alcohol withdrawal
   - Malnutrition
   - Preoperative evaluation
   - Medication reconciliation and polypharmacy
   - "Second opinions"

7. **How does an internist perform a consultation for "multiple medical problems"?**
   By initially focusing on the most significant problem for the patient and referring physician. Most patients with "multiple problems" usually have an extensive past medical history of many inactive illnesses. By setting the priorities, the internist can then focus care toward the acute, active, or neglected medical issues that can be effectively treated during the patient's hospitalization. The consultant may also help return (or start, if necessary) the care to a primary care physician in the outpatient setting.

8. **What are key issues that a consultant should review prior to seeing a patient in consultation?**
   - Any previous evaluation of the identified medical problem, including review of past diagnostic tests and the most recent notes summarizing the diagnostic work-up to date.
   - The patient's most important underlying diagnosis, which may not be the reason the consultation was requested. For example, a patient with advanced Alzheimer disease or other terminal diagnosis may need supportive care instead of extended testing or new medical or surgical

interventions. A patient with a fractured hip is more likely in urgent need of repair instead of surgical delay to diagnose a possible history of asymptomatic chronic obstructive lung disease (COPD).

- Review of home and hospital medications to ascertain that the patient is receiving his or her usual medications in the hospital, if appropriate.

9. **How does the consultant succinctly document the findings of a medical consultation?**
By answering the question(s) posed by the requesting physician with *concise* and *specific* recommendations.

Example of appropriate **initial** consultation note:

- Impression: A 72-year-old diabetic man with resolving sepsis following revision total hip arthroplasty. Diabetes remains suboptimally controlled with sugars 250–300 mg/dL contributing to risk of reinfection. Hypertension also not yet at goal. He needs overall further adjustment of chronic medications for these diseases.
- Recommendations:
  1. Increase insulin glargine to 40 units nightly subcutaneously.
  2. Add premeal insulin aspart 5 units prior to meals subcutaneously.
  3. Increase labetalol to 100 mg twice daily by oral route.
  4. Follow patient daily.

Example of appropriate **follow-up** consultation note:

- Impression: His diabetes is much improved following insulin adjustment. Hypertension now appears controlled with systolic pressures 130–140 mm Hg. He is noting some new pain in his left ankle and has a history of gout in this area; exam shows tenderness and mild induration. This could be a gout exacerbation. His creatinine is normal.
- Recommendations:
  1. Continue current dosages of insulin.
  2. Continue current dosages of antihypertensive medication.
  3. Order uric acid level. (Order entered today. I will review result.)
  4. Empirically treat for gout with indomethacin 50 mg three times daily by oral route.

PREOPERATIVE ASSESSMENT

10. **In general, how risky is surgery?**
Overall mortality rates are highest for emergent, vascular surgery procedures such as repair of a ruptured abdominal aortic aneurysm (AAA), for which mortality rates may exceed 40%. Vascular surgery is associated with the highest risk of death; rates for elective procedures such as open, surgical repair of an asymptomatic AAA may be as high as 5% in highest-risk patients. Most nonvascular hospital surgery mortality rates are 1% or less. Mortality rates are lowest for ambulatory surgery and approach less than 0.01%. Operative risk can also be described in terms of invasiveness and bleeding risk. Procedures with the highest invasiveness and greatest risk of bleeding (>1500 mL) are cardiothoracic, intracranial, major orthopedic and spinal reconstruction, major gastrointestinal (pancreatic resection), genitourinary surgery (radical prostatectomy and cystectomy), and vascular procedures. Procedures with mild to moderate invasiveness and bleeding of typically 500–1500 mL include arthroscopies, laparoscopic cholecystectomies, inguinal herniorrhaphies, hysterectomies, and hip and knee replacements. Procedures with minimal invasiveness and little to no associated bleeding risk are cystoscopies, breast biopsies, and bronchoscopy.

11. **What are the three phases of general anesthesia (GA)?**
Induction, maintenance, and emergence

12. **What are the complications associated with each phase?**
- **Induction:** Hypotension, bradycardia, nausea, and vomiting
- **Maintenance:** Hepatic necrosis with some volatile anesthetics (halothane) and vitamin B_{12} inactivation with use of nitrous oxide
- **Emergence:** Hypertension, tachycardia, bronchospasm, and laryngospasm

13. **What is monitored anesthesia care (MAC)?**
    Monitoring and appropriate treatment by an anesthesiologist of a patient during a procedure that usually uses a local anesthetic. The patient is not fully sedated and may have some awareness of the procedure.

14. **Is spinal or epidural anesthesia safer than GA?**
    Probably not. In spinal anesthesia, the anesthetic agent is inserted into the subarachnoid space, and in epidural anesthesia, into the epidural space. There still may be complications of hypotension and respiratory depression with these techniques, and there is less airway control because the patients are not intubated. Both can be combined with GA for lower extremity procedures.

15. **What tests are routinely indicated prior to surgery?**
    None. Routinely ordered tests fail to help physicians predict perioperative complications, are expensive, can delay needed surgery, and can result in further morbidity if additional unnecessary and invasive confirmatory testing is performed. Preoperative tests should be ordered to address the acuity or stability of a medical problem or to investigate an abnormal symptom or physical sign detected during the preoperative assessment of a patient's risks for surgery. Approximately $30 billion is spent yearly in the United States on "routine" preoperative testing alone; 60–70% of this testing is unnecessary because it rarely changes preoperative management.
    Roisen MF. More preoperative assessment by physicians and less by laboratory tests. *N Engl J Med.* 2000;342:204–205.

16. **How do internists assess patients in preparation for surgery?**
    By reviewing the patient's risk factors and identifying those risk factors that require modification prior to the scheduled procedure. The internists also determine the likelihood and nature of specific complications that may occur during and after the surgery.

17. **What are the specific goals of preoperative assessment?**
    To reduce perioperative morbidity, mortality, and unnecessary evaluations by:
    - Optimizing chronic diseases such as COPD, diabetes, and congestive heart failure.
    - Identifying specific, modifiable risks and interventions including thromboembolic disease, pneumonia, and infection.
    - Correcting medication errors or omissions in the hospital record.
    - Reducing delays and costs of unnecessary testing and additional consultations through expeditious and appropriate referral to subspecialists, avoiding unnecessary referral in patients who show no signs of medical decompensation.

18. **Which physicians should play a role in preoperative assessment?**
    - **Primary care physician**
      - Provides the best source of information regarding patient's baseline health status.
      - Can address comorbid conditions prior to making a referral for elective surgery and incorporate them into the consultation request.
    - **Surgeon**
      - Assesses if the procedure is indicated.
      - Discusses risks and benefits with the patient.
    - **Anesthesiologist**
      - Synthesizes medical and surgical management to assess risks of anesthesia.
      - Decides between general and regional anesthetic agents.
      - Detects recent changes in chronic illness.
    - **Consultant** (internist, cardiologist, or pulmonologist)
      - Answers specific questions about the patient's risks for surgery.

19. **Which patients are most likely to benefit from preoperative assessment?**
    Those who:
    - Appear to be medically unstable.
    - Are likely to have a complicated postoperative course.
    - Are likely to require medical consultation perioperatively to assist in managing significant cardiopulmonary diseases or other disorders that could directly impact postoperative infection risk or wound healing (e.g., diabetes).

- Have a "past medical history" that actually describes suboptimal treatment of an active problem list, which is particularly important to recognize in patients awaiting elective or cosmetic surgical procedures.
- Have symptoms, signs, or current and past illnesses that are known to be associated with increased risk for myocardial infarction (MI), pneumonia, thromboembolic event, stroke, infection, delirium, and uncontrolled bleeding.

20. **Which medical conditions are most important to identify preoperatively because they may be contraindications to surgery?**
    - Cardiac
      - Unstable angina
      - MI within the past 30 days with persistent chest pain
      - Recurrent pulmonary edema with associated ischemic cardiomyopathy
      - Symptomatic ventricular arrhythmias such as ventricular tachycardia
      - Second- or third-degree atrioventricular (AV) block
      - Severe aortic or mitral stenosis or other severe valvular disease
      - Bradycardia associated with syncope
      - Unexplained chest pain
    - Pulmonary
      - Pneumonia
      - COPD or asthma exacerbation
      - Recent deep venous thrombosis or pulmonary embolism (PE)
      - Unexplained dyspnea
    - Miscellaneous
      - Recent stroke
      - Uncontrolled diabetes
      - Cellulitis
      - Endovascular infections
      - Thyrotoxicosis

KEY POINTS: PREOPERATIVE ASSESSMENT

1. There are no laboratory tests that should be done before all surgeries. Preoperative testing should be based on an individual patient's risk factors.
2. The patient and family history is the best predictor of potential bleeding risk during surgery.
3. Much of the preoperative consultation involves identifying and managing acute illness or exacerbations of chronic illness.
4. Patients with unstable or significant underlying disease (particularly cardiac disease, pulmonary disease, and diabetes) are most likely to benefit from preoperative assessment.

21. **Describe the features of a preoperative medical interview.**
    The preoperative interview is an example of focused, targeted history taking. The physician should identify specific medical conditions or symptoms that may be associated with perioperative morbidity. The internist then documents how these conditions were diagnosed, what records substantiate the diagnosis, what treatments have been effective (or ineffective), and whether further diagnostic or follow-up testing is needed to better clarify these diagnoses. The interview usually does not focus on the illness requiring surgery; rather, the "history of present illness" becomes a discussion of concomitant or chronic illnesses that impact upon the perioperative period. The consultant does not simply document that a patient has hypertension and diabetes; instead, she or he documents the chronicity of the hypertension diagnosis, the presence of any end-organ damage (i.e., congestive heart failure, retinopathy, and nephropathy), the patient's baseline blood pressure (BP), the medication regimen, and the presence of any symptoms of decompensation (i.e., edema, dyspnea, curtailment of physical activity, unusual headaches, and chest pain). The consultant should focus on:
    - **Medication reconciliation** by recording the names and dosages of prescription and nonprescription medications taken by the patient, particularly nonsteroidal anti-inflammatory drugs (NSAIDs) and complementary or alternative supplements and medications. Medication reconciliation is crucial to reduce the likelihood of medication errors of omission (a chronically prescribed

medication that is omitted during the perioperative period) or commission (an incorrect dosage of a medication that is prescribed during the hospitalization).

- **Any history of abnormal bleeding,** particularly difficult-to-control bleeding during previous surgical or dental procedures that may indicate an undiagnosed inherited disorder of hemostasis (such as von Willebrand disease). (See Chapter 14, Hematology.)
- **Any history of adverse reactions to anesthesia.** If a patient has never undergone prior surgery, the consultant can inquire about a family history of unexplained or sudden intraoperative death or muscle disorders. Unexpected death or muscle disorders associated in the patient or patient's family suggest malignant hyperthermia, a genetic, autosomal dominant skeletal muscle disorder in which patients develop severe fever and organ damage when exposed to anesthetic agents. The incidence of malignant hyperthermia is estimated at 1:50,000 adults and 1:15,000 children and is fatal in 10% of patients. If necessary, genetic testing and a skeletal muscle contracture test can be used for diagnosis in asymptomatic patients with an appropriate family history.
- **The patient's baseline functional status.** Instead of inquiring about theoretical functional limits (e.g., "Could you climb a flight of stairs if you needed to?") or questions about ability to perform activities that require minimal effort (e.g., "Can you dress yourself?"), physicians should instead ask a patient about his or her daily physical routine to detect physical limitations brought on by dyspnea, chest pain, or other signs of decompensated disease.
- **A detailed cardiopulmonary review of systems** including history of chest pain, angina with description of typical pattern, shortness of breath, dyspnea on exertion, orthopnea, paroxysmal nocturnal dyspnea, wheezing, and peripheral edema. Most adult patients referred to an internist for preoperative assessment will have some degree of chronic organ impairment. In the United States, ischemic heart disease and COPD are common and viewed by surgeons as impediments to a successful operative course.

22. What are some appropriate indications for tests that can be ordered as part of a preoperative assessment?
See Table 3.1.

23. Which medications can be safely continued preoperatively?
See Table 3.2
Most medications are safely taken with a small amount of water the morning of surgery. Patients with severe hypertension or recurrent angina are advised to take their usual medications as scheduled before surgery. Abrupt withdrawal of antihypertensive or antianginal medications could lead to unstable BP or chest pain. Diuretics such as furosemide and hydrochlorothiazide are customarily discontinued while the patient is fasting owing to concerns about dehydration or hypokalemia, but the evidence supporting this practice is limited. Aspirin, warfarin, direct oral anticoagulants, and heparin are often discontinued preoperatively, but it is crucial that physicians understand the specific diagnosis that led to the prescription of these medications. For patients at high risk of perioperative deep venous thrombosis (DVT), PE, or stroke, anticoagulation should be discontinued for the minimum time possible and may require "bridging" with subcutaneous heparin. For patients at high risk for intracoronary thrombotic events but at low risk for catastrophic surgical bleeding, it may be advisable to continue antiplatelet medications (such as aspirin) perioperatively. Subspecialty consultation with the patient's cardiologist, hematologist, or neurologist (depending upon the diagnosis prompting anticoagulation) is recommended. Diabetic patients who are insulin-dependent or require insulin to maintain glucose control should continue to receive basal (long-acting) insulin while fasting, but at a lower dose, with more frequent monitoring and with hydration to prevent hypoglycemia. Diabetic patients who are non–insulin-requiring should avoid taking sulfonylureas the morning of surgery because these drugs could precipitate hypoglycemia while fasting.

PERIOPERATIVE MANAGEMENT OF CARDIAC DISEASE

24. Should the BP reach target goals in patients with known or newly diagnosed hypertension prior to scheduled surgery?
No. Consistently elevated BP in a patient without symptoms of malignant hypertension is consistent with chronically undertreated hypertension. Rapid correction with medication may induce myocardial and cerebral ischemia and is of no proven benefit. Diastolic BPs of > 110 mm Hg should probably be lowered prior to elective surgery.

Table 3.1. Indications for Preoperative Tests

TEST	SUGGESTED INDICATION IN ASYMPTOMATIC PATIENTS AWAITING SURGERY	COMMON INDICATIONS IN SYMPTOMATIC PATIENTS OR THOSE WITH CHRONIC DISEASE
Electrocardiogram	Age ≥ 40 yr; diabetes, hypertension	Chest pain, coronary artery disease, dysrhythmia
Creatinine	Age > 65 yr	Prescribed diuretics, ACE inhibitors, potassium supplements, chronic kidney disease, hypertension
Glucose	Age > 65 yr	Prescribed steroids; diabetes (consider hemoglobin A_{1c} as better verification of diabetic control)
Serum electrolytes	Not routinely indicated	Prescribed diuretics, ACE inhibitors, potassium supplements; chronic kidney disease, hypertension
Hemoglobin or hematocrit	Age > 65 yr	Prescribed warfarin, NSAIDs; estimated blood loss with surgery > 500 mL; menstruating
Urine human chorionic gonadotropin (hCG)	Childbearing age	Uncertain menstrual history
Prothrombin time	Not routinely indicated	Prescribed warfarin; chronic liver disease, metastatic cancer, alcoholism, neurosurgical procedures
Liver function tests	Not routinely indicated	Prescribed warfarin; chronic liver disease, metastatic cancer, alcoholism
Chest x-ray	Age > 65 yr and never performed	Dyspnea, cough, fever
Urinalysis	Not routinely indicated	Genitourinary procedures, joint prostheses
Pulmonary function tests	Not routinely indicated	Thoracic or upper abdominal surgery; questionable history of COPD/asthma; unexplained dyspnea
Echocardiogram	Not routinely indicated	Unexplained dyspnea, orthopnea, or other features suggestive of heart failure: heart murmur suggesting significant valvular disease

ACE, angiotensin-converting enzyme; COPD, chronic obstructive pulmonary disease; NSAIDs, nonsteroidal anti-inflammatory drugs.

Table 3.2. Medications That Are Safe to Continue Preoperatively

DRUG NAME	CLASS	HOLD OR CONTINUE?	SPECIFIC CONCERNS
Chlorthalidone Hydrochlorothiazide Indapamide	Thiazide diuretics	Continue until the day prior to surgery; hold the morning of surgery[1]	For all diuretics: hypokalemia, hypovolemia, hypotension
Bumetanide Furosemide Torsemide	Loop diuretics	Continue until the day prior to surgery; hold the morning of surgery[1]	For patients taking diuretics for heart failure: optimize fluid status prior to surgery
Spironolactone	Potassium-sparing diuretics	Continue until the day prior to surgery; hold the morning of surgery[1]	Resume diuretics when patient resumes oral fluid intake

Table 3.2. Medications That Are Safe to Continue Preoperatively *(Continued)*

DRUG NAME	CLASS	HOLD OR CONTINUE?	SPECIFIC CONCERNS
Benazepril Captopril Enalapril Fosinopril Lisinopril Ramipril	Angiotensin-converting enzyme inhibitor (ACE inhibitor)	Continue ACE inhibitor or ARB perioperatively[2]	For both ACE inhibitors and ARBs: hypotension after surgery
Candesartan Irbesartan Losartan Valsartan	Angiotensin receptor blocker (ARB)		For patients taking an ACE inhibitor/ARB for heart failure or hypertension: Continue perioperatively as benefit of ACE/ARB outweighs risk If ACE-inhibitor/ARB is held, resume as soon as clinically feasible
Clonidine	Alpha-2 agonist	Continue perioperatively[2,3]	For patients stable on clonidine, withdrawal There is no benefit starting clonidine to prevent postoperative cardiovascular outcomes; clonidine should NOT be started preoperatively for this indication[3]
Amlodipine	Dihydropyridine calcium channel blocker (CCB)	Continue perioperatively[2]	There is no interaction between CCBs and anesthetic agents; bleeding risk is negligible[4]
Diltiazem Verapamil	Non-dihydropyridine CCB	Continue perioperatively[2,4]	
Isosorbide dinitrate Isosorbide mono-nitrate	Nitrates	Continue perioperatively[1]	For patients with no oral intake, use of transdermal nitrate may be indicated[1]
Amiodarone Digoxin Dofetilide Dronedarone Sotalol	Antiarrhythmic	Continue perioperatively[2]	The risk of holding an antiarrhythmic should be evaluated according to the risk of inducing a life-threatening arrhythmia
Atorvastatin Lovastatin Pravastatin Simvastatin Rosuvastatin	HMG-CoA reductase inhibitor ("statin")	Continue perioperatively[2]	Statins are beneficial in both cardiac and noncardiac surgery; statins could be initiated perioperatively[2]
Warfarin Direct oral anticoagulants (DOACs):	Vitamin K antagonist	Hold warfarin 5 days prior to surgery[5]	For all anticoagulants, the risk of holding therapy perioperatively must be evaluated according to the risk of thrombosis Perioperative bridging, in the setting of atrial fibrillation, has shown increased risk of bleeding[7]
Apixaban Edoxaban Rivaroxaban	Factor Xa inhibitor	Hold DOACs according to renal function[6]: Apixaban, edoxaban, rivaroxaban: CrCl ≥ 50 mL/min: hold 24 hr CrCl 30–49 mL/min: hold 36 hr CrCl 15–29 mL/min: hold 48 hr	
Dabigatran	Direct thrombin inhibitor	Dabigatran: CrCl ≥ 50 mL/min: hold 36 hr CrCl 30–49 mL/min: hold 48 hr CrCl 15–29 mL/min: hold 72 hr	Perioperative bridging in the setting of mechanical heart valves is recommended[5]

Continued

DRUG NAME	CLASS	HOLD OR CONTINUE?	SPECIFIC CONCERNS
Aspirin (ASA)	Antiplatelet	If patients take ASA for primary prevention and are deemed low cardiac risk: hold ASA for 7 days prior to surgery[1]	Bleeding If held, resume ASA and/or $P2Y_{12}$ receptor antagonist as soon as clinically stable
Clopidogrel Prasugrel Ticagrelor	$P2Y_{12}$ receptor antagonist	If patients take ASA for secondary prevention: continue[2] For urgent, noncardiac surgery 4–6 wk after placement of bare metal stent or drug-eluting stent: continue ASA + $P2Y_{12}$ receptor antagonist [2] If $P2Y_{12}$ receptor antagonist must be stopped: continue ASA[2] If $P2Y_{12}$ receptor antagonist must be stopped: hold clopidogrel and ticagrelor 5 days prior to surgery; hold prasugrel 7 days prior to surgery[2]	Patients should delay elective surgery until 30 days after implantation of bare metal stents and 365 days after placement of drug-eluting stents[2]
Glipizide Glyburide Metformin Pioglitazone Linagliptin Sitagliptin Dapagliflozin	Sulfonylurea Biguanide Thiazolidinedione (TZD) Dipeptidyl peptidase-IV (DPP-IV) inhibitor Sodium-glucose co-transporter 2 (SGLT2) inhibitor	Continue all oral antidiabetic medications until the morning of surgery; hold medications the morning of surgery[8]	Monitor glucose every 4–6 hr while NPO (nothing by mouth); dose with short-acting insulin as needed Glucose target in the perioperative period is 80–180 mg/dL[8] Resume sulfonylurea when oral intake is resumed Metformin should not be resumed until renal function is stable TZDs should not be resumed in setting of heart failure, fluid retention, abnormal liver function tests
NPH Lantus Regular insulin Aspart insulin Exenatide Liraglutide Pramlintide	Insulin Incretin mimetic; glucagon-like petide-1 (GLP-1) analog Synthetic analog of amylin	Continue until the morning of surgery On the morning of surgery[8]: Omit the dose of short- or rapid-acting insulin Give half of the NPH, intermediate-, or long-acting insulin dose Give the usual dose of basal insulin for patients on an insulin pump Continue until the morning of surgery; hold the morning of surgery[8]	For short procedures, subcutaneous insulin may be continued. For long procedures, IV insulin may be required

1. Spell NO. Med Clin North Am 2001;85(5):1117–1128.
2. Fleisher LA et al. Circulation 2014;130:e278–e333.
3. Devereaux PJ et al. NEJM 2014;370:1504–1513.
4. Duminda N et al. Anesth Analg 2003;97:634–641.
5. Douketis JD et al. CHEST 2012;141(2)(Suppl):e326s–e350s.
6. Heidbuchel H et al. Europace 2013;15:625–651.
7. Douketis JD et al. NEJM 2015;373:823–833.
8. Cefalu WT et al. Diabetes Care 2016;39(Suppl 1):1–119.

Table 3.3. Risk Factors for Perioperative Cardiovascular Events (Myocardial Infarction, Heart Failure, and Death)

MAJOR	INTERMEDIATE	MINOR
Unstable coronary syndrome	Mild angina pectoris	Advanced age
Acute MI (<7 days) or recent MI (within past 7–30 days) and evidence of ischemia by symptoms or noninvasive testing	Previous MI by history of pathologic Q wave on ECG	Abnormal ECG
	Compensated or prior heart failure	Rhythm other than sinus
Decompensated heart failure		Low functional capacity
Significant arrhythmias	Diabetes mellitus (particularly if insulin-dependent)	History of stroke
High-grade atrioventricular block	Renal insufficiency	Uncontrolled hypertension
Symptomatic ventricular arrhythmia in patients with heart disease		
SVT with uncontrolled ventricular rate		
Severe valvular disease		

ECG, electrocardiogram; MI, myocardial infarction; SVT, supraventricular tachycardia.
Adapted from Fleisher LA, Beckman JA, Brown KA, et al: ACC/AHA 2006 guideline update on perioperative cardiovascular evaluation for noncardiac surgery: focused update on perioperative beta-blocker therapy. A report of the American College of Cardiology/American Heart Association Task Force on Practice Guidelines (Writing Committee to Update the 2002 Guidelines on Perioperative Cardiovascular Evaluation for Noncardiac Surgery). *J Am Coll Cardiol.* 2006;47:2347.

25. **Which noncardiac procedures have low, intermediate, and high risk of cardiac death or nonfatal MI?**
    - **Low** (<1%): Endoscopic and superficial procedures, cataract surgery, breast procedures, and ambulatory surgery
    - **Intermediate** (1–5%): Intraperitoneal, intrathoracic, head and neck, orthopedic, and prostate surgeries and carotid endarterectomy
    - **High** (<5%): Vascular surgeries

26. **Which patients should undergo preoperative cardiac testing?**
    Those with historical and physical findings suggesting a high likelihood of serious coronary artery disease (CAD) that may require prompt intervention, even if the patient were not scheduled for upcoming surgery (Table 3.3). Specific syndromes include:
    - Unstable coronary syndrome
    - Decompensated heart failure or new-onset heart failure
    - Significant arrhythmias
    - Severe valvular disease

27. **What are the risks of preoperative cardiac testing?**
    Unnecessarily delayed urgent surgery or complications caused by invasive procedures. Performing routine cardiac "stress tests" on patients does not improve perioperative morbidity or mortality rates.

28. **Which patients should receive evaluation for preoperative coronary revascularization?**
    Those who have angina or other symptoms likely due to CAD.
    Fleisher LA, Fleischmann KE, Auerbach AD, et al. 2014 ACC/AHA guideline on perioperative cardiovascular evaluation and management of patients undergoing noncardiac surgery: executive summary: a report of the American College of Cardiology/American Heart Association Task Force on Practice Guidelines. *Circulation.* 2014;130:2215–2245.

29. **What specific perioperative complications may develop in patients with aortic stenosis (AS)?**
    - Hypotension
    - Pulmonary edema
    - MI
    - Cardiogenic shock

30. **In what situations does the current evidence most clearly support use of beta blockers for patients in the perioperative period?**
For patients already taking beta blockers with high cardiac risk as identified by ischemia on preoperative testing.

31. **In what other situations might perioperative beta blocker use be considered?**
Possibly for those with multiple cardiac risks, but this use remains controversial.

PERIOPERATIVE MANAGEMENT: PULMONARY DISORDERS

32. **Which factors are commonly associated with perioperative pulmonary complications?**
    - Cigarette smoking
    - Upper abdominal or thoracic surgery
    - Surgery lasting > 3 hours
    - Active respiratory tract infection
    - Chronic sleep apnea

33. **What are the goals of preoperative assessment of a patient with chronic lung disease?**
    - Evaluate and stabilize acute exacerbations.
    - Advise and implement smoking cessation techniques
    - Review and verify that the patient is receiving appropriate maintenance therapy.
    - Review any use of corticosteroids within the previous year.
    - Review influenza and pneumococcal immunization status.

34. **What degree of impairment from pulmonary function tests (PFTs) precludes safe surgical intervention?**
None, unless a patient is being considered for partial lung resection. PFT results do not preclude surgery. Forced expiratory volume in 1 second (FEV_1) or forced vital capacity (FVC) < 70%, FEV_1/FVC < 65%, and arterial carbon dioxide pressure ($PaCO_2$) > 45 mm Hg suggest that patients are at higher risk for pulmonary complications, but there is no prohibitive threshold for surgery.

35. **What are some specific ways to lower the risk of perioperative pulmonary complications in patients with chronic lung diseases?**
    - Stop smoking 8 weeks preoperatively.
    - Continue bronchodilators and/or steroids throughout the perioperative period.
    - Treat respiratory infection, and postpone elective surgery if possible until infection resolved.
    - Prescribe *lung expansion maneuvers* (preoperative education for either deep breathing or incentive spirometry, which are equally effective).
    - Initiate or continue continuous positive airway pressure (CPAP) for patients with known or suspected sleep apnea.
    - Prescribe perioperative venous thromboembolism (VTE) prophylaxis to prevent DVT and PE, if indicated.

36. **Which patients are at high risk for postoperative VTE?**
Those with:
    - Major orthopedic procedures such as repair of pelvic, hip, or leg fractures
    - Multiple major trauma
    - Spinal cord injury
    - Abdominal or pelvic malignancy undergoing resection (e.g., colectomy for colorectal cancer; hysterectomy for endometrial or ovarian cancer)
    - Prior history of DVT and PE
    - Known thrombophilia (such as factor V Leiden, protein deficiencies, and antiphospholipid antibody syndrome)
    - Critical illness with major comorbid conditions (decompensated heart failure, pneumonia requiring intubation, sepsis, and burns)
    - Prolonged periods of immobilization before or after surgery

Table 3.4. General Guidelines for Postoperative Prevention of Venous Thromboembolism

RISK OF DVT	Pharmacologic Prophylaxis				MECHANICAL PROPHYLAXIS†
	LMWH	LDUH	VKA	FONDAPARINUX*	
Low	No	No	No	No	None, but early and frequent ambulation
Moderate	Yes	Yes	No	Yes	Yes, if bleeding risk is high
High	Yes	No	Yes	Yes	Yes, if bleeding risk or as adjunctive therapy

*Not U.S. Food and Drug Administration (FDA) approved for nonorthopedic procedures.
†Includes graduated compression stockings and intermittent compression devices.
DVT, deep venous thrombosis; LDUH, low-dose unfractionated heparin; LMWH, low-molecular-weight heparin; VKA, vitamin K antagonists.
From Geerts WH, Bergqvist D, Piineo GF, et al: Prevention of venous thromboembolism. American College of Chest Physicians Evidence-Based Clinical Practice Guidelines (8th ed). *Chest.* 2006;133:381S–453S.

37. **Which patients should receive VTE prophylaxis?**
Most undergoing procedures with a moderate to high risk of VTE, including general surgical, open gynecologic and urologic procedures, knee or hip arthroplasty, hip fracture surgery, trauma, and spinal cord surgery.

38. **What are the methods of VTE prophylaxis?**
   - Early and frequent ambulation when appropriate
   - Graduated elastic compression stockings
   - Sequential compression devices
   - Low-molecular-weight heparin (LMWH)
   - Low-dose unfractionated heparin (LDUH)
   - Vitamin K antagonists (warfarin) to maintain INR between 2 and 3
   - Factor Xa inhibitor (fondaparinux)
   - Inferior vena cava filter

39. **How does one choose the appropriate method of VTE prophylaxis?**
The exact method of prophylaxis will depend on the patient's risk factors for VTE, the VTE risk associated with the procedure, and the risk of postoperative bleeding. Current guidelines from the American College of Chest Physicians recommend that institutions establish clearly written thromboprophylaxis policies for all patients. Physicians should first identify whether their hospital has such guidelines. A complete description of the indications of the methods is available in the reference. See Table 3.4 for general guidelines.
   Geerts WH, Bergqvist D, Pineo GF, et al. Prevention of venous thromboembolism. American College of Chest Physicians Evidence-Based Clinical Practice Guidelines (8th ed). *Chest.* 2006;133:S381–453.

40. **If a patient is on warfarin, how long before surgery is warfarin stopped to allow normalization of the INR? Direct anticoagulants?**
5 days for warfarin and usually 2–3 days for direct anticoagulants, but timing may depend upon renal function.

41. **When can warfarin be restarted after surgery?**
Within 12–24 hours if there are no bleeding complications.

42. **How is perioperative anticoagulation managed in outpatients at high risk of an embolic event if the anticoagulation is stopped?**
"Bridging" therapy is prescribed consisting of LMWH administered subcutaneously. LMWH should be started 3 days before surgery. The last dose is given 24 hours before surgery as one half of the total daily dose. The postoperative resumption of LMWH depends on the bleeding risks.

43. **What antithrombotic drugs require adjustment for renal function?**
LMWH, apixaban, edoxaban, rivaroxaban, dabigatran, and fondaparinux. See Table 3.5.

Table 3.5. Perioperative Stress Doses of Glucocorticoids

	Intravenous Hydrocortisone Dose (mg)	
PROCEDURE RISK	**PREOPERATIVE**	**POSTOPERATIVE**
Minor	None	None
Moderate	50	25 q8h × 1–2 days
Major	100	50 q8h × 2–3 days

44. **How soon before surgery should aspirin and other antiplatelet agents (i.e., clopidogrel and prasugel) be stopped?**
Usually 7–10 days, but patients at risk for thrombotic events may need to continue the antiplatelet agent. Patients who are on aspirin for secondary prevention (e.g., have had an MI, stroke, or intracoronary stent) should continue 81 mg aspirin daily during the perioperative period unless specifically contraindicated.

PERIOPERATIVE MANAGEMENT: ENDOCRINOLOGY

45. **How should diabetes be treated during the perioperative period? Is "tight control" important?**
    - Patients with well-controlled diabetes should resume their customary regimen as soon as they can eat normally.
    - Patients with type 1 (insulin-dependent) diabetes must continue to receive basal (long-acting) insulin even while fasting to protect them from developing diabetic ketoacidosis and require frequent monitoring with blood glucose checks at least every 4 hours while fasting. The insulin dose is customarily reduced by 50% while fasting while at the same time hydration with parenteral dextrose and normal saline is provided to protect against dehydration and hypoglycemia.
    - Patients with poorly controlled type 2 diabetes (hemoglobin A_{1c} greater than 7.5%) treated with basal insulin should continue basal insulin and only hold prandial insulin.
    - "Tight" control of glucose (80–110 mg/dL) has been shown in some studies to reduce the risk of perioperative infection, wound healing, and cardiovascular complications, but subsequent studies have failed to replicate these results and the practice remains controversial. The optimal range for control of glucose has not been well established but 140 mg/dL to 180 mg/dL is acceptable based on observational studies.
    - Do NOT use "sliding scales" or "correction" doses of regular (short-acting) insulin alone to treat patients with poorly controlled diabetes.

46. **How are patients taking metformin managed when undergoing imaging studies or procedures that involve iodinated contrast media?**
By discontinuing the medication before or at the time of the procedure and not resuming until normal renal function is confirmed by measurement of blood urea nitrogen (BUN) and creatinine 48 hours later. Patients can develop acute renal failure in this setting.

47. **Is metformin also withheld during surgery?**
Yes. Metformin should be stopped before surgery and not restarted until the patient has usual oral intake and normal renal function is confirmed by laboratory testing.
See Table 3.2.

48. **How are patients taking chronic glucocorticoids managed in the perioperative period?**
By monitoring closely for signs of adrenal insufficiency postoperatively. The routine use of "stress doses" of glucocorticoids perioperatively is questionable. Those patients at high risk for adrenal suppression during major surgery should probably receive stress doses, though. (See Chapter 16, Endocrinology.)

49. **When indicated, how are stress doses of glucocorticoids given?**
See Table 3.5.

50. What are the risks of surgery in patients with thyroid disease?

Patients with **hypothyroidism** on stable thyroid replacement doses should continue the medication perioperatively. Patients with newly diagnosed severe hypothyroidism or myxedema should have surgery delayed if possible. Patients with **hyperthyroidism** should have this adequately treated before surgery.

PERIOPERATIVE MANAGEMENT: MISCELLANEOUS

51. When should patients receiving dialysis be dialyzed?

Generally the day before surgery with nephrology consultation for postoperative dialysis.

52. Do all patients with anemia need to be transfused before elective surgery?

Not for mild anemia, but those with hemoglobin < 8 mg/dL may benefit from transfusion, depending on the cause of the anemia. Anemia is associated with increased risk of perioperative complications.

53. Which patients with liver disease are at highest risk of perioperative complications?

Those with:
- Acute viral hepatitis
- Acute alcoholic hepatitis
- Cirrhosis

54. What are the complications of liver disease associated with surgery?

Bleeding, encephalopathy, hypotension, sepsis, and worsening of liver dysfunction.

55. How can these complications be prevented?

With preoperative endoscopy, if indicated for possible variceal bleeding; correction of abnormal prothrombin time (PT) with vitamin K or fresh frozen plasma; replacement of electrolytes when indicated; cessation of alcohol use; ascites treatment as appropriate; postponement of elective surgery in unstable patients; and minimal sedative use.

BIBLIOGRAPHY

1. Gross RJ, Caputo JM. *Kammerer and Gross' Consultation: The Internist on Surgical, Obstetric, and Psychiatric Services.* Philadelphia: Lippincott Williams & Wilkins; 1998.

CHAPTER 4

CARDIOLOGY

Gabriel Habib, Sr., MS, MD, FACC, FCCP, FAHA

Her blood pressure was on the low side. I felt her pulse in the carotid artery in her neck; it was weak, difficult to detect. Unlike the usual thumping carotid artery, her pulse rose only reluctantly to the examining finger. At the base of her neck, on the chest wall, there was an easily felt shudder, a rough vibration with each pulse, like a cat's purr. When I listened to her heart, ... I heard a gruff, harsh sound like the clearing of a throat. ... It was no great Oslerian feat of diagnosis on my part to suspect that she had severe aortic stenosis.

John Stone (1936–2008)
"The Long House Calls" from
In the Country of Hearts: Journeys in the Art of Medicine, 1990

PHYSICAL EXAMINATION

1. **Explain normal splitting of the second heart sound (S_2).**
   S_2 is normally split into aortic (A_2) and pulmonary (P_2) components caused by the closing of the two respective valves. The degree of splitting varies with the respiratory cycle or physiologic splitting. With inspiration, the negative intrathoracic pressure leads to increased venous return to the right side of the heart and a decrease to the left side. The increased venous return to the right atrium (RA) causes P_2 to occur slightly later and A_2 to occur slightly earlier, leading to a widening of the S_2 split. With expiration, the negative intrathoracic pressure is eliminated and A_2 and P_2 occur almost simultaneously. The largest contributor to the physiologic third heart sound (S_3) split is the respiratory variation in the timing of the pulmonary closure sound.

2. **What is paradoxical splitting of S_2?**
   A widening of the split of A_2 and P_2 with expiration and shortening of the split with inspiration (the opposite of normal).

3. **What causes paradoxical splitting of S_2?**
   Usually aortic insufficiency, aortic stenosis, and hypertrophic cardiomyopathy (HCM). In paradoxical splitting, P_2 precedes A_2 during expiration and is usually due to conditions that delay A_2 by delaying ejection of blood from the left ventricle (LV) and, therefore, aortic valve closure. Other causes include, myocardial infarction (MI), left bundle branch block (LBBB), and a right ventricular pacemaker.

4. **What causes fixed and wide splitting of S_2?**
   Atrial septal defects (ASDs), right ventricular dysfunction, or both, resulting in an interval between A_2 and P_2 that is wider than normal and does *not* change with the respiratory cycle. The wide and fixed S_2 split occurs because:
   - A_2–P_2 is wider than normal owing to shunting of blood from the left atrium (LA) to the RA, resulting in a greater right ventricular filling and a resulting delay in the timing of the pulmonary closure sound P_2; and
   - A_2–P_2 splitting is fixed and does *not* increase with inspiration. The fixed splitting occurs because the extra filling of the right ventricle (RV) that normally occurs during inspiration is small relative to the above-described increase in right ventricular filling due to interatrial shunting and thus does *not* significantly delay P_2.

5. **What does a loud P_2 signify?**
   Pulmonary hypertension (HTN), whether primary or secondary to chronic pulmonary disease.

6. **What is S_3?**
   A low-frequency sound heard just after S_2; also called a *ventricular gallop.*

7. **What is a physiologic S_3?**
   An S_3 found in young patients without cardiac disease.

8. **How is S_3 best heard?**
   With the stethoscope bell. Unlike a physiologically split A_2–P_2, the A_2–S_3 interval does not change during respiration. Associated physical findings of congestive heart failure (CHF), such as pulmonary rales, distended neck veins, or edema, are usually present along with an S_3.

9. **What is a pathologic S_3?**
   An S_3 occurring in a variety of pathologic conditions including CHF, mitral valve prolapse (MVP), thyrotoxicosis, coronary artery disease (CAD), cardiomyopathies, pericardial constriction, mitral or aortic insufficiency, and left-to-right shunts.

10. **Describe the mechanism behind an S_3.**
    The mechanism behind an S_3 is controversial, but it may be due to an increase in the velocity of blood entering the ventricles (rapid ventricular filling). When present, an S_3 usually represents myocardial decompensation associated with heart disease.

11. **What is the fourth heart sound (S_4)?**
    A sound occurring just before S_1; also called an *atrial gallop.* An S_4 reflects decreased ventricular compliance (a stiff ventricle) and is associated with CAD, pulmonary or aortic valvular stenosis, HTN, and ventricular hypertrophy from any cause.

12. **What is an opening snap (OS)?**
    A high-frequency early diastolic sound associated with mitral or tricuspid valve opening. A diastolic rumble at the apex confirms the physical diagnosis of mitral stenosis.

13. **Summarize the pathophysiology and significance of an OS in patients with mitral stenosis.**
    An OS is typically present only when the mitral valve leaflets are pliable, and it is, therefore, usually accompanied by an accentuated first heart sound (S_1). Diffuse calcification of the mitral valve can be expected when an OS is absent. If calcification is confined to the tip of the mitral valve, an OS is still commonly present. The interval between the aortic closure sound and the OS (A_2–OS) is inversely related to the mean LA pressure. A short A_2–OS interval is a reliable indicator of severe mitral stenosis; however, the converse is not necessarily true.

14. **What is the differential diagnosis of an abnormal early diastolic sound heard at the apex and lower left sternal border?**
    - Loud P_2
    - S_3 gallop
    - OS
    - Pericardial knock
    - Tumor plop (atrial myxoma)
    An early diastolic sound may be due to wide splitting of S_2, with or without a loud pulmonary closure sound. An ASD causes wide and fixed splitting of S_2.

15. **What causes a pericardial knock?**
    The sudden slowing of left ventricular filling in early diastole associated with the restriction of a rigid pericardium acting as a "rigid shell," such as in chronic constrictive pericarditis.

16. **What is a tumor plop?**
    The sound heard with cardiac auscultation caused by obstruction of blood flow by an atrial myxoma protruding through the mitral valve during diastole leading to sudden cessation of left ventricular filling. Cardiac auscultation in various positions helps to detect a tumor plop; likewise, cardiac symptoms in these patients are often related to body position.

17. **What is a hyperdynamic precordial impulse?**
    A thrust of exaggerated height that falls away immediately from the palpating fingers and is typically found in patients with a large stroke volume. (Stroke volume is the amount of blood ejected with each contraction.) The clinical conditions with a large stroke volume include thyrotoxicosis, anemia, beriberi, atrioventricular (AV) shunts or grafts, exercise, or mitral regurgitation (MR). A hyperdynamic precordial impulse should be differentiated from the sustained

apical impulse, a graphic equivalent of a heave, detected in the presence of LV hypertrophy due to HTN or aortic stenosis.

18. **What are the classifications of and physical findings associated with heart murmurs?**
See Table 4.1. Systolic murmurs are classified from grade 1 to grade 6. Diastolic murmurs are classified from grade 1 to grade 4. Murmurs rarely exceed grade 4. Systolic murmurs grade 3 or greater are more likely to be clinically significant.

Table 4.1. Classification of Heart Murmurs

GRADE (CLASSIFICATION)	PHYSICAL EXAMINATION FINDINGS
1	Heard only with concentration in a quiet room
2	Soft, low-intensity audible murmur
3	Loud murmur
4	Loud murmur with a palpable chest vibration ("thrill")
5	Loudest murmur heard with stethoscope touching the chest
6	Murmur loud enough to be heard with the stethoscope off the chest

19. **What is the likely cause of a systolic ejection murmur, best heard at the second right intercostal space, in an 82-year-old asymptomatic man?**
Aortic **sclerosis,** not aortic **stenosis.** Aortic sclerosis is characterized by thickening or calcification of the aortic valve and, unlike valvular aortic stenosis, is typically *not* associated with any significant transvalvular systolic pressure gradient.

20. **How is aortic stenosis differentiated from aortic sclerosis by physical examination?**
The following clinical findings are **present** in patients with **aortic stenosis** but **absent** with **aortic sclerosis:**
   • Diminished carotid arterial upstroke (i.e., the rate of rise of the carotid pulse is less steep)
   • Diminished peripheral arterial pulses (a finding consistent with moderate to severe aortic stenosis)
   • Late peaking of systolic murmur (as aortic stenosis worsens in severity, the systolic murmur peak becomes more delayed)
   • Loud or audible (or both) S_4
   • Syncope, angina, or heart failure signs or symptoms
   • Loud systolic murmur associated with a systolic thrill

21. **How do standing, squatting, and leg-raising affect the intensity and duration of the systolic murmur heard on dynamic auscultation in a patient with HCM?**
Standing increases the murmur intensity, and leg-raising and squatting decrease the murmur intensity. In HCM, a decrease in the size of the LV increases the dynamic LV outflow obstruction, leading to an increased intensity of the murmur. A decrease in LV volume occurs on standing. In contrast, **leg-raising** and **squatting** increase venous return and thereby increase LV volume, decreasing the dynamic LV obstruction and the murmur intensity.

22. **What are the physical examination findings in MR?**
   • An apical holosystolic murmur with variation of intensity and radiation depending on the cause and severity of the MR
   • S_3
   • Quick upstroke and short duration of peripheral pulses
   • Widened pulse pressure
   • Hyperdynamic precordium

23. List the peripheral arterial signs of chronic aortic regurgitation (AR).
    - **de Musset sign:** bobbing of the head with each heartbeat
    - **Corrigan pulse:** abrupt distention and quick collapse of femoral pulses (also called *water-hammer pulse*)
    - **Traube sign:** booming, "pistol-shot" systolic and diastolic sounds heard over the femoral pulse
    - **Müller sign:** systolic pulsations of the uvula
    - **Duroziez sign:** systolic murmur over the femoral artery when compressed proximally and diastolic murmur when compressed distally
    - **Quincke sign:** capillary pulsations of the fingertips
    - **Hill sign:** popliteal cuff systolic pressure exceeding brachial cuff pressure by > 60 mm Hg

24. How do you measure the jugular venous pulse (JVP) as an estimate of central venous pressure (CVP) at the bedside?
    - Elevate the head of the bed until the patient's chest is at the point at which the venous pulsations are maximally visualized (usually 30–45 degrees).
    - Measure the height of this oscillating venous column above the sternal angle (angle of Louis) (Fig. 4.1).
    - Estimate the CVP by adding 5 cm to the measurement. The sternal angle is about 5 cm from the RA regardless of the elevation angle. Normal CVP is 5–9 cm H_2O.

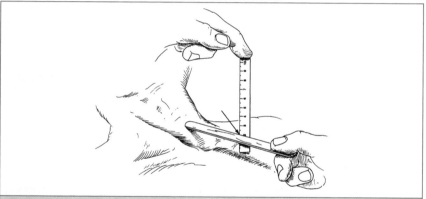

Fig. 4.1. Measurement of venous jugular pressure at the bedside. *(From Adair OV, Havranek EP. Cardiology Secrets. Philadelphia: Hanley & Belfus; 1995, p 6.)*

25. Name the three waves composing the JVP.
    - **A wave:** produced by RA contraction, occurring just before S_1
    - **C wave:** caused by bulging upward of the closed tricuspid valve during RV contraction (often difficult to see)
    - **V wave:** caused by RA filling just before opening of the tricuspid valve

26. What are "cannon" A waves?
    Very large and prominent A waves occurring when the atria contract against a closed tricuspid valve. Irregular "cannon" A waves are seen in AV dissociation or ectopic atrial beats. Regular "cannon" A waves are seen in a junctional or ventricular rhythm in which the atria are depolarized by retrograde conduction.

27. Define *pulsus paradoxus*.
    A decrease of > 10 mm Hg in the systolic blood pressure (BP) during normal inspiration, first described by Adolf Kussmaul in 1873. Kussmaul originally described the disappearance of the pulse during inspiration, though.

28. **Describe the mechanism of a pulsus paradoxus.**

Pulsus paradoxus can occur when the fall in intrathoracic pressure during inspiration is rapidly transmitted through a pericardial effusion, resulting in an exaggerated increase in venous return to the right side of the heart. The increased venous return causes bulging of the interventricular septum toward the LV, resulting in a smaller LV volume and a smaller LV stroke volume. The decreased LV stroke volume results in a lower cardiac output and lower systolic BP during inspiration. A drop in systolic BP is a normal physiologic finding as long as this drop does *not* exceed 10 mm Hg. In contrast, an exaggerated drop in systolic BP > 10 mm Hg is a pathologic finding characteristic of cardiac tamponade.

29. **What medical diseases present with pulsus paradoxus?**
    - Cardiac tamponade (classic finding but may be absent with severe volume contraction, dehydration, or hypotension)
    - Severe chronic obstructive pulmonary disease (COPD)
    - Chronic constrictive pericarditis (very rarely)

30. **Describe the *y* descent of the JVP waveform tracing in chronic constrictive pericarditis.**

The *y* descent of the JVP waveform tracing corresponds to the rapid early RA emptying phase or the rapid early ventricular filling phase. In patients with chronic constrictive pericarditis, early ventricular filling is unimpeded. During the very early filling, the RV is very small and its filling is enhanced by the sudden "pouring" of blood as the tricuspid valve opens. During this early filling phase, the ventricle is too small and has not yet "perceived" the constricting effect of the calcified or thickened pericardium, and, thus, filling is unimpeded. Once the ventricle meets the thick or calcified "noncompliant" pericardium, ventricular filling suddenly slows and corresponds to the "pericardial knock" sound. Although found in chronic constrictive pericarditis, the steep *y* descent rarely occurs in cardiac tamponade. At the same time that the steep *y* descent occurs, the RV early filling occurs and there is a "dip" or sudden decrease in RV pressure. Once the ventricular filling is suddenly slowed or halted by the thick or calcified noncompliant pericardium, the RV pressure rises to a plateau. The "dip-and-plateau" RV pressure waveform, just like the steep *y* descent of the RA pressure waveform, is a distinctive finding in chronic constrictive pericarditis and helps to differentiate chronic constrictive pericarditis from cardiac tamponade.

31. **What is cardiac tamponade?**

The sudden accumulation of fluid within the pericardial sac under pressure. When the clinical triad of cardiac tamponade was first described by Claude Beck in 1935, he noted hypotension, elevated systemic venous pressure, and a small, quiet heart. The condition was commonly due to penetrating cardiac injuries, aortic dissection, or intrapericardial rupture of an aortic or cardiac aneurysm. Today, the most common causes are neoplastic disease, idiopathic pericarditis, acute MI, and uremia.

32. **Summarize the physical examination findings in cardiac tamponade.**
    - **Jugular venous distention:** almost universally present except in patients with severe hypovolemia.
    - **Pulsus paradoxus:** defined as a decrease in systolic BP > 10 mm Hg during quiet inspiration. Pulsus paradoxus is difficult to elicit in volume-depleted patients.
    - **Tachycardia with a thready peripheral pulse:** sometimes severe cardiac tamponade may restrict LV and RV filling enough to cause hypotension, but a thready and rapid pulse is almost invariably present.

33. **What is the Kussmaul sign?**

An inspiratory increase in systemic venous pressure commonly present in chronic constrictive pericarditis but rarely detected in acute cardiac tamponade.

ELECTROCARDIOGRAPHY

34. **What is the normal range for PR and QT intervals on a 12-lead electrocardiogram (ECG)? Do these intervals vary with heart rate or age?**
    - **PR interval:** 0.12–0.20 seconds with no variation due to heart rate or age.

- **QT interval:** Varies with heart rate but not with age. As the heart rate increases, the QT interval shortens. To help evaluate a QT interval independent of heart rate, the corrected QT interval (QTc) can be calculated:

QTc (in ms) = measured QT (in ms) /square root of the R − R interval (in seconds)

The normal range for the QTc is 0.36–0.44 seconds. A prolonged QTc is defined as QTc > 0.44 seconds.

35. **What are the congenital causes of a prolonged QT interval?**
    - **With deafness:** Jervell and Lange-Nielsen syndrome
    - **Without deafness:** Romano-Ward syndrome

36. **List the acquired causes of a prolonged QT interval.**
    - **Electrolyte abnormalities:** low K^+, low Ca^{2+}, low Mg^{2+}. In clinical practice, the most common electrolyte abnormality causing a prolonged QT interval is hypokalemia, often in a patient receiving a thiazide or loop diuretic.
    - **Drugs:** class IA/IC antiarrhythmics, tricyclic antidepressants, antipsychotics (haloperidol, phenothiazines), anti-infectives (fluoroquinolone and macrolide antibiotics), azoles (antifungals), donepezil, and opioids (methadone)
    - **Hypothermia**
    - **CAD**
    - **Cardiomyopathy**
    - **Central nervous system injury:** least common cause

37. **Why is a prolonged QT interval clinically significant?**
    Because a prolonged QT interval is associated with an increased risk of sudden cardiac death due to a ventricular tachyarrhythmia such as ventricular tachycardia (VT) or ventricular fibrillation (VF). A distinctive type of VT associated with a prolonged QT interval is torsades de pointes (turning of the points) or more descriptively called "polymorphic VT."

38. **In the frontal plane, is a QRS axis of +120 degrees compatible with a diagnosis of left anterior hemiblock (LAHB)?**
    No. The diagnosis of LAHB requires the presence of a QRS of −60 to −90 degrees in the frontal plane. A frontal plane QRS axis of +120 degrees is consistent with right axis deviation and is, therefore, not compatible with a diagnosis of LAHB (left anterior fascicular block).

39. **List the diagnostic criteria for left anterior fascicular block.**
    - QRS axis −60 to −90 degrees
    - Small Q wave in lead I
    - Small R wave in lead III

40. **Describe the ECG manifestations of RV hypertrophy.**
    - R wave > S wave in V_1 or V_2
    - R wave > 5 mm in V_1 or V_2
    - Right axis deviation
    - Persistent rS pattern (V_1–V_6)
    - Normal QRS duration

41. **Describe the three phases of the ECG evolution of an acute MI.**
    - **Tall upright or inverted T waves:** Typically seen in the first hour or two of MI evolution and are thus called "hyperacute T waves" but are not a common ECG presentation in patients with MI. Inverted T waves are more frequent and usually appear after the first 8–12 hours of MI symptom onset and may persist for an indeterminate length of time (days, weeks, or years). An ECG characterized by pathologic Q waves and inverted T waves is called "MI, age indeterminate."
    - **ST-segment elevations:** Found in ECG leads facing the infarcted myocardial wall with reciprocal **ST-segment depressions** in opposite ECG leads. ST-segment changes are the most common acute ECG signs of MI. ST-segment elevations appear immediately at onset of an MI and usually resolve after the first 2–3 days and rarely persist longer than 2 weeks except in patients with a ventricular aneurysm.

- **New pathologic Q waves:** Usually starting anywhere from 8–12 hours to several days after MI symptom onset. Some patients may not develop pathologic Q waves but develop a significant > 25% decrease in R-wave amplitude (Fig. 4.2).

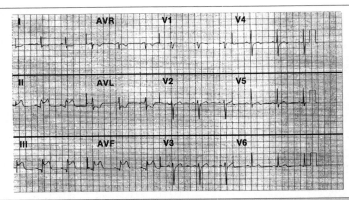

Fig. 4.2. Acute myocardial infarction (MI) localized to inferior leads (II, III, and aVF). The electrocardiogram (ECG) shows ST-segment elevation with hyperacute peaked T waves and the early development of significant Q waves. Reciprocal ST-segment depression is also seen (leads I and aVL). *(From Seelig CB.* Simplified ECG Analysis. *Phila-delphia: Hanley & Belfus; 1997, p 13.)*

42. **What is a pseudoinfarction? What is its differential diagnosis?**
An ECG pattern with changes similar to an MI without definitive evidence of ischemia. The differential diagnosis includes:

LV or RV hypertrophy	Wolff-Parkinson-White	HCM
Hyperkalemia	(WPW) syndrome	Intracranial hemorrhage
LBBB	Cardiac sarcoid or	
Early repolarization	amyloid	

43. **What are the ECG manifestations of atrial infarction?**
Depressed or elevated PR segment and atrial arrhythmias such as atrial flutter, atrial fibrillation (AF), or AV nodal rhythms.

44. **Which arrhythmias can be detected by 24-hour ECG monitoring in young patients without apparent heart disease?**
- Severe sinus bradycardia (≤40 beats per minute [bpm])
- Sinus pauses of up to 2 seconds
- Nocturnal AV nodal block
  Frequent premature atrial or ventricular beats were not commonly found.
  Brodsky M, Wu D, Denes P, et al. Arrhythmias documented by 24-hour continuous electrocardiographic monitoring in 50 male medical students without apparent heart disease. *Am J Cardiol.* 1977;39:390–395.

45. **What ECG findings help distinguish AF from other supraventricular tachycardias (SVTs)?**
AF differs from all other SVTs by having totally disorganized atrial depolarization without effective atrial contractions. An ECG may occasionally show fine or coarse irregular waves of variable amplitude and morphology, occurring at a rate of 350–600/min, but these are often difficult to recognize on a routine 12-lead ECG. A distinctive finding in AF is an irregular ventricular rhythm resulting from random and erratic transmission of the wave of depolarization from the atria to the ventricles via the AV conduction system. When untreated, patients with AF will usually have fast ventricular rates > 100 bpm, often in the 150–200 bpm range. The finding of AF with a slow ventricular rate < 60 bpm in a patient *not* receiving any AV nodal blocking

drugs is suggestive of severe AV nodal structural disease (due to degenerative or calcific disease or due to CAD) and prompts immediate cardiology consultation for possible pacemaker placement.

46. **How do you differentiate atrial tachycardia and atrial flutter from AF?**
Unlike AF, atrial tachycardia (or paroxysmal atrial tachycardia [PAT]) and atrial flutter demonstrate a regular ventricular rhythm and are characterized by regular and slower atrial rhythms (Table 4.2). The flutter rate (i.e., the atrial rate) in atrial flutter ranges between 250 and 350 bpm. The most common flutter rate is 300 bpm, and the most common ventricular rates are 150 and 75 bpm, respectively. Atrial tachycardias have slower atrial rates, ranging from 150 to 250 bpm. The most common cause of atrial tachycardia with block is digitalis toxicity.

Table 4.2. Comparison of Supraventricular Tachycardias

MEASUREMENT	ATRIAL FIBRILLATION	ATRIAL FLUTTER	ATRIAL TACHYCARDIA
Atrial rate (bpm)	>400	240–350	100–240
Atrial rhythm	Irregular	Regular	Regular
AV block	Variable	2:1, 4:1, 3:1, or variable	2:1, 4:1, 3:1, or variable
Ventricular rate (bpm)	Variable	150, 75, 100, or variable	Variable

AV, atrioventricular; bpm, beats per minute.

47. **What is the significance of capture and fusion beats on ECG in differentiating between VT and SVT with aberrancy?**
Capture beats, fusion beats, and AV dissociation are virtually pathognomonic of VT (Table 4.3). A capture beat is a normally conducted sinus beat interrupting a wide-complex tachycardia. A fusion beat has a QRS morphology intermediate between a normally conducted narrow beat and a wide-complex ventricular beat. The clinical hallmark of AV dissociation is the presence of intermittent cannon waves in the jugular neck veins.

Table 4.3. Distinguishing Features of Wide-Complex Ventricular Tachycardia and Supraventricular Tachycardia

FEATURE	VT	SVT
History of MI	+	−
Ventricular aneurysm	+	−
Fusion beats	+	−
Capture beats	+	−
Complete AV dissociation	+	−
Similar QRS complex when in sinus rhythm	−	+
RBBB + QRS > 0.14 sec	+	−
LBBB + QRS > 0.16 sec	+	−
Positive concordance in V_1–V_6	+	−
LBBB + right QRS axis	+	−
Intermittent cannon waves	+	−

+, present; −, absent; AV, atrioventricular; LBBB, left bundle branch block; MI, myocardial infarction; RBBB, right bundle branch block; SVT, supraventricular tachycardia; VT, ventricular tachycardia.

48. **What are the types of AV blocks?**
    - **First-degree:** Prolongation of the PR interval due to a conduction delay at the AV node.
    - **Second-degree:** Presence of dropped beats in which a P wave is not followed by a QRS complex (no ventricular depolarization and, therefore, no ventricular contraction). There are three types of second-degree AV blocks:
        - **Type I** (Wenckebach phenomenon): PR interval lengthens with each successive beat until a beat is dropped and the cycle repeats itself.
        - **Type II:** PR intervals are prolonged but do not gradually lengthen until a beat is suddenly dropped. The dropped beat may occur regularly, with a fixed number (X) of beats for each dropped beat (called an *X:1 block*). Type II is much less common than type I and is commonly associated with bundle branch blocks.
        - **2:1 AV block:** Every other P wave is followed by a QRS complex alternating with P wave NOT followed by any QRS complex.
    - **Third-degree** (complete heart block): Separate pacemaker control of the atria and ventricles. The ECG shows widening of the QRS complex and a ventricular rate of 35–50 bpm.

49. **What ECG changes are seen first in hyperkalemia?**
    Tall, peaked, symmetrical T waves with a narrow base (so-called tented T wave) that usually are present in leads II, III, V_2, V_3, and V_4. As hyperkalemia progresses, the following may occur:
    - Shortened QT interval
    - Widened QRS complex
    - Depressed ST segment
    - Flattened P wave
    - Prolonged PR interval
    Eventually, the P waves disappear and the QRS complexes assume a configuration similar to a sine wave, eventually degenerating into VF. Widening of the QRS complex can assume a configuration consistent with atypical right bundle branch block (RBBB) or LBBB, making the recognition of hyperkalemia more difficult. Unlike typical RBBB, hyperkalemia often causes prolongation of the entire QRS complex.

50. **Summarize the sequence of ECG changes in experimental hyperkalemia.**
    See Table 4.4.

Table 4.4. Electrocardiogram Changes in Experimental Hyperkalemia

SERUM K⁺ (MEQ/L)	ECG FINDING
>5.7	Tall, symmetrical T waves
>7.0	Reduced P wave amplitude
>7.0	Prolongation of PR interval
>8.4	Disappearance of P waves
9–11	Widening of QRS interval
>12	Ventricular fibrillation

ECG, electrocardiogram.

51. **What ECG signs suggest hypercalcemia? Are similar changes seen in other conditions?**
    Shortened QT interval (particularly the interval between the beginning of the QRS complex and the peak of the T wave) and an abrupt slope to the peak of the T wave. Digitalis toxicity also causes shortened QT interval.

52. **Patients maintained on digitalis commonly exhibit some changes on ECG referred to as the "digitalis effect." What are these changes?**
    Sagging of the ST segment and flattening and inversion of the T waves typically occurring in the inferolateral ECG leads that occur when administered in therapeutic doses. Digitalis can cause a variety of other ECG abnormalities depending on the serum digoxin level.

53. **How do the ECG changes of "digitalis effect" compare with the ECG changes in myocardial ischemia?**
Typically, horizontal or downsloping ST-segment depression, sharp-angled ST-T junctions, and U wave inversion are present in patients with subendocardial ischemia (coronary insufficiency). Less commonly, tall T waves may be a subtle ECG sign of myocardial ischemia.

54. **Where does the venous *a* wave appear in the cardiac cycle and to what specific component of the cardiac cycle does it correspond?**
During the course of the cardiac cycle, the electrical events (corresponding to various ECG components of the PQRST complex) initiate and, therefore, precede the mechanical (pressure) events, and, in turn, mechanical events are followed by auscultatory events (normal and extra heart sounds). Shortly after the ECG P wave, the atria contract to produce the *a* wave, which may at times be visible by careful inspection of the jugular pressure waveform. In patients with longstanding systemic HTN, this atrial contraction may be "stronger" and a larger contributor to the total filling of the ventricle, and, as a result, a loud extra sound called *atrial gallop* or S_4 *heart sound* may be audible by cardiac auscultation in patients with HTN.

55. **Where does an S_3 occur in relation to the QRS complex?**
The QRS complex initiates ventricular systole, followed shortly by LV contraction and the rapid buildup of LV pressure. Almost immediately, LV pressure exceeds LA pressure to close the mitral valve and produces S_1. When LV pressure exceeds aortic pressure, the aortic valve opens, and when aortic pressure is once again greater than LV pressure, the aortic valve closes to produce S_2 and terminate ventricular ejection. The decreasing LV pressure drops below LA pressure to open the mitral valve, and a period of rapid ventricular filling commences. During this time, an S_3 may be heard (Fig. 4.3).

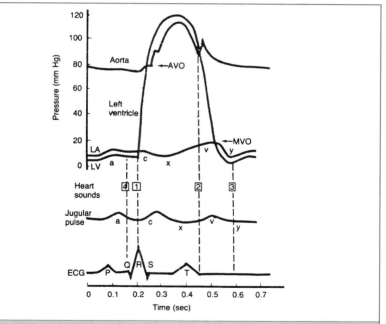

Fig. 4.3. Production of first through fourth heart sounds (S_1, S_2, S_3, and S_4) in the cardiac cycle. For simplification, right-sided heart pressures have been omitted. AVO, aortic valve opens; MVO, mitral valve opens. *(From Andreoli TE, Cecil RL, editors. Cecil Essentials of Medicine. 2nd ed. Philadelphia: WB Saunders; 1990, p 8.)*

DIAGNOSIS

56. **What are the cardiac and noncardiac causes of chest pain, and what are their characteristics?**
See Tables 4.5 and 4.6.

Table 4.5. Cardiovascular Causes of Chest Pain

CONDITION	LOCATION	QUALITY	DURATION	AGGRAVATING/ RELIEVING FACTORS	ASSOCIATED SIGNS AND SYMPTOMS
Angina	Retrosternal region; radiates to or occasionally isolated to neck, jaw, epigastrium, shoulder, or arms (left common)	Pressure, burning, squeezing, heaviness, indigestion	<2–10 min	Precipitated by exercise, cold weather, or emotional stress; relieved by rest or nitroglycerin; atypical (Prinzmetal) angina may be unrelated to activity, often early morning	S_3 or murmur of papillary muscle dysfunction during pain
Rest or crescendo angina	Same as angina	Same as angina but may be more severe	Usually <20 min	Same as angina, with decreasing tolerance for exertion or at rest	Similar to stable angina, but may be pronounced; transient heart failure can occur
Myocardial infarction	Substernal and may radiate like angina	Heaviness, pressure, burning, constriction	>30 min but variable	Unrelieved by rest or nitroglycerin	Shortness of breath, sweating, weakness, nausea, vomiting
Pericarditis	Usually begins over sternum or toward cardiac apex and may radiate to neck or left shoulder; often more localized than the pain of myocardial infarction	Sharp, stabbing, knifelike	Lasts many hours to days; may wax and wane	Aggravated by deep breathing, rotating chest, or supine position; relieved by sitting up and leaning forward.	Pericardial friction rub
Aortic dissection	Anterior chest; may radiate to back, abdomen	Excruciating, tearing, knifelike	Sudden onset, unrelenting	Usually occurs in setting of hypertension or predisposition, such as Marfan syndrome	Murmur of aortic insufficiency, pulse or blood pressure asymmetry; neurologic deficit

Pulmonary embolism (chest pain often not present)	Substernal or over area of pulmonary infarction	Pleuritic (with pulmonary infarction) or like angina	Sudden onset; minute to < 1 hr	May be aggravated by breathing	Dyspnea, tachypnea, tachycardia, hypotension, signs of acute right ventricular failure, and pulmonary hypertension with large emboli; rales, pleural rub, hemoptysis with pulmonary infarction
Pulmonary hypertension	Substernal	Pressure, oppressive	Similar to angina	Aggravated by effort	Pain usually associated with dyspnea; signs of pulmonary hypertension

S_3, third heart sound.

From Goldman L. Approach to the patient with possible cardiovascular disease. In Goldman L, Ausiello D, editors. *Cecil Medicine*. 23rd ed. Philadelphia: WB Saunders; 2007.

Table 4.6. Noncardiac Causes of Chest Pain

CONDITION	LOCATION	QUALITY	DURATION	AGGRAVATING/ RELIEVING FACTORS	ASSOCIATED SIGNS AND SYMPTOMS
Pneumonitis and pleurisy	Localized over involved area	Pleuritic, localized	Brief or prolonged	Painful breathing	Dyspnea, cough, fever, dull to percussion, bronchial breath sounds, rales, occasional pleural rub
Spontaneous pneumothorax	Unilateral	Sharp, well localized	Sudden onset, lasts many hours	Painful breathing	Dyspnea, hyperresonance, and decreased breath and voice sounds over involved lung
Musculoskeletal disorders	Variable	Aching	Short or long duration	Aggravated by movement, history of muscle exertion or injury	Tender to pressure or movement
Herpes zoster	Dermatomal in distribution	Burning, itching	Prolonged	None	Vesicular rash appears in area of discomfort
Esophageal reflux	Substernal, epigastric	Burning, visceral discomfort	10–60 min	Aggravated by large meal, postprandial recumbency; relief with antacid	Water brash
Peptic ulcer	Epigastric, substernal	Visceral burning, aching	Prolonged	Relief with food, antacid	
Gallbladder disease	Epigastric, right upper quadrant	Visceral	Prolonged	May be unprovoked or follow meals	Right upper quadrant tenderness may be present
Anxiety	Often localized over precordium	Variable; location often moves from place to place	Varies; often fleeting	Situational	Sighing respirations, often chest wall tenderness

From Goldman L. Approach to the patient with possible cardiovascular disease. In Goldman L, Ausiello D, editors. *Cecil Medicine.* 23rd ed. Philadelphia: WB Saunders; 2007.

57. **Is exercise treadmill ECG testing helpful in confirming the diagnosis of exertional angina?**
    Yes. Exercise tolerance testing (ETT) is the most common provocative test used by clinicians to confirm the clinical diagnosis of exertional angina pectoris. An exercise ECG test is considered positive for CAD if it shows at least a 1-mm horizontal or downsloping ST-segment depression during exercise. Myocardial ischemia is induced in these patients by an increase in myocardial O_2 demand, primarily due to the increase in heart rate with exercise.

58. **How does Bayes theorem help determine the value of ETT in the detection of CAD?**
    By allowing prediction of the presence or absence of CAD in a patient based on the prevalence of CAD in the population and the sensitivity and specificity of the diagnostic test. Bayes theorem is the calculation that allows one to predict the posttest probability of a diagnosis based on the likely probability expected prior to performance of the diagnostic test. In general, the ability of noninvasive stress tests (treadmill ETT, treadmill thallium myocardial scintigraphy, treadmill or dobutamine echocardiography, or bicycle exercise radionuclide ventriculography) to predict the presence or absence of CAD in patients with a very low or very high pretest probability of CAD is poor. With either a high or a low pretest probability (based on clinical history), noninvasive testing does not help the clinician decide whether or not to perform a definitive diagnostic test, such as coronary arteriography. Conversely, patients with an intermediate pretest probability of CAD (30–70%) are good candidates for noninvasive stress testing (Table 4.7). In the patient with typical exertional angina pectoris and two or more coronary risk factors (associated with ≥ 80% pretest probability of CAD), a negative ETT and thallium myocardial scintigram predict < 30% probability of CAD. However, a positive treadmill thallium test in the same patient predicts a 90% probability of CAD. In such patients, coronary angiography is recommended in the latter case (positive treadmill thallium test) but not in the former.

Table 4.7. Probability of Coronary Artery Disease

PRETEST PROBABILITY (%)	AFTER TREADMILL ECG (%)		AFTER TREADMILL THALLIUM (%)
80	Positive test: 95	→	Positive test: 99
		→	Negative test: 85
	Negative test: 60	→	Positive test: 90
		→	Negative test: 30

ECG, electrocardiogram.

59. **What are the medical contraindications to ETT?**

    Acute or pending MI
    Acute coronary syndrome (ACS)
    Acute myocarditis or pericarditis

    Left main CAD
    Severe aortic stenosis
    Uncontrolled HTN
    Uncontrolled cardiac arrhythmias

    Second- or third-degree AV block
    Acute noncardiac illness

60. **A 31-year-old man complains of a sudden onset of sharp left chest pain, increased by deep inspiration and coughing. Physical findings, chest radiograph, and ECG are normal. What is your differential diagnosis?**
    - Acute pleuritis (coxsackievirus A, B)
    - Acute pericarditis (coxsackievirus B)
    - Pneumonia (viral, bacterial)
    - Pulmonary embolus or infarction
    - Pneumothorax
    In this patient, the most likely clinical diagnosis causing pleuritic chest pain in the presence of normal physical, chest x-ray, and ECG findings is **acute viral pleuritis** or **pericarditis**.

61. A 56-year-old man presents to the emergency department with acute onset of squeezing and diffuse anterior chest pain associated with diaphoresis and dyspnea. What is your differential diagnosis?
    - Acute MI
    - Angina pectoris
    - Acute pericarditis
    - Acute pulmonary embolus
    - Acute aortic dissection
    - Pneumothorax

62. Which tests will help confirm your clinical suspicions?
    12-lead ECG, cardiac enzymes, and chest radiograph. Among these diagnoses, the first three are most common and should be carefully considered in the diagnostic work-up of this patient. A **12-lead ECG** is performed to look for ST-segment elevations (evidence of acute myocardial injury due to infarction or pericarditis), ST-segment depressions (evidence of subendocardial ischemia), or T-wave changes. Determination of **serial cardiac enzymes** (troponin I or T or creatine kinase and CK MB isoenzyme) over the first 24–48 hours of hospitalization will help to confirm a diagnosis of acute MI. The absence of any ECG changes of acute MI or ischemia in a patient with severe anterior chest pain radiating to the back should suggest the clinical diagnosis of acute aortic dissection. Finally, a **chest radiograph** is helpful in the work-up of patients with acute chest pain to look for evidence of pneumothorax, cardiac enlargement suggestive of cardiac failure, or wedge-shaped pulmonary consolidation suggestive of acute pulmonary embolus.

63. An 89-year-old woman was found unconscious in her backyard. She "woke up" a few minutes after arrival at the emergency department. Physical, neurologic, ECG, laboratory, and chest x-ray findings are all normal. She feels fine and demands to be released. Would you admit her to the hospital?
    Yes. Syncope, defined as a transient loss or impairment of consciousness, can be due to a wide variety of causes, both cardiovascular and noncardiovascular. Patients most likely to have cardiovascular syncope are older and may or may not have a prior history of documented cardiac disease (manifested by angina pectoris, MI, or resuscitated sudden cardiac death). Patients at high risk for cardiovascular syncope (similar to this elderly patient) should be hospitalized because they have a worse prognosis and may have potentially life-threatening complications of their underlying cardiovascular disease (CVD).

64. List the common cardiovascular causes of syncope.
    - **Tachyarrhythmias:** VT or SVT (AF, atrial flutter, or paroxysmal SVT).
    - **Bradyarrhythmias:** second- or third-degree AV block, AF with a slow ventricular response rate, or sinus bradycardia due to sick sinus syndrome.
    - **LV outflow obstruction:** due to fixed lesions (valvular, subvalvular, or supravalvular aortic stenosis) or dynamic obstruction such as HCM. Characteristically, these patients present with syncope during or immediately after exercise.
    - **LV inflow obstruction:** due to severe mitral stenosis or a large LA myxoma.
    - **Primary pulmonary HTN**

HYPERTENSION

See also Chapter 2, General Medicine and Ambulatory Care, and Chapter 18, Geriatrics.

65. How do you classify or stage HTN severity?
    HTN is classified into two stages:
    - **Stage 1:** BP range 140–150/90–99 mm Hg
    - **Stage 2:** BP range ≥ 160/≥100 mm Hg

    This new classification or staging of HTN is simpler than prior staging based on various ranges of diastolic and systolic BP values and was first recommended by the Seventh Report of the Joint National Committee on Prevention, Detection, Evaluation, and Treatment of High Blood Pressure (JNC 7) consensus report. The new staging emphasizes the importance of starting **two** antihypertensive drugs as initial treatment in patients with stage 2 HTN.

Chobanian AV, Bakris GL, Black HR, et al. The Seventh Report of the Joint National Committee on Prevention, Detection, Evaluation, and Treatment of High Blood Pressure: the JNC 7 report. *JAMA.* 2003;289:2560–2572.

66. **How does the initial HTN stage predict treatment response?**
Patients with stage 2 HTN are rarely controlled to a goal BP of < 140/90 mm Hg on a single BP-lowering drug. The Antihypertensive and Lipid-Lowering Treatment to Prevent Heart Attack Trial (ALLHAT) as well as several other trials have shown that at least two or more drugs are needed in two thirds of hypertensive patients and one third require three antihypertensives to achieve target BP.
ALLHAT Officers and Coordinators for the ALLHAT Collaborative Research Group. Major outcomes in high-risk hypertensive patients randomized to angiotensin-converting enzyme inhibitor or calcium channel blocker vs. diuretic: the Antihypertensive and Lipid-Lowering Treatment to Prevent Heart Attack Trial (ALLHAT). *JAMA.* 2002;288:2981–2997.

67. **Which antihypertensive drugs are recommended for patients with chronic kidney disease (CKD) and HTN? Are different antihypertensive drugs recommended in blacks or diabetics in the presence of CKD?**
Angiotensin-converting enzyme (ACE) inhibitors and angiotensin receptor blockers (ARB).
The renoprotective benefit of these medications in patients with CKD has been widely recognized and confirmed in many randomized controlled clinical trials. Both ACE inhibitors and ARBs have been proved to be effective in preventing progression of renal disease in patients with CKD regardless of presence or absence of diabetes mellitus and are recommended as first-line drugs in CKD and HTN by both JNC 7 and JNC 8. The JNC 8 evidence-based guidelines recommend ACE inhibitors or ARBs as initial therapy in hypertensive patients with CKD, regardless of age, race, or concomitant diabetes mellitus.

68. **What antihypertensive drugs are recommended as first-line agents in black or nonblack hypertensive patients with or without diabetes mellitus?**
The recent JNC 8 evidence-based report differs from the JNC 7 consensus report in recommending any of the four classes of antihypertensive drugs in diabetic nonblack hypertensive patients: thiazide type diuretic, calcium channel blocker, ACE inhibitor, or ARB. However, in the general black hypertensive population with or without diabetes mellitus, initial antihypertensive treatment recommended by JNC 8 report should include a thiazide-type diuretic or a calcium channel blocker.

69. **How effective are diuretics?**
Very effective. Thiazide diuretics appear to be unsurpassed in preventing cardiovascular complications of HTN and were recommended by the JNC 7 consensus report as preferred initial antihypertensive drug therapy in uncomplicated HTN. However, the more recent evidence-based JNC 8 report recommends any of four antihypertensive drugs as first-line therapy in hypertensive patients: a thiazide-type diuretic, a calcium channel blocker, an ACE inhibitor, or an ARB regardless of age.
Chobanian AV, Bakris GL, Black HR, et al. The Seventh Report of the Joint National Committee on Prevention, Detection, and Treatment of High Blood Pressure: the JNC 7 report. *JAMA.* 2003;289:2560–2572. Available at: www.nhlbi.nih.gov/guidelines/hypertension.
James PA, Oparil S, Carter BL, et al. 2014 evidence-based guideline for the management of high blood pressure in adults: report from the panel members appointed to the Eighth Joint National Committee (JNC 8). *JAMA.* 2014;311:507–520.

70. **Does antihypertensive therapy in older patients reduce the risk of MI and stroke?**
Yes. The Systolic Hypertension in the Elderly Program (SHEP) demonstrated that a thiazide-based antihypertensive regimen (chlorthalidone, 12.5–25 mg/day, alone or combined with atenolol, 25–50 mg/day) reduces stroke risk by 36% and nonfatal MI plus coronary death by 27% in older (>60 years) patients with isolated systolic HTN (systolic BP > 160 mm Hg/diastolic BP < 90 mm Hg). Major cardiovascular events were reduced by 32%. As a result, overall all-cause mortality rate was 13% lower. Similar studies in younger hypertensive patients have shown a smaller beneficial effect or no effect of antihypertensive drug therapy on CAD events.
The recent JNC 8 evidence-based report has recommended any of four antihypertensive drugs as first-line agents in hypertensive patients regardless of age: a thiazide-type diuretic, a calcium channel blocker, an ACE inhibitor, or an ARB.

SHEP Cooperative Research Group. Prevention of stroke by anti-hypertensive drug treatment in older persons with isolated systolic hypertension. Final results of the Systolic Hypertension in the Elderly Program (SHEP). *JAMA*. 1991;265:3255–3264.

71. **What are the two key take-home messages from ALLHAT?**
    - Control of HTN frequently requires multiple antihypertensive drugs used in combination. The JNC 7 report recommends initiation of two antihypertensive drugs whenever BP > 160/100 mm Hg (now called *stage 2 HTN*).
    - More effective reduction of systolic BP in a high-risk older hypertensive patient results in more effective cardiovascular disease prevention.

    Cushman WC, Ford CE, Cutler JA, et al. For the ALLHAT Collaborative Research Group: Success and predictors of blood pressure control in diverse North American settings: the Antihypertensive and Lipid-Lowering to Prevent Heart Attack Trial (ALLHAT). *J Clin Hypertens*. 2002;4:393–404.

72. **Are calcium channel blockers as effective as diuretics in treating isolated systolic HTN in older patients? If so, can a calcium channel blocker be used as a first-line drug in older hypertensive patients?**
    Yes. A multicenter clinical trial, the Systolic Hypertension in Europe (Syst-Eur) Trial, showed the same reduction in cardiac and stroke events in older (>60 years) patients with systolic HTN (systolic BP > 160 mm Hg) and normal or mildly elevated diastolic BP (<95 mm Hg) with a long-acting dihydropyridine calcium channel blocker, alone or in combination with an ACE inhibitor. However, it has *not* yet been shown whether a dihydropyridine calcium channel blocker or a thiazide diuretic is *more* potent in reducing cardiovascular complications of HTN.

    The most recent Joint National Committee Report (JNC 8) recommended a thiazide type diuretic, a calcium channel blocker, an ACE inhibitor, or an ARB as first-line drugs regardless of the patient's age.

    Staessen JA, Fagard R, Thijs L, et al. Randomised double-blind comparison of placebo and active treatment for older patients with isolated systolic hypertension. The Systolic Hypertension in Europe (Syst-Eur) Trial Investigators. *Lancet*. 1997;350:757–764.

73. **What are the goals of HTN treatment?**
    See also Chapter 8, Nephrology.
    Reducing elevated BP levels to prevent various complications of systemic HTN such as stroke, heart attacks, heart failure, and renal disease. The best predictor of the efficacy in preventing various cardiorenal complications is the degree of reduction of BP. The risk of death from ischemic heart disease or stroke *in cohort longitudinal studies* is lowest at a BP of approximately 115/75 mm Hg and doubles beginning at 115/75 mm Hg with each 20 mm Hg increment in systolic BP. Although BP less than 120/80 mm Hg is associated in observational cohort studies with the lowest risk of death from ischemic heart disease and stroke, the goal of BP treatment recommended by JNC 8 is a BP < 140/90 mm Hg in patients 60 years of age and < 150/90 mm Hg in patients older than 60 years. Targeting a systolic BP < 120 mm Hg as compared with < 140 mm Hg in patients with type 2 diabetes mellitus did not reduce the rate of a composite outcome of fatal and nonfatal major cardiovascular events in the Action to Control Cardiovascular Risk in Diabetes (ACCORD) BP trial. However, SBP < 120 mm Hg did significantly reduce stroke risk, a secondary study endpoint. *Thus, it is NOT recommended at this time to target systolic BP < 120 mm Hg in type 2 diabetic patients.* However, targeting a systolic BP < 120 mm Hg compared to < 140 mm Hg in patients at high risk for cardiovascular events but without diabetes in the more recently published Systolic Blood Pressure Intervention Trial (SPRINT) resulted in lower rates of fatal and nonfatal major cardiovascular events and death from any cause, although significantly higher rates of some adverse events were observed in the intensive-treatment group. The SPRINT trial was published in 2015 after the JNC 8 report (December 2014) and may affect future National Hypertension Management Guidelines.

    ACCORD Study Group, Cushman WC, Evans GW, et al. Effects of intensive blood pressure control in type 2 diabetic. *N Engl J Med*. 2010;362:1575–1578.

    James PA, Oparil S, Carter BL, et al. Treatment of hypertension in the prevention and management of ischemic heart disease: a scientific statement from the American Heart Association Council for High Blood Pressure Research and the Councils on Clinical Cardiology and Epidemiology and Prevention. *Circulation*. 2007;115:2761–2788.

SPRINT Research Group, Wright JT Jr, Williamson JD, et al. A randomized trial of intensive versus standard blood pressure control. *N Engl J Med.* 2015;373:2103–2116.

74. **Which hypertensive patients may benefit from beta blocker treatment?**
Those with a past history of an MI, compensated heart failure, or CAD. These patients derive significant improvement in major cardiovascular outcomes with beta blocker treatment. Contraindications to beta blockers must be carefully weighed against their potential therapeutic benefits. For example, a beta blocker should be avoided in a patient admitted to the hospital with acutely decompensated heart failure but may be started at lower doses and then gradually increased in patients with well-compensated and stable heart failure. Withdrawal of beta blockers—particularly in patients with CAD—should be done gradually to avoid rebound increase in anginal symptoms upon their discontinuation. Beta blockers are strongly recommended in several national guidelines in patients with CHF with reduced ejection fraction (EF) and in patients with CAD with MI or prior MI.

75. **Is an ARB equally effective as an ACE inhibitor in preventing cardiovascular complications of HTN?**
Yes. Until recently, the evidence supporting the importance of ARB as an effective and safe BP-lowering drug class was quite limited. Recently, large prospective, randomized clinical trials have shown that an ARB is at least as effective as a beta blocker and as effective as an ACE inhibitor in preventing major cardiovascular complications. The largest clinical trials that support these conclusions are the Losartan Intervention For Endpoint reduction in hypertension (LIFE) trial and ONgoing Telmisartan Alone and in combination with Ramipril Global Endpoint Trial (ONTARGET).
ARBs are also one of the first-line antihypertensive drugs recommended by JNC 8 in addition to calcium channel blockers, ACE inhibitors, and diuretics.
The ONTARGET Investigators. Telmisartan, ramipril or both in patients at high risk for vascular events. *N Engl J Med.* 2008;358:1547–1559.

76. **A 45-year-old hypertensive woman has been treated with amlodipine, a calcium channel blocker, for chronic stable angina pectoris and HTN. She complains of ankle edema that worsened after her dose was recently increased. Are diuretics indicated?**
No. Ankle edema is a common side effect of dihydropyridine calcium channel blockers, occurring in 7–20% of patients treated. Edema is a dose-dependent side effect and readily responds to lowering of the calcium channel blocker dose. Another novel strategy to minimize the occurrence of ankle edema combines calcium channel blockade with ACE inhibition. This combination is more effective than monotherapy with either drug in lowering BP and is associated with lower prevalence of any dose-related side effects, including ankle edema.

CORONARY ARTERY DISEASE AND ANGINA SYNDROMES

77. **Define *angina*.**
The symptom complex that occurs during myocardial ischemia. Angina is typically described as a pressure or bandlike sensation in the middle of the chest that is precipitated by exertion and relieved by rest. Angina may also present with left arm or jaw pain and fatigue. Symptoms in women may be atypical and include dyspnea and palpitations.

78. **What is Prinzmetal or variant angina?**
Sudden localized spasm of a coronary artery that usually occurs near an atherosclerotic plaque that was described by Myron Prinzmetal in 1955. Typical ischemic ST-segment changes (elevation) occur during the spasm.

79. **Is treadmill ETT helpful in confirming the diagnosis of variant angina?**
No. In patients with variant angina, myocardial ischemia is primarily due to a decrease in O_2 supply rather than to an increase in O_2 demand. Exercise testing is thus of limited diagnostic value in these patients and may show ST-segment elevation, ST-segment depression, or no change in ST segments during exercise.

80. **Do nitrates differ in efficacy when used in the management of variant angina compared with classic effort angina?**
No. Patients with both forms of angina respond promptly to nitrates.

81. **Do beta blockers differ in efficacy and safety when used in the management of variant angina compared with classic effort angina?**
Yes. Although the response of patients with effort angina to beta blockers is uniformly good, the response of patients with vasospastic or Prinzmetal angina is variable. In some patients with vasospastic angina, the duration of episodes of angina pectoris may be prolonged during therapy with propranolol, a noncardioselective beta blocker. In others, especially those with associated fixed atherosclerotic lesions, beta blockers may reduce the frequency of anginal episodes. Noncardioselective beta blockers may, in some patients with vasospastic angina, leave a receptor-mediated coronary arterial vasoconstriction unopposed and thereby worsen anginal symptoms.

82. **Do calcium channel blockers differ in efficacy and safety when used in the management of variant angina compared with classic effort angina?**
No. In contrast to beta blockers, calcium blockers are quite effective in reducing the frequency and duration of episodes of vasospastic angina. Along with nitrates, calcium channel blockers are the mainstay of treatment of vasospastic angina because of their proven efficacy and safety.

83. **A 78-year-old asthmatic man has stable exertional angina of 3 years' duration. His past medical history reveals intermittent claudication after walking 50 yards. What is your approach to medical management of his anginal symptoms?**
This elderly man has three medical problems: asthma, intermittent claudication, and chronic stable angina. Of the available antianginal drugs, beta blockers are contraindicated because of the presence of asthma. Cardioselective beta blockers, such as metoprolol or atenolol, may be used cautiously in low doses in asthma, but noncardioselective beta blockers are not safe in this patient. However, the presence of peripheral vascular disease, manifested by intermittent claudication, also is a contraindication for the use of any beta blocker. Calcium channel blockers or nitrates are thus the antianginal drugs of choice in this patient.

84. **What is the high-density lipoprotein hypothesis?**
The observation that elevated high-density lipoprotein (HDL) cholesterol levels reduce the risk of coronary heart disease. Historically, the first hint of the validity of this "HDL hypothesis" was the finding of the Helsinki Heart Study that a 10% increase in HDL cholesterol levels induced by gemfibrozil accounted for the 15% larger reduction in CAD mortality rate compared with the first Lipid Research Clinic Coronary Primary Prevention Trial (LRC-CPPT) that used cholestyramine, a bile acid sequestrant resin. Both cholestyramine and gemfibrozil reduce low-density lipoprotein (LDL) cholesterol modestly by 10% but only gemfibrozil raises HDL cholesterol levels by as much as approximately 10%. More recent clinical trials have further supported an independent role of HDL in mediating coronary heart disease risk.

Frick MH, Elo O, Haapa K, et al. Helsinki Heart Study: primary prevention trial with gemfibrozil in middle-aged men with dyslipidemia. Safety of treatment, changes in risk factors, and incidence of coronary heart disease. *N Engl J Med.* 1987;371:1237–1245.

ACUTE CORONARY SYNDROME

85. **Define *acute coronary syndrome* (ACS).**
A clinical syndrome characterized by *chest pain suggestive of cardiac ischemia* that is further classified by ECG and cardiac biomarker findings as:
- Unstable angina (UA)
  - ECG: may or may not show ST-segment depression, transient ST-segment elevation, or new T-wave inversion
  - Cardiac biomarkers: not elevated (no evidence of cardiac injury)
- Non–ST-segment elevation myocardial infarction (NSTEMI)
  - ECG: may or may not show ST-segment depression, transient ST-segment elevation, or new T-wave inversion
  - Cardiac biomarkers: elevated
- ST-segment elevation myocardial infarction (STEMI)
  - ECG: ST-segment elevation or depression
  - Cardiac biomarkers: elevated

86. **How common is ACS?**
Very common. ACS is a common, potentially life-threatening medical condition. In 2003, it accounted for over 750,000 hospital admissions in the United States.

87. **Is aspirin effective in the treatment of UA?**
Yes. Unequivocal evidence from two clinical trials, the Veterans Administration (VA) and Canadian Cooperative Trials, indicates that aspirin reduces subsequent MI and mortality rate in UA patients. Both mortality rate and MI are reduced by approximately 50% in aspirin-treated patients. Aspirin should be administered immediately when UA is suspected. There is less evidence to suggest a beneficial effect of aspirin in chronic stable angina pectoris.

   Cairns JA, Gent M, Singer J, et al. Aspirin, sulfinpyrazone, or both in unstable angina: results of a Canadian multicenter trial. *N Engl J Med*. 1985;313:1369–1375.

   Lewis HD, Davis JW, Archibald DG, et al. Protective effects of aspirin against acute myocardial infarction and death in men with unstable angina: results of a Veterans Administration Cooperative Study. *N Engl J Med*. 1983;309:396–403.

88. **Is clopidogrel recommended in patients admitted with UA or NSTEMI already treated with aspirin?**
Yes. The American Heart Association/American College of Cardiology (AHA/ACC) guidelines recommend clopidogrel in patients admitted with ACS with no ST-segment elevation in addition to aspirin therapy. This recommendation is based on the Clopidogrel in Unstable Angina to Prevent Recurrent Events (CURE) trial, which showed a significant reduction in recurrent cardiac events with the addition of clopidogrel to standard therapy including aspirin, beta blockers, and statins.

   Anderson JL, Adams CD, Antman EM, et al. ACC/AHA 2007 Guidelines for the Management of Patients With Unstable Angina/Non–ST-Elevation Myocardial Infarction. A Report of the American College of Cardiology/American Heart Association Task Force on Practice Guidelines (Writing Committee to Revise the 2002 Guidelines for the Management of Patients With Unstable Angina/Non–ST-Elevation Myocardial Infarction) developed in collaboration with the American College of Emergency Physicians, the Society for Cardiovascular Angiography and Interventions, and the Society of Thoracic Surgeons endorsed by the American Association of Cardiovascular and Pulmonary Rehabilitation and the Society for Academic Emergency Medicine. *J Am Coll Cardiol*. 2007;50:1–157.

   Yusuf S, Zhao F, Mehta SR, et al. Clopidogrel in Unstable Angina to Prevent Recurrent Events Trial Investigators. Effects of clopidogrel in addition to aspirin in patients with acute coronary syndrome without ST segment elevation. *N Engl J Med*. 2001;345:494–502.

89. **Is clopidogrel equally effective in all patients?**
No. Recent studies showed that approximately 3% of the population are poor metabolizers of clopidrogel; therefore, the drug is less effective. The incidence among the Chinese population may be as high as 14%. Patients who take proton pump inhibitors (PPIs) and clopidrogel also have an increased risk of rehospitalization after MI or coronary stent placement, suggesting PPIs affect efficacy.

   Mega JL, Close SL, Wiviott SD, et al. Cytochrome P-450 polymorphisms and response to clopidogrel. *N Engl J Med*. 2009;360:354–362.

   Simon T, Verstuyft C, Mary-Krause M, et al. Genetic determinants of response to clopidogrel and cardiovascular events. *N Engl J Med*. 2009;360:363–375.

   Stocki KM, Le L, Zahkaryan A, et al. Risk of rehospitalization for patients using clopidogrel with a proton pump inhibitor. *Arch Intern Med*. 2010;170:704–710.

90. **Based on clinical assessments, which patients with ACS are at highest risk for death or recurrent MI?**
Those with:
   - Age ≥ 65 years
   - Presence of at least three risk factors for CAD
   - Prior coronary stenosis ≥ 50%
   - ST-segment deviation on ECG at presentation
   - History of at least two anginal events in prior 24 hours
   - Use of aspirin in prior 7 days
   - Elevated serum cardiac markers

The scoring system listed (Thrombosis in Myocardial Infarction [TIMI] trial) counts one point for the presence of each characteristic and can be easily obtained at the bedside on initial evaluation of any patient with acute chest pain in the emergency department. In validation studies of the TIMI risk scoring variables, cardiovascular event rates increased significantly as the TIMI risk score increased (Table 4.8).

Antman EM, Cohen M, Bernik PJLM, et al. The TIMI risk score for unstable angina/non–ST elevation MI: A method for prognostication and therapeutic decision making. *JAMA.* 2000;284:835–842.

Table 4.8. Cardiovascular Event Rates by Thrombosis in Myocardial Infarction Score

TIMI SCORE	EVENT RATE INCREASE (%)
0–1	4.7
2	8.3
3	13.2
4	19.9
5	26.2
6–7	40.9

TIMI, Thrombosis in Myocardial Infarction (trial).

91. **Which patients with UA should undergo cardiac catheterization?**
Those with:
- UA refractory to medical management
- Prior revascularization, including percutaneous coronary intervention (PCI [balloon angioplasty or coronary stent placement or both]) or coronary artery bypass surgery (CABG)
- Depressed LV function (left ventricular ejection fraction [LVEF] < 50%)
- Life-threatening "malignant" ventricular arrhythmias
- Persistent or recurrent angina/ischemia
- Inducible myocardial ischemia (provoked by exercise, dobutamine, adenosine, or dipyridamole) at a low exercise level

However, despite the above risk stratification of patients with UA, it has been a fairly widely accepted standard of care to recommend a diagnostic cardiac catheterization in most if not all patients who require hospitalization for UA to better define the coronary anatomy and provide the patient with a variety of treatment options spanning from optimal medical management to PCI and CABG.

92. **Describe the pathophysiologic mechanisms of NSTEMI and STEMI.**
In NSTEMI, the coronary artery is intermittently or incompletely occluded or both by platelet-rich white thrombus that is recently formed from platelet aggregation at the site of a damaged inner surface of a coronary artery. The trigger for this platelet aggregation is usually rupture of an atherosclerotic plaque in an artery with < 50% stenosis and causes acute subendocardial ischemia. Subendocardial ischemia may present with ST-segment depression or T-wave changes on ECG that are transient or dynamic in nature. This white thrombus is in sharp contrast to the mature red blood cell and fibrin-rich red thrombus, which is the hallmark pathologic finding in patients with STEMI. Unlike the platelet-rich thrombus, a mature thrombus results in a complete or persistent coronary artery occlusion or both resulting in severe transmural ischemia characterized by acute ST-segment elevation on ECG.

93. **Are the treatments different for NSTEMI and STEMI?**
Yes. For patients with STEMI, thrombolytic or "clot-busting" drugs such as alteplase (tPA), tenecteplase (TNK-tPA), and reteplase (rPA) are also indicated either as primary treatment or prior to PCI such as balloon angioplasty with or without coronary stent placement. PCI should be attempted if available as soon as possible after initial emergency room (ER) presentation. For

NSTEMI, patients can be initially treated with potent platelet aggregation inhibitors such as aspirin in addition to more potent platelet aggregation inhibitors such as glycoprotein (GP) IIb/IIIA inhibitors (such as eptifibatide) or a platelet P2Y12 receptor blocker such as clopidogrel or both. Beta blockers are also indicated for NSTEMI patients. For some, calcium channel blockers, ARBs, and potassium and magnesium replacement should be considered. Current standard of care is to recommend a diagnostic cardiac catheterization in patients with STEMI within the first 30–60 minutes and as soon as possible after ER presentation and in patients with NSTEMI in the first 2–3 days of hospitalization. However, the decision to recommend a diagnostic cardiac catheterization should be carefully considered in the context of the possible benefits and risks as well as in the context of the patient's personal preferences. Coronary angiography is usually indicated and recommended by the 2014 AHA/ACC Guideline for the Management of Patients With Non–ST-Elevation Acute Coronary Syndromes who have recurrent symptoms or ischemia despite adequate medical therapy or who are at high risk as categorized by clinical findings (heart failure or serious ventricular arrhythmias), noninvasive test findings (significant left ventricular dysfunction with a depressed LVEF < 40%, large anterior or multiple perfusion defects or wall motion abnormalities on echocardiography, high-risk Duke treadmill score ≤ −11), high-risk TIMI scores, or markedly elevated troponin levels. Patients with NSTEMI or ACS who have had previous PCI or CABG should also be considered for early coronary angiography, unless prior coronary angiography data indicate that no further revascularization is feasible. The general indications for coronary angiography and revascularization should also take into consideration individual patient characteristics and preferences using a patient-centered approach to decision making. For instance, very frail older adults and those with serious comorbid conditions (e.g., severe hepatic, pulmonary, or renal failure; active or inoperable cancer) might not be candidates for coronary revascularization and thus are not appropriate candidates for an invasive diagnostic cardiac catheterization.

Amesterda EA, Wenger NK, Brindis RG. 2014 AHA/ACC Guideline for the management of patients with non–ST-elevation acute coronary syndromes: a report of the American College of Cardiology/American Heart Association Task Force on Practice Guidelines. *J Am Coll Cardiol.* 2014;64:e139–e228.

94. **What are the contraindications to thrombolytic therapy in patients with STEMI?**
    - Bleeding disorders
    - Severe uncontrolled HTN (BP > 180/120 mm Hg)
    - Recent history of thromboembolic cerebrovascular accident (within 2 months)
    - Any prior history of a hemorrhagic cerebrovascular accident
    - Prolonged cardiopulmonary resuscitation (>10 minutes)
    - Active bleeding from a peptic ulcer or other noncompressible source
    - Known brain metastasis or cerebrovascular arteriovenous malformation (AVM) or aneurysm

    Kushner FG, Hand M, Smith SC Jr, et al. 2009 focused updates: ACC/AHA Guidelines for the Management of Patients With ST-Elevation Myocardial Infarction (updating the 2004 Guideline and 2007 Focused Update) and ACC/AHA/SCAI Guidelines on Percutaneous Coronary Intervention (updating the 2005 Guideline and 2007 Focused Update). A report of the American College of Cardiology Foundation/American Heart Association Task Force on Practice Guidelines. *Circulation.* 2009;20:2271–2306.

95. **Does early administration of thrombolytic therapy after STEMI decrease mortality rate?**
    Yes. Thrombolysis is the most effective lifesaving pharmacologic therapy in acute MI, saving approximately 40 lives for every 1000 treated patients and reducing 30-day and 1-year mortality rates by about 25%. In the GISSI (Gruppo Italiano per lo Studio della Sopravivenza nell' Infarto Miocardio) trial published in 1986, 11,806 patients with acute MI presenting within 12 hours of symptom onset were randomly assigned to receive intravenous (IV) streptokinase (SK) or placebo. The hospital mortality rate was significantly reduced in patients treated with SK within the first 6 hours. Most important, there was a remarkable 50% reduction in hospital mortality rate in patients treated within 1 hour of symptom onset. Subsequent clinical trials of various thrombolytic drugs—including SK, tPA, rPA, TNK-tPA—confirmed the consistent improvement in survival with thrombolytic therapy in patients with acute STEMI.

    Gruppo Italiano per lo Studio della Streptochinasi nell'Infarto Miocardico (GISSI) Trial: Effect of time to treatment on reduction in hospital mortality observed in streptokinase-treated patients. *Lancet.* 1986;1:397–401.

96. **Which drug is more effective in achieving successful reperfusion of a thrombosed coronary artery: SK, tPA, rPA, or TNK-tPA?**
    tPA. In the TIMI trial, tPA resulted in approximately twice as many successful reperfusions (due to clot lysis) as SK. In the Global Utilization of Streptokinase and Tissue Plasminogen Activator for Occluded Coronary Arteries (GUSTO) trial, tPA was more effective than SK in opening coronary arteries and preventing death in the first 30 days after acute MI. In the Reteplase (rPA) Angiographic Phase II International Dose-finding Study (RAPID) I and RAPID II trials, approximately 60% of rPA-treated patients experienced complete reperfusion at 90 minutes compared with about 50–55% of patients treated with tPA. In the large-scale GUSTO III trial, however, despite the higher TIMI flow grade 3 in patients treated with rPA, survival was similar in patients who received tPA or rPA. Angiographic trials of TNK-tPA showed similar coronary angiographic success compared with tPA, and the Assessment of the Safety and Efficacy of a New Thrombolytic (ASSENT-2) trial confirmed the equivalent efficacy of both agents in improving survival. Recent mortality trials of TNK-tPA showed no survival benefit over tPA. In summary, tPA is clearly angiographically superior to SK in opening arteries and saving lives, whereas the newer rPA and TNK-tPA thrombolytics are not clearly superior to tPA in overall efficacy but are more convenient to administer as a bolus (single bolus for TNK-tPA and double boluses, 30 minutes apart, for tPA).

    GUSTO Angiographic Investigators. The effects of tissue plasminogen activator, streptokinase, or both on coronary-artery patency, ventricular function and survival after acute myocardial infarction. *N Engl J Med.* 1993;329:1615–1622.

97. **What are the third-generation thrombolytic drugs?**
    - Recombinant tissue plasminogen activator (rPA): reteplase
    - TNK tissue plasminogen activator (TNK-tPA): tenecteplase
    - Novel plasminogen activator (nPA): lanoteplase

      Third-generation thrombolytics (better called *fibrinolytics,* because they basically degrade fibrin) are mutants of wild-type tissue plasminogen activator. Only rPA and TNK-tPA are currently Food and Drug Administration (FDA)-approved and commercially available; nPA was found to cause an unacceptably high risk of intracranial hemorrhage and is not approved by the FDA for general use in the United States.

98. **Explain the advantages of the third-generation thrombolytics.**
    These drugs lack the finger moiety of wild-type tPA that makes the drug less "sticky" to the fibrin on the surface of the clot and potentiates the clot-dissolving effect of rPA and nPA. The ability of the drug to "stick" to the outer clot surface is called *fibrin affinity.* The main advantages of third-generation thrombolytic drugs are:
    - **Efficacy:** Greater clot lysis effect.
    - **Convenience:** Longer half-life allowing for bolus injection. Both rPA and TNK-tPA have longer half-lives than tPA and can be given as bolus injections; rPA is administered as a double bolus (10 units IV q30min), and TNK-tPA is administered as a single 5-second IV bolus.
    - **Fibrin specificity:** More than 80-fold for TNK-tPA.
    - **Resistance to plasminogen activator inhibitor 1 (PAI-1):** With less making it more resistant to breakdown of TNK-tPA by naturally occurring inhibitors of plasminogen activator. This is the case for TNK-tPA.

99. **How successful is the combination of thrombolysis and GP IIb/IIIa inhibitors for patients with acute coronary occlusion?**
    Not very. This combination is not routinely recommended. Three clinical trials have evaluated the angiographic results of thrombolysis in combination with an inhibitor of the platelet glycoprotein GP IIb/IIIa receptor: the TIMI 14, Strategies for Patency Enhancement in the Emergency Department (SPEED), GUSTO, and the INtegrelin and low dose ThRombolysis in Acute Myocardial Infarction (INTRO-AMI) trials. All three specifically evaluated angiographic outcome at 60 and 90 minutes after thrombolytics when combined with a platelet glycoprotein GP IIb/IIIa receptor. The TIMI 14 SPEED and GUSTO trials revealed that the proportion of patients who completely reperfuse (as evidenced by a TIMI flow grade 3) is significantly higher with the combination of half-dose tPA or rPA with the platelet glycoprotein GP IIb/IIIa receptor inhibitor abciximab (Reopro). The INTRO-AMI trial confirmed these results using the platelet glycoprotein GP IIb/IIIa receptor inhibitor eptifibatide (Integrelin) and showed a similar increase in rate and extent of thrombolysis at 90 minutes after thrombolysis is initiated. However, despite these

promising angiographic results, none of the mortality trials showed any survival advantages for the combination of lysis + GP IIb/IIIa inhibitors.

Antman EM, Giugliano RP, Gibson CM, et al, for the TIMI 14 Investigators. Abciximab facilitates the rate and extent of thrombolysis: results of the Thrombolysis in Myocardial Infarction (TIMI) 14 trial. *Circulation.* 1999;99:2720–2732.

Trial of abciximab with and without low-dose reteplase for acute myocardial infarction: Strategies for Patency Enhancement in the Emergency Department (SPEED) Group. *Circulation.* 2000;101:2788–2794.

KEY POINTS: PLATELET AGGREGATION

1. Platelet aggregation is the key pathophysiologic mechanism causing non–ST-segment elevation acute coronary syndrome.
2. Strategies specifically targeting the inhibition of platelet aggregation, such as aspirin, low-molecular-weight or unfractionated heparin, and clopidogrel, are routinely recommended.
3. The use of more potent platelet aggregation inhibitors (the glycoprotein IIB/IIIA inhibitors such as tirofiban, eptifibatide, or abciximab) are reserved for patients with acute coronary syndromes at substantially high risk for major cardiovascular complications because of greater bleeding risk.
4. Patients may have genetic characteristics that make clopidogrel less effective.
5. Clopidogrel may have less efficacy in patients taking proton pump inhibitors.

100. **Is a PCI such as primary angioplasty using a balloon-tipped catheter as effective as pharmacologic reperfusion therapy with a thrombolytic drug in patients with STEMI?**

Yes. The Primary Angioplasty in Myocardial Infarction (PAMI) trial is the first published clinical trial designed specifically to compare balloon angioplasty with thrombolysis as the primary reperfusion therapy in patients with acute STEMI. Survival rates (at 30 days and at 2 years) after primary angioplasty were similar to those with thrombolysis in acute MI, but angioplasty conferred greater freedom from recurrent ischemia, reinfarction, and need for readmission to the hospital. Another important advantage of balloon angioplasty over thrombolytic drug therapy is reduced risk of intracranial hemorrhage, a dreadful complication of thrombolysis, particularly in elderly patients. Several subsequent trials using more modern and effective revascularization techniques such as coronary stenting have consistently demonstrated a clinical survival advantage of primary coronary intervention (coronary balloon angioplasty ± stent placement) over thrombolysis as well as lower risk of intracranial hemorrhage. In clinical practice and included in the most current recommendations of the ACC, mechanical coronary reperfusion with primary stenting is recommended as a preferred reperfusion strategy in STEMI patients over thrombolytic therapy in clinical settings in which PCI is feasible. Subsequently many randomized controlled clinical trials have compared primary stenting to thrombolytic therapy in STEMI and meta-analyses have clearly demonstrated the clinical superiority of primary stenting over thrombolytic therapy as the preferred initial revascularization strategy of choice. Thrombolytic therapy is now reserved to the rare patient with STEMI who has no access to an interventional cardiologist who can perform a primary coronary stenting procedure in a timely manner.

Kushner FG, Hand M, Smith SC Jr, et al. 2009 Focused Updates: ACC/AHA Guidelines for the Management of Patients With ST-Elevation Myocardial Infarction (updating the 2004 Guideline and 2007 Focused Update) and ACC/AHA/SCAI Guidelines on Percutaneous Coronary Intervention (updating the 2005 Guideline and 2007 Focused Update): a report of the American College of Cardiology Foundation/American Heart Association Task Force on Practice Guidelines. *Circulation.* 2009;54:2205–2241.

Levine GN, Bates ER, Blankenship JC, et al. 2015 ACC/AHA/SCAI Focused Update on Primary Percutaneous Coronary Intervention for Patients with ST-Elevation Myocardial Infarction: An Update of the 2011 ACCF/AHA/SCAI Guideline for Percutaneous Coronary Intervention and the 2013 ACCF/AHA/SCAI Guidelines for Percutaneous Coronary Intervention and the 2013 ACCF/AHA Guideline for the Management of ST-Elevation Myocardial Infarction. *J Am Coll Cardiol.* 2015;67:1235–1250.

Nunn CM, O'Neill WW, Rothbaum D, et al. Long-term outcome after primary angioplasty: Report from the Primary Angioplasty in Myocardial Infarction (PAMI-I) trial. *J Am Coll Cardiol.* 1999;33:640–646.

101. **How common is restenosis after balloon angioplasty bare metal noncoated coronary stent placement and coated coronary stent placement?**

About 40–45% of patients undergoing balloon angioplasty and about 25–35% of patients undergoing bare metal noncoated coronary stent placement develop restenosis. Restenosis occurs in only 5–7% of patients undergoing a coated coronary stent placement.

KEY POINTS: PERCUTANEOUS CORONARY INTERVENTION

1. Restenosis is the most common complication of PCA.
2. The incidence of restenosis is significantly reduced with PCA and bare metal coronary artery stents.
3. The incidence is even more reduced with PCA and sirolimus- or paclitaxel-coated drug-eluting coronary artery stents.
4. However, coated drug-eluting stents are more prone to thrombosis than bare metal stents and require a longer period of treatment with the platelet inhibitor clopidogrel.
5. Restenosis is most common in the first 6 months after balloon angioplasty or stent placement and presents with recurrent angina; stent thrombosis can occur up to several years after a coronary stent placement and presents with an acute myocardial infarction.

PCA, percutaneous coronary balloon angioplasty.

102. **Are drug-eluting coronary stents more or less likely to be complicated by restenosis compared with bare metal stents?**

Less likely. Two types of drug-eluting stents, sirolimus- and paclitaxel-eluting stents, have been extensively investigated in patients with CAD. These two coated stents have been developed specifically to inhibit proliferation of vascular smooth muscle cells, the primary mechanism for restenosis over the first 6 months after stent placement. Both drug-eluting coronary stents have now been demonstrated in large randomized clinical trials to cause significantly less restenosis than the so-called bare metal stents. Overall, restenosis occurs in 2–6% of patients receiving a drug-eluting coronary stent compared with about 25–35% with bare metal stents. Coated stents are also associated with substantially decreased need for readmission with recurrent angina and repeat coronary interventions.

Colombo A, Drzewiecki J, Banning A, et al. for the TAXUS II Study Group. Randomized study to assess the effectiveness of slow- and moderate-release polymer-based paclitaxel-eluting stents for coronary artery lesions. *Circulation.* 2003;108:788–794.

Moses JW, Leon MB, Popma JJ, et al. for the SIRIUS investigators. Sirolimus-eluting stents versus standard stents in patients with stenosis in a native coronary artery. *N Engl J Med.* 2003;349:1315–1323.

Schofer J, Schluer M, Gershlick AH, et al. for the E-SIRIUS Investigators. Sirolimus-eluting stents for treatment of patients with long atherosclerotic lesions in small coronary arteries: Double-blind, randomized controlled trial (E-SIRIUS). *Lancet.* 2003;362:1093–1099.

103. **Why should IV ACE inhibitors be avoided in the first 24 hours after acute MI?**

Because they may cause a potentially harmful acute decrease in BP with a resultant reduction in coronary blood flow.

Swedberg K, Held P, Kjekshus J, et al. Effects of the early administration of enalapril on mortality in patients with acute myocardial infarction: Results of the Cooperative New Scandinavian Enalapril Survival Study II (CONSENSUS-II). *N Engl J Med.* 1992;327:678–684.

104. **Should oral nitrates be administered routinely to all patients with uncomplicated MI?**

No. IV, transdermal, or oral nitrates or a combination has traditionally been used routinely in all patients admitted with suspected acute MI. However, despite the encouraging results of early small clinical studies, two large multicenter clinical trials, International Study of Infarct Survival (ISIS)-4 and GISSI-3, consisting of about 78,000 patients, showed no significant benefit of early oral nitrates on survival, infarct size, or ventricular function. Nitrate administration should be limited to patients with well-established indications for nitrates, such as postinfarction angina, ischemia, or CHF.

Gruppo Italiano per lo Studio della Sopravivenza nell' Infarto Miocardio (GISSI-3). Effects of lisinopril and transdermal glyceryltrinitrate singly and together on 6-week mortality and ventricular function after acute myocardial infarction. *Lancet.* 1994;343:1115–1122.

ISIS-4 (Fourth International Study of Infarct Survival) Collaborative Group: A randomized factorial trial assessing early oral captopril, oral mononitrate, and intravenous magnesium sulphate in 58,050 patients with suspected acute myocardial infarction. *Lancet.* 1995;345:669–685.

Morris JL, Zaman AG, Smyllie JH, Cowan JC. Nitrates in myocardial infarction: Influence on infarct size, reperfusion, and ventricular remodeling. *Br Heart J.* 1995;73:310–319.

105. Do ACE inhibitors improve survival in patients recovering from acute MI?
Yes. Long-term oral ACE inhibitors started 3–16 days after acute MI and maintained for about 3 years reduce mortality rate by about 19% in patients with asymptomatic LV systolic dysfunction (LVEF < 40%), as demonstrated in the Survival and Ventricular Enlargement (SAVE) Trial. Subsequent trials (ISIS-4 and GISSI-3) specifically showed that even a short 6-week course of an ACE inhibitor started within 24 hours of infarct onset decreases 6-week mortality rate by 7–12%, corresponding to 5 deaths prevented for every 1000 treated patients.

Gruppo Italiano per lo Studio della Sopravivenza nell' Infarto Miocardio (GISSI-3): Effects of lisinopril and transdermal glyceryltrinitrate singly and together on 6-week mortality and ventricular function after acute myocardial infarction. *Lancet.* 1994;343:1115–1122.

ISIS-4 (Fourth International Study of Infarct Survival) Collaborative Group: A randomized factorial trial assessing early oral captopril, oral mononitrate, and intravenous magnesium sulphate in 58,050 patients with suspected acute myocardial infarction. *Lancet.* 1995;345:669–685.

Pfeffer MA, Braunwald E, Moye LA, et al. Effect of captopril on mortality and morbidity in patients with left ventricular dysfunction after myocardial infarction. Results of the Survival and Ventricular Enlargement Trial. *N Engl J Med.* 1992;327:669–677.

106. What is the most common cause of death in the first 48 hours after an acute MI?
VF. Other causes of death include cardiac rupture, pump failure due to massive infarction, acute mechanical complication such as ventricular septal rupture or acute MR, and cardiogenic shock.

107. Cardiac rupture is almost always a fatal complication of acute MI. List the three risk factors for its development.
Female sex, HTN, and first MI.

108. List the clinical features of cardiac rupture.
- Occurs more often in LV than in RV in a 7:1 ratio.
- Seen in anterior or lateral wall MI.
- Usually occurs with large MI.
- Usually occurs within 3–6 days after MI.
- Rarely occurs with LV hypertrophy or good collateral vessels.

109. What complication of acute inferior wall MI typically presents with hypotension, elevated neck veins, clear lungs, and a normal cardiac silhouette on chest radiograph?
RV MI. The diagnosis can be confirmed by demonstrating at least 1-mm ST-segment elevation in right-sided chest leads V_3R or V_4R. Further confirmation of RV MI can be derived from noninvasive assessment of RV systolic function using radionuclide techniques or, more commonly, bedside two-dimensional echocardiography. A **right-sided ECG** should be done in **every** patient presenting to an emergency department with an acute inferior wall MI. Studies have shown that inferior wall MI patients with RV infarction are sicker, are more likely to die, and have an increased incidence of major cardiac complications of their inferior wall MI. Thus, these patients should be readily identified at initial clinical presentation and aggressively treated. Clinical management consists of volume expansion in combination with IV dopamine. In these patients, diuretics or preload-reducing drugs such as nitrates worsen the low cardiac output state and hypotension and should be avoided.

110. **What is the differential diagnosis of a new systolic murmur and acute pulmonary edema appearing 3 days after an acute anterior wall MI?**
Acute MR due to papillary muscle rupture and interventricular septal rupture. Both are potentially fatal complications and are most common 3–6 days after infarction. Rupture of the posteromedial papillary muscle, associated with inferior wall MI, is more common than rupture of the anterolateral papillary muscle. Unlike rupture of the interventricular septum, which occurs with large infarcts, papillary muscle rupture occurs with a small infarction in approximately 50% of cases.

111. **How do you differentiate between acute MR and ventricular septal rupture?**
With two-dimensional and Doppler echocardiography (which can be done at the bedside), which will demonstrate the presence and severity of MR and localize the site of a ventricular septal defect (VSD). Further confirmation of the presence of a left-to-right shunt across a VSD can be obtained by a step-up in blood oxygen saturation from the RA to the pulmonary artery, documented by blood sampling using a Swan-Ganz catheter.

112. **What is the most likely cause of a persistent ST-segment elevation several weeks after recovery from a large transmural anterolateral wall MI?**
LV aneurysm. Persistent ST-segment elevation is not an uncommon complication of a large anterolateral, transmural MI and may represent dyskinesis of the thinned-out, infarcted myocardium. However, persistent ST-segment elevations should suggest the presence of an **LV aneurysm,** and noninvasive confirmation of this diagnosis by two-dimensional echocardiography or radionuclide ventriculography should be sought.

113. **Which MIs are most commonly complicated by LV aneurysms?**
Acute transmural MI, developing in 12–15% of survivors. Aneurysms range from 1–8 cm in diameter and are four times more common at the apex and anterior wall than in the inferoposterior wall. Patients with larger infarcts are more likely to develop LV aneurysms, and the mortality rate is about six times higher in patients with an LV aneurysm than in those with comparable global LV function. Death is often sudden, suggesting an increased risk of sustained VT and VF in these patients.

114. **What is Dressler syndrome?**
Post-MI chest pain *not* due to coronary insufficiency. The syndrome was first described in 1854 and its exact cause remains unclear. Dressler syndrome occurs in 3–4% of MI patients 2–10 weeks after the event and is characterized by inflammation of the pericardium and surrounding tissues. Corticosteroids and nonsteroidal anti-inflammatory drugs (NSAIDs) are effective treatments.

115. **Summarize the current guidelines for use of an ACE inhibitor, an ARB, and an aldosterone antagonist in patients recovering from a STEMI.**
The current guidelines for the management of patients with STEMI recommend the routine use of an ACE inhibitor in patients with no contraindications for an ACE inhibitor. An ARB is recommended for those intolerant of an ACE inhibitor who have heart failure or LV dysfunction defined as an LVEF < 40%. Aldosterone antagonists are recommended in patients who recovered from a STEMI without substantial renal dysfunction (defined as creatinine < 2.5 mg/dL in men and < 2.0 mg/dL in women) or hyperkalemia who already are receiving an ACE inhibitor, have LVEF < 40%, and have symptomatic heart failure or diabetes mellitus.
Kushner FG, Hand M, Smith SC Jr, et al. 2009 focused updates: ACC/AHA Guidelines for the Management of Patients With ST-Elevation Myocardial Infarction (Updating the 2004 Guideline and 2007 Focused Update) and ACC/AHA/SCAI Guidelines on Percutaneous Coronary Intervention (Updating the 2005 Guideline and 2007 Focused Update). A report of the American College of Cardiology Foundation/American Heart Association Task Force on Practice Guidelines. *Circulation.* 2009;120:2271–2306.
Wright RS, Anderson JL, Adams CD, et al. 2011 ACCF/AHA Focused Update of the Guidelines for the Management of Patients with Unstable Angina and Non ST Elevation Myocardial Infarction. *J Am Coll Cardiol.* 2011;57:1920–1959.

116. **Which lipid-lowering drug was shown in a prospective placebo-controlled clinical trial to reduce cardiovascular mortality in MI survivors with "average" blood cholesterol levels?**
Pravastatin, a potent 3-hydroxy-3-methylglutaryl coenzyme A (HMG-CoA) reductase inhibitor, was evaluated in MI patients in the Cholesterol and Recurrent Events (CARE) Trial. In this double-blind

trial, 3583 men and 576 women who had survived a recent MI and had plasma total cholesterol levels below 240 mg/dL and LDL levels of 115–174 mg/dL received pravastatin (40 mg/day) or placebo for 5 years. The primary endpoint was a fatal coronary event or a nonfatal MI. The frequency of the primary endpoint was 10.2% in the pravastatin group and 13.2% in the placebo group (24% reduction in risk). Subgroup analysis revealed that most of the benefit occurred in patients with baseline serum LDL cholesterol levels > 125 mg/dL. In practical terms, patients with LDL cholesterol > 125 mg/dL and prior MI should receive an HMG-CoA reductase inhibitor for at least 5 years. More recently, the Pravastatin or Atorvastatin Evaluation and Infection Therapy (PROVE-IT) trial has demonstrated the superiority of a more potent statin, atorvastatin, over pravastatin in preventing cardiovascular complications of an MI. Based on the PROVE-IT and other recent statin clinical trials, the goal of lipid lowering in patients with ACS has been changed from < 100 mg/dL to a more optimal—yet still "optional"—goal LDL of < 70 mg/dL.

Cannon CP, Braunwald E, McCabe CH, et al. For the Pravastatin or Atorvastatin Evaluation and Infection Therapy—Thrombolysis in Myocardial Infarction: Intensive versus moderate lipid lowering with statins after acute coronary syndromes. *N Engl J Med.* 2004;350:1495–1504.

Sacks FM, Pfeffer MA, Moye LA, et al. for the Cholesterol and Recurrent Events Trial Investigators: The effect of pravastatin on coronary events after myocardial infarction in patients with average cholesterol levels. *N Engl J Med.* 1996;335:1001–1009.

117. **Do statins help prevent MI and stroke in patients with CAD (or other vascular disease) or diabetes mellitus or both, regardless of the LDL cholesterol level?**
Yes. The Heart Protection Study (HPS) investigated the effect of simvastatin (40 mg/day) on fatal or nonfatal coronary heart disease events in about 20,000 patients, aged 40–79 years, with vascular disease and/or diabetes mellitus and a mildly elevated LDL cholesterol level of approximately 130 mg/dL. This trial showed the same overall 24% reduction in cardiovascular mortality rate and 30–35% reduction in coronary heart disease events and stroke in the 3800 patients with a baseline LDL cholesterol of < 100 mg/dL as in patients with higher LDL cholesterol levels (100–130 mg/dL or > 130 mg/dL). These results indicate that patients aged 40–79 years with known vascular disease or diabetes mellitus should receive statin therapy, regardless of the LDL cholesterol level. A study of atorvastatin (10 mg/day) in diabetics aged 40–79 years reported similar results. As a result, the American Diabetes Association has recommended statin therapy in all diabetics 40 years and older regardless of LDL unless total cholesterol is < 135 mg/dL.

Colhoun HM, Betteridge DJH, Durrington PN, et al. Primary prevention of cardiovascular disease with atorvastatin in type 2 diabetes in the Collaborative Atorvastatin Diabetes Study (CARDS): multicentre randomised placebo-controlled trial. *Lancet.* 2004;364:686–696.

Heart Protection Study Investigators. MRC/BHF Heart Protection Study of cholesterol lowering with simvastatin in 20,536 high-risk individuals: a randomised placebo-controlled trial. *Lancet.* 2002;360:7–22.

118. **Beta blockers are effective in the treatment of stable exertional angina pectoris. Should you recommend routine administration of oral beta blockers in MI survivors who are angina-free?**
Yes. Several large-scale, multicenter clinical trials conducted in the United States and abroad have shown a consistent reduction in total and cardiovascular mortality rate in survivors of acute transmural MI treated with oral beta blockers for 1–3 years. The largest published U.S. trial is the Beta-Blocker Heart Attack Trial, which randomized 3837 MI survivors to either propranolol (180 or 240 mg/day) or placebo. At 3 years of follow-up, a 26% reduction in mortality rate was found in patients treated with propranolol compared with placebo-treated patients. Thus, regardless of the presence or absence of angina, oral beta blockers such as propranolol (180–240 mg), timolol (10 mg twice a day), or metoprolol (100 mg twice a day) should be routinely started 5–21 days after MI and continued for at least 7 years.

Beta-Blocker Heart Attack Trial Research Group. A randomized trial of propranolol in patients with acute myocardial infarction: 1. Mortality results. *JAMA.* 1982;247:1707–1714.

119. **A 67-year-old man has stayed in bed for the past 3 days with flulike symptoms. A 12-lead ECG reveals new Q waves in leads V_1–V_6 and ST-segment elevation of 3 mm in leads V_2–V_5, I, and aVL. What do you suspect in this patient?**
Anterolateral MI. This patient has ECG changes indicative of the recent evolution of an extensive anterolateral MI evidenced by (1) 3-mm ST-segment elevations in anterolateral leads V_2–V_5, I, and aVL and (2) new Q waves in all anterolateral chest leads. The most likely clinical diagnosis is an acute, extensive anterolateral MI that occurred 3–4 days ago, when he first complained of flulike symptoms.

120. **Is plasma creatine kinase (CK) likely to be high in this patient?**
No. The laboratory confirmation of MI is routinely done by measuring serum CK containing M and B subunits (CKMB) and CK levels at 6-hour intervals for 24–48 hours. Serum CKMB and CK levels are elevated starting at 4–8 hours after symptom onset, peak at 18–24 hours, and normalize within 3–4 days. Thus, serum CKMB and CK levels in this patient are likely to be normal.

121. **What other laboratory tests are helpful in establishing the diagnosis of MI?**
Cardiac troponins T and I, which are newer, more specific enzymatic markers of MI that remain elevated up to 10–14 days after an MI. Troponins T and I are now routinely obtained in patients with chest pain syndromes and are of particular value in diagnosing MI in patients presenting late (>12–24 hours) after MI symptom onset as well as in risk-stratifying patients presenting with ACSs.

122. **A 48-year-old man presents with acute severe epigastric pain, anorexia, nausea, vomiting, and diaphoresis. Which myocardial wall is likely affected? Explain the rationale for such an unusual clinical presentation.**
Inferior wall. Patients with an **acute inferior wall MI** sometimes present with epigastric pain associated with gastrointestinal (GI) symptoms. Less commonly, they present with hiccupping, which may at times be intractable. These unique clinical manifestations are thought to be related to increased vagal tone and irritation of the diaphragm by the adjacent infarcted inferior wall.

CONGESTIVE HEART FAILURE

See also Chapter 2, General Medicine and Ambulatory Care.

123. **Name the types of cardiomyopathies.**
See Table 4.9.

Table 4.9. Characteristics of Cardiomyopathies

CHARACTERISTICS	Cardiomyopathy		
	HYPERTROPHIC	DILATED	RESTRICTIVE
Causes	Genetic Secondary to pressure overload (e.g., hypertension, aortic stenosis)	Myocarditis Chronic Genetic Arrhythmogenic right ventricular dysplasia	Infiltrative or storage diseases Endomyocardial (e.g., Löffler syndrome, carcinoid)
Ejection fraction (normal > 55%)	>60%	<50%	>55%
Left ventricular diastolic dimension (normal < 55 mm)	Often decreased	≥60 mm	<60 mm
Left ventricular wall thickness	Increased	Decreased	Normal or increased
Atrial size	Increased	Increased	Increased; may be massive
Valvular regurgitation	Mitral regurgitation	Mitral first during decompensation; tricuspid regurgitation in late stages	Frequent mitral and tricuspid regurgitation, rarely severe
Common first symptoms*	Exertional intolerance; may have chest pain	Exertional intolerance	Exertional intolerance, fluid retention

Table 4.9. Characteristics of Cardiomyopathies (Continued)

CHARACTERISTICS	Cardiomyopathy		
	HYPERTROPHIC	DILATED	RESTRICTIVE
Congestive symptoms*	Primary exertional dyspnea	Left before right, except right prominent in young adults	Right often exceeds left
Risk for arrhythmia	Ventricular tachyarrhythmias, atrial fibrillation	Tachyarrhythmias; atrial fibrillation; conduction block in Chagas disease, giant cell myocarditis, and some families	Atrial fibrillation; ventricular, tachyarrhythmias uncommon except in sarcoidosis; conduction block in sarcoidosis and amyloidosis

*Left-sided symptoms of pulmonary congestion: dyspnea on exertion, orthopnea, paroxysmal nocturnal dyspnea. Right-sided symptoms of systemic venous congestion: discomfort on bending, hepatic and abdominal distention, peripheral edema.

124. List common signs and symptoms of CHF in order of decreasing specificity.

Right-Sided Heart Failure	Left-Sided Heart Failure
Jugular vein distention	Chest radiograph showing redistribution of perfusion or interstitial edema
Hepatomegaly	
Pleural effusion	S_3
Decreased albumin	Cardiomegaly
Abdominal discomfort	Paroxysmal nocturnal dyspnea, orthopnea
Anorexia	
Proteinuria	Dyspnea on exertion
Increased prothrombin time	
Peripheral edema	
Increased aspartate aminotransferase (AST), bilirubin	

125. What is the differential diagnosis of the cause of CHF symptoms?

Isolated Right-Sided Heart Failure	Left-Sided or Biventricular Failure
Pulmonary embolus	Aortic stenosis
Tricuspid stenosis	Aortic insufficiency
Tricuspid regurgitation	Mitral stenosis
RA tumor	MR
Cardiac tamponade	Most cardiomyopathies
Constrictive pericarditis	Acute MI
Pulmonary insufficiency	Myxoma
RV infarction	Hypertensive heart disease
Intrinsic lung disease	Myocarditis
Ebstein anomaly	Supraventricular arrhythmias
High cardiac output states	LV aneurysm
(e.g., anemia, systemic fistulas, beriberi, Paget disease, carcinoid, thyrotoxicosis)	Cardiac shunts
	High cardiac output states

126. What factors can precipitate an exacerbation of formerly well-controlled chronic CHF?

Increased consumption of salt	Renal failure	Elevated BP
	Pregnancy	High environmental temperature
Fluid overload	Paget disease	
Pulmonary emboli	Poor compliance with medications	Cardiac ischemia or MI
Fever, infection		Thyrotoxicosis
Anemia	Arrhythmias	

When patients with well-controlled, chronic CHF experience a sudden exacerbation, the precipitating factors must be sought.

127. A 68-year-old man with HTN presents with a 2-week history of progressive exertional dyspnea, orthopnea, and paroxysmal nocturnal dyspnea. What is the differential diagnosis of CHF in hypertensive patients?
- CAD
- Heart failure with normal EF (diastolic dysfunction) associated with HTN
- Dilated cardiomyopathy (idiopathic or alcoholic)
- Valvular heart disease (MR, aortic stenosis, aortic insufficiency)
- Restrictive heart disease (amyloidosis)
- HCM

128. What are the less common causes of GI symptoms in patients with CHF?
Passive hepatic congestion or ascites. Differentiation of the various causes of nausea and vomiting in such patients, on clinical grounds alone, can be difficult.

129. Which drugs are available for the treatment of CHF?
- **Venous vasodilators:** nitrates to relieve pulmonary congestive symptoms
- **Arteriolar dilators:** ACE inhibitors or ARBs to reduce afterload, improve cardiac performance, and reduce progressive ventricular dilatation or "remodeling"
- **Inotropic drugs:** digoxin to reduce ventricular response to concomitant AF or improve cardiac performance
- **Diuretics:** loop diuretics to relieve congestive signs and symptoms of left- and right-sided CHF

130. Which drug classes have been proved to decrease mortality in patients with CHF?
- ACE inhibitor: enalapril
- ARBs: valsartan and candesartan
- Beta blockers: metoprolol succinate, carvedilol, bisoprolol, and nebivolol

These medications have been shown in a number of major clinical trials to reduce cardiovascular mortality in patients with systolic New York Heart Association (NYHA) functional classes II–IV and are now considered the standard treatment in patients with CHF. Generally, ARBs are recommended in patients who are intolerant of ACE inhibitors (particularly due to cough).

Cohn JN, Tognomi G. A randomized trial of the angiotensin-receptor blocker valsartan in chronic heart failure. *N Engl J Med.* 2001;345:1667–1675.

Consensus Trial Study Group. Effects of enalapril on mortality in severe congestive heart failure: Results of the Cooperative North Scandinavian Enalapril Survival Study (CONSENSUS). *N Engl J Med.* 1987;316:1429–1435.

Foody JM, Farrell MH, Krumholz HM. Beta-blocker therapy in heart failure: Scientific review. *JAMA.* 2002;287:883–889.

Hunt SA, Abraham WT, Chin MH, et al. 2009 focused update incorporated into the ACC/AHA 2005 Guidelines for the Diagnosis and Management of Heart Failure in Adults: A report of the American College of Cardiology Foundation/American Heart Association Task Force on Practice Guidelines: Developed in collaboration with the International Society for Heart and Lung Transplantation. *Circulation.* 2009;119:e391–e479.

SOLVD Investigators, Yusuf S, Pitt B, Davis CE, et al. Effect of enalapril on survival in patients with reduced left ventricular ejection fractions and congestive heart failure. *N Engl J Med.* 1991;325:293–302.

131. What classes of antihypertensive drugs are recommended in a patient with CHF?
    - ACE inhibitors (captopril, enalapril, lisinopril, ramipril, or monopril).
    - ARBs (losartan, irbesartan, valsartan, candesartan, or telmisartan) if ACE inhibitors are not well tolerated or contraindicated.
    - Vasodilators (hydralazine) if ACE inhibitors or ARBs if not tolerated. In African Americans with CHF, a combination of hydralazine plus isosorbide dinitrate is recommended in addition to an ACE inhibitor to prevent cardiovascular complications of CHF.
    - Diuretics (furosemide). Loop diuretics are recommended in patients with CHF and clinical evidence of overt decompensated CHF with volume overload and should be titrated to minimize congestive symptoms without unduly reducing intravascular volume and worsening renal function.

132. Which drugs should be usually avoided in patients with acutely decompensated CHF?
    - Calcium channel blockers of the nondihydropyridine class (verapamil, diltiazem)
    - Beta blockers (propranolol, metoprolol, atenolol)
      These drugs have negative inotropic effects and should generally be avoided, particularly in patients with acutely decompensated CHF.

133. How is acute pulmonary edema managed?
    - IV diuresis
    - IV, cutaneous, or oral preload-reducing drug therapy
    - IV digitalization (in patients with acute pulmonary edema particularly with associated AF)
    - Oxygen therapy (depending on results of arterial oxygen saturation)
    - Bed rest and salt restriction
    - Afterload-reducing drugs

134. Describe the effect of IV diuresis in heart failure patients.
    A loop diuretic, such as furosemide given as 20–60 mg IV push, lowers venous tone and thus lowers pulmonary wedge pressure even before inducing effective diuresis.

135. Which drugs are useful for reducing preload?
    Nitrates by acting as effective venodilators. In single oral doses of 40–60 mg (to be repeated three to four times daily), they are effective in lowering pulmonary capillary wedge pressure and, thus, improving congestive symptoms of heart failure: dyspnea, orthopnea, paroxysmal nocturnal dyspnea, and nocturnal cough.

136. Describe the effects of afterload-reducing drugs.
    Afterload-reducing drugs are effective in alleviating the signs and symptoms of CHF. ACE inhibitors such as captopril, enalapril, or lisinopril are effective afterload- and preload-reducing drugs and can be administered orally in patients with overt CHF. Unlike other drugs that effectively improve the symptoms of heart failure (such as diuretics and digoxin), ACE inhibitors (and ARBs in ACE inhibitor–intolerant patients) have been proved—in a large number of randomized, placebo-controlled clinical trials—to reduce cardiovascular mortality in patients with heart failure and depressed LV systolic function.

137. Are all calcium channel blockers contraindicated in patients with heart failure?
    No. Calcium channel blockers are not all created equal. Dihydropyridine calcium channel blockers such as amlodipine and felodipine have no clinically significant negative inotropic effects; have been evaluated in large, prospective, placebo-controlled clinical trials in patients with heart failure; and can be used safely in patients with impaired systolic function and CHF if there is an additional clinical indication for a calcium blocker, such as HTN or angina pectoris.

138. Do beta blockers ever have a role in treating patients with heart failure?
    Yes. Although beta blockers are generally contraindicated in patients with acute or decompensated heart failure or both, a large number of prospective, randomized clinical trials with beta blockers such as carvedilol, metoprolol, and bucindolol at low and gradually titrated doses support a beneficial long-term effect in patients of NYHA functional classes II and III (mild to moderate symptomatic heart failure). Even low-dose beta blocker initiation in patients with heart failure should be done cautiously because a significant proportion (as high as 30–40%) of these patients may experience symptomatic hypotension and worsening heart failure symptoms in the first 4 weeks of beta blocker initiation.

139. **Why are digoxin, diuretics, and nitrates still used to treat CHF?**
Because they decrease the number of hospitalizations for acute CHF exacerbations and reduce mortality in patients with CHF.

140. **What is the mechanism of action of digitalis?**
Inhibition of Na^+-K^+-ATPase activity (the sodium pump) that blocks the transport of sodium and potassium across cell membranes, leading to an intracellular increase in sodium and decrease in potassium. The increase in intracellular sodium in turn leads to an exchange for calcium. The increased intracellular calcium, the contractile element of muscle, leads to increased contractility (positive inotropic effect). The antiarrhythmic effects of cardiac glycosides are probably not due to any direct effect of the drugs. Rather, they are mediated by an increase in vagal tone in the atria and AV junction.

141. **A 78-year-old man with a longstanding history of CHF and chronic AF presents with increasing generalized weakness, anorexia, nausea, and vomiting for the last few days. He has been receiving increasing digoxin doses up to 0.5 mg/day to slow the ventricular response to his AF and furosemide 120 mg twice a day to relieve his pulmonary congestive symptoms. What clinical diagnosis should you suspect in this patient?**
Digitalis toxicity. Any patient receiving digitalis who presents with GI symptoms, such as anorexia, nausea, or vomiting, should be suspected of having digitalis toxicity. The nausea and vomiting are thought to be mediated by stimulation of the area postrema in the medulla oblongata of the brainstem rather than by any direct effects of digitalis on the GI mucosa. These GI manifestations may occur in patients receiving excessive oral or IV doses of digitalis for the management of heart failure or rapid AF or both. Another diagnosis to consider in an elderly man receiving digoxin and with known peripheral vascular disease presenting with worsening GI symptoms is acute mesenteric ischemia, which is precipitated or worsened by digoxin's mesenteric vasoconstrictor effect. Early clinical suspicion and diagnosis followed by prompt and effective treatment of acute mesenteric ischemia are critically important to improve the clinical outcome. Acute mesenteric ischemia is a life-threatening vascular emergency associated with a 60–80% mortality rate and is almost uniformly fatal if unsuspected and not effectively and promptly treated.
Oldenbure QA, Lau LL, Rosenberg TJ, et al. Acute mesenteric ischemia: a clinical review. *Arch Intern Med.* 2004;164:1054–1062.

142. **List other manifestations of digitalis toxicity.**
    - **Neurologic symptoms:** headache, neuralgia, confusion, delirium, seizures
    - **Visual symptoms:** scotomata, halos, altered color perception
    - **Cardiac toxicity:** ventricular or junctional tachyarrhythmias, AV block
    - **Miscellaneous:** gynecomastia, skin rash

143. **What factors contribute to digitalis toxicity?**
    - Hypokalemia
    - Hypercalcemia
    - Hypomagnesemia
    - Renal insufficiency (digoxin)
    - Hepatic insufficiency (digitoxin)
    - Drugs (quinidine, verapamil, amiodarone, others)

144. **What arrhythmias are frequently found as complications of digitalis toxicity?**
    - Paroxysmal atrial tachycardia (PAT) with AV block
    - Junctional tachycardia with or without AV block
    - First-degree or Mobitz I second-degree AV block

    Any arrhythmia can be a manifestation of digitalis intoxication. The coexistence of increased automaticity or ectopic pacemakers with impaired AV conduction is also highly suggestive of digitalis intoxication. Cardiac manifestations are by far the most life-threatening complications of digitalis intoxication.

145. **What laboratory test helps confirm the diagnosis of digitalis toxicity?**
Digoxin level. However, even serum digoxin levels in the "therapeutic range" may be toxic in elderly patients and patients with hypokalemia, hypercalcemia, acid-base disorders, or thyroid disorders.

146. Which patients with CHF should be considered for implantable cardioverter-defibrillator (ICD) placement to prevent sudden cardiac death? For cardiac resynchronization therapy (CRT)?
Those with an LVEF < 35% and NYHA class II or III symptoms of ACC/AHA stage B or C. Patient with either ischemic or nonischemic cardiomyopathy should be evaluated for ICD. CRT may be needed for patients with NYHA III or IV symptoms and ventricular dyssynchrony (intraventricular conduction delays or LBBB).
McAliser FA, Ezekowitz J, Hooton N, et al. Cardiac resynchronization therapy for patients with left ventricular systolic dysfunction: a systematic review. *JAMA.* 2007;297:2502–2514.

147. How is the B-type natriuretic peptide (BNP) used in the evaluation of CHF?
The BNP is elevated in patients with CHF and is most useful clinically in evaluating patients with acute symptoms of possible heart failure. CHF is unlikely in a patient in the acute setting with BNP < 100 pg/mL. The test is currently under investigation for management of chronic CHF.
Maisel AS, Krishnaswamy P, Nowak RM, et al. Rapid measurement of B-type natriuretic peptide in the emergency diagnosis of heart failure. *N Engl J Med.* 2002;347:161–167.

ARRHYTHMIAS, CONDUCTION DISTURBANCES, AND PACEMAKERS

148. What arrhythmia is most commonly found in clinical practice?
AF.

149. Why is the diagnosis of AF important?
Becauses AF is a strong risk factor for embolic stroke. AF is common among middle-aged and older patients, and embolic stroke can be prevented by effective oral anticoagulation with warfarin or novel oral anticoagulants (NOACs) such as dabigatran, rivaroxaban, apixaban, or edoxaban.

150. How is AF treated?
In most patients with AF with fast heart rates, effective rate control can be achieved by the use of AV nodal blocking drugs such as a beta blocker, a heart rate lowering nondihydropyridine calcium channel blocker (such as diltiazem or verapramil), digoxin, and amiodarone. Some patients are candidates for rhythm control with conversion to normal sinus rhythm with medications or direct-current cardioversion. Ablation therapy is also now used for patients with AF who may benefit from rhythm control. All patients with AF should be assessed for long-term anticoagulation with warfarin or NOAC to prevent embolic stroke.
Wilber DJ, Pappone C, Neuzil P, et al. Comparison of antiarrhythmic drug therapy and radiofrequency catheter ablation in patients with paroxysmal atrial fibrillation: A randomized controlled trial. *JAMA.* 2010;303:333–340.

151. Is anticoagulation recommended before elective cardioversion of a patient with AF?
Yes. A 4-week course of adequate anticoagulation decreases the risk of thromboembolic events during and shortly after cardioversion planned in a patient with chronic sustained AF. The risks and benefits of cardioversion and anticoagulation, however, must be weighed very carefully prior to elective cardioversion. The most important consideration is the urgency of cardioversion. Patients with AF presenting with markedly elevated ventricular response rate complicated by systemic hypotension or significant systemic hypoperfusion or signs of "hemodynamic instability" should undergo emergency cardioversion without the need for preceding anticoagulation. In patients with a recent onset of newly developed AF, a transesophageal echocardiogram (TEE) is recommended, and if no clots are detected in the left atrial appendage, cardioversion can be performed preferably within the next 24 hours without the need for a precardioversion anticoagulation period.

152. Is anticoagulation similarly required in a patient with AF with a fast ventricular rate of 230 bpm and systolic BP of 70 mm Hg?
No. With clinical evidence of hemodynamic compromise (such as CHF, hypotension or systemic hypoperfusion, acute anginal symptoms, or acute MI), urgent cardioversion should be administered immediately, regardless of LA or LV size, systolic LV function, or prior anticoagulation. Thus, in a patient with AF complicated by a fast ventricular response rate of 230 bpm and severe

hypotension with a systolic BP of 70 mm Hg, emergency cardioversion absolutely should not be delayed until anticoagulation has been initiated or has successfully achieved desirable anticoagulation targets.

153. **What is the ECG triad of WPW syndrome?**
    - Short PR interval (<0.12 second)
    - Wide QRS complex (>0.12 second)
    - Delta wave or slurred upstroke of QRS complex (Fig. 4.4)

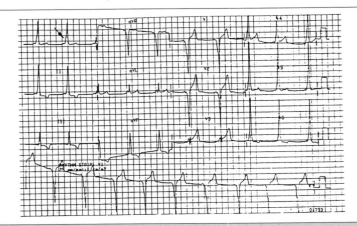

Fig. 4.4. Right anteroseptal accessory pathway in Wolff-Parkinson-White (WPW) syndrome. The 12-lead ECG characteristically exhibits a normal to inferior axis. The delta wave is negative in V_1 and V_2; upright in leads I, II, aVL (augmented voltage for left arm), and aVF (augmented voltage for the foot); isoelectric in lead III; and negative in aVR (augmented voltage for the right arm). The *arrow* indicates delta wave (lead I). *(From Braunwald E, editor. Heart Disease: A Textbook of Cardiovascular Medicine. 3rd ed. Philadelphia: WB Saunders; 1988, p 686.)*

154. **Discuss the mechanism underlying sudden cardiac death in patients with WPW syndrome.**
    AF with antegrade conduction along the accessory pathway. This tachycardia presents a serious risk because of its propensity to degenerate into VF due to very rapid conduction over the accessory pathway. Patients with accessory pathways and short refractory periods (<200 ms) are at highest risk for this antegrade conduction AF and, therefore, sudden cardiac death.

155. **Are patients with intermittent preexcitation during sinus rhythm at risk for sudden cardiac death?**
    No. Intermittent preexcitation during sinus rhythm and loss of conduction along the accessory pathway during exercise or during administration of ajmaline or procainamide suggest that the refractory period of the accessory pathway is long (>250 ms). These patients are not at risk of developing very rapid ventricular rates when AF or atrial flutter occurs and are, therefore, not at risk for sudden cardiac death.

156. **What is the holiday heart syndrome?**
    Supraventricular arrhythmias following an acute alcoholic binge, sometimes associated with holiday parties or long weekends. These arrhythmias are often transient and do not require long-term antiarrhythmic drug therapy. The most common arrhythmias are AF and atrial flutter. Digitalis and beta blockers produce an effective and rapid therapeutic response. Supportive care is also essential to prevent alcohol withdrawal symptoms in these patients.

157. **Describe the three-letter code used to indicate the essential functions of a cardiac pacemaker.**
    - **First letter:** chamber(s) paced (A = atrial, V = ventricle, D = dual chamber)
    - **Second letter:** chamber(s) sensed (A = atrial, V = ventricle, D = dual chamber)

- **Third letter:** mode of response to sensed event (0 = no response, I = inhibition, T = triggering, and D = dual response)

158. What are the two most commonly used pacemakers today?
   - **VVI:** A pacemaker that can pace and sense the RV (VV) and has an inhibited mode of response (I).
   - **DDD:** The so-called dual-chamber AV sequential pacemaker can pace and sense either RV or RA (DD) and has both inhibited and triggered modes of response (D).

159. What do the different modes of response indicate?
   - **I = inhibited:** When a spontaneous depolarization (atrial or ventricular) is sensed by the pacemaker, pacing does not occur. Following a fixed interval, if no spontaneous depolarization is sensed, pacing occurs. The inhibited mode of response is most commonly used.
   - **T = triggered:** Pacing occurs shortly after a spontaneous depolarization is sensed. After a fixed interval, pacing will occur if no spontaneous depolarization is sensed.
   - **D = dual-response:** Pacing occurs with both inhibited and triggered modes of response.

160. Who generally receives dual-chamber pacemakers (DDD)?
   Patients who are not good candidates for ventricular-demand pacemakers. DDD pacemakers are more expensive, are more difficult to implant, and require greater expertise from the clinician in charge of the patient's follow-up compared with ventricular-demand pacemakers (VVI). Examples of patients who benefit from DDD pacemakers include older patients, those with CHF, those with LV hypertrophy, and physically active young adults who would not tolerate fixed-rate ventricular pacing.

161. Who is not a good candidate for dual-chamber pacemakers?
   Patients who have a history of recurrent SVT are not good candidates for any pacing modality that involves atrial sensing, such as dual-chamber pacemakers. They are better served by a simpler VVI pacemaker.

162. Describe the manifestations and pathophysiology of pacemaker syndrome.
   Dizziness, palpitations, a pounding sensation in the chest or neck, or dyspnea associated with ventricular pacing in patients who had symptomatic bradyarrhythmias. The underlying mechanism is the loss of the normal AV synchrony during ventricular pacing.

163. How is pacemaker syndrome managed?
   By changing from ventricular to dual-chamber or AV sequential pacing. An improvement in cardiac output has been documented in various studies when the pacing modality was changed. Patients with LV hypertrophy or LV failure or older patients who have a large atrial contribution to LV filling are most prone to develop pacemaker syndrome and may be better candidates for AV sequential pacing using a DDD pacemaker.

AORTIC DISEASES

164. What are the causes of acute, severe AR?
   - Infective endocarditis
   - Dissecting aneurysm
   - Rupture or prolapse of aortic leaflet(s)
   - Traumatic rupture
   - Spontaneous rupture of myxomatous valve
   - Spontaneous rupture of leaflet fenestrations
   - Sudden sagging of a "normal" leaflet
   - Faulty incision of a stenotic aortic valve postoperatively
      Morganroth J, Perloff JK, Zeldis SN, et al. Acute severe aortic regurgitation: pathophysiology, clinical recognition, and management. *Ann Intern Med.* 1977;87:223–232.

165. Why is a wide pulse pressure, typically present in chronic severe AR, frequently absent in patients with acute AR?
   Because of the much higher left ventricular end-diastolic pressure (LVEDP) in the acute form. The acute development of a severe aortic valvular leak causes a much higher LVEDP in the normal-sized LV of patients with acute AR. Patients with chronic AR commonly have a dilated LV

with increased compliance capable of accommodating large blood volumes without a significant rise of LVEDP.

166. Explain the effects of the rapid elevation of LVEDP in acute AR.

A much shorter and softer diastolic rumble results from the rapid elevation of LVEDP in acute AR and its rapid equilibration with aortic pressure. Another auscultatory manifestation of the rapid rise of LVEDP is premature mitral valve closure that is also considered a reliable echocardiographic sign of acute AR.

167. Summarize the hemodynamic features of AR.

See Table 4.10.

Table 4.10. Hemodynamic Features of Severe Aortic Regurgitation

MEASUREMENT	ACUTE	CHRONIC
LV compliance	Not ↑	↑
Regurgitant volume	↑	↑
LV end-diastolic pressure	Markedly ↑	May be normal
LV ejection velocity	Not significantly ↑	Markedly ↑
Aortic systolic pressure	Not ↑	↑
Aortic diastolic pressure	→ to ↑	Markedly
Systemic arterial pulse pressure	Slightly to moderately ↑	Markedly ↑
Ejection fraction	Not ↑	↑
Effective stroke volume	↓	↔
Effective cardiac output	↓	↔
Heart rate	↑	↔
Peripheral vascular resistance	↑	Not ↑

↔, unchanged; ↑, increased; ↓, decreased; LV, left ventricular.
Data from Morganroth J, Perloff JK, Zeldis SN, et al. Acute severe aortic regurgitation: pathophysiology, clinical recognition, and management. *Ann Intern Med.* 1977;87:223–232.

168. What are the hemodynamic signs of chronic AR?
- Dilated LV due to longstanding volume overload
- Large stroke volume
- Wide pulse pressure causing the peripheral arterial auscultatory signs

INFECTIONS

See also Chapter 12, Infectious Diseases.

169. What are the indications for surgical intervention in infectious endocarditis?
- Severe or progressive heart failure due to valvular regurgitation
- Perivalvular abscess
- Fungal endocarditis
- Persistent bacteremia despite appropriate antibiotic therapy
- Vegetations > 10 mm
- More than one systemic embolic event despite appropriate therapy

Bonow RO, Carabello BA, Chatterjee K, et al. ACC/AHA 2006 guidelines for the management of patients with valvular heart disease. A report of the American College of Cardiology/American Heart Association Task Force on Practice Guidelines (Writing Committee to Revise the 1998 Guidelines for the Management of Patients with Valvular Heart Disease). *J Am Coll Cardiol.* 2006;48:e1–e142.

170. **What does the new onset of conduction system abnormalities in the setting of endocarditis imply?**
Perivalvular or myocardial abscesses or both. Surgical drainage and valve replacement are usually necessary.

171. **Explain the pathophysiology of the so-called immunologic manifestations of subacute bacterial endocarditis (SBE).**
Immunologic manifestations of infective endocarditis are believed to be mediated by the deposition of immune complexes within extracardiac structures, such as the retina, joints, fingertips, pericardium, skin, and kidney, rather than direct bacterial invasion. Interestingly, these immunologic manifestations of endocarditis are reported almost exclusively in patients with a prolonged course of SBE.

172. **List examples of the immunologic manifestations of SBE.**
- **Roth spots:** cytoid bodies in the retina
- **Osler nodes:** tender nodular lesions in the terminal phalanges
- **Janeway lesions:** painless macular lesions on palms and soles
- **Petechiae and purpuric lesions**
- **Proliferative glomerulonephritis**

173. **What are the most common causes of acute pericarditis in the outpatient setting?**
Idiopathic, although many of these cases are probably due to viral infections or autoimmune reactions.

174. **What are the most common causes of acute pericarditis in the inpatient setting?**
- **T**rauma
- **U**remia
- **M**yocardial infarction (acute and post)
- **M**edications (e.g., hydralazine and procainamide)
- **O**ther infections (bacterial, fungal, tuberculous)
- **R**heumatoid arthritis and other autoimmune disorders
- **R**adiation
These causes can be remembered easily with the mnemonic TUM(M)OR(R), which also serves as a reminder that metastatic cancer is a frequent cause of pericarditis and pericardial effusion in hospitalized patients.

175. **What is the major cardiac finding in Lyme disease?**
AV conduction abnormalities, such as first-degree AV block, second-degree AV block, complete heart block, fascicular block, or bundle branch block. Complete heart block is often associated with syncope because of concomitant depression of ventricular escape rhythms. Temporary pacing is indicated (the AV block usually resolves), as is antibiotic treatment with high-dose IV penicillin or oral tetracycline. A mild myopericarditis may also occur. Cardiac findings are seen in about 1 in 10 patients.

CONGENITAL HEART DISEASE

176. **Which congenital heart disease (CHD) lesions most often present in adulthood?**
- Bicuspid aortic valve
- ASD, which accounts for about 30% of all CHD in adults
Congenital cyanotic cardiac lesions rarely present in adulthood.

177. **List the types and frequencies of ASDs.**
- Ostium secundum: 70%
- Ostium primum: 15%
- Sinus venosus: 15%

178. **What is the difference between ostium secundum ASD and ostium primum ASD?**
Ostium secundum ASD occurs near the fossa ovalis in the atrial septum and ostium primum ASD occurs in the inferior portion of the septum.

179. *Coeur en sabot* ("boot-shaped heart") is a term coined in 1888 by a French scientist in his first report of a congenital cardiac disease. In which CHD is this heart configuration found?
Tetralogy of Fallot, a term first coined by E. L. Fallot that described the typical configuration of the cardiac silhouette on chest radiograph in affected patients. The four components of this malformation are:
- VSD
- Obstruction to RV outflow
- Overriding of the aorta
- RV hypertrophy

180. Summarize the radiographic findings in tetralogy of Fallot.
RV hypertrophy, which results in a fairly classic boot-shaped (or wooden shoe–shaped) configuration of the cardiac silhouette, with prominence of the RV and a concavity in the region of the underdeveloped RV outflow tract and main pulmonary artery.

181. Which cardiac disease most commonly presents in adulthood with RBBB, first-degree AV block, and left-axis deviation on ECG?
Ostium primum ASD. Because of hypoplastic changes in the left anterior fascicle, patients with ostium primum ASD have left-axis QRS deviation. Thus, the combination of RBBB and left-axis QRS deviation is a fairly distinctive feature of ostium primum ASD, and it is often accompanied by first-degree AV block.

182. What are the most common sites of aortic coarctation?
In descending order of frequency:
- Postductal (adult-type coarctation)
- Localized juxtaductal coarctation
- Preductal (infantile-type coarctation)
- Ascending thoracic aorta
- Distal descending thoracic aorta
- Abdominal aorta

183. Which congenital cardiac lesions are associated with coarctation of the aorta?
- Bicuspid aortic valve
- Patent ductus arteriosus
- VSD
- Berry aneurysms of circle of Willis

184. What is the "figure 3" sign?
A finding on chest radiograph described as a characteristic "3" sign resulting from poststenotic dilatation of the descending aorta and the dilated left subclavian artery. A barium swallow may reveal a reverse "3" sign. Along with rib notching, the presence of the "3" sign is almost pathognomic for **aortic coarctation.**

OTHER CARDIAC SYNDROMES

185. Identify the types of shock and their causes.
See Table 4.11.

186. How common are cardiac manifestations of ankylosing spondylitis?
3–10%, depending on the duration of the disease.

187. What valvular dysfunction is commonly encountered in ankylosing spondylitis?
Dilatation of the aortic valve ring and the sinuses of Valsalva as well as inflammatory changes in the aortic valve ring. The resultant clinical hallmark is aortic root dilatation and AR, often rapidly progressive and ultimately requiring aortic valve replacement. Echocardiography is the diagnostic technique of choice in the evaluation and follow-up of these patients.

Table 4.11. Classification, Mechanism, and Etiology of Shock

Hypovolemic		Cardiogenic		Extracardiac Obstructive		Distributive	
MECHANISM	ETIOLOGY	MECHANISM	ETIOLOGY	MECHANISM	ETIOLOGY	MECHANISM	ETIOLOGY
Hemorrhage	Trauma, gastrointestinal, retroperitoneal	Myopathic	Myocardial infarction (left ventricle, right ventricle) Myocardial contusion (trauma) Myocarditis Cardiomyopathy Postischemic myocardial stunning Septic myocardial depression Pharmacologic (anthracycline, calcium channel blockers)	Impaired diastolic filling	Vena cava obstruction (tumor) Tension pneumothorax Mechanical ventilation Asthma Constriction pericarditis Cardiac tamponade	Septic	Bacterial Viral Fungal Rickettsial
Fluid depletion (nonhemorrhagic)	Dehydration Vomiting Diarrhea Polyuria	Mechanical	Valvular failure (stenotic or regurgitant) Hypertrophic cardiomyopathy Ventricular septal defect	Impaired systolic contraction	Pulmonary embolism Acute pulmonary hypertension Aortic dissection	Toxic shock syndrome	
Interstitial fluid redistribution	Thermal injury Trauma Anaphylaxis	Arrhythmic	Bradycardia Tachycardia				
Increased vascular capacitance (venodilation)	Sepsis Anaplylaxis Toxins/drugs					Anaphylactic Anaphylactoid	
						Neurogenic Endocrinologic	Spinal shock Adrenal crisis Thyroid storm
						Toxic	Nitroprusside Bretylium

From Parrillo JE. Approach to the patient with shock. In Goldman L, Ausiello D, editors. Cecil Medicine. 23rd ed. Philadelphia: WB Saunders; 2007.

188. **What is Marfan syndrome?**
A generalized disorder of connective tissue that is inherited as an autosomal dominant trait. Cardiac abnormalities occur in over 60% of patients and are almost always responsible for early death when present.

189. **What is the most common cardiac lesion in Marfan syndrome?**
Dilatation of the aortic ring, sinuses of Valsalva, and ascending aorta that leads to progressive AR. Acute aortic complication may occur and the risk of dissection is markedly increased during pregnancy.

190. **Describe another common valvular dysfunction in Marfan syndrome.**
MR due to a redundant myxomatous mitral valve (called *floppy* prolapsed mitral valve). In contrast to adults, children with Marfan syndrome are much more likely to have severe isolated MR than aortic root or aortic valve disease.

191. **To what does the term *Marfan syndrome–forme fruste* refer?**
Mitral valve prolapse (MVP) in the absence of other systemic manifestations of Marfan syndrome because of the similar pathologic appearance of the myxomatous mitral valve in both disorders. Isolated MVP is more common than Marfan syndrome.

192. **Which of the cardiac chambers is most frequently involved in an atrial myxoma?**
    - **LA:** 86%
    - **RA:** 10%
    - **LV:** 2%
    - **RV:** 2%
    - **Multiple locations:** 10%

193. **What surgical technique is used to prevent recurrence of myxoma?**
Wide resection of the fossa ovalis area of the interatrial septum. The most common site of origin of atrial myxomas is the fossa ovalis.

194. **What is the most common cause of chronic MR in the United States?**
MVP, which has replaced rheumatic heart disease (the most common cause of chronic MR in the 1950s and 1960s).

195. **How is MR treated medically? Surgically?**
Medically:
    - Afterload reduction (to maximize "forward" cardiac output)
    - Salt restriction
    - Diuretics (with symptoms of CHF)
    - Digitalis (with AF)
Surgically:
    - Mitral valve repair or valvuloplasty (particularly for patients with MVP or rheumatic heart disease)
    - Mitral valve replacement
    Surgical mitral valve repair or replacement should be performed in patients refractory to medical management before they enter the severely symptomatic stage, or in asymptomatic patients before they develop irreversible ventricular dysfunction as evidenced by LVEF < 40% or progressive ventricular dilatation.

DRUG THERAPY

196. **In primary prevention trials aimed at reducing cardiovascular mortality with cholesterol-lowering statin drugs, which drugs have been shown to lower the risk of death from cardiac causes?**
    - Pravastatin
    - Lovastatin
    - Atorvastin
    - Rosuvastatin

Three primary coronary prevention trials—the West of Scotland Coronary Prevention Study (WOSCOPS), the Air Force/Texas Coronary Atherosclerosis Prevention Study (AFCAPS/TexCAPS), and the Anglo-Scandinavian Cardiac Outcome Trial (ASCOT)—have demonstrated that pravastatin, lovastatin, and atorvastatin reduce coronary and cardiovascular fatal and nonfatal events in patients with baseline LDL cholesterol levels ranging from 130–190 mg/dL. These three clinical trials provide compelling evidence that reduction of LDL cholesterol to ≤ 100 mg/dL is effective in preventing heart disease and stroke in patients with no known vascular disease. More recently, the Justification for the Use of Statins in Primary Prevention: An Intervention Trial Evaluating Rosuvastatin (JUPITER) trial showed efficacy in reducing major CVD in patients without hyperlipidemia but with elevated CRP (C-reactive protein). The FDA approved rosuvastatin for primary prevention of CVD in these patients.

Downs JR, Clearfield M, Weis S, et al. Primary prevention of acute coronary events with lovastatin in men and women with average cholesterol levels: results of AFCAPS/TexCAPS. Air Force/ Texas Coronary Atherosclerosis Prevention Study. *JAMA*. 1998;279:1615–1622.

Sever PS, Dahlof B, Poulter NR, et al. for the ASCOT Investigators. Prevention of coronary and stroke events with atorvastatin in hypertensive patients who have average or lower-than-average cholesterol concentrations, in the Anglo-Scandinavian Cardiac Outcomes Trial–Lipid Lowering Arm (ASCOT-LLA): a multicentre randomised controlled trial. *Lancet*. 2003;361:1149–1158.

Ridker PM, Danielson E, Fonseca FAH, et al. Rosuvastatin to prevent vascular events in men and women with elevated C-reactive protein. *N Engl J Med*. 2008;359:2195–2207.

197. **Which classes of lipid-lowering drugs are most effective in reducing LDL fraction and in reducing cardiovascular complications in patients with known CAD?**
A variety of lipid-lowering drug classes reduce total and LDL cholesterol levels. These lipid-lowering drug classes include:

- **Bile acid resin sequestrants** (cholestyramine and colestipol): Reduce LDL cholesterol by approximately 10%. The LRC-CPPT demonstrated a 20% reduction in CAD events but no change in total mortality rate during a 10-year treatment with cholestyramine in patients with no previous known CAD.

- **Niacin and nicotinic acid:** Reduce LDL cholesterol by 15–25% and have been shown to reduce cardiovascular complications in clinical prospective trials.

- **Fibrates** (gemfibrozil and fenofibrate): Reduce LDL cholesterol by approximately 10%. Gemfibrozil has been shown to reduce cardiovascular complications in patients without and patients with previous known CAD. A prospective placebo-controlled, randomized clinical trial of fenofibrate failed to show an overall reduction in fatal and nonfatal CAD complications in diabetic patients.

- **Statins:** Achieve reductions of LDL of up to 60% unsurpassed by any other lipid-lowering class. Recent statin trials have suggested a clinical benefit related to both the reduction in LDL cholesterol and the reduction in CRP, suggesting a non–LDL-dependent mechanism possibly mediated by the anti-inflammatory or endothelial protective benefits of statins.

Frick MH, Elo O, Happa K, Heinonen OP. Helsinki Heart Study: primary prevention trial with dyslipidemia. *N Engl J Med*. 1987;317:1237–1245.

Grundy S, Cleeman CN, Brewer HB, et al. Implications of recent clinical trials for the National Cholesterol Education Program Panel III Guidelines. *J Am Coll Cardiol*. 2004;44:720–732.

Lipid Research Clinics Program. The Lipid Research Clinics Coronary Primary Prevention Trial results: Reduction in incidence of coronary heart disease. *JAMA*. 1984;251:351–364.

Rubins HB, Robins SJ, Collins D, et al. Gemfibrozil for the secondary prevention of coronary heart disease in men with low levels of high-density lipoprotein cholesterol. Veterans Affairs High-Density Lipoprotein Cholesterol Intervention Trial Study Group. *N Engl J Med*. 1999;341:410–418.

Sever P, Dahlof B, Poulter NR, et al. Prevention of coronary and stroke events with atorvastatin in hypertensive patients who have average or lower-than-average cholesterol concentrations, in the Anglo-Scandinavian Cardiac Outcomes Trial—Lipid Lowering Arm (ASCOT-LLA): a multicentre randomised controlled trial. *Lancet*. 2003;361:1149–1158.

198. **Are statins recommended in diabetic patients, and have they been proved to prevent cardiovascular complications in such patients?**
Yes. Two leading recent randomized, placebo-controlled clinical trials have provided important insight into the role of statins in diabetics: the Heart Protection Study (HPS) of simvastatin and

the Collaborative Atorvastatin Diabetes Study (CARDS) of atorvastatin. The HPS consisted of 5963 diabetic patients (33% of whom had prior CAD) randomized to simvastatin 40 mg/day versus placebo and prospectively followed up for 4.8 years for the primary composite study outcome of MI or coronary death. LDL cholesterol levels were reduced from 125 to 85 mg/dL. Primary outcome was significantly reduced by 27%, and stroke risk was reduced by 24% ($P < .0001$, both comparisons). An important observation in this trial was that diabetics with no CAD or other vascular disease at baseline had a 33% reduction in coronary heart disease independently of baseline LDL cholesterol levels.

CARDS was the first prospective, randomized, placebo-controlled clinical trial of a statin, namely atorvastatin, in a population composed solely of adult-onset diabetic patients with *no* known vascular disease. This CARDS trial randomized 2838 diabetics with at least one other cardiovascular risk factor to atorvastatin 10 mg or placebo. This trial was prematurely terminated 2 years early, after a median follow-up of 3.9 years because of the large statin benefit. It was noted that LDL cholesterol levels were reduced from 118 to 82 mg/dL. The primary study outcome (major coronary events, revascularization, UA, resuscitated cardiac arrest, and stroke) was reduced by 37% ($P = .001$) and stroke risk was reduced by 48%.

The more recent Action to Control Cardiovascular Risk in Diabetes (ACCORD) trial, though, did not find that intensive treatment of cholesterol with fenofibrate in addition to simvastatin reduced combined occurrence of MI, strokes, or cardiovascular death in patients with diabetes.

ACCORD Study Group, Ginsberg HN, Elam MB, et al. Effect of combination lipid lowering therapy in type 2 diabetes mellitus. *N Engl J Med.* 2010;362:1563–1574.

Colhoun HM, Betteridge DJ, Durrington PN, et al. on behalf of the CARDS Investigators. Primary prevention of cardiovascular disease with atorvastatin in type 2 diabetes in the Collaborative Atorvastatin Diabetes Study (CARDS): multicentre randomized placebo-controlled trial. *Lancet.* 2004;364:685–696.

Collins R, Armitage J, Parish S, et al. on behalf of the Heart Protection Study Collaborative Group: MRC/BHF Heart Protection Study of cholesterol-lowering with simvastatin in 5963 people with diabetes: a randomized placebo-controlled trial. *Lancet.* 2003;361:2005–2016.

199. What does "cardioselectivity" of a beta blocking drug mean? Summarize the clinical implications of this pharmacologic property.
That the drug predominantly blocks the beta$_1$-adrenergic receptors, which are mostly present in the heart. Cardioselective beta blockers, in low doses, have minimal blocking effects on beta$_2$ receptors, the predominant beta receptors in the lungs. However, cardioselectivity is only relative; when drugs are administered in large doses, cardioselectivity is markedly diminished. Despite these limitations, cardioselective beta blockers are much safer than noncardioselective beta blockers in patients with obstructive lung disease. There are three commercially available cardioselective beta blockers: atenolol, metoprolol, and acebutolol.

200. What is the importance of intrinsic sympathomimetic activity (ISA) as it applies to beta blockers?
ISA refers to the partial beta-adrenergic agonist properties of some beta blockers. When sympathetic activity is low (at rest), these beta blockers produce low-grade beta stimulation. However, under conditions of stress (exercise), beta blockers with ISA behave essentially as conventional beta blockers without ISA. The clinical significance of ISA is not clearly established.

201. Which beta blockers possess ISA?
Pindolol and acebutolol. All other beta blockers currently available have no significant ISA. Beta blockers with ISA are rarely used today and are, in fact, contraindicated in patients recovering from a recent MI because they are not proved to be "cardioprotective," that is, effective in reducing the risk of a recurrent MI, cardiovascular death, or sudden cardiac death.

WEBSITES

1. American College of Cardiology: www.acc.org
2. American Heart Association: www.americanheart.org

BIBLIOGRAPHY

1. Kasper SL, Fauci DL, Hauser SL, et al., eds. *Harrison's Principles of Internal Medicine.* 19th ed. New York: McGraw-Hill; 2014.
2. Mann DL, Zipes D, Libby R, et al., eds. *Braunwald's Heart Disease: A Textbook of Cardiovascular Medicine.* 10th ed. Philadelphia: Elsevier; 2015.
3. Wagner GS. *Marriott's Practical Electrocardiography.* 11th ed. Philadelphia: Lippincott Williams & Wilkins; 2008.

CHAPTER 5

VASCULAR MEDICINE

Timothy R.S. Harward, MD, FACS

> *... Dr. DeBakey suspected that he was not having a heart attack ... but ... that the inner lining of the [thoracic aorta] had torn, known as a dissecting aortic aneurysm. ... [A]s a younger man, he devised the operation to repair such torn aortas, a condition virtually always fatal.*
>
> *The New York Times, December 25, 2006*

GENERAL EVALUATION

1. **Describe the evaluation of a patient for arterial diseases.**
   - History. Ask the patient:
     - Do your symptoms get better or worse with activity?
     - Do you have a history of diabetes?
       - High blood pressure (BP)?
       - Heart disease, angina, or heart attack?
       - High cholesterol?
     - Does anyone in your family have a history of blood vessel aneurysms?
       - Strokes?
       - Surgeries on blood vessel in the neck, arm, or leg?
       - Amputation of a leg or arm?
   - Physical examination:
     - Examine all bilateral pulses including carotid, brachial, radial, femoral, popliteal, dorsalis pedis, and posterior tibial.
     - Listen for bruits at carotid pulse and any other pulse with abnormal palpation.
     - Examine for pulsatile masses at the abdomen, groin, and popliteal areas.
     - Listen for bruits in all quadrants of the abdomen.

2. **What tests can be used to evaluate blood flow if pulses are not palpable?**
   - Noninvasive vascular laboratory evaluation
     - BP measurements in upper arm, thigh, and lower leg to determine ankle-brachial index (ABI) and differences between BP on left and right sides
     - Doppler waveform analysis that evaluates velocity of blood flow
     - Ultrasound imaging that visualizes the arterial anatomy, morphology of any lesions seen, and hemodynamics of the blood flow
   - Computed tomography (CT) scan or magnetic resonance (MR) angiography that allows visualization of vascular anatomy through contrast injection into the venous system
   For initial evaluation of nonpalpable pulses, the noninvasive evaluation is preferable because of lower cost, less risk, and provision of both anatomic and hemodynamic data.

3. **How are noninvasive vascular laboratory tests interpreted?**
   By comparing BP measurements at different locations, analyzing waveforms representing the blood flow, and viewing ultrasound. All pressure measurements are compared with the arm BP. By dividing the ankle BP by the highest arm BP measurement, one can calculate an ABI. Values > 0.9 are considered normal, values < 0.4 are consistent with severe ischemia, whereas values of 0.5–0.8 are consistent with complaints of claudication. These measurements are difficult to interpret in the diabetic patient because the arteries become very stiff secondary to calcification in the artery wall. Fortunately, toe pressures are still accurate in this setting for determining overall ischemia but do not help locate the site of obstruction. The addition of Doppler waveform analysis markedly increases the accuracy in determining the level of disease. A triphasic waveform is normal, whereas a monophasic waveform is consistent with a severe upstream obstruction. Finally, ultrasound helps detect aneurysms and delineate stenoses from occlusions. Overall, these criteria are 92–95% accurate in detecting the location and severity of arterial disease.

4. **When are noninvasive vascular laboratory tests indicated?**
When a clinician considers a peripheral arterial disease (PAD) diagnosis. In some cases, nothing other than the noninvasive study is needed to diagnose the problem and to plan treatment. In addition, the noninvasive study provides a baseline objective examination that can be repeated at no risk to the patient should the clinical situation change. In addition, the information learned will help steer future testing and intervention. After intervention, noninvasive vascular laboratory evaluation is used to follow the progress or regression of the intervention because the disease process has not been cured, only temporarily arrested.

ANEURYSM DISEASE

5. **What is an aneurysm?**
A dilatation of all three layers of the arterial wall measuring at least 50% larger than the expected normal diameter. When the dilatation is < 50% of the expected normal diameter, the artery is described as "ectatic."

6. **What are the most common sites for aneurysms?**
   - Infrarenal aorta: 65%
   - Isolated thoracic aorta: 16%
   - Infrarenal aorta with extension into the common iliac artery: 13%
   - Peripheral aneurysms: <3%

7. **Among *peripheral* arteries, which are the most frequent sites for aneurysms?**
   - Popliteal (70% of peripheral arterial aneurysms)
   - Common femoral
   - Carotid (rare)
   - Mesenteric (rare)

8. **How does one detect an aneurysm?**
By a detailed physical examination with palpation of the aortic, femoral, and popliteal arteries. When an aneurysm is present, the pulsation feels broad and prominent. When a patient is obese, abdominal aortic and iliac artery aneurysms may not be palpable and are detected when an ultrasound or CT scan is performed for other reasons such as low back pain or gallbladder disease. When an aneurysm is suspected, CT or ultrasound confirms its presence. After an aneurysm is diagnosed, CT is used to follow the growth of a small abdominal aneurysm that is not yet large enough to warrant repair. For peripheral artery aneurysms, follow-up is done using ultrasound.

9. **What are the risks of an abdominal aortic aneurysm (AAA) or thoracic aneurysm?**
Rupture leading to death. The larger the diameter of the aneurysm, the greater the risk of rupture.

10. **How does the size of the AAA correlate with risk of rupture?**
Exponentially with increasing maximal diameter. A 3.0- to 4.4-cm-diameter aneurysm has a 2%/year risk of rupture, whereas a 4.5- to 5.9-cm-diameter aneurysm has a 10%/year risk of rupture. If the patient's aneurysm ruptures outside the hospital setting, overall mortality rate is approximately 80–90%. Of these patients, 50% die at the scene of the rupture, 50% who make it to the hospital die in the operating room, and 50% of those who survive the operation die of other comorbid conditions prior to hospital discharge.
    Brewster DC, Cronenwett JL, Hallett JW Jr, et al. Guidelines for the treatment of abdominal aortic aneurysms. Report of a subcommittee of the Joint Council of the American Association for Vascular Surgery and Society for Vascular Surgery. *J Vasc Surg*. 2003;37:1106–1117.
    Thomas PR, Stewart RD. Abdominal aortic aneurysm. *Br J Surg*. 1988;75:733–736.

11. **What are the recommended methods of treating aortic aneurysms?**
Open surgical replacement or endovascular repair. Traditional therapy is open surgical replacement of the aneurysmal segment with an artificial conduit. Hospital stay is 5–7 days, whereas 30-day mortality rate is 1–5% depending on comorbid conditions. More recently, endovascular repair has become increasingly used. Under a light general anesthetic, this

method utilizes a catheter delivery system to place a covered stent graft inside the aneurysm. Hospital stay is 1 day and operative mortality rate < 1%; however, 30-day mortality rate is the same as for the open repair. More recent studies have found, though, that endovascular repair is associated with more late complications, higher late mortality rate, and higher cost than open surgical repair.

The United Kingdom EVAR Trial Investigators, Greenhalgh RM, Brown LC, Powell JT, et al. Endovascular versus open repair of abdominal aortic aneurysm. *N Engl J Med.* 2010;362: 1863–1871.

12. Are there reasons why all patients do not undergo endovascular repair?
Yes. The aortic or aneurysm anatomy precludes the proper placement of the stent graft by endovascular repair in 5–10% of patients.

13. Which vasculitides are associated with thoracic aortic disease?
- Giant cell arteritis
- Takayasu arteritis
- Behçet disease

14. What genetic disorders are most often associated with increased risk of thoracic aortic disease?
- Marfan syndrome (connective tissue disorder)
- Loeys-Dietz syndrome (characterized by arterial aneurysms, hypertelorism, and cleft palate)
- Turner syndrome (characterized by genotype 45,X)
- Ehlers-Danlos, type IV (characterized by easy bruising, thick skin, characteristic facial features, and rupture of arteries, uterus, and intestines)
  Hiratzka LF, Bakris GL, Beckman JA, et al. 2010 ACCF/AHA/AATS/ACR/ASA/SCA/SCAI/SIR/STS/ SVM guidelines for the diagnosis and management of patients with thoracic aortic disease. *J Am Coll Cardiol.* 2010;55:e27–e129.

15. Should these patients with genetic disorders be followed regularly?
Yes. Aortic imaging should be done at the time the genetic syndrome is identified and periodically as indicated for follow-up.

16. What are the characteristics of the pain associated with acute thoracic aortic dissection (AoD)?
- Abrupt onset
- Severe intensity
- Sharp or stabbing in nature
- Usually in the chest but also occurs in the back and abdomen depending on origin and progression of the dissection
- May be asymptomatic with presenting symptoms of syncope, stroke, or congestive heart failure

17. What are the physical examination findings?
- Hypotension, hypertension, or normotension
- Pulse deficits
- Neurologic deficits
- Symptoms of cardiac tamponade
- Aortic insufficiency murmur

18. How is a thoracic AoD diagnosed?
By thoracic CT scan, MR angiography, or transesophageal echocardiogram (TEE).

19. What are the two commonly used classification systems for thoracic AoD and their descriptions?
- DeBakey (Fig. 5.1)
  - Type I: Begins in the ascending aorta (proximal to the brachiocephalic artery) and propagates distally to at least the aortic arch. The descending aorta may also be involved.
  - Type II: Begins in and remains confined to the ascending aorta.
  - Type III: Begins in the descending aorta and propagates distally.
  - Type IIIa: Limited to descending thoracic aorta.
  - Type IIIb: Extends below the diaphragm.

- Stanford
  - Type A: Involves the ascending aorta without regard to site of initial dissection.
  - Type B: All other dissections that do not involve the ascending aorta.

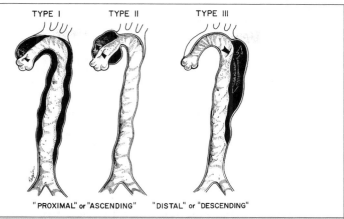

Fig. 5.1. DeBakey classification of aortic dissection. *(From Braunwald E, editor.* Heart Disease: A Textbook of Cardiovascular Medicine. *3rd ed. Philadelphia: WB Saunders; 1988, p 1554.)*

20. **Which dissections should be considered for surgical repair?**
Type I and type II for the DeBakey classification and type A for Stanford. Type III/type B dissection with persistent pain, pleural fluid, or false lumen > 3 cm should be considered for emergent thoracic endovascular aortic repair (TEVAR) with a stent graft.

21. **Which dissections should be considered for medical treatment?**
Type III (DeBakey) and type B (Stanford).

22. **Describe the medical management of thoracic AoD.**
- Heart rate control with intravenous (IV) beta blockade to achieve a heart rate of < 60 beats per minute (bpm), if no contraindications to beta blockers. Non-dihydropyridine calcium channel blockers can be used for patients unable to receive beta blockers.
- IV vasodilators (i.e., angiotensin-converting enzyme [ACE] inhibitors) if systolic BP remains > 120 mm Hg **after adequate beta blockade.**
- Pain control with IV opiates.

KEY POINTS: THORACIC AORTIC DISSECTION

1. Patients with thoracic aortic dissection may have symptoms suggestive of myocardial ischemia.
2. Aortic dissection should be considered in all patients presenting with chest and upper back pain.
3. Improvement in pain does not rule out a thoracic aortic dissection.
4. Relatives of patients with thoracic aortic disease are at increased risk and should have appropriate screening.

23. **Who should be screened for thoracic aortic disease?**
- Patients with identified genetic syndromes that have an increased risk
- First-degree relative of patients with diagnosed thoracic aortic aneurysm or dissection
- Patients with a bicuspid aortic valve
- First-degree relatives of patients with bicuspid aortic valve
  Hiratzka LF, Bakris GL, Beckman JA, et al. 2010 ACCF/AHA/AATS/ACR/ASA/SCA/SCAI/SIR/STS/ SVM guidelines for the diagnosis and management of patients with thoracic aortic disease. *J Am Coll Cardiol.* 2010;55:e27–e129.

24. **Do peripheral arterial aneurysms frequently rupture?**
No. Only about 2% of peripheral arterial aneurysms rupture; however, peripheral arterial aneurysms can lead to distal embolization of intraluminal clot. Embolization can occur insidiously without symptoms until significant obstruction of smaller arteries is present. At this point, the upstream popliteal artery aneurysm thromboses, producing severe ischemic rest pain. In addition, peripheral aneurysm can enlarge sufficiently to compress the accompanying adjacent vein and nerve, producing distal swelling and a burning discomfort, as typically seen in patients with venous disease.

25. **When should peripheral arterial aneurysms be repaired?**
When the aneurysm becomes > 2 cm in diameter or contains intraluminal clot. If a peripheral aneurysm clots and the patient develops rest pain, 20–30% will require an amputation.

26. **What is the treatment for peripheral arterial aneurysms?**
Treatment methods differ based on the artery involved. Common femoral artery aneurysms are resected and replaced with a new prosthetic graft. Popliteal artery aneurysms are left in place but excluded from the circulation by ligating the artery above and below the aneurysm and constructing a bypass graft. With newer techniques, a flexible intraluminal stent graft can be inserted if tibial artery runoff is adequate.

27. **What other arteries can become aneurysmal? How are they treated?**
Carotid, renal, superior mesenteric, splenic, and subclavian arteries. Carotid artery aneurysms are very rare but should be resected and repaired when found. Splenic artery aneurysms are more common and can rupture during pregnancy owing to hormonal and hyperdynamic changes in blood flow and BP. Splenic artery rupture can be fatal to both mother and fetus and requires resection. The renal artery aneurysm is treated much as the splenic artery aneurysm. Superior mesenteric artery (SMA) aneurysms are frequently mycotic or associated with infection and require removal and repair. Subclavian artery aneurysms may be associated with thoracic outlet syndrome. Symptoms of finger tip ulcers can occur from microemboli. Subclavian artery aneurysms are not true aneurysms but poststenotic arterial dilatation generated by disturbed blood flow.

PERIPHERAL ARTERIAL OCCLUSIVE DISEASE

28. **What is the clinical spectrum of chronic PAD?**
    - Asymptomatic
    - Intermittent claudication
    - Rest pain
    - Nonhealing ulcers
    - Gangrene

29. **What is intermittent claudication?**
A cramping pain or discomfort associated with activity that is relieved by rest, yet returns with resumption of activity. Claudication should not be confused with nocturnal cramps that have no association with PAD. The location of claudication discomfort suggests the level of the arterial obstruction. The disease is usually one level proximal to the discomfort. For example, calf claudication is associated with thigh level arterial obstruction.

30. **What is neurogenic claudication?**
Calf discomfort with activity that is both reproducible and relieved by rest and occurs in a patient with normal arterial circulation but with lumbar spine stenosis. The calf discomfort does not go away with just stopping activity. To make the discomfort dissipate, the patient must relieve pressure on the spine by either sitting or lying down. Noninvasive vascular laboratory testing is frequently normal. Imaging evaluation of the lumbar spine shows lumbar spinal stenosis, often from protrusion of an intravertebral disk. This process often requires surgical decompression to relieve nerve compression.

31. **Describe the significance of rest pain, nonhealing ulcers, and gangrene.**
Ischemic rest pain, nonhealing ulcers, and gangrene develop with worsening of PAD and occur when the level of tissue perfusion is unable to maintain normal tissue viability, usually at approximately 40% or less of normal blood flow. Nonhealing ulcers and gangrene also suggest limb-threatening ischemia.

32. **What are the causes of claudication and tissue loss in the upper extremity?**
    - Focal stenosis or total occlusion of the left subclavian artery due to atherosclerotic plaque
    - Thoracic outlet syndrome
    - Chronic trauma
    - Giant cell arteritis (in women > 50–60 years old)

33. **What causes claudication, rest pain, and tissue loss in the lower extremity?**
    - Atherosclerotic occlusive disease
    - Popliteal artery entrapment due to an unusual anatomic location
    - Adventitial cystic disease due to a mucin-secreting cell rest in the arterial wall

34. **Are there any medical therapies to help treat PAD?**
    Yes. Risk modification can slow the progression of atherosclerotic arterial disease. Foremost is cessation of smoking. Smoking increases the incidence of PAD 16-fold.
    Control of hypertension and diabetes mellitus also decreases progression of PAD. The ratio of total cholesterol to high-density lipoprotein (HDL) cholesterol is a strong predictor of developing PAD. Dietary modification to lower fat intake in combination with exercise improves this ratio. Statin medications help modify serum cholesterol levels. In addition, statins seem to have a protective effect unrelated to cholesterol control. This effect may be due to stabilization of the atherosclerotic plaque. Finally, pentoxifylline and cilostazol are medications used to increase pain-free walking distance in patients with claudication. Unfortunately, pentoxifylline does not work any better than placebo, but recent studies suggest that cilostazol may improve walking distance up to 200%. Antiplatelet therapy with aspirin is also helpful, particularly for the secondary prevention of cardiac and cerebrovascular disease, which are frequently concurrent (and sometimes without symptoms) in these patients.

    Hirsch AT, Haskal ZJ, Hertzer NR, et al. ACC/AHA 2005 Practice Guidelines for the management of patients with peripheral arterial disease (lower extremity, renal, mesenteric, and abdominal aortic): A collaborative report from the American Association for Vascular Surgery/Society for Vascular Surgery, Society for Cardiovascular Angiography and Interventions, Society for Vascular Medicine and Biology, Society of Interventional Radiology, and the ACC/AHA Task Force on Practice Guidelines (Writing Committee to Develop Guidelines for the Management of Patients With Peripheral Arterial Disease): endorsed by the American Association of Cardiovascular and Pulmonary Rehabilitation; National Heart, Lung, and Blood Institute; Society for Vascular Nursing; TransAtlantic Inter-Society Consensus; and Vascular Disease Foundation. *Circulation.* 2006;113:e463–e654.

    Sobel M, Verhaeghe R. Antithrombotic therapy for peripheral artery occlusive disease. *Chest.* 2008;133:1–38.

35. **Should patients with PAD receive anticoagulants?**
    Generally no for patients with intermittent claudication. Anticoagulation is indicated for the initial treatment of acute arterial emboli or thrombosis.

36. **What are the surgical interventions used to improve arterial blood flow?**
    Endarterectomy or bypass. Endarterectomy is done by removing the atherosclerotic plaque. This technique works well for short, focal lesions, but longer segments of disease are prone to early recurrent stenoses produced by development of both scar tissue and recurrent atherosclerotic plaque. Bypass is accomplished using a new conduit to redirect blood around an area of extensive arterial disease. This is best done using the patient's saphenous vein for the smaller arteries of the leg, whereas artificial conduits can be used for the larger arteries of the abdomen/pelvis. To ensure success of these techniques, one must originate the bypass in an area free of disease. The distal target artery needs to also be free of obstruction and have good runoff into the distal circulation.

37. **What are the endovascular procedures used to improve arterial blood flow?**
    These newer percutaneous techniques focus on recanalizing the arterial lumen using balloon dilatation to fracture the atherosclerotic plaque away from the arterial wall followed by insertion of a stent to reexpand the arterial lumen. This technique was initially utilized only to treat short focal stenoses or occlusion (<5–10 cm in length). As stenting technology has evolved, longer and more complex segments of disease are being treated. More recently, drug-eluting balloons and stents can emit a chemotherapeutic agent that slows recurrent disease. Final data of long-term effects are still pending, but preliminary data are quite promising.

38. **What aspects of an open surgical intervention for treatment of PAD convey the greatest risk?**

   General anesthesia and infection from a skin incision. In addition, both of these maneuvers (anesthesia and incision) stress the patient and increase the risk of myocardial infarction (MI), stroke, and death secondary to underlying comorbid conditions that are common in this patient population; therefore, surgical intervention is reserved for patients with incapacitating symptoms (short-distance claudication < 100 yards or signs and symptoms of limb-threatening ischemia [rest pain, nonhealing ulcers, gangrene]). Appropriate patient selection and preoperative preparation produce perioperative mortality rates < 2% for inflow procedures such as aortic bypass, renal artery endarterectomy, and mesenteric artery bypasses, whereas outflow procedures to improve blood flow into the lower leg and foot have 30-day mortality rates of 4–5%.

39. **Are percutaneous endovascular procedures less risky than open surgical procedures?**

   Yes. The endovascular procedure is performed with a light sedation and requires only local anesthetic at the skin puncture site. Major risks consist of allergic reactions to the iodine contrast agent used to visualize arteries, potential renal failure created by the toxic effects of the iodine contrast material in the renal tubules, and local arterial trauma secondary to the initial puncture and wire insertion where a dissection plane is created that leads to arterial thrombosis and embolization of the atherosclerotic plaque downstream during the balloon and stenting portion of the procedure.

40. **How do results of open surgical procedures compare with percutaneous endovascular interventions?**

   Short-term results in appropriately selected patients are excellent for both procedures. With endarterectomy or bypass, the 30-day patency rates exceed 95%, whereas 30-day patency rates for the majority of endovascular recanalization procedures are greater than 80%; however, these endovascular results vary depending on the location, length, and severity of the disease treated. Shorter, more focal disease responds much better than longer, more diffuse disease. Long-term results for both surgical and endovascular procedures are excellent for aortoiliac PAD. Five-year patency rates for both techniques are above 90%; therefore, balloon angioplasty and stenting have become the standard of care for this disease. For outflow artery PAD, surgical bypass is much better. If an adequate saphenous vein is used, 5-year patency rates are 70–80%. Unfortunately, even with the use of stenting, many arterial segments treated with endovascular repair develop recurrent disease within 6–12 months. Some reports suggest > 50% recurrence rates, but this topic is still under close study. The question of using drug-eluting coronary artery stents has been considered and preliminary study results are quite promising. In summary, the surgical bypass works better over the long term but carries higher upfront risk, whereas endovascular recanalization procedures are less risky but, at the present time, do not produce equivalent long-term results.

41. **Do medical therapies alter the outcome of surgical or endovascular procedures?**

   Yes. Smoking cessation dramatically improves maintenance of patency of both procedures. The use of statin drugs has been shown to improve patency of surgical bypass grafting and is being evaluated with endovascular recanalization procedures. At present, patients who have stents placed are started on clopidogrel, an antiplatelet adhesion medication. This decreases the incidence of stent thrombosis until the struts of the stent are covered. In addition, the use of aspirin or warfarin or both has been shown to improve long-term patency of leg bypass grafts, especially in patients requiring a second or third redo procedure; however, this advantage must be weighed against the risk of bleeding in an elderly population.

CAROTID DISEASE

42. **What causes carotid disease?**

   Atherosclerotic plaque in the proximal common carotid artery at the aortic arch (8%) or at the bifurcation extending into the internal carotid artery (ICA) (92%).

43. **How does carotid disease present clinically?**

   When symptomatic, with a transient ischemia attack (TIA) (80%) or a stroke (20%) as the initial symptom. These are known as *hemispheric signs and symptoms,* usually secondary to cholesterol or platelet or both and thrombus emboli breaking off of a friable atherosclerotic plaque.

44. What are the symptoms of a TIA due to small emboli?
- Unilateral blindness in the eye ipsilateral to the carotid disease
- Arm numbness or weakness or both contralateral to the carotid plaque
- Leg numbness or weakness or both contralateral to the carotid plaque (may occur in association with arm symptoms)
- Speech difficulties such as aphasia if the left side is involved or dysphasia if the right side is involved

   Events may last only seconds or hours, and neuroimaging will not show any sign of ischemia.

45. What is the initial evaluation for a patient presenting with a TIA?
- BP measurement and monitoring.
- Head CT scan to evaluate for intracerebral bleed.
- Duplex scanning (high-resolution ultrasound and Doppler) of the carotid arteries. This test allows one to diagnose the offending plaque without risk to the patient and is >94% accurate.
- Patients with TIAs require urgent evaluation and treatment to prevent complications of stroke. See also Chapter 17, Neurology.

   Luengo-Fernandez R, Gray AM, Rothwell PM. Effect of urgent treatment of transient ischaemic attack and minor stroke on disability and hospital costs (EXPRESS study): a prospective population-based sequential comparison. *Lancet*. 2009;8:235–243.

46. What is the natural history of symptomatic carotid disease if not treated?
An increased risk of stroke. The NASCET (North American Symptomatic Carotid Endarterectomy Trial) study provided these data. Phase I evaluated symptomatic patients with ≥70% stenosis and demonstrated a 12.5% stroke/year with only medical therapy. Phase II evaluated symptomatic patients with 50–69% stenosis. This group of patients still presented with an unacceptable stroke rate of approximately 5%/year. The natural history was shown to be dramatically altered by surgical intervention.

   North American Symptomatic Carotid Endarterectomy Trial: Methods, patient characteristics, and progress. *Stroke*. 1991;22:711–720.

47. What is the treatment for patients with symptomatic carotid disease?
If the duplex scan identifies a stenosis ≥ 50%, carotid endarterectomy is indicated. If the stenosis is < 50%, the patient should be treated with antiplatelet medications and followed closely with serial duplex scans. The only exception is when there is a significant ulcer in the atherosclerotic plaque. This situation is also an indication for surgical repair. However, if the patient is high risk for surgery (i.e., severe heart disease, prior neck irradiation or radical neck surgery, or is undergoing a repeat operation), the patient should be considered for a carotid artery balloon angioplasty and stenting.

48. How should patients with asymptomatic carotid artery disease be treated?
With regular follow-up with carotid duplex scanning. If the percentage of stenosis becomes > 60–70%, the surgeon can perform a carotid endarterectomy with a stroke rate < 3%, and if the patient's life expectancy is at least 3 years, then prophylactic carotid endarterectomy should be performed. Antiplatelet therapy with aspirin and use of statin medications for cholesterol control are also important. These patients may also have asymptomatic coronary artery disease.

49. What are the risks of carotid endarterectomy?
Mainly perioperative stroke. This is usually due to intraoperative embolization but can be due to postoperative thrombosis usually caused by an operative technical defect. More common but less dramatic are cranial nerve injuries that can occur in approximately 10%. Most common of these is marginal mandibular nerve bruising that produces numbness around the ipsilateral mouth associated with droopiness. Other risks include bleeding and infection, both of which are moderately uncommon.

50. Where does carotid angioplasty and stenting fit into the treatment of this disease?
At this time, angioplasty is approved only for high-risk patients. The technique is still considered experimental for all other situations, and current trial results continue to be analyzed. The risk for periprocedure stroke from angioplasty and stenting is still higher than that for endarterectomy, and its cost is more than twice that of surgical intervention. Still, for high-risk patients, the benefit outweighs the risk and cost.

Brott TG, Hobson RW II, Howard G, et al. Stenting versus endarterectomy for treatment of carotid-artery stenosis. *N Engl J Med.* 2010;360:11–23.

51. **What are nonhemispheric TIAs?**
TIAs with signs and symptoms of drop attacks, dysarthria, ataxia, blurred vision secondary to bilateral eye involvement, dizziness, and, occasionally, headaches. These events are due to ischemia in the posterior circulation distribution that includes the cerebellum and brainstem. They are usually due to vertebral artery pathology but can be due to generalized global ischemia when both ICAs are > 90% stenotic. In the latter situation, carotid endarterectomy will resolve these TIAs, especially if the posterior communicating artery off the circle of Willis is patent.

52. **What are crescendo TIA and stroke-in-evolution?**
Crescendo TIAs occur when the patient experiences several transient neurologic events within 24 hours, and a stroke-in-evolution is an acute neurologic deficit of mild to moderate degree that is progressive. Both entities can be associated with a severe carotid artery stenosis due to a friable, unstable atherosclerotic plaque. Emergent carotid endarterectomy or carotid balloon angioplasty and stenting are indicated for both these syndromes for qualifying patients.

53. **When is repair of an occluded carotid artery associated with a stroke indicated?**
Never. Complete occlusion should be treated with anticoagulation alone. Surgical procedures that attempt to reopen the artery are associated with possible progression of the stroke and an accompanying perioperative mortality rate of > 20%.

VENOUS DISEASE

54. **What is Virchow's triad?**
- Stasis of flow
- Hypercoaguable state
- Vein wall injury
The presence of these conditions increases the risk of deep venous thrombosis (DVT).
Surgical procedures under general anesthesia, prolonged inactivity in patients suffering a neurologic event (e.g., strokes, brain surgery), severe diffuse trauma, orthopedic pelvic/knee surgery, and pelvic procedures all augment this situation and increase the risk for DVT development.

55. **What are the physical findings of DVT?**
Physical findings may be present in as few as 50% of patients with acute DVT. If present, unilateral leg swelling, warmth, pitting edema, or engorged superficial veins may be seen. Physical examination should not be relied upon to confirm or refute the suspected diagnosis.

56. **How is DVT diagnosed?**
The physical findings of DVT are nonspecific with an overall accuracy of 50%. This inaccuracy led to the development of noninvasive methods for detecting thrombosis. The examination includes both Doppler analysis of venous flow dynamics and ultrasonic imaging of the lower extremity veins. Intraluminal thrombus is detected when the vein is noncompressible and hemodynamic flow analysis shows a delay in flow with distal tissue compression due to upstream obstruction by clot.

57. **What are the complications of DVT?**
Pulmonary emboli, which are associated with a high mortality rate. Untreated DVT can also lead to chronic venous insufficiency with resultant swelling and predisposition to leg ulcerations.

58. **What is the standard therapy for DVT?**
Immediate anticoagulation with heparin and warfarin. Heparin should always accompany warfarin (Coumadin) administration initially to prevent warfarin skin necrosis. The heparin may be given by subcutaneous injections for 4–5 days while warfarin takes effect and increases the international normalized ratio (INR). Anticoagulation is maintained for 3–6 months to allow for autolysis and recanalization of the thrombus; then it is discontinued. After 3–6 months, the risk of the warfarin causing bleeding outweighs the risk of recurrent clot or pulmonary embolus. Currently, other oral anticoagulants are under investigation for prevention and treatment of DVT.

59. **What is postphlebitic syndrome?**
Venous hypertension created by destruction of intraluminal valves during an initial thrombotic event with associated symptoms.

60. **What are the symptoms of postphlebetic syndrome?**
- Lower extremity swelling: 95%
- Rust-colored skin discoloration (called *venous stasis dermatitis*): 50%
- Ulcerations located in the "gaiter zone" of the lower calf and ankle region: 5%

61. **Describe a venous insufficiency ulcer.**
An ulcer usually located on the medial leg with surrounding pigmentation of hemosiderin. The involved leg is usually swollen.

62. **When does postphlebitic syndrome occur?**
Usually insidiously 5–10 years after the initial DVT.

63. **How is postphlebitic syndrome treated?**
With external compression stockings to decrease soft tissue venous hypertension and to control lower extremity edema. Unfortunately, this treatment is for life. Valves cannot be repaired or replaced. Ulcerations may need débridement and attentive wound care in addition to compression.

64. **What is May-Thurner syndrome?**
A proximal left common iliac vein narrowing or occlusion caused by an anatomic abnormality. Normally, the left common iliac vein passes under the right common iliac artery as it joins the contralateral right common iliac vein to form the inferior vena cava (IVC). Constant pulsation of the artery causes fibrosis of the underlying left common iliac vein, producing severe narrowing or total occlusion. When occlusion occurs, the entire left iliac venous system usually thromboses, and these patients are usually diagnosed as having an iliofemoral DVT. Treatment with thrombolysis can dissolve the clot and uncover the underlying disease. If a wire can cross the narrowing, the area is treated with balloon angioplasty and stent placement. In addition, these patients still require anticoagulation.

65. **What is venous claudication?**
Pain with walking after short distances in which the patient has normal arterial circulation but a chronic, severe venous obstruction in either the iliac or the femoral veins or both. In addition, there are also few draining collaterals around the chronic obstruction.

66. **What is an IVC filter?**
A metallic device inserted into the flow stream of the IVC below the renal veins. It allows blood to pass through its interstices while having the ability to trap blood clots passing up from the pelvis/lower extremities and preventing pulmonary emboli. Original filters were permanent, but recent changes have produced a filter that can be removed 2–4 weeks after placement.

67. **What are the indications for placement of an IVC filter?**
Absolute indications are development of DVT in patients with contraindications to anticoagulation; recurrent pulmonary embolization despite proper anticoagulation; complications of anticoagulation forcing discontinuation of anticoagulant therapy; and chronic pulmonary embolism associated with pulmonary hypertension and cor pulmonale. Relative indications include free-floating clot in the iliofemoral region.

68. **What is Takayasu arteritis?**
A chronic, large vessel vasculitis. The cause of Takayasu arteritis is unknown. Women are affected in nearly 90% of cases and are usually aged between 10 and 40 years.

69. **What arteries are involved?**
- Aortic arch and brachiocephalic vessels (type I)
- Thoracoabdominal aorta and renal arteries (type II)
    Type III Takayasu arteritis has features of type I and type II involvement. Patients with Takayasu arteritis may also have accelerated atherosclerosis of other blood vessels such as the carotid arteries.

70. **Describe the clinical prodrome associated with Takayasu arteritis.**
Initially, these patients have systemic symptoms such as fever, fatigue, anorexia, weight loss, and arthralgias. Later in the disease, classic symptoms of arterial occlusive disease develop such as lack of palpable pulses, cool extremities, and upper or lower extremity claudication.

71. **Do these patients need revascularization procedures?**
Not always. Usually treatment with glucocorticoids or agents such as methotrexate and azothioprine may help abate the progression, although it remains a chronic disease. Revascularization procedures (either open repair or angioplasty with stent placement) are indicated in the presence of significant occlusion but may have increased risks of restenosis. Aortic valve surgery is sometimes needed to repair aortic regurgitation.

LYMPHEDEMA

72. **What is the difference between primary and secondary lymphedema?**
Primary disease occurs when the lymphatic system is insufficient from birth (Milroy disease) or puberty (lymphedema praecox), and secondary disease is from destruction of lymphatic channels as a result of trauma (usually surgical), radiation therapy, tumor invasion, and recurrent infections (bacteria and parasites).

73. **How does lymphedema present?**
Usually with unilateral, extensive swelling, worse at the distal end of the involved limb where one typically finds digit involvement. Late findings are verrucous skin changes. In severe cases caused by tropical filiaria infection, elephantiasis develops.

74. **Are there any specific diagnostic tests to perform to verify lymphedema?**
Yes. Lymphoscintigraphy with radiolabeled colloid is often used to verify lymphedema. In this test, the colloid is injected into the subcutaneous tissue. Normally, the colloid will move up into the abdomen within hours, but with lymphatic obstruction, the colloid never ascends but becomes trapped in the interstitial space of the lower limb.

75. **What is the treatment for lymphedema?**
Reduction of swelling with pneumatic compression pumps and stockings. Adjuvant therapies include weight control, exercise, and massage. Antibiotics are given whenever there are recurrent episodes of cellulitis. Lymphatic bypass procedures and reduction procedures are mentioned only to condemn them because of poor results.

WEBSITE

1. www.vascularweb.org

BIBLIOGRAPHY
1. Cronenwett JL, Johnston W, eds. *Rutherford's Vascular Surgery.* 8th ed. Philadelphia: Elsevier; 2014.
2. Moore WD. *Vascular and Endovascular Surgery: A Comprehensive Review.* 8th ed. Philadelphia: Elsevier; 2014.

PULMONARY MEDICINE

Abbas Shahmohammadi, MD, Adriano R. Tonelli, MD, and Eloise M. Harman, MD

The orderly spoke of my father as a little man, but he was not, not until his black lung made its final assault. In a space of a few short weeks, he had shrunk, literally collapsing around his lungs as they became the entire focus of his being.

Homer Hickam, *October Sky*

ANATOMY

1. Describe the main airway structure.
   - **Trachea:** C-shaped cartilage with dorsal smooth muscle
   - **Main bronchi:** Semicircular cartilage
   - **Bronchi:** Irregularly shaped cartilage plates
   - **Bronchioles:** No cartilage support, surrounded by muscular layer

2. What are the components of the alveolar-capillary surface?
   Surfactant, alveolar epithelium (type 1 and type 2 alveolar cells, the latter producing surfactant), interstitium, and endothelium.

3. Describe the respiratory muscles.
   - **Diaphragm:** Innervated by C3–C5, and in supine position, provides more work than other muscles
   - **Inspiratory accessory:** External intercostal, scalene, and sternocleidomastoid muscles
   - **Expiratory accessory:** Internal intercostal and abdominal muscles

PHYSIOLOGY AND PATHOPHYSIOLOGY

4. What part of the brain generates spontaneous breathing?
   The medulla, which integrates information from higher brain centers and reflexes from arterial, central chemoreceptors, lung, airways, and other components of the respiratory system.

5. What size particles can reach the small airways?
   Particles 2–5 μm in size. **Particles > 10 μm are stopped in the upper airways.** Particles 5–10 μm in size impact on the carina or main bronchi.

6. What is the difference between lung volumes and capacities and how are they measured?
   - **Lung volumes:** amount of air at specific points in the respiratory cycle
   - **Lung capacities:** the summation of volumes (Fig. 6.1)
   In general, lung volumes and capacities are measured by either helium equilibration or body plethysmography. Both methodologies allow the calculation of functional residual capacity (FRC). The rest of the volumes and capacities are then calculated using spirometric values. Helium equilibration may underestimate the FRC in patients with severe airflow limitation (trapped gas may not communicate with the airways).

7. What is the main determinant of airway resistance?
   The radius of the medium-sized bronchi. The airway smooth muscle is mainly controlled by the autonomic nervous system including:
   - **Parasympathetic:** responsible for bronchoconstriction and mucus secretion
   - **Sympathetic (beta$_2$):** responsible for bronchodilatation and inhibition of glandular secretion

8. What is lung compliance?
   The change in lung volume generated by a change in pressure. Compliance is the inverse of elasticity. In a compliant lung, a small change in pressure will generate a large change in volume.

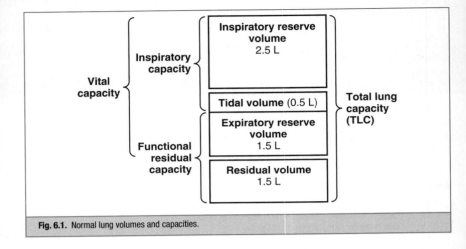

Fig. 6.1. Normal lung volumes and capacities.

9. Give examples of respiratory diseases associated with high and low compliance.
   - High compliance: emphysema
   - Low compliance: interstitial lung disease (ILD), acute respiratory distress syndrome (ARDS), chest wall stiffness

10. What is the difference between minute and alveolar ventilation?
    - **Minute ventilation:** tidal volume × respiratory rate
    - **Alveolar ventilation:** (tidal volume − dead-space volume) × respiratory rate
      Dead space is the air that remains in the conducting airways and does not participate in gas exchange (1 mL/lb).

11. How is the alveolar pressure of oxygen (P_{AO_2}) calculated?

$$P_{AO_2} = P_{IO_2} - P_{aCO_2}/RQ$$

$$P_{IO_2} = F_{IO_2} (P_{ATM} - P_{H_2O})$$

F_{IO_2} = fraction of inspired oxygen; P_{aCO_2} = arterial partial pressure of carbon dioxide; P_{ATM} = atmospheric pressure; P_{H_2O} = water vapor pressure; P_{IO_2} = partial pressure of inspired oxygen; RQ = respiratory quotient.

12. What are the two extremes of the ventilation/perfusion relationship?
    Alveolar dead space (ventilation without perfusion) and right-to-left shunt (perfusion without ventilation). Ventilation and perfusion must match for optimal gas exchange.

13. How is O_2 transported in the blood?
    Mainly through combination with hemoglobin, but a small amount of oxygen is dissolved in the blood. The dissolved portion contributes to the arterial partial pressure of oxygen (P_{aO_2}).

14. Why is the oxygen-hemoglobin dissociation curve important?
    The oxygen-hemoglobin curve is the relation between percent saturation hemoglobin (S_{O_2}) and P_{aO_2} and explains how blood carries and releases O_2. An important measure is P50, defined as the P_{aO_2} at which the hemoglobin is 50% saturated. An increase in P50 indicates a shift to the right of the standard curve, or decreased affinity of the hemoglobin for oxygen (Fig. 6.2).

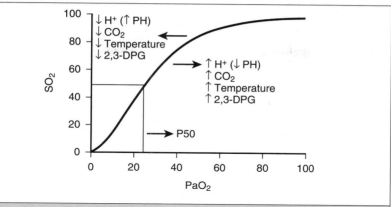

Fig. 6.2. Oxygen-hemoglobin dissociation curve.

15. What is the relationship between PaO_2 and aging?
    With aging, effective alveoli are decreased with a resultant decline in PaO_2. The expected PaO_2 can be calculated by the formula:

$$PaO_2 \text{ (sea level)} = 100.1 - 0.32 \times \text{age (in yr)}$$

16. Describe the mechanisms of arterial hypoxemia and give examples.
    * **Low inspired O_2:** high altitude, air flight, and hypoxia inhalation test ($FiO_2 = 15\%$)
    * **Hypoventilation:** central nervous system (CNS) depressant drugs, cerebrovascular accident (CVA), and head injury
    * **Diffusion impairment:** ILD, emphysema, pulmonary embolism (PE), pulmonary hypertension, and lung resection
    * **Mismatch:** chronic obstructive pulmonary disease (COPD), atelectasis, ARDS, and pulmonary edema
    * **Right-to-left-shunt:** Eisenmenger syndrome and pulmonary arteriovenous malformation

17. What is the value of measuring $PAO_2 - PaO_2$?
    The alveolar-arterial difference in partial pressure of O_2 is measured by the formula:

$$[FiO_2 \, (PATM - PH_2O) - PaCO_2/RQ] - PaO_2$$

    This equation allows the calculation of the shuntlike component in the lungs (due to shunting, diffusion, and $\dot{V}/\dot{Q}$ abnormalities). The normal value when breathing room air at sea level is <10–15. Generalized alveolar hypoventilation without $\dot{V}/\dot{Q}$ abnormalities will have normal $PAO_2 - PaO_2$.

18. What is the best way of estimating the severity of hypoxemia in patients receiving supplemental O_2?
    By calculating the PaO_2/FiO_2 ratio. In the new definition of ARDS, PaO_2/FiO_2 ratios of ≤ 300 are considered mild, ≤ 200 moderate, and ≤ 100 severe.
    The ARDS Definition Task Force. Acute respiratory distress syndrome: the Berlin Definition. *JAMA.* 2012;307:2526–2533.

SIGNS AND SYMPTOMS

19. What physical examination maneuvers can help distinguish among pneumonia, atelectasis, pleural effusion, and pneumothorax?
    See Table 6.1.

Table 6.1. Physical Examination Maneuvers and Findings of Common Pulmonary Disorders

MANEUVER	PNEUMONIA	ATELECTASIS	PLEURAL EFFUSION	PNEUMOTHORAX
Inspection	↓ Chest wall movement	↓ Chest wall movement	↓ Chest wall movement	↓ Chest wall movement
Percussion	Dull	Dull	Dull	↑ Resonance
Fremitus	↑	↓	↓	↓
Auscultation	Crackles, bronchial breath sounds, whispered pectoriloquy, and egophony	↓ Breath sounds	↓ Breath sounds	↓ Breath sounds

20. **What are the most common causes of dyspnea?**
    - **Respiratory:** COPD, asthma, and ILD
    - **Cardiac:** congestive heart failure (CHF) and coronary artery disease (CAD)
    - **Other:** metabolic acidosis, anemia, deconditioning, and anxiety

21. **What is the difference between orthopnea and platypnea?**
    - **Orthopnea:** Dyspnea increases on *recumbency* as found in CHF, COPD, and respiratory muscle weakness.
    - **Platypnea:** Dyspnea increases in the *upright* position as found in right-to-left shunts, $\dot{V}/\dot{Q}$ mismatch, hepatopulmonary syndrome, and PE.

22. **What is the definition of chronic cough?**
    A cough that has been present > 8 weeks.

23. **What are the most common causes of chronic cough?**
    - Gastroesophageal reflux disease (GERD)
    - Rhinitis or sinusitis
    - Asthma
    - Chronic bronchitis primarily related to cigarette smoking
    - Angiotensin-converting enzyme (ACE) inhibitor use
    - Bronchiectasis
    - Bronchogenic carcinoma
    - ILD
    - Upper airway cough syndrome (UACS; previously named "*postnasal drip syndrome*")
    - Nonasthmatic eosinophilic bronchitis (NAEB)
    - Hair or cerumen tickling the tympanic membrane ("ear-cough")
    - Aspirated foreign bodies
    - Chronic aspiration
    - Hyperactive cough reflex
    - Psychogenic cough

24. **How is a chronic cough evaluated?**
    Initially with history, physical examination, and chest radiograph which may reveal a likely cause such as ACE inhibitor use or smoking. Discontinuing the offending agent can improve the cough. Other causes identified initially include asthma, UACS, and GERD. These disorders can be treated empirically and cough symptoms reevaluated. Asthma can be further evaluated with spirometry, demonstrating bronchodilator reversibility. NAEB can be confirmed by the finding of sputum eosinophilia. If none of these more common causes is found, additional testing may include 24-hour esophageal pH monitoring (GERD), swallow evaluation (aspiration), sinus radiographs (sinusitis), high-resolution computed tomography scan (HRCT; lung lesions), bronchoscopy (endobronchial lesions and aspirated foreign bodies), and evaluation for environmental exposures.
    Irwin RS, Baumann MH, Bolser DC, et al. Diagnosis and management of cough. Executive Summary: ACCP Evidence-Based Clinical Practice Guidelines. *Chest*. 2006;129:S1–S23.

25. What are the most common causes of wheezing?
Asthma, COPD, CHF, vocal cord dysfunction (VCD), and UACS. The wheezing of UACS originates from the extrathoracic airway (most likely vocal cords). Wheezing lacks sensitivity and specificity for the diagnosis of asthma. Asthma can present without wheeze, and wheezing can be seen in other conditions that mimic asthma.

26. What is massive hemoptysis and pseudohemoptysis?
Massive hemoptysis is the expectoration of ≥600 mL of blood within 24–48 hours. The most common causes of massive hemoptysis are bronchiectasis (as in cystic fibrosis [CF]), bronchogenic carcinoma, arteriovenous malformations, aortobronchial fistulas, PE with infarction, aspergilloma, invasive aspergillosis, cavitary lung disease (as in tuberculosis), necrotizing pneumonia, and diffuse alveolar hemorrhage. **Pseudohemoptysis** is the expectoration of blood coming from a source other than the respiratory tract, including the posterior pharynx or gastrointestinal (GI) tract.

27. How is massive hemoptysis managed?
Initially, the uninvolved lung must be protected from aspiration of blood because blood can flood the airway and cause asphyxia and death. Maneuvers that keep the bleeding lung dependent can help. In severe cases, selective bronchial intubation or the use of endobronchial balloons to occlude the bleeding bronchus may be needed. Tamponade of tracheoarterial fistulas in patients with tracheostomies can sometimes be achieved by overinflation of the cuff of an endotracheal tube and applying forward pressure to the tube to compress the innominate artery. Definitive management of massive hemoptysis may require angiographic bronchial artery embolization or surgical resection. In cases of bleeding from endobronchial lesions, such as tumor, argon plasma coagulation (APC) via bronchoscopy may be utilized.

THORACIC IMAGING

28. What are the common diseases of the tracheobronchial tree?
- **Tracheal stenosis:** narrowing of the trachea
- **Tracheobronchomalacia:** weakness of airway walls with excessive expiratory collapse
- **Tracheobronchopathia osteochondroplastica:** calcified nodules on anterolateral walls of the trachea
- **Amyloidosis:** concentric or nodular thickening of the trachea
- **Relapsing polychondritis:** thickening of the anterolateral tracheal wall (occurs in approximately half of these patients)
- **Wegener granulomatosis:** usually lung nodules with or without cavitation but rarely circumferential tracheal thickening
- **Tracheobronchomegaly (Mounier-Kuhn syndrome):** diffuse dilatation (>3 cm) of the trachea and main bronchi

29. What are the radiographic findings in the posteroanterior chest x-ray study of atelectasis in different lung lobes?
See Fig. 6.3.

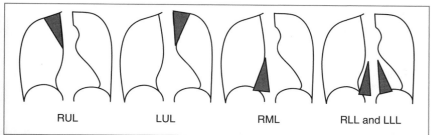

RUL   LUL   RML   RLL and LLL

Fig. 6.3. Diagram showing atelectases of different lung lobes. Right upper lobe (RUL) atelectasis results in the elevation of the right hilum and minor fissure. Left upper lobe (LUL) atelectasis obliterates the left heart border. The right middle lobe (RML) collapse obscures the right heart border. Right lower lobe (RLL) collapse exposes the major fissure and the RLL pulmonary artery is obscured. Left lower lobe (LLL) collapse shifts the hilum downward with opacification behind the heart (sail sign) and obscuration of the left hemidiaphragm.

30. **What diseases can be found in the different regions of the mediastinum?**
    See Table 6.2.

Table 6.2. Locations and Types of Mediastinal Masses

	Mediastinal Location*	
ANTERIOR	**MIDDLE**	**POSTERIOR**
Thymomas	Lymphomas	Neurogenic neoplasms
Lymphomas	Metastases	Esophageal lesions
Germ cell tumors	Sarcoidosis	Extramedullary hematopoiesis
Thyroid goiter or tumors	Mediastinal cysts	Descending aortic aneurysm
Morgagni hernia	Vascular lesions	Bochdalek hernia

*Anterior mediastinum: from the sternum to the anterior aspect of the heart and great vessels; middle mediastinum: between anterior and posterior compartments; posterior mediastinum: from the posterior heart border and trachea to the posterior aspect of the vertebral bodies.

31. **What are the most common lesions found on chest radiograph in the right cardiophrenic angle?**
    Prominent fat, lipoma, pericardial cyst, and Morgagni hernia. Most lesions in this area are benign.

32. **How is a solitary pulmonary nodule (SPN) defined, and what are the characteristics of a benign lesion?**
    A well-circumscribed single lung lesion that measures < 3 cm in diameter. Most common causes of SPN include granulomas, intrapulmonary lymph nodes, benign and malignant tumors, and vascular malformations. Characteristics of benign nodules include stability over time, presence of fat, and calcifications characterized as central, laminated, or popcorn-like.

33. **What are the most common HRCT patterns and the associated diseases?**
    See Table 6.3.

Table 6.3. Patterns of Pulmonary Disease on High-Resolution Computed Tomography Scan

PATTERN	DISORDERS	ANATOMY
Linear	Pulmonary edema, lymphangitic spread	Due to thickening of interlobular septa (Kerley lines)
Reticular	Pulmonary fibrosis, idiopathic pulmonary fibrosis, asbestosis, and collagen vascular disease	May appear as honeycombing
Nodular		Multiple nodules < 1 cm
Perilymphatic	Sarcoidosis, pneumoconiosis, lymphangitic carcinomatosis	Peribronchovascular interstitium and interlobular septa
Centrilobar	Hypersensitivity pneumonitis, infections	Center of pulmonary lobule
Randomly located	Metastatic disease, chronic histoplasmosis	
Ground-glass opacities	Pulmonary edema, *Pneumocystis jiroveci* pneumonia, hemorrhage, alveolar proteinosis	Hazy opacity that does not obscure pulmonary vessels
Cystic	Lymphangioleiomyomatosis, Langerhans cell histiocytosis	Thin walled cysts < 1 cm in diameter

34. **What are tree-in-bud opacities, and in what conditions may they be seen?**
Dilated terminal bronchioles with impacted mucus that are often seen in atypical mycobacterial infections and aspiration but may also be seen in bacterial or viral infections, collagen vascular disease, fungal infections, collagen diseases, CF, or toxic inhalations. This abnormality is best seen on HRCT and is typical of bronchiectasis.

35. **What is positron-emission tomography (PET) scanning, and how is it useful for assessment of pulmonary nodules?**
PET scanning uses a D-glucose analog labeled with ^{18}F to image the tissues. Metabolically active lesions will have increased uptake of this molecule. The degree of uptake is measured using a standardized uptake ratio (SUV). Typically, lung cancers will have an SUV > 2.5, and lesions with increased metabolism are highly likely to be malignant. False-positive results are found in infectious and inflammatory lesions, including sarcoidosis and atypical mycobacterial infections. False-negative results may be observed in broncholoalveolar carcinoma, well-differentiated malignancies, carcinoid, and small lesions (<1 cm).

CHRONIC OBSTRUCTIVE PULMONARY DISEASE

36. **Define COPD.**
A preventable and treatable disease state characterized by chronic airflow limitation that is not fully reversible and is usually progressive. The airflow limitation is usually associated with an enhanced chronic inflammatory response of the airways and the lung to noxious substances or gases. COPD traditionally comprises chronic bronchitis and emphysema. **Chronic bronchitis** is characterized by productive cough for at least 3 consecutive months in 2 consecutive years. **Emphysema** is an abnormal enlargement of the air spaces distal to the terminal bronchioles with destruction of their walls.
Global Strategy for the Diagnosis, Management and Prevention of COPD. Global Initiative for Chronic Obstructive Lung Disease (GOLD). Available at: www.goldcopd.org.

37. **What are the main risk factors for COPD?**
Exposure to cigarette smoke, indoor air pollution from biomass cooking and heating, and longstanding asthma. Other risk factors include alpha$_1$-antitrypsin deficiency (AATD), low socioeconomic status, and exposure to particulate matter.

38. **What is the prevalence of COPD?**
In the United States, >16 million people have COPD that frequently leads to hospitalization, increased mortality rate, and rising health costs. The prevalence and burden of COPD are projected to increase.

39. **What are the comorbid conditions frequently encountered in COPD patients?**
Weight loss, nutritional abnormalities, and skeletal muscle dysfunction. COPD patients also have an increased risk of CAD, osteoporosis, respiratory infection, lung cancer, diabetes, depression, sleep disorders, glaucoma, and anemia.

40. **What are the Global Initiative for Chronic Obstructive Lung Disease (GOLD) guidelines on stages for classifying COPD severity based on postbronchodilator FEV_1 (forced expiratory volume in 1 second)?**
- **Stage I** (mild): FEV_1/FVC (forced vital capacity) < 0.7 and $FEV_1 \geq 80\%$ of predicted
- **Stage II** (moderate): FEV_1/FVC < 0.7 and FEV_1 50–80% of predicted
- **Stage III** (severe): FEV_1/FVC < 0.7 and FEV_1 30–50% of predicted
- **Stage IV** (very severe): FEV_1/FVC < 0.7 and FEV_1 < 30% of predicted

41. **What characteristics help differentiate between asthma and COPD?**
See Table 6.4. However, patients with COPD can have features of asthma and vice versa. Patients with asthma may develop fixed airflow limitation. Subjects with COPD can have a mixed inflammatory pattern with increased eosinophils.

Table 6.4. Characteristics Useful to Distinguish Between Asthma and Chronic Obstructive Pulmonary Disease

CHARACTERISTIC	ASTHMA	COPD
Airflow limitation	Largely reversible	Largely irreversible
Airway inflammation	CD4+ T lymphocytes and eosinophils	CD8+ T lymphocytes, macrophages, and neutrophils
Onset	Early in life	Midlife
Symptoms	Vary from day to day and are worse at night or early morning	Slowly progressive
Risk factors	Family history of asthma	History of tobacco abuse

COPD, chronic obstructive pulmonary disease.

42. What is asthma-COPD overlap syndrome (ACOS)?

Symptoms in which patients have a component of persistent airflow limitation along with one or more features associated with asthma, such as wheezing, a component of reversible airflow obstruction, bronchial hyperresponsiveness, or sputum eosinophilia.

GINA-GOLD Diagnosis of disease of chronic airflow limitation: Asthma, COPD and asthma-COPD overlap syndrome (ACOS), 2015m. Available at www.ginasthma.org.

Postma DS, Rabe KF. The asthma-COPD overlap syndrome. *N Engl J Med.* 2015;373:1241–1249.

43. What are the risk factors for the development of COPD?

- Tobacco smoke
- Occupational dusts
- Indoor air pollution (biomass cooking and heating)
- Outdoor air pollution
- Genetic inheritance (AATD)
- Impaired lung growth and development (reduced maximal attained lung function)
- Older age and female gender (women may be more susceptible)
- Oxidative stress
- Low socioeconomic status
- Recurrent infections

44. What features are associated with a poorer prognosis in COPD?

- Decreased FEV_1
- Cigarette smoking
- Low body mass index (BMI $\leq$ 21)
- Human immunodeficiency virus (HIV) infection
- Decreased exercise tolerance and peak O_2 consumption
- High airway bacterial load and C-reactive protein (CRP)
- Advanced age
- Need for supplemental O_2
- Elevated BODE index

45. What is the BODE index?

An index used to calculate the 4-year survival of patients with COPD based on:

- **B**MI
- Airway **o**bstruction (FEV_1)
- Degree of **d**yspnea (based on Medical Research Council dyspnea score)
- **E**xercise capacity (6-minute walk distance)

The 4-year survival decreases as the number of points increases (e.g., the 4-year survival is only 18% when the score is 7–10 points).

Celli BR, Cote CG, Marin JM, et al. The body-mass index, airflow obstruction, dyspnea and exercise capacity index in chronic obstructive pulmonary disease. *N Engl J Med.* 2004;350:1005–1012.

46. **What are the steps for managing COPD according to the GOLD guidelines?**
    - Assess and monitor disease:
        - Consider COPD in any patient with dyspnea, chronic cough, or sputum production or a history of exposure to risk factors for COPD.
        - Confirm the diagnosis with spirometry.
        - Consider arterial blood gas (ABG) analysis in patients with $FEV_1 < 50\%$ of predicted or clinical signs suggestive of respiratory or right-sided heart failure.
        - Consider hereditary emphysema (AATD) in Caucasian patients who develop COPD at age < 50 years or have a strong family history for COPD.
        - Actively identify comorbid conditions.
    - Reduce risk factors: Counsel about smoking cessation and reduce exposure to pollution and occupational hazards.
    - Encourage regular physical activity.
    - Manage stable COPD: Assess severity of airflow limitation, and evaluate symptoms and frequency of exacerbations. Use pharmacotherapy to decrease symptoms and complications.
    - Manage exacerbations: Prescribe inhaled bronchodilators, oral or intravenous (IV) steroids. Add antibiotics if needed for infection. Use noninvasive mechanical ventilation (NIV) for hypercapnic respiratory failure. Use of NIV reduces need for endotracheal intubations, length of hospital stay, and mortality rate.

47. **What is the basic treatment for COPD?**
    Bronchodilators such as beta$_2$-agonists or anticholinergics or both in short-acting and long-acting forms with addition of:
    - Inhaled steroids in patients with symptomatic COPD, repeated exacerbations, and $FEV_1 < 60\%$ of predicted
    - Combinations of inhaled corticosteroid (ICS) and inhaled long-acting beta$_2$-agonists (LABAs): More effective than either individual component in improving lung function and reducing exacerbations
    - Phosphodiesterase-4 inhibitor Roflumilast (Daliresp): For frequent exacerbations in patients with severe airflow limitation and chronic bronchitis, treatment with the phosphodiesterase-4 inhibitor Roflumilast (Daliresp) may reduce exacerbations.
    - Long-term administration of continuous O_2 (>15 hours/day): Indicated in patients with chronic hypoxemic respiratory failure, characterized by a $Pao_2 \le 55$ mm Hg or O_2 saturation $\le 88\%$ on room air. If the patient also has evidence of PH, CHF, or polycythemia, oxygen is indicated for a $Po_2 \le 59$ mm Hg or oxygen saturation of $\le 89\%$. Oxygen therapy has been shown to prolong survival in patients who meet these criteria.
    - Seasonal influenza vaccine annually
    - Both types of pneumococcal vaccine: Pneumonia polysaccharide vaccine (PPSV23) and pneumonia conjugate vaccine (PCV13)
    - Pulmonary rehabilitation
    - Consideration of alpha-1 antitrypsin augmentation therapy in AATD patients
    - Consideration of lung volume reduction surgery (LVRS) in selected patients with upper lobe emphysema and low exercise capacity
    - Consideration of lung transplantation for patients who fail other therapies and have no significant comorbid conditions

48. **What bacterial pathogens are most commonly involved in COPD exacerbations?**
    - *Streptococcus pneumoniae*
    - *Haemophilus influenzae*
    - *Moraxella catarrhalis*
        If the patient does not respond within 3–7 days of appropriate empirical antibiotic therapy for these organisms, consider sputum culture.

49. **What are the indications for hospital admission in COPD exacerbation?**
    - Marked increase in symptoms
    - Severe underlying COPD
    - Increased oxygen requirement
    - Failure of initial management as outpatient or in emergency department (ED)

- Significant comorbid conditions
- Older age
- Insufficient home support
- New findings on physical examination or imaging
- Frequent exacerbations

50. **What signs and symptoms of COPD suggest that intensive care unit (ICU) admission is indicated?**
    - Severe dyspnea, poorly responsive to initial therapy
    - Change in mental status
    - Persistent or worsening hypoxemia or hypercapnia or worsened respiratory acidosis (pH < 7.25)
    - Patient uncooperative with or failing to improve with NIV
    - Need for invasive mechanical ventilation
    - Need for vasopressors

51. **When is a hospitalized patient with COPD exacerbation ready for discharge?**
    The following criteria should be met prior to discharge:
    - Return to baseline use of inhaled short-acting beta$_2$-agonists (SABAs), or their as-needed use less frequently than every 4 hours
    - Return to baseline level of function or consideration of posthospital rehabilitation
    - Stable blood gases or oxygen saturation for 12–24 hours
    - Able to maintain ventilation without continuous assistance BiPAP (bilevel positive airway pressure)
    - Acceptance by patient and caregiver of the discharge plan of care and follow-up arrangements

ASTHMA

52. **Define *asthma*.**
    A complex disorder characterized by variable and recurring symptoms, airflow obstruction, bronchial hyperresponsiveness, and underlying inflammation. This disease appears to be due to a combination of genetic and environmental factors (e.g., airborne allergens, viral infections, tobacco smoke, air pollution, and diet) as well as a dominant T helper 2 (T$_H$2)–type cytokine response of the innate immunity.
    National Asthma Education and Prevention Program. Expert Panel Report 3 (EPR-3): Guidelines for the Diagnosis and Management of Asthma—Summary Report 2007. *J Allergy Clin Immunol.* 2007;120:S94–S138.

53. **How is the diagnosis of asthma established?**
    By the identification of recurrent symptoms of airflow obstruction or airway hyperresponsiveness, the demonstration that the airflow obstruction is at least partially reversible on spirometry after administration of bronchodilator, and the exclusion of other diagnoses. Reversibility on pulmonary function testing is defined as 12% or 200 mL improvement in FEV$_1$ after bronchodilator. Asthma symptoms include cough that is typically worse at night, wheezing, dyspnea, and chest tightness. In general, the symptoms occur or worsen during exercise, viral infection, inhalation of allergens or irritants, change in weather, stress, and menstrual cycles. The finding of a negative bronchoprovocation challenge with methacholine practically excludes asthma.

54. **What is exhaled nitrous oxide (NO)? How may it be used in the diagnosis of asthma?**
    A gas produced by cells in the lung that is a smooth muscle relaxer, vasodilator, and possibly bronchodilator. Fractional concentration of exhaled nitric oxide (FENO) is increased in eosinophilic asthma but also can be increased in other conditions. Therefore, measuring FENO is currently not recommended for diagnosing asthma in adults. Measurement of FENO may be helpful in the diagnosis of asthma in children ages 1–5 years as normal values have been established.

55. **What other conditions can be confused with asthma?**
    - Vocal cord dysfunction (VCD)
    - Allergic rhinitis and sinusitis
    - COPD

- CHF
- PE
- Mechanical airway obstruction
- Cough secondary to use of ACE inhibitors

KEY POINTS: VOCAL CORD DYSFUNCTION

1. Symptoms are similar to asthma, including wheezing and stridor that may or may not be in response to irritants.
2. Can occur in patients who also have asthma and exercise-induced asthma.
3. Diagnosis is made by flow volume loops that show inspiratory cut-off.
4. Treatment includes speech therapy and behavior modification, NOT corticosteroids.

56. What steps are followed for asthma management?
- Assess and monitor disease through the evaluation of:
  - Severity and control of asthma.
  - Response to treatment.
- Educate patient to:
  - Develop asthma action plan.
  - Understand the difference between long-term control and quick-relief medications.
  - Use medications correctly.
  - Avoid environmental exposures.
  - Self-monitor disease.
  - Control environmental factors and comorbid conditions.
- Use medications based on asthma severity with frequent adjustment based on control.
  National Asthma Education and Prevention Program. Expert Panel Report 3 (EPR-3): Guidelines for the diagnosis and management of asthma—Summary Report 2007. *J Allergy Clin Immunol.* 2007;120:S94–138.

57. How is asthma classified according to sign and symptom severity?
See Table 6.5.

Table 6.5. Asthma Classification Based on Sign and Symptom Severity

SIGNS AND SYMPTOMS	INTERMITTENT	MILD	MODERATE	SEVERE
			Persistent*	
Symptoms	≤2 days/wk	>2 days/wk	Daily	Throughout the day
Nighttime awakenings	≤2 nights/mo	3–4 nights/mo	>1 night/wk	Almost every night
SABA use	≤2 days/wk	>2 days/wk	Daily	Several times a day
Interference with normal activity	None	Minor limitation	Some limitation	Severely limited
Lung function	Normal FEV$_1$ between exacerbations	FEV$_1$ 80%	FEV$_1$ 60–80% FEV$_1$/FVC reduced < 5%	FEV$_1$ < 60% FEV$_1$/FVC reduced > 5%
Need for systemic steroids	0–1/yr	≥2/yr	≥2/yr	≥2/yr

*The level of severity is determined by assessing impairment (previous 2–4 weeks) and risk. Assign severity to the most severe category in which any feature occurs.
FEV$_1$, forced expiratory volume in 1 second; FVC, forced vital capacity; SABA, short-acting beta$_2$ agonist.
Adapted from Expert Panel Report 3 (EPR-3). Guidelines for the Diagnosis and Management of Asthma-Summary Report 2007. *J Allergy Clin Immunol.* 2007;120:S94–S138.

58. What comorbid conditions can complicate asthma management?
- GERD (even in the absence of suggestive GERD symptoms)
- Rhinitis or sinusitis (interrelationship between upper and lower airway)
- Obesity (weight loss may improve asthma control)
- Stress and depression
- Obstructive sleep apnea (OSA)
- Allergic bronchopulmonary aspergillosis (ABPA)

KEY POINTS: DIAGNOSTIC FEATURES FOR ALLERGIC BRONCHOPULMONARY ASPERGILLOSIS

1. Asthma
2. Serum IgE > 1000 IU/mL
3. Positive skin test for *Aspergillus fumigatus* or positive RAST (radioallergosorbent test) for *A. fumigatus*
4. Elevated serum *A. fumigatus* specific antibody levels (IgG)
5. Central bronchiectasis, mucoid impaction
6. Eosinophilia (typically seen and support diagnosis but not required)

> Patterson K, Strek ME. Allergic bronchopulmonary aspergillosis. *Proc Am Thorac Soc.* 2010;7:237–244.

59. What medications are used for long-term control and quick relief of asthma?
See Table 6.6.

Table 6.6. Asthma Medications Used for Long-Term Control and Immediate Symptom Relief

LONG-TERM CONTROL	IMMEDIATE SYMPTOM RELIEF
Inhaled corticosteroids (most effective)	SABAs
LABAs (not to be used as monotherapy)	Ipratropium bromide
Leukotriene modifiers (adjunctive therapy)	Systemic corticosteroids (short course)
Omalizumab (anti-IgE) (in patients with elevated IgE, documented allergy, and persistent asthma despite inhaled corticosteroids and LABA)	
Methylxanthines (theophylline)	
Tiotropium (persistent symptoms)	
Mepolizumab or reslizumab (refractory asthma with peripheral eosinophilia)	

IgE, immunoglobulin E; LABAs, long-acting beta$_2$ agonists; SABAs, short-acting beta$_2$ agonists.

60. Describe the stepwise approach for asthma management in adults.
See Table 6.7.
1. Short-acting bronchodilator (SABA) as needed for intermittent asthma
2. Low-dose ICS
3. Low-dose ICS + LABA or medium-dose ICS
4. Medium-dose ICS + LABA
5. High-dose ICS + LABA ± tiotropium
6. High-dose ICS + LABA + tiotropium, ± omalizumab or mepolizumab, reslizumab or oral corticosteroid
   Omalizumab (anti-IgE) is a subcutaneous (SQ) drug added in severe persistent allergic asthma, with elevated IgE levels and documented allergy, that is not controlled with maximum inhaler therapy.

Mepolizumab (anti-IL-5) is an SQ drug and reslizumab is an IV drug added in severe persistent asthma with peripheral eosinophila that is not controlled with maximum inhaler therapy.

Leukotriene receptor antagonist (LTRA) or low-dose theophylline can be added as an alternative or additional therapy in steps 2–6.

Table 6.7. Stepwise Approach for Asthma Management in Adult*

STEP	PREFERRED MEDICATION
1	SABA as needed for intermittent asthma
2	Low-dose ICS†
3	Low-dose ICS + LABA or medium-dose ICS†
4	Medium-dose ICS + LABA†
5	High-dose ICS + LABA‡
6	High-dose ICS + LABA + oral corticosteroid‡

*Step up if poor control and step down if good control for ≥ 3 months.
†Consider subcutaneous allergen immunotherapy in patients with allergic asthma.
‡Consider omalizumab for patients with allergies.
ICS, inhaled corticosteroid; LABA, long-acting beta$_2$ agonist; SABA, short-acting beta$_2$ agonist.
Adapted from Expert Panel Report 3 (EPR-3). Guidelines for the Diagnosis and Management of Asthma-Summary Report 2007. *J Allergy Clin Immunol.* 2007;120:S94–S138.

Global Initiative for Asthma. Available at www.ginaasthma.org.

61. **What symptoms and objective clinical findings help determine whether a patient with an acute asthma exacerbation can receive treatment as an outpatient or in the hospital?**
The decision to admit a patient to the hospital incorporates the evaluation of signs and symptoms, pulse oximetry (SpO$_2$), and lung function measurements.
- **Mild exacerbations:** Dyspnea with activity and peak expiratory flow (PEF) ≥ 70% of personal best can be treated at home.
- **Moderate exacerbations:** Dyspnea with usual activity and PEF 51–69% of personal best will require office or ED visit.
- **Severe exacerbations:** Dyspnea at rest and PEF ≤ 50% of personal best will require ED visit and likely hospitalization.
- **Life-threatening exacerbation:** Inability to speak, sweating, and PEF < 25% of personal best will require hospitalization and ICU admission.

In general, patients who have a good response after treatment in the ED as demonstrated by a sustained response after 60 minutes, no respiratory distress, normal physical examination, and PEF ≥ 70% can be discharged home. Those with poor response to ED treatment who exhibit severe symptoms, confusion, PaCO$_2$ ≥ 42 mm Hg or PEF < 40% generally need ICU admission.

62. **Which patients are at high risk of asthma-related death?**
Those with:
- Previous severe exacerbation requiring intubation and mechanical ventilation
- Asthma-related hospitalizations or ED visit within past 12 months
- Nonuse or nonadherence to ICS
- Current oral corticosteroid use or recently discontinued oral corticosteroid use
- More than one SABA canister use per month
- Lack of asthma action plan, poor adherence with treatments
- Food allergy
- Low socioeconomic status, illicit drug use, major psychosocial problems or psychiatric disease
- Comorbid conditions
  www.ginareport.com.

63. **What is exercise-induced asthma?**
Asthma symptoms (cough, dyspnea, chest tightness, or wheezing) that occur during exercise or immediately after exercise. A 15% decrease in FEV$_1$ after exercise (defined as 5-minute intervals of exercise for 20–30 minutes) will establish the diagnosis.

64. **How is exercise-induced asthma managed?**
    Usually with pretreatment with inhaled beta$_2$ agonists before exercise. (SABA may last for 2–3 hours, whereas LABAs may protect for up to 12 hours.) If the symptoms are frequent or severe, initiate or step up long-term control medications. A warm-up period before exercise and the use of a mask or scarf over the mouth for patients with cold- and exercise-induced asthma may attenuate this condition. Leukotriene modifiers may also block exercise-induced bronchospasm but are less effective than beta agonists.

65. **How is asthma managed during pregnancy?**
    With SABA (albuterol) and ICSs (budesonide) because more safety data during pregnancy are available for these medications. Asthma control during pregnancy is important for the well-being of the mother and the baby. Uncontrolled asthma increases perinatal mortality, preterm birth, low-birth-weight infants, and preeclampsia. Classically, asthma during pregnancy improves in one third of the patients and worsens in another third.

COMMUNITY-ACQUIRED PNEUMONIA

See also Chapter 12, Infectious Diseases.

66. **How is the diagnosis of community-acquired pneumonia (CAP) made?**
    By the presence of suggestive clinical features and a demonstrable infiltrate by an imaging technique, with or without supporting microbiologic data. Patients should be evaluated for an etiologic diagnosis with pretreatment blood cultures, urinary antigens for *Legionella pneumophila* and *S. pneumoniae*, and expectorated sputum culture when there is suspicion that these results may alter the empirical management or if there are concerns for unusual pathogens or antibiotic resistance.

67. **List the risk factors for CAP associated with specific pathogens.**
    See Table 6.8.

Table 6.8. Risk Factors for Pneumonia Associated with Specific Pathogens

RISK FACTOR	PATHOGEN(S)
Alcoholism	*Streptococcus pneumoniae*, oral anaerobes, *Klebsiella pneumoniae*
Aspiration	Gram-negative enteric pathogens, oral anaerobes
Exposure to bat/bird droppings	*Histoplasma capsulatum*
Exposure to birds	*Chlamydophila psittaci*
Exposure to rabbits	*Francisella tularensis*
Hotel/cruise ship stay	*Legionella* spp.
Travel to southwestern United States	*Coccidioides* spp., *Hantavirus*
Injection drug use	*Staphylococcus aureus*, anaerobes, *Mycobacterium tuberculosis*
Bioterrorism	*Bacillus anthracis*, *Yersinia pestis*, *F. tularensis*

From Mandell LA, Wunderink RG, Anzueto A, et al. Infectious Diseases Society of America/American Thoracic Society consensus guidelines on the management of community-acquired pneumonia in adults. *Clin Infect Dis.* 2007;44:S27–S72.

68. **What is a CURB-65 score?**
    A prognostic index that helps to identify which patients require hospital admission for CAP. The score uses five variables and assigns one point for the presence of each variable. The variables are:
    - **C**onfusion: defined as disorientation to person, place, and time
    - **U**rea (blood urea nitrogen [BUN]): >20 mg/dL
    - **R**espiratory rate: >30 breaths/min
    - **B**lood pressure: systolic < 90 mm Hg or diastolic < 60 mm Hg
    - Age > **65** years

Patients with a score of 2 generally require hospital admission and patients with scores 3 and above should be considered for ICU admission. Other prognostic models include the Pneumonia Severity Index (PSI) that includes 20 different variables, which limits its practicality. All models should be supplemented by consideration of other factors such as the ability to take oral medications and have adequate outpatient support.

Fine MJ, Auble TE, Yealy DM, et al. A prediction rule to identify low-risk patients with community-acquired pneumonia. *N Engl J Med.* 1997;336:243–250.

Lim WS, van der Ferden MM, Laing R, et al. Defining community acquired pneumonia severity on presentation to hospital: an international derivation and validation study. *Thorax.* 2003;58:377–382.

69. **When do patients with CAP require ICU admission?**
When they need mechanical ventilation or vasopressors. ICU care is usually also required if patients meet at least three of the following criteria:
- Respiratory rate $\geq$ 30 breaths/min
- $PaO_2/FiO_2 \leq 250$
- Multilobar infiltrates
- Confusion
- BUN $\geq$ 20 mg/dL
- White blood cell (WBC) count 4000 cells/mm^3
- Platelets < 100,000 cells/mm^3
- Hypothermia (<36° C)
- Hypotension requiring aggressive fluid resuscitation

Mandell LA, Wunderink RG, Anzueto A, et al. Infectious Diseases Society of America/American Thoracic Society consensus guidelines on the management of community-acquired pneumonia in adults. *Clin Infect Dis.* 2007;44:S27–S72.

70. **What are the recommended empirical antibiotics for CAP?**
See Table 6.9.

Table 6.9. Recommended Empirical Antibiotic Treatment for Pneumonia

OUTPATIENT	INPATIENT (NON-ICU)	INPATIENT (ICU)
Healthy and no antibiotics in previous 3 mo:	• Respiratory fluoroquinolone	• Beta-lactam‡ + macrolide or respiratory fluoroquinolone
• Macrolide	• Beta-lactam +macrolide	• Respiratory fluoroquinolone + aztreonam
• Doxycycline		
Comorbid conditions*:		
• Respiratory fluoroquinolone†		
• Beta-lactam + macrolide		

If pseudomonas is a consideration, use (piperacillin-tazobactam, cefepime, imipenem, or meropenem) + ciprofloxacin or levofloxacin (750 mg) or aminoglycoside. If community-acquired MRSA is a consideration, add vancomycin or linezolid. For patients requiring admission, the first dose of antibiotic should be given within 4 hours of admission to the emergency department.
*Comorbid conditions include heart, lung, liver, or renal disease; diabetes; alcoholism; malignancy; asplenia; immunosuppressing conditions; and use of immunosuppressing drugs.
†Respiratory fluoroquinolones include moxifloxacin, gemifloxacin, and levofloxacin.
‡Cefotaxime, ceftriaxone, or ampicillin-sulbactam.
ICU, intensive care unit; MRSA, methicillin-resistant *Staphylococcus aureus*.
Adapted from Mandell LA, Wunderink RG, Anzueto A, et al. Infectious Diseases Society of America/American Thoracic Society consensus guidelines on the management of community-acquired pneumonia in adults. *Clin Infect Dis.* 2007;44:S27–S72.

71. **When can antibiotics be switched from IV to oral?**
When the following criteria are met:
- Temperature ≤ 37.8° C oral
- Heart rate ≤ 100 beats per minute (bpm)
- Respiratory rate ≤ 24 breaths/min
- Systolic blood pressure ≥ 90 mm Hg
- So_2 ≥ 90% on room air
- Able to maintain oral intake
- Mental status normal or approaching prehospital state
  Mandell LA, Wunderink RG, Anzueto A, et al. Infectious Diseases Society of America/American Thoracic Society consensus guidelines on the management of community-acquired pneumonia in adults. *Clin Infect Dis.* 2007;44:S27–S72.

INTERSTITIAL LUNG DISEASES

72. **How are ILDs classified?**
- **Identified cause:** Drugs and collagen vascular diseases
- **Granulomatous:** Sarcoidosis
- **Other forms:** Lymphangioleiomyomatosis (LAM) and Langerhans cell histiocytosis (LCH)
- **Idiopathic**
  - Idiopathic pulmonary fibrosis (IPF)
  - Others
    o Desquamative interstitial pneumonia
    o Acute interstitial pneumonia
    o Nonspecific interstitial pneumonia (NSIP)
    o Respiratory bronchiolitis-associated ILD
    o Cryptogenic organizing pneumonia (COP)
    o Lymphocytic interstitial pneumonia (LIP)
  American Thoracic Society, European Respiratory Society. American Thoracic Society/European Respiratory Society International Multidisciplinary Consensus Classification of the Idiopathic Interstitial Pneumonias. *Am J Respir Crit Care Med.* 2002;165:277–304.
  Bradley B, Branley HM, Egan JJ, et al. Interstitial lung disease guideline: The British Thoracic Society in collaboration with the Thoracic Society of Australia and New Zealand and the Irish Thoracic Society. *Thorax.* 2008;63:v1–v58.

73. **What is the initial evaluation of ILD?**
History and physical examination, chest radiography, and lung function testing, looking for specific causes such as collagen vascular disease, environmental exposures, or drugs. If a cause is not found from the initial evaluation, HRCT is helpful, followed by transbronchial or surgical lung biopsy, if needed.

74. **What is IPF?**
A distinct type of chronic fibrosing interstitial pneumonia of unknown cause, limited to the lung. An interstitial pneumonia pattern is usually present on biopsy. On occasion, the diagnosis of IPF can be made without lung biopsy if the clinical setting and radiographic findings are consistent with IPF. In general, patients with IPF have no other known cause of ILD and are > 50 years old with insidious onset of unexplained dyspnea or cough or both that evolves over > 3 months. Examination finds bibasilar inspiratory crackles. HRCT shows predominantly bibasilar reticular abnormalities with minimal ground-glass opacities, associated with honeycombing, traction bronchiectasis, and volume loss. On pulmonary function tests, the total lung capacity (TLC) is reduced with decreased diffusing capacity of lung for carbon monoxide (D_{LCO}).

75. **What is the prognosis of IPF?**
Generally poor with a median length of survival from the time of diagnosis of 2.5–3.5 years. A decline in oxygen saturation during 6-minute walk test and a D_{LCO} < 40% indicate advanced disease. During the course of the disease, patients can have episodes of rapid decline that may represent accelerated disease. A drop in the FVC ≥ 10% or in D_{LCO} ≥ 15% in the first 6–12 months indicates a poorer prognosis.

76. **What is the treatment of IPF?**
    Nintedanib (from the INPULSIS-1 and INPULSIS-2 trials) and pirfenidone (from the ASCEND [A Study of Cardiovascular Events iN Diabetes] trial) have been shown to decrease disease progression with reducing decline of FVC. Additional management includes oxygen supplementation, antireflux therapy, pulmonary rehabilitation, participation in clinical trials evaluating new therapies, and lung transplantation.
    King TE Jr, Bradford WZ, Castro-Bernardini S, et al. A phase 3 trial of pirfenidone in patients with idiopathic pulmonary fibrosis. *N Engl J Med.* 2014;370(22):2083–2092.
    Richeldi L, du Bois RM, Raghu G, et al. Efficacy and safety of nintedanib in idiopathic pulmonary fibrosis. *N Engl J Med.* 2014;370:2071–2082.

77. **What ILD(s) are associated with tobacco smoking?**
    - IPF
    - Desquamative interstitial pneumonitis
    - Respiratory bronchiolitis-associated ILD
    - LCH
    Smokers are less likely to have hypersensitivity pneumonitis (HP) or sarcoidosis.

78. **What is HP?**
    A lung disorder caused by repeated exposure to a sensitizing agent (organic and inorganic particles) and classified as acute, subacute, and chronic. The acute form is characterized by respiratory symptoms that occur in a few hours after a heavy exposure. The other forms occur with ongoing lower-level exposure. Patients with the chronic type have diffuse pulmonary fibrosis that may resemble IPF or NSIP. The features of acute and subacute HP on chest computed tomography (CT) scan include diffuse pulmonary nodules, ground-glass opacities, and mosaic attenuation. Treatment includes avoidance of the causative antigen and corticosteroids in severe or progressive disease.

79. **Which connective tissue diseases (CTDs) are most commonly associated with ILD?**
    - Rheumatoid arthritis (RA)
    - Systemic sclerosis (SSc)
    - Polymyositis/dermatomyositis

SARCOIDOSIS

80. **What is sarcoidosis?**
    A granulomatous disease with systemic involvement whose cause is unknown. Affected groups include young and middle-aged adults, women, and African Americans. Sarcoidosis is postulated to occur in genetically susceptible individuals exposed to certain unknown environmental agents.
    Dempsey OJ, Paterson EW, Kerr KM, et al. Sarcoidosis. *BMJ.* 2009;339:b3206.

81. **Which organs are affected by sarcoidosis?**
    In general, the disease can affect any organ, although the most commonly involved organs are:
    - **Lungs** (>90%): Hilar adenopathy, ILD, and nodules
    - **Skin** (24%): Erythema nodosum, maculopapular lesions, and lupus pernio
    - **Liver** (18%): Elevated liver enzymes, hepatosplenomegaly, intrahepatic cholestasis
    - **Eyes** (12%): Uveitis, conjunctival nodules, and lacrimal gland enlargement
    - **Kidney** (5%): Renal calculi, nephrocalcinosis, and interstitial nephritis
    Nonspecific constitutional symptoms such as fever, fatigue, malaise, and weight loss are observed in up to one third of the patients. The disease can be asymptomatic in up to half of the patients. Mode of presentation and severity of disease are influenced by race and gender.

82. **What are the five radiographic stages of thoracic involvement?**
    - **Stage 0:** No visible thoracic finding
    - **Stage 1:** Bilateral hilar adenopathy
    - **Stage 2:** Bilateral hilar adenopathy + parenchymal infiltrates
    - **Stage 3:** Parenchymal infiltrates
    - **Stage 4:** Advanced fibrosis
    Stage 1 usually improves spontaneously or stabilizes. Spontaneous remission occurs less often as the disease stage progresses.

83. **What is Löfgren syndrome?**
A presentation of sarcoidosis with specific features, usually seen in women. Löfgren syndrome has an excellent prognosis, and patients usually recover spontaneously.

84. **What are the features of Löfgren syndrome?**
- Erythema nodosum
- Arthralgia
- Malaise
- Bilateral hilar adenopathy

85. **How is sarcoidosis diagnosed?**
When patients present with Löfgren syndrome, a clinical diagnosis of sarcoidosis is appropriate. In the remaining patients without this classic presentation, a tissue diagnosis is required. Most commonly, the diagnosis is made by EBUS-TBNA (endobronchial ultrasonography-guided transbronchial needle aspiration), endobronchial or transbronchial biopsy, mediastinal lymph node biopsy, biopsy of skin lesions, or less commonly, conjunctival or lacrimal gland biopsy. With the advance in bronchoscopic procedures, EBUS-TBNA has been shown to have high yield and may be preferred over other bronchoscopic procedures in obtaining diagnosis.

> von Bartheld MB, Dekkers OM, Szlubowski A, et al. Endosonography vs conventional bronchoscopy for the diagnosis of sarcoidosis: the GRANULOMA randomized clinical trial. *JAMA.* 2014;309:2457–2464.

86. **Are noncaseating granulomas pathognomonic of sarcoidosis?**
No. The characteristic lesion of sarcoidosis is a discrete, noncaseating epithelioid cell granuloma. However, noncaseating granulomas can be encountered in other diseases such as fungal and mycobacterial infections, foreign bodies, berylliosis, and common variable immunodeficiency. Any biopsy tissues obtained are routinely stained to exclude mycobacterial or fungal infections. In sarcoidosis, granulomas either resolve or lead to fibrotic changes.

87. **What is the utility of measuring ACE serum levels in sarcoidosis?**
Limited. ACE levels have low sensitivity and specificity and are not helpful for monitoring patients for disease progression. Pulmonary function tests and chest CT scans monitor disease progression more effectively.

88. **What is the differential diagnosis of sarcoidosis?**
- Tuberculosis
- Atypical mycobacteria
- Cryptococcosis
- Aspergillosis
- Coccidioidomycosis
- Blastomycosis
- *Pneumocystis jiroveci* infection
- Brucellosis
- Toxoplasmosis
- Cat-scratch disease
- Lymphomas
- Drug reaction (interferon alpha)
- Granulomatous lesions of unknown significance (GLUS)

89. **Which pneumoconiosis resembles sarcoidosis?**
Chronic beryllium lung disease. Berylliosis develops after a usual latent period of years following a low-level exposure to beryllium. The treatment is removal from further exposure to beryllium and steroids. Other hard metal–induced lung diseases due to aluminum and cobalt exposure are also characterized by the presence of sarcoid-like granulomas.

90. **What is the prognosis of sarcoidosis?**
Generally good. Many patients are asymptomatic, and spontaneous resolution occurs in up to two thirds of them. Risk factors for poor prognosis include age $\geq$ 40 years at onset of symptoms, African-American race, lupus pernio, chronic uveitis, chronic hypercalcemia, nephrocalcinosis, progressive pulmonary sarcoidosis, neurosarcoidosis, myocardial compromise, and the presence of cystic bony lesions.

91. **What is the treatment of sarcoidosis?**
    Oral steroids, although treatment is usually not indicated in patients who are asymptomatic or
    in those with mild pulmonary function abnormalities. Steroid therapy is started in patients with
    progressive radiographic findings or moderate symptoms; hypercalcemia; and neurologic, cardiac,
    or ocular involvement. Treatment duration is 6–24 months. Other medications used in patients who
    cannot tolerate steroids or have progressive disease on steroid therapy include hydroxychloroquine,
    methotrexate, azathioprine, and biologic agents (e.g., leflunomide).

    Baughman RP, Culver AD, Judson MA. A concise review of pulmonary sarcoidosis. *Am J Respir Crit Care Med.* 2011;183:573–581.

    Statement on sarcoidosis. Joint Statement of the American Thoracic Society (ATS), the European
    Respiratory Society (ERS) and the World Association of Sarcoidosis and Other Granulomatous
    Disorders (WASOG) adopted by the ATS Board of Directors and by the ERS Executive Committee,
    February 1999. *Am J Respir Crit Care Med.* 1999;160:736–755.

PULMONARY THROMBOEMBOLIC DISEASE

92. **What are the predisposing factors for the development of venous
    thromboembolism (VTE)?**
    - Age > 40
    - Prior VTE
    - Prolonged anesthesia (>30 minutes)
    - Prolonged immobilization
    - CHF
    - CVA
    - Cancer
    - Fracture of the pelvis, hip, or tibia
    - Hip or knee replacement
    - Pregnancy and postpartum period
    - Estrogen-containing medications
    - Tamoxifen
    - Obesity
    - Inflammatory bowel disease
    - Genetic or acquired thrombophilia: lupus anticoagulant, factor V Leiden, anticardiolipin antibody
      syndrome, protein S or C deficiency, antithrombin III deficiency, prothrombin 20210A mutation

93. **Describe the initial evaluation of possible PE.**
    Clinical grounds are insufficient for diagnosis and confirmation of PE. Clinical prediction tools, such
    as the Wells criteria, may be helpful in determining the clinical probability of PE and the need for
    further evaluation. In patients with a low or moderate clinical probability of PE, the D-dimer assay
    may be a useful screening tool. (D-dimers are cross-linked fibrin fragments that are released from
    thrombi soon after they are formed.) About 95% of patients with PE have an abnormal D-dimer
    level, depending on the assay used. However, an elevated D-dimer level may be seen in many
    other conditions, such as malignancy or recent surgical procedures. D-dimer can also increase with
    age. Use of age-adjusted D-dimer levels may reduce unnecessary testing. In those patients with
    a low or moderate probability of PE, a D-dimer level < 500 ng/mL by quantitative enzyme-linked
    immunosorbent assay (ELISA) or semiquantitative latex agglutination is sufficient evidence to rule
    out PE. Helical (spiral) chest CT scan performed with contrast is often used to confirm the diagnosis
    of PE, but may miss small PEs. CT scan has the potential to identify other diagnoses that may
    explain the patient's symptoms. In patients with allergy to contrast agent or who have renal failure,
    a nuclear medicine V̇/Q̇ scan and compression ultrasonography of the lower extremity veins may be
    performed. The V̇/Q̇ scan is very sensitive but nonspecific.

    Righini M, Van Es J, Den Exter PL, et al. Age-adjusted d-dimer cutoff levels to rule out
    pulmonary embolism: the ADJUST-PE study. *JAMA.* 2014;311:1117–1124.

94. **What is the Wells formula for predicting the clinical probability of PE?**
    PE is unlikely with a score ≤ 4 and likely with a score > 4. Points are assigned as follows:
    - Clinical symptoms of deep venous thrombosis (DVT): 3
    - Other diagnoses more likely than PE: 3
    - Heart rate > 100 bpm: 1.5

- Immobilization ≥ 3 days: 1.5
- Surgery in previous 4 weeks: 1.5
- Previous DVT or PE: 1.5
- Hemoptysis: 1
- Malignancy: 1

vanBelle A, Buller HR, Huisman MV, et al. Effectiveness of managing suspected pulmonary embolism using an algorithm combining clinical probability, D-dimer testing, and computed tomography. *JAMA.* 2006;295:172–179.

95. **Summarize the chest radiograph findings associated with PE.**
Frequently chest radiographs in patients with PE are "normal," although subtle nonspecific abnormalities can be found. Examples of abnormal findings include differences in diameters of vessels that should be similar in size, abrupt cut-off of a vessel followed distally, increased radiolucency in some areas, regional oligemia (Westermark sign), a peripheral wedge-shaped density over the diaphragm (Hampton hump), or an enlarged right descending pulmonary artery (Palla sign).

96. **What are the new long-term medications for VTE?**
Novel oral anticoagulants (NOACs) include dabigatran, rivaroxaban, apixaban, and edoxaban that may be used for treatment of VTE in addition to warfarin and low-molecular-weight heparin (LMWH). Dabigatran is a direct thrombin inhibitor, and the rest are factor Xa inhibitors. Rivaroxaban and apixaban do not require bridging with parenteral anticoagulation. Dabigatran and edoxaban require bridging with parenteral anticoagulation.

97. **What is the treatment of PE?**
Treatment depends upon severity. Severity may be categorized into three groups: massive PE (hypotension, shock), submassive PE (signs of right ventricular strain, elevated NT-proBNP [N-terminal pro brain natriuretic peptide], and elevated troponin), and low-risk PE.

Massive PE: Systemic thrombolytic therapy is indicated for patients without contraindications (see later). In selected patients with massive PE who cannot undergo systemic thrombolysis, catheter-directed thrombolysis should be considered.
Submassive PE: Anticoagulation with IV unfractionated heparin (UH) and careful monitoring of hemodynamics, as some of these patients can progress to massive PE. After monitoring with period of stability, long-term anticoagulation can be started.
Low-risk PE: NOACs (preferred over warfarin or LMWH for long-term treatment). Low-risk patients without significant comorbid conditions may be treated as outpatients with rivaroxaban or apixaban. For initial management of VTE in patients whose continued therapy will be warfarin, dabagatrin, or edoxaban, parenteral anticoagulation with IV UH or SQ LMWH is indicated for at least 5 days.

98. **What is the recommended treatment and duration of anticoagulation for VTE?**
- For patients with PE or proximal leg DVT without history of cancer, NOACs are preferred over warfarin or LMWH.
- For patients with cancer and VTE, LMWH such as enoxaparin is preferred over warfarin or NOACs.
- In patients with provoked VTE, recommended duration of treatment is 3 months.
- In patients with unprovoked VTE, recommended duration of treatment is at least 3 months and after this period the patient should be assessed and considered for long-term anticoagulation, depending on an analysis of risk and benefit.
- Patients at high risk for recurrent PE may require lifelong anticoagulation.
- If warfarin is selected for treatment, it should be dosed to achieve an international normalized ratio (INR) between 2 and 3. Heparin can be discontinued after 5 days and once the INR target is achieved for two consecutive measurements, 24 hours apart.

Kearon C, Akl EA, Ornelas J, et al. Antithrombotic therapy for VTE disease: chest guideline and expert panel report. *Chest.* 2016;149:315–352.

99. **What are contraindications to thrombolytic therapy?**
The **absolute contraindications** include:
- History of intracranial hemorrhage
- Brain tumor (primary or metastatic)

- Recent intracranial surgery or trauma
- Recent ischemic stroke in the last 3 months
- Recent or active internal bleeding.
- Bleeding diathesis
  Relative contraindications include:
- Uncontrolled hypertension
- Thrombocytopenia
- Bleeding tendency
- Recent surgery or invasive procedure
- Pericarditis or pericardial effusion
- Pregnancy
- Age > 75 years old
  Kearon C, Akl EA, Ornelas J, et al. Antithrombotic therapy for VTE disease: chest guideline and expert panel report. Chest 2016;49:315–352.

100. **What is the mortality rate for PE?**
PEs occur in over 600,000 people per year, resulting in over 100,000–200,000 deaths.

101. **How common is pulmonary infarction?**
Approximately 1 in 10 PEs results in pulmonary infarction.

102. **What findings are associated with pulmonary infarction?**
Pleuritic chest pain, hemoptysis, and low-grade fever. Pulmonary infarction is classically described as a wedge-shaped infiltrate that abuts the pleura (Hampton hump) and is often associated with a small pleural effusion that is usually exudative and hemorrhagic.

103. **List the causes of nonthrombotic PE.**
- Fat embolism (following bone trauma or fracture)
- Amniotic fluid embolism
- Air embolism
- Tumor emboli
- Trophoblastic emboli

104. **What are the clinical manifestations of fat embolism?**
Altered mental status, respiratory decompensation, anemia, thrombocytopenia, and petechiae that usually occur 12–36 hours after the inciting trauma.

PULMONARY HYPERTENSION

105. **Define *pulmonary hypertension* (PH).**
A mean pulmonary artery pressure (PAP) ≥ 25 mm Hg. The normal resting PAP is 8–20 mm Hg. The previous criterion of mean PAP ≥ 30 mm Hg during exercise has been updated.

106. **How is PH classified?**
As five groups based on cause. Group 1 is referred to as pulmonary arterial hypertension (PAH), and is distinct from the remaining four, which are referred to as PH. In addition, pulmonary veno-occlusive disease (PVOD) is considered group 1′ and persistent PH of the newborn (PPHN) as group 1″ to indicate they are similar to but distinct from PAH (group 1).
- **Group 1 PAH:** Idiopathic, heritable (*BMPR2* mutations), drug- and toxin-induced (e.g., fenfluramine), and associated with CTD, HIV, portal hypertension, congenital heart disease, schistosomiasis
  - Group 1′ PAH: PVOD
  - Group 1″ PAH: PPHN
- **Group 2 PH:** Due to left-sided heart disease
- **Group 3 PH:** Due to sleep apnea, lung diseases or hypoxia, or both
- **Group 4 PH:** Chronic thromboembolic PH (CTEPH)
- **Group 5 PH:** Due to multiple associations including splenectomy, sickle cell disease, myelo-proliferative disorders, LAM, sarcoidosis, pulmonary LCH, thyroid disorders, and chronic renal failure on hemodialysis

107. **What is the gold standard for the diagnosis of PH?**
Right-sided heart catheterization with the definition of mean PAP ≥ 25 mm Hg. Doppler echocardiography can estimate the systolic PAP, though it has intrinsic and operator-related limitations. A tricuspid insufficiency jet > 2.8 m/sec that corresponds to an estimated systolic PAP of 36 mm Hg is also considered PH.

108. **What factors predict poor prognosis in PH?**
Presence of New York Heart Association (NYHA) CHF functional class III or IV, BNP level ≥ 150 pg/mL, inability to walk more than 250 m in 6 minutes, low peak oxygen consumption, high right atrial pressure, low cardiac index, lack of response to acute vasodilator therapy, presence of pericardial effusion, right atrial and ventricular dilatation, and low tricuspid annular pansystolic excursion are some of the variables that predict worse outcome in PH.

109. **What is the treatment of PAH?**
In general, these patients should be treated by a physician with expertise in the condition. Supportive measures includes diuretics and oxygen therapy. Pulmonary rehabilitation should be considered. An acute vasodilator response to inhalation of nitric oxide or administration of IV prostacyclin at the time of right-sided heart catheterization supports the use of calcium channel blockers. Treatment decisions are based on the patient's functional class and degree of PH. Classes of medication include phosphodiesterase inhibitors type 5 (sildenafil or tadalafil), endothelin receptor antagonists (bosentan, macitentan, ambrisentan), and prostacyclin analogs (epoprostenol, treprostinil, iloprost, selexipag). In group 1 PAH with NYHA CHF functional classes 2–3, combination therapy (such as ambrisentan and tadalafil) is superior to monotherapy. Treatment of CTEPH includes anticoagulation, riociguat (guanylate cyclase stimulant), or IV therapy with a prostanoid. Pulmonary thromboendarterectomy can be curative in selected CTEPH patients.
    Galie JA, Barbera AE, Frost HA, et al. Initial use of ambrisentan plus tadalafil in pulmonary arterial hypertension. *N Engl J Med*. 2015;373:834–844.

110. **Which CTDs have an association with PH?**
Scleroderma carries the highest risk of PH. The prevalence of PH in scleroderma is between 7 and 12%, and its presence is associated with markedly poorer outcomes. The prevalence of PH is less common in systemic lupus erythematosus (SLE), mixed CTD (MCTD), Sjögren syndrome, polymyositis, or RA.

111. **What percentage of patients with acute PE develop CTEPH?**
Up to 4% of patients. These patients may benefit from pulmonary thromboendarterectomy. This intervention is considered in centers with experience for patients with central obstruction of the pulmonary arteries who have abnormal hemodynamic findings and a small number of comorbid conditions.

PLEURAL DISEASES

112. **What is the difference between primary spontaneous pneumothorax (PSP) and secondary spontaneous pneumothorax (SSP)?**
PSP occurs in patients without apparent underlying lung disease (usually tall, thin subjects). **SSP** occurs in patients with underlying lung disease. Other types of pneumothoraces are:
- **Catamenial pneumothorax:** occurs in conjunction with menstruation
- **Traumatic pneumothorax:** classified as iatrogenic (central line placement) and noniatrogenic (blunt or penetrating chest injury)
  Noppen M, De Keukelseir T. Pneumothorax. *Respiration*. 2008;76:7–15.

113. **What is the management of PSP?**
- If the pneumothorax < 20% or < 3 cm (from the lung edge to the chest wall) and the patient has few symptoms, the suggested approach is observation ± oxygen supplementation with appropriate follow-up.
- If the pneumothorax > 20% or > 3 cm or the patient is symptomatic, air evacuation by aspiration or small catheter placement is needed.
- If the pneumothorax occurred more than once, the recommended approach is recurrence prevention with thoracoscopy with talc insufflation or mechanical pleurodesis or chest tube drainage with chemical pleurodesis.

114. **Which diseases are most commonly associated with SSP?**
- Emphysema
- CF

- *P. jiroveci* pneumonia
- Tuberculosis
- IPF
- Sarcoidosis
- LCH
- LAM
- Marfan syndrome
- Lung cancer

115. What is the management of SSP?

Immediate evacuation of the air in the pleural space and recurrence prevention at the first episode. All patients should be hospitalized.

116. What is the difference between transudative and exudative pleural effusions?

The differentiation between these two types of effusions is important because it helps narrow the diagnostic possibilities. **Transudative effusions** are usually due to an imbalance in the hydrostatic or oncotic pressures or both (e.g., CHF, hepatic hydrothorax, nephrotic syndrome, and atelectasis). **Exudative effusions** have a broader differential diagnosis and are generally caused by inflammation, infection, malignancy, and lymphatic abnormalities. According to **Light's criteria** the pleural fluid is an **exudate** if one of the following is present:

- Pleural fluid protein-to-serum protein ratio > 0.5
- Pleural fluid lactate dehydrogenase (LDH)–to–serum LDH ratio > 0.6
- Pleural fluid LDH > two thirds the upper limit of normal serum LDH
  Other criteria for exudative effusion include at least one of the following:
- Pleural fluid cholesterol > 45 mg/dL
- Pleural fluid protein > 2.9 g/dL
- Pleural fluid LDH > 0.45 times the upper limit of normal LDH
  Patients with CHF who are undergoing diuretic therapy may be falsely classified as having an exudative effusion by Light's criteria. The serum to effusion albumin gradient > 1.2 g/dL correctly classifies this effusion as transudative.

  Bielsa S, Porcel JM, Castellote J, et al. Solving the Light's criteria misclassification rate of cardiac and hepatic transudates. *Respirology*. 2012;17:721–726.

117. Describe the most relevant characteristic of the following exudative causes of pleural effusions.

See Table 6.10.

Table 6.10. Disorders Associated With Exudative Pleural Effusions and Pleural Fluid Characteristics

DISORDER	PLEURAL FLUID CHARACTERISTICS
Complicated parapneumonic effusion	pH < 7.2, positive Gram stain or culture
Chylothorax	Triglycerides > 110 mg/dL, presence of chylomicrons
Hemothorax	Hematocrit in fluid > 50% of blood
Tuberculosis	Lymphocyte/neutrophil ratio > 0.75, adenosine deaminase > 50 IU/L, lysozyme > 15 mg/dL, <5% mesothelial cells, positive AFB or culture
Rheumatoid pleurisy	Glucose < 30 mg/dL, pH ~7, LDH > 1000 IU/L
Malignancy (most commonly, lung and breast)	Positive cytologic finding, low glucose concentration in chronic effusion
Esophageal rupture	pH ~6 and high salivary amylase
Peritoneal dialysis	Protein 0.5 g/dL, glucose 300 mg/dL
Pancreatitis	Pleural fluid/serum amylase 3–6:1

AFB, acid-fast bacilli; LDH, lactate dehydrogenase.
Adapted from Sahn SA. The value of pleural fluid analysis. *Am J Med Sci.* 2008;335:7–15.

118. **What are the diseases that can present with a predominantly lymphocytic exudate?**
    - Tuberculosis
    - Lymphoma
    - Malignancy
    - Sarcoidosis
    - Post–coronary artery bypass grafting (CABG)
    - Chylothorax
    - Yellow nail syndrome (triad of yellow nails, lymphedema, and pulmonary symptoms more commonly seen in women and associated with abnormal lymphatics)
    - RA

119. **What are the diseases that can present with eosinophilic exudate (>10% eosinophils)?**
    - Hydropneumothorax
    - Hemothorax
    - Benign asbestos effusions
    - Drug-induced effusions
    - Churg-Strauss syndrome
    - Fungal diseases
    - Parasitic diseases

120. **What are the diseases that can present with pleural fluid acidosis (pH < 7.3)?**
    - Parapneumonic effusion or empyema
    - Esophageal rupture
    - RA
    - Malignancy
    - Lung cancer
    See also Chapter 15, Oncology.

121. **How common is lung cancer?**
    Lung cancer is the second most common cancer after skin cancer but is the leading cause of cancer death in both men and women. More men than women die from lung cancer, but the gap in mortality is steadily narrowing. Lung cancer occurrence is 45% higher among African-American men than among white men. This neoplasia occurs more often in the poor and less educated and has marked regional variation. Interestingly, in developed countries, the frequency of adenocarcinoma has increased while that of squamous carcinoma has decreased.

122. **What is the cause of lung cancer?**
    The risk of lung cancer is based on the interrelationship between the exposure to etiologic agents and individual susceptibility (genetic factors). In the United States, smoking is responsible for 90% of lung cancer. Compared with never smokers, smokers have an approximately 20-fold increase in lung cancer risk. The risk for lung cancer increases with the duration and number of cigarettes smoked per day. The risk of lung cancer decreases among those who quit smoking but remains increased above that of nonsmokers for years after the quit date. Asbestos and cigarette smoking act synergistically to increase the risk of lung cancer. Cigar and pipe smoking are also established causes of lung cancer.

123. **What is asbestosis, and how is it diagnosed?**
    ILD caused by exposure to asbestos fibers is diagnosed by:
    - History of asbestos exposure
    - Presence of latency period (20–30 years) between exposure and symptoms
    - Interstitial fibrosis on chest radiograph or CT scan
    - Symptoms and signs of breathlessness, bibasilar inspiratory crackles, and clubbing
    - Restrictive pattern on pulmonary function testing with reduced D_{LCO}
    - Exclusion of other pneumoconioses
    - Presence of interstitial pneumonia pattern with asbestos bodies on biopsy (if needed)

124. **Is there any benefit in screening patients at high risk for lung cancer?**
    Yes. Early studies showed that screening with chest radiographs and sputum cytology did not decrease lung cancer mortality rate; however, more recent studies (National Lung Screening Trial [NLST]) demonstrated that an annual low-dose CT scan decreases mortality rate. Lung cancer

screening is currently recommended for patients in good health between ages 55 and 80 with 30 pack-years of smoking who are currently smoking or have quit in the past 15 years.

Church TR, Black WC, Aberle DR, et al. Results of initial low-dose computed tomographic screening for lung cancer. *N Engl J Med*. 2014;368:1980–1991.

The National Lung Screening Trial Research Team, Aberle DR, Adams AM, Berg CD, et al. Reduced lung-cancer mortality with low-dose computed tomographic screening. *N Engl J Med*. 2011;365:395–409.

U.S. Preventive Services Task Force. Recommendation Statement: Screening for Lung Cancer Available at: www.uspreventiveservicestaskforce.org/uspstf13/lungcan/lungcanfinalrs.htm. [accessed 09.09.16].

125. What are the clinical predictors for malignancy of SPNs?
Older age, current or past smoking history, history of extrathoracic cancer > 5 years before nodule detection, larger nodule diameter, spiculation, and upper lobe location.

126. What is the management of an SPN?
Initially, to review previous imaging tests to evaluate growth. If the nodule is growing, tissue diagnosis should be obtained unless contraindicated by the presence of significant comorbid conditions. If the nodule has been stable for at least 2 years, no additional diagnostic evaluation is generally needed. An exception to the 2-year rule is adenocarcinoma in situ (formerly known as bronchioloalveolar carcinoma), which may be slow growing and present as nodular ground-glass opacities. At the time a nodule is found, if it has a clear-cut benign pattern, such as complete calcification, no additional evaluation is needed. PET scan is indicated in patients with low to moderate pretest probability and nodule(s) > 8–10 mm. If PET is positive or the patient has a high pretest probability (>60%) of cancer, then consider surgery.

Currently lung nodules are managed per Fleischner Society guidelines. Guidelines should be used for patients who are ≥35 years old and those without history of cancer or not suspected to have cancer.
For low-risk patients
- Nodules ≤ 4 mm, no follow-up needed
- Nodules > 4–6 mm, repeat CT at 12 months, no further follow-up indicated if no change
- Nodules > 6–8 mm, repeat CT at 6-12 months, and then 18–24 months
- Nodules > 8 mm, consider PET or biopsy or repeat CT at 3, 9, and 24 months
For high-risk patients (smoking history, asbestos or other substance exposure increasing risk of lung cancer, first-degree relative with lung cancer)
- Nodules ≤ 4 mm, repeat CT in 12 months, no further follow-up if not changed
- Nodules > 4–6 mm, repeat CT at 6–12 months and then at 18–24 months
- Nodules > 6–8 mm, repeat CT at 3–6 months, then 9–12 months, then 24 months
- Nodules > 8 mm, consider PET or biopsy or repeat CT at 3, 9, and 24 months

MacMahon H, Austin JH, Gamsu G, et al. Guidelines for management of small pulmonary nodules detected on CT scans: a statement from the Fleischner Society. *Radiology*. 2005;237:395–400.

127. Which SPNs can be followed?
Indeterminate nodules > 8–10 mm can be followed by CT scan if the clinical probability of cancer is very low (<5%) or low (<30%) and:
- PET scan is negative for malignancy,
- Needle biopsy is nondiagnostic and PET is negative, or
- Patient prefers a nonaggressive approach.
Serial CT scans should be repeated at 3, 6, 12, and 24 months.

Alberts WM, American College of Chest Physicians. Diagnosis and management of lung cancer executive summary: ACCP evidence-based clinical practice guidelines (2nd ed). *Chest*. 2007;132:1S–422S.

128. What is the difference between small cell carcinoma (SCLC) and non–small cell carcinoma (NSCLC) of the lung?
- **SCLC:** High-grade, mitotically active, undifferentiated carcinomas that derive from neuroendocrine cells. SCLC usually presents as disseminated disease and is capable of secreting bioactive peptides.
- **NSCLC:** Some degree of cytoplasmic differentiation. Depending on the type, the carcinoma can have glandular features, cytoplasmatic mucin, and extracellular keratin. Adenocarcinoma and squamous cell and large cell carcinomas are classified as NSCLC.

129. **What is hypertrophic osteoarthropathy?**
A systemic disorder characterized by painful symmetrical arthropathy of the ankles, wrists, and knees with periosteal new bone formation in the distal long bones of the limbs, usually associated with clubbing.

130. **Which antibody is associated with paraneoplastic neurologic syndromes?**
Type 1 antineuronal nuclear antibodies (anti-Hu antibodies).

131. **Does the presence of paraneoplastic syndrome modify the treatment strategy?**
No. Patients with any of the paraneoplastic syndromes, and otherwise potentially treatable lung cancer, should not be excluded from potentially curative therapies.

CYSTIC FIBROSIS

132. **What are the clinical features of CF?**
    - **Chronic sinopulmonary disease:** Chronic productive cough, nasal polyps, digital clubbing, bronchiectasis, and colonization or infection with *Staphylococcus aureus*, mucoid and nonmucoid *Pseudomonas aeruginosa*, *Stenotrophomonas maltophilia,* and *Burkholderia cepacia*
    - **GI and nutritional abnormalities:** Distal intestinal obstruction syndrome (DIOS), rectal prolapse, pancreatic insufficiency, chronic hepatic disease, and failure to thrive
    - **Salt loss syndromes**
    - **Obstructive azoospermia**

133. **How is the diagnosis of CF made?**
By analysis of sweat chloride by the quantitative pilocarpine iontophoresis sweat test. Sweat chloride levels are abnormally high (>60 mM) in > 90% of patients with CF. With recognition of the genetic basis of CF, analysis may also be done for the CF mutation (cystic fibrosis transmembrane conductance regulator [CFTR]). The most common mutation is ΔF508. Genetic analysis is usually done in patients suspected of having CF who have a normal or borderline sweat chloride test. Also in those patients with confirmed diagnosis, genetic analysis also helps identify patients with a unique mutation that may benefit from new CF specific therapies. The diagnosis of CF is usually made early in life (such as in newborns who undergo screening), but the increasing awareness of the spectrum of disease has led to more frequent diagnosis of CF in adults. Patients diagnosed in adulthood usually have chronic respiratory symptoms, milder lung disease, fewer *Pseudomonas* infections, and more frequent pancreatic sufficiency than patients diagnosed during childhood.

134. **What is the treatment of CF?**
    - Airway clearance
    - Antibiotic therapy: for acute exacerbations and chronic antibiotic suppression (aerosolized tobramycin, aztreonam, and oral azithromycin for selected patients)
    - Mucolytic agents: recombinant human DNase, hypertonic saline
    - Bronchodilators
    - Anti-inflammatory agents: ibuprofen. Inhaled steroids are recommended in selected patients with asthma or ABPA.
    - Oxygen supplementation when indicated
    - Pancreatic enzyme and vitamin supplements
    - Control of hyperglycemia
    - Nutritional support

135. **What are the new targeted therapies for CF patients with selected genotypes?**
New medications have been approved that provide great hope for the future management of patients with CF. This class of medication is called *CFTR modulators.* Currently there are two medications in this class. Ivacaftor is approved for CF patients with G551D mutation (<5% of CF patients have this mutation) and other gating mutations and may result in dramatic improvement. Lumacaftor-ivacaftor is approved for patients who have homozygous mutation ΔF508 and has less significant benefit. Both drugs are extremely expensive.

Mogayzel PJ Jr, Naureckas ET, Robinson KA, et al. Pulmonary Clinical Practice Guidelines Committee. Cystic fibrosis pulmonary guidelines. Chronic medications for maintenance of lung health. *Am J Respir Crit Care Med.* 2013;187:680–689.

MECHANICAL VENTILATION

136. **What are the main modes of mechanical ventilation (MV)?**

Volume-controlled (VC) or pressure-controlled (PC) with assist control (AC) or synchronized intermittent mandatory ventilation (SIMV). In VC ventilation, the volume (based on patient height and ideal body weight) and flow rate or inspiratory time are set. In PC ventilation, the pressure above positive end-expiratory pressure (PEEP) and inspiratory time are set. In PCV, the volume delivered depends upon compliance and is variable. Both VC and PC breaths may be delivered by AC or SIMV. In both modes, patients may trigger breaths. In AC, the patient receives a set number of ventilator breaths and, with self-initiated breaths, receives the same volume or pressure parameters set for ventilator-controlled breaths. In SIMV, patients receive a fixed number of ventilator breaths synchronized to their effort. If the patient breathes between ventilator breaths, some pressure support is provided which augments the spontaneous breath volume. The patient may also be allowed to breathe spontaneously with pressure support and continuous positive airway pressure (CPAP), often as a transition to weaning.

137. **What interventions on the respirator can increase oxygenation?**

Increase in inspired oxygen concentration (FIO_2), increase in the PEEP, and increase in the inspiratory time. Sometimes a change to a more complex ventilator mode such as APRV (airway pressure relief ventilation) or ventilating the patient in the prone position will improve oxygenation.

138. **What ventilator changes can decrease hypercapnia?**

Increasing the minute ventilation by increasing the respiratory rate or tidal volume can decrease hypercapnia.

139. **Why is plateau pressure important?**

Ventilator-associated lung injury may occur with high plateau pressures. The goal is to maintain plateau pressures < 30 cm H_2O. Change in peak or plateau pressure above set limits may be a clue to important problems in the patient or with the ventilator and repeated high pressure alarms require assessment. When only the peak inspiratory pressure increases, consider bronchospasm, obstruction of the endotracheal tube by secretions, or the patient biting the tube. Elevation in both peak and plateau pressures can be caused by abnormalities at several sites, including the lung parenchyma (pulmonary edema or pneumonia), pleural space (pneumothorax or large effusion), chest wall (obesity), or abdomen (obesity and ascites). High pressures can cause barotrauma such as pneumothorax and pneumomediastinum.

140. **In what setting does auto-PEEP occur?**

Auto-PEEP occurs when there is incomplete exhalation prior to the next ventilator breath, resultant air trapping, and hyperinflation. This occurs most commonly in the setting of obstructive lung disease or severe asthma. Risk factors include high respiratory rates, high tidal volumes, short exhalation times, and expiratory airflow obstruction. Auto-PEEP can cause increased intrathoracic pressure resulting in hypotension and increased work of breathing related to difficulty in triggering the ventilator. Blood pressure will improve if the ventilator is briefly disconnected. The ventilator should then be adjusted to increase the expiratory time. Sometimes the application of small amounts of extrinsic PEEP will be beneficial.

Brochard L. Intrinsic (or auto) positive end expiratory pressure during spontaneous and assisted ventilation. *Intensive Care Med.* 2002;10:1376–1378.

141. **What conditions should be met before discontinuation of a patient from MV?**

The patient should be alert and hemodynamically stable and able to cough and handle oral secretions and the underlying cause of the respiratory failure should be improved or resolved. The inspired oxygen concentration should be $< 50\%$, and the patient should tolerate a spontaneous breathing trial for 30 minutes to 2 hours.

142. **What are the indications of using noninvasive positive-pressure ventilation (NIPPV)?**

Patients who are awake and able to handle oral secretions and have:
- Acute hypercapnic respiratory failure, particularly in COPD
- Cardiogenic pulmonary edema
- Acute hypoxic respiratory failure (use of high-flow nasal cannula may be preferred)
- Postextubation respiratory failure (use with caution). COPD patients may benefit, but in other patients use of NIPPV for postextubation respiratory failure may increase mortality risk.

Consider conventional MV if the NIPPV has not resulted in clear improvement of the condition in 2 hours.

143. **What are the main characteristics of ARDS?**
The definition of ARDS was recently revised by a multidisciplinary group (The Berlin Definition) and includes:
- Onset occurs within 7 days of an insult such as sepsis, pneumonia, aspiration, or massive transfusion.
- Chest radiograph will show bilateral opacifications not fully explained by another process such as lobar collapse or pleural effusions.
- The respiratory failure must not be fully explained by cardiogenic pulmonary edema or fluid overload.
- There is significant impairment of oxygenation with severity based on the PaO_2/FIO_2 ratio. Severity is defined as follows:
  - Mild: $PaO_2/FIO_2 > 200$ but ≤ 300 on 5 cm H_2O or more of CPAP
  - Moderate: $PaO_2/FIO_2 > 100$ but ≤ 200 on 5 cm H_2O or more of CPAP
  - Severe: PaO_2/FIO_2 of < 100 on 5 cm H_2O or more of CPAP
  ARDS mortality rate is about 30% for those with mild ARDS and 46% for severe ARDS.
The ARDS Definition Task Force. Acute respiratory distress syndrome: the Berlin Definition. *JAMA*. 2012;307:2526–2533.

144. **What is the recommended strategy to ventilate patients with acute ARDS?**
Low tidal volumes (6 mL/kg of ideal body weight based on patient's height). The ARDSNet study showed this application reduced inflammation, lung injury, and duration of MV and improved survival.
The Acute Respiratory Distress Syndrome Network, Brower RG, Matthay MA, Morris A, et al. Ventilation with lower tidal volumes as compared with traditional tidal volumes for acute lung injury and the acute respiratory distress syndrome. *N Engl J Med*. 2000;342:1301–1308.

MISCELLANEOUS

145. **What is the alveolar hemorrhage syndrome?**
The occurrence of bleeding into the alveolar spaces due to disorders that disrupt the alveolar-capillary basement membrane. Alveolar hemorrhage syndrome is diagnosed by progressive reddening of fluid aliquots on bronchoalveolar lavage (BAL) or presence of $> 20\%$ hemosiderin-laden macrophages on BAL.

146. **Which diseases are associated with alveolar hemorrhage syndrome?**
- **Immunologic:** Goodpasture syndrome, renal-pulmonary syndromes, glomerulonephritis, SLE, graft vs. host disease
- **Toxic:** crack cocaine, abciximab, penicillamine
- **Traumatic**
- **Increased vascular pressure:** mitral stenosis

147. **Which are the pulmonary complications of HIV infection?**
See Table 6.11. Early in the course of disease, patients with HIV have respiratory disorders similar to those in the general population. As the disease progresses, opportunistic infections may occur. The CD4+ lymphocyte count is the most reliable marker for the risk of opportunistic infection.

Table 6.11. Infectious Agents in Pulmonary Complications of Human Immunodeficiency Virus Infection

PULMONARY COMPLICATION	INFECTIOUS AGENT
Focal infiltrate	Bacteria, *Mycobacterium tuberculosis*, *Pneumocystis jiroveci*
Diffuse infiltrate	*P. jiroveci*, *M. tuberculosis*, Kaposi sarcoma
Diffuse nodules	Kaposi sarcoma, *M. tuberculosis*, fungi
Pneumothorax	*P. jiroveci*, *M. tuberculosis*
Pleural effusion	Bacteria, *M. tuberculosis*, Kaposi sarcoma
Mediastinal adenopathy	*M. tuberculosis*, atypical mycobacteria, Kaposi sarcoma
Cavities	*M. tuberculosis*, *P. jiroveci*, *Pseudomonas aeruginosa*

Adapted from Rosen MJ. Pulmonary complications of HIV infection. *Respirology*. 2008;13:181–190.

148. What are the main characteristics of LAM?

Smooth muscle infiltration and cystic destruction of the lung due to mutations in tuberous sclerosis genes. LAM is rare and found almost exclusively in women. Up to a third of the cases are associated with the tuberous sclerosis complex of seizures, brain tumors, and cognitive impairment. Clinically, LAM patients have progressive dyspnea, recurrent pneumothoraces, lymphadenopathy, chylothorax, and abdominal angiomyolipomas and lymphangiomyomas. Sirolimus, an mTOR inhibitor, has been shown to stabilize lung function, reduce symptoms, and improve quality of life.

McCormack FX, Inoue Y, Moss J, et al. Efficacy and safety of sirolimus in lymphangioleiomyomatosis. *N Engl J Med.* 2011;364:1595–1606.

Meraj R, Wikenheiser-Brokamp KA, Young LR, et al. Lymphangioleiomyomatosis: new concepts in pathogenesis, diagnosis, and treatment. *Semin Respir Crit Care Med.* 2012;33:486–497.

149. What are the main characteristics of pulmonary LCH?

Focal Langerhans cell granulomas that infiltrate and destroy terminal bronchioles. Imaging studies show a combination of nodules (with or without cavitation) and thick- and thin-walled cysts. Pulmonary LCH is a rare disorder of unknown cause that predominantly affects young smokers. The diagnosis usually requires lung biopsy showing the characteristic granulomas. Treatment consists of smoking cessation, steroids, and cytotoxic agents. Many patients recover or remain stable after smoking cessation.

Tazi A. Adult pulmonary Langerhans' cell histiocytosis. *Eur Respir J.* 2006;27:1272–1285.

150. What is high-altitude pulmonary edema (HAPE)?

A noncardiogenic form of pulmonary edema that usually occurs 2–3 days after rapid ascent to altitudes < 8500 feet. Hypoxic pulmonary vasoconstriction causes PH with capillary stress fractures, release of inflammatory mediators, and decreased nitric oxide synthesis, leading to edema. HAPE can be prevented by a slow ascent, nifedipine, phosphodiesterase inhibitors (tadalafil, sidenafil), acetazolamide, and salmeterol. Treatment includes immediate descent to lower altitude, O_2, nifedipine, phosphodiesterase inhibitors, and dexamethasone.

151. What determines if a patient with respiratory disease will need oxygen during air travel?

- Spo_2 on room air > 95%: No oxygen.
- Spo_2 on room air < 92%: Oxygen supplementation.
- Spo_2 on room air between 92% and 95% with risk factors: Perform a hypoxic challenge. Oxygen will be needed if Pao_2 < 50 mm Hg on Fio_2 of 15%.

The airplane cabin pressure is maintained at pressures that correspond to altitudes < 8000 feet. At this altitude, the Pao_2 is equivalent to an Fio_2 of 15.1%. Patients cannot carry their own oxygen tank on commercial flights but can use their own battery-powered O_2 concentrators. Patients already on oxygen can increase O_2 flow by 1–2 L.

152. What is the difference between arterial gas embolism (AGE) and decompression sickness (DS) in divers?

- **AGE:** Caused by air retention in the lungs that expands during ascent with rupture of alveoli and adjacent vessels. The air bubbles embolize and can reach the brain. Treatment includes 100% O_2 inhalation and hyperbaric oxygen recompression.
- **DS:** Caused by bubble formation on the tissues during rapid ascent because of inability of the nitrogen gas to leave the tissue in an orderly fashion. Patients have different symptoms such as pruritus, joint pain, paralysis, or unconsciousness. Treatment includes 100% O_2, aspirin, fluids, and hyperbaric oxygen recompression.

SLEEP

See also Chapter 2, General Medicine and Ambulatory Care, and Chapter 17, Neurology.

153. What changes occur in the respiratory system during sleep?

Decreased Pao_2 and increased $Paco_2$ because the hypercapnic and hypoxic ventilator responses decrease when compared with responses during wakefulness. The decreased responses become more prominent during rapid eye movement (REM) sleep. In addition, the upper airway dilator muscle tone decreases, favoring the development of upper airway obstruction in susceptible individuals.

154. **Define *apnea* and *hypopnea*.**
   - **Apnea:** Cessation or near cessation of airflow to < 20% of baseline for at least 10 seconds.
   - **Hypopnea:** A 30% decrease in airflow for at least 10 seconds accompanied by at least a 4% decline in oxygen saturation. The apnea-hypopnea index (AHI) is the number of apneas plus hypopneas in 1 hour of sleep. This index defines the severity as:
     - Mild: 5–15
     - Moderate: 16–30
     - Severe: >30

155. **How are apneas classified?**
   - **Obstructive:** Inspiratory effort is present.
   - **Central:** Inspiratory effort is absent.
   - **Mixed:** A central event is followed by an obstructive one.

156. **What are the risk factors for developing obstructive sleep apnea (OSA)?**
   - Male gender
   - Menopause
   - Older age
   - Obesity
   - Use of tobacco and alcohol
   - Hypothyroidism
   - Acromegaly
   - Neuromuscular disorders
   - Stroke
   - Increased neck circumference
   - Mandibular hypoplasia
   - Enlarged tonsils and adenoids
   - Medications (e.g., muscle relaxants)

157. **What are the consequences of having OSA?**
   - Increased mortality rate
   - Insulin resistance
   - CAD
   - CHF
   - CVA
   - Cardiac arrhythmias
   - Hypertension
   - PH
   - Mood disorders (depression or anxiety or both)
   - Erectile dysfunction
   - GERD

158. **What is the treatment of OSA?**
   - **General measures:** Sleep hygiene, appropriate positioning during sleep, safety counseling, weight loss, and avoidance of muscle relaxants and alcohol
   - **Positive airway pressure:** CPAP, BiPAP, and autotitrating positive airway pressure (APAP)
   - **Oral devices:** Mandibular repositioners and tongue-retainers
   - **Upper-airway surgery:** Uvulopalatopharyngoglossoplasty, maxillomandibular advancement, tracheostomy and upper airway stimulator in selected patients
     Strollo PJ Jr, Soose RJ, Maurer JT, et al. Upper-airway stimulation for obstructive sleep apnea. *Sleep Medicine Pearls.* 2nd ed. *N Engl J Med.* 2014;370:139–149.

159. **How is central sleep apnea (CSA) classified?**
   - **Hypercapnic:** decreased responsiveness to hypercapnias seen in neuromuscular disorders and use of opioids
   - **Nonhypercapnic:** increased response to hypercapnia as seen in idiopathic CSA, Cheyne-Stokes respiration, and high-altitude periodic breathing

160. **What is the treatment of CSA?**
   - Avoidance of respiratory depressants
   - Correction of underlying conditions such as heart failure

- Positive airway pressure (CPAP, BiPAP, adaptive seroventilation [ASV]). Selection is based on type of CSA and patient's tolerance.
- Supplemental oxygen for patients who failed PAP therapy or who remain hypoxic with PAP therapy, patients with hyperventilatory type CSA

161. What are the main characteristics of narcolepsy?
Excessive sleepiness, cataplexy (episodes of muscle atonia/hypotonia precipitated by intense emotions), sleep paralysis, and sleep hallucinations (at sleep onset or on awakening). **Cataplexy is the only pathognomonic characteristic of narcolepsy.** Not all patients have all the components, and narcolepsy is usually diagnosed by history. Polysomnography followed by multiple sleep latency is required when cataplexy is absent. Treatment includes sleep hygiene and combination of modafinil or other stimulants, hypnotic agents, or sodium oxybate, and REM sleep suppressants (selective serotonin reuptake inhibitors [SSRIs] and tricyclic antidepressants).

162. What are parasomnias?
Physical or experiential phenomena that occur in association with both non–REM (NREM) and REM sleep. NREM parasomnias are confusional arousals, sleep terrors (abrupt awakening with intense fear and autonomic discharge), and sleepwalking. REM parasomnias include nightmares and REM sleep behavioral disorder ("dream-enacting").

163. What is restless leg syndrome (RLS)?
An unpleasant sensation or urge to move in the legs that increases with inactivity and at night and improves transiently with movement. RLS may be associated with anemia, uremia, pregnancy, aging, Parkinson disease, diabetes mellitus, alcohol intake, and certain medications. Polysomnography is rarely needed because the diagnosis is obtained by clinical history. Treatment includes iron if ferritin < 50 μg/L and dopaminergic agents such as pramipexole and ropinirole. Treatment is not indicated for asymptomatic periodic limb movement during sleep.

WEBSITES

1. American College of Chest Physicians: www.chestnet.org
2. National Heart, Lung, and Blood Institute: www.nhlbi.nih.gov
3. American Thoracic society: www.thoracic.org
4. Global Initiative for COPD: www.goldcopd.org
5. Global Initiative for asthma: www.ginaasthma.org

BIBLIOGRAPHY

1. Berry RB, Wagner MH. *Sleep Medicine Pearls.* 2nd ed. Philadelphia: Elsevier; 2003.
2. Strauss M, Aksenov I. *Diving Science.* Champaign, IL: Human Kinetics; 2004.
3. West JB. *Pulmonary Pathophysiology: The Essentials.* 8th ed. Philadelphia: Lippincott Williams & Wilkins; 2008.

CHAPTER 7

GASTROENTEROLOGY

Rhonda A. Cole, MD, FACG, Nisreen Husain, MD, and Yamini Natarajan, MD

I had opportunities for the examination of the interior of the stomach, and its secretions, which have never before been so fully offered to any one.

William Beaumont (1785–1853) and Andrew Combe (1797–1847)
"Experiments and Observations on the Gastric Juice and the Physiology of Digestion"

GASTROINTESTINAL BLEEDING

1. **How does gastrointestinal (GI) bleeding present?**
   - **Hematemesis:** Vomiting of blood, which may appear bright red or similar to coffee grounds (bleeding originating proximal to ligament of Treitz)
   - **Melena:** Black, tarry, foul-smelling stool (90% originate proximal to ligament of Treitz)
   - **Hematochezia:** Bright red blood per rectum, blood mixed with stool, bloody diarrhea or clots
   - **Occult GI blood loss:** Normal-appearing stool that is FIT (fecal immunochemical test) positive
   - **Symptoms only:** Syncope, dyspnea, angina, palpitation, confusion, dizziness, or shock

2. **Describe the initial care of the patient with acute GI bleeding.**
   - Resuscitation!
   - Assess patient's hemodynamic stability by measuring blood pressure (including orthostatic readings, if appropriate) and pulse.
   - Obtain venous access with a large-bore intravenous (IV) cannula.
   - Begin crystalloid infusion, preferably with normal saline.
   - Obtain appropriate laboratory tests: complete blood count (CBC), prothrombin time (PT), international normalized ratio (INR), platelets, and routine chemistry including liver function tests such as alanine aminotransferase (ALT/SGPT) and aspartate aminotransferase (AST/SGOT).
   - Type and cross-match for blood transfusion.

3. **Describe the management of a hemodynamically unstable patient with GI bleeding.**
   - Immediate fluid infusion with normal saline
   - Blood transfusion (see next question)
   - Placement of a nasogastric (NG) tube to assess for evidence of an upper GI source and, if present, to document the rapidity of bleeding
   - Close monitoring of vital signs and urinary output in an intensive care unit (ICU) setting
   - Assessment of other underlying disease involving the cardiovascular, GI (especially liver), renal, pulmonary, and central nervous systems

4. **Cite a good rule of thumb for determining the use of blood transfusions.**
   Transfuse the blood as quickly as the patient loses or has lost blood. For example, if the patient presents with massive hematochezia and is hemodynamically compromised, packed red blood cells (RBCs) should be given immediately. Conversely, if the patient presents with iron-deficiency anemia, hemoccult positive stools, and stable vital signs, blood transfusions may not be needed. The decision to transfuse must be individualized. Evidence supports refraining from transfusing patients unless their hemoglobin is <7 g/dL (including those patients with stable coronary artery disease).

5. **What information in the patient's medical history may suggest a potential bleeding source?**

Medical History	Potential Source
Chronic liver disease	Varices or portal hypertensive gastropathy
Aortic graft, abdominal aortic aneurysm	Aortoenteric fistula
Renal disease, aortic stenosis, hereditary hemorrhagic telangiectasia	Angiodysplasias
Helicobacter pylori infection	Peptic ulcer disease, malignancy
Nonsteroidal anti-inflammatory drug (NSAID) use	Peptic ulcer disease
Tobacco abuse	Peptic ulcer disease, malignancy
Alcohol abuse	Malignancy, varices or portal hypertensive gastropathy
Gastroenteric anastomosis, bariatric surgery	Marginal ulcers

6. **List the common causes of upper GI bleeding.**
   - Peptic ulcer disease (duodenal and gastric)
   - Esophageal or gastric varices
   - Severe or erosive esophagitis
   - Nonspecific mucosal abnormalities
   - Angiodysplasia (vascular ectasia)
   - Tumors or mass lesions
   - Mallory-Weiss tears (most commonly seen in patients with forceful vomiting)
   No lesion is identified in ~10–15% patients.

7. **What is the recommended approach to patients who present with a bleeding peptic ulcer and are *H. pylori* positive (Table 7.1)?**
   To treat the *H. pylori* infection and confirm eradication. Treatment of *H. pylori* has been found to significantly reduce the risk of rebleeding. See later questions for treatment recommendations.

Table 7.1. Skin Findings in Conditions That Cause GI Bleeding

DISEASE	ASSOCIATED SKIN FINDINGS
Peutz-Jeghers syndrome	Pigmented macules on lips, palms, soles
Malignant melanoma	Melanoma
Hereditary hemorrhagic telangiectasias	Telangiectasias on lips, mouth, palms, soles (Osler-Weber-Rendu syndrome)
Blue rubber bleb nevus	Dark, blue soft nodules
Bullous pemphigoid	Oral and skin bullae
Neurofibromatosis	Café au lait spots, axillary freckles, neurofibromas
Cronkhite-Canada syndrome	Alopecia; hyperpigmentation of creases, hands, and face
Cirrhosis	Spider angiomas, Dupuytren contracture
Neoplasm	Acanthosis nigricans
Kaposi sarcoma	Cutaneous Kaposi sarcoma
Ehlers-Danlos syndrome	Skin fragility, keloids, paper-thin scars
Pseudoxanthoma elasticum	Yellow "chicken fat" papules and plaques in flexural areas
Turner syndrome	Webbing of neck, purpura, skin nodules

From Berger T, Silverman S. Oral and cutaneous manifestations of gastrointestinal disease. In Sleisenger MH, Fordtran JS, editors. *Gastrointestinal Disease*. 5th ed. Philadelphia: WB Saunders; 1994, pp 268–285.

8. **What are clinical predictors of poor outcome in patients presenting with bleeding ulcers?**
   - Age > 60 years
   - Presence of fresh blood per NG tube or rectum
   - Hemodynamic instability despite aggressive resuscitative measures
   - Presence of four or more comorbid illnesses (e.g., cardiac disease, liver disease, diabetes, chronic obstructive pulmonary disease [COPD], sepsis, or renal failure)

9. **What are the indications for surgery in a patient with upper GI bleeding?**
   - Two failed attempts at endoscopic therapy
   - Perforation, obstruction, or bleeding from a cancer
   - GI bleeding that is not responsive to resuscitative measures
   - Rehospitalization for peptic ulcer bleeding

10. **List the more common causes of lower GI bleeding.**
    - Hemorrhoids (most common under the age of 50)
    - Ischemia
    - Neoplasms (polyps and cancer)
    - Diverticulosis with bleeding from either the right or the left colon
    - Vascular ectasias
    - Colitis
    - Small bowel or upper GI bleeding source

11. **Does melena indicate a right-sided colonic source and hematochezia a left-sided source?**
    Not always. The stool color depends on colonic transit time. If the stool remains in contact with intestinal bacteria that degrade hemoglobin, the resulting stool is melanotic. Although right-sided lesions are usually associated with melena (dark, tarry stools) and left-sided lesions with hematochezia (the passage of bright red blood per rectum), the opposite can also be seen. Therefore, the evaluation of a patient with hematochezia must include examination of the proximal colon.

12. **What causes esophageal varices?**
    Any condition that elevates the pressure in the hepatic portal system leads to varices. The normal portal venous pressure is approximately 10 mm Hg but increases to >20 mm Hg in portal hypertension.

13. **What is the most common cause of esophageal varices in the Western world?**
    Alcohol-related cirrhosis.

14. **What factors predict that esophageal varices will likely bleed?**
    - Location of varices: Gastroesophageal junction
    - Size of varices: Larger size >> small size
    - Appearance of varices: "Red color signs"
    - Clinical features of patient: Higher Child classification, previous variceal bleed
    - Variceal pressure:
      - ≤13 mm Hg (0% chance)
      - >15 and ≤16 mm Hg (50% chance)
      - >16 mm Hg (70% chance)

15. **Is there a role for proton pump inhibitors (PPI) in a patient presenting with peptic ulcer bleeding?**
    Yes. PPIs have been shown to decrease the risk of rebleeding, decrease the need for repeated endoscopic therapy, and decrease the need for surgery. Certain select studies have also shown that PPIs improve mortality rates. Best results have been confirmed when PPIs are administered intravenously as an 80-mg IV bolus followed by 8 mg/hr continuous infusion for 48–72 hours.

16. **What is Meckel diverticulum? What is its role in GI bleeding?**
    A true diverticulum of the small intestine formed from incomplete obliteration of the vitelline duct that is the most common congenital anomaly of the GI tract. GI bleeding related to Meckel diverticulum is caused by ulceration of the small bowel due to acid secretion by ectopic gastric mucosa within the diverticulum.

17. **What is the classic description of Meckel diverticulum?**
The "Rule of Twos":
- Occurs in 2% population
- 2:1 male:female ratio
- Located within 2 feet from the ileocecal valve
- Can be 2 inches in length (although this varies)
- ~2–4% patients will develop a complication typically by the age of 2
- If bleeding occurs, the Meckel diverticulum is usually lined by two different types of mucosa (most commonly intestinal and gastric mucosae)

18. **What are potential causes of bleeding in patients with suspected small bowel bleeding (previously known as *obscure* GI bleeding)?**
- In patients age < 40: Inflammatory bowel disease (IBD), Dieulafoy lesion, Meckel diverticulum, neoplasia, polyposis syndrome
- In patients age > 40: Angiodysplasia, Dieulafoy lesion, neoplasia, NSAID ulcers

LIVER DISEASE AND HEPATITIS

19. **What are the common blood tests used to assess liver function?**
- ALT/SGPT: Relatively specific for liver injury
- AST/SGOT: Less specific for liver injury because it is also found in skeletal muscles, cardiac muscles, and other organs
- Alkaline phosphatase (ALP): Increased in cholestatic disease but can also be released from bone
- γ-Glutamyltransferase (GGT): An enzyme of intrahepatic biliary canaliculi, more specific marker for cholestasis than ALP
- Bilirubin: Can be separated into direct (or conjugated) or indirect (unconjugated). Direct bilirubin is more specific for liver disease and diseases blocking the bile ducts.
- PT and albumin: Markers of liver synthetic function

20. **Which type of viral hepatitis is a major health concern?**
Hepatitis C virus (HCV). Currently, 130–150 million people are infected with HCV worldwide, and approximately 3.2 million people are infected with HCV in the United States. Veterans enrolled for care at the Veterans Administration have higher rates (5.4%) of HCV infection than the general U.S. population (1.8%). In addition to the known sources of risk and exposure, at least one third of all infected patients have no known exposures for this potentially debilitating illness.

21. **What complications are associated with HCV?**
- Cirrhosis
- Hepatocellular carcinoma (HCC)
- Decompensated liver disease requiring liver transplantation

22. **What are the differences among hepatitis A, B, and C?**
Hepatitis A, called *infectious hepatitis,* is easily spread by the fecal/oral route. The hepatitis A virus (HAV) causes a short-lived, acute hepatitis that is not followed by chronic liver disease. Immunoglobulin G (IgG) antibodies to HAV remain positive for life. To determine whether the hepatitis is acute, one must look for IgM antibodies in the serum.
    Hepatitis B, called *serum hepatitis,* is contracted by contact with blood or other bodily secretions from an infected individual, usually through a break in the skin, sexual contact, perinatal transmission, use of a contaminated needle in IV drug users, or accidental needlestick in health care workers. Transmission through blood transfusions is less common when blood donors are volunteers and are screened for hepatitis B surface antigen (HBsAg). Unlike HAV, hepatitis B virus (HBV) infection may cause chronic disease and cirrhosis *and* predisposes to HCC. A carrier state occurs when infected patients demonstrate persistent HBsAg without clinically evident disease and are able to transmit the disease.
    Hepatitis C is the form of hepatitis most commonly contracted by contact with blood or other bodily secretions from an infected individual. HCV infection is the most common viral cause of chronic liver disease in the United States and increases the patient's risk for HCC.

23. **Who should receive the HAV vaccine?**
- All children 1 year of age (12–23 months old)
- Travelers to endemic areas

- Military personnel and others with occupational exposure
- Users of illegal injectable and noninjectable drugs
- People with high-risk sexual practices (e.g., men who have sex with men)
- Children and adolescents in communities with routine HAV vaccination due to high incidence
- Patients with clotting factor disorders
- Patients with chronic liver disease
- People who work with infected primates or in an HAV research laboratory

24. **Summarize the usual serologic response to naturally acquired HBV infection.**
See Fig. 7.1.

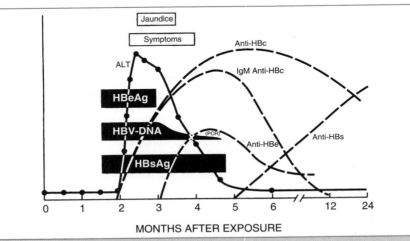

Fig. 7.1. Clinical and serologic course of a typical case of acute hepatitis B. ALT, alanine aminotransferase; anti-HBC, antibody to hepatitis B core antigen; anti-HBe, antibody to HBeAg; anti-HBs, antibody to HbsAg; HBeAg, hepatitis Be antigen; HBsAg, hepatitis B surface antigen; HBV-DNA, hepatitis B virus DNA; PCR, polymerase chain reaction. *(From Hoofnagle JH. Acute viral hepatitis. In Mandell GL, Bennett JE, Dolin R, et al, editors.* Principles and Practice of Infectious Diseases. *4th ed. New York: Churchill Livingstone; 1995, p 1143.)*

25. **How should you treat a health care worker with a recent (<48 hours) needlestick exposure to HBV?**
By administering hepatitis immunoglobulin, 0.06 mL/kg intramuscularly (IM), as soon as possible within 7 days of exposure. If the health care worker has not previously received the HBV vaccine, the vaccination program should be initiated with the usual three doses—the first dose within 14 days after exposure and again at 1 and 6 months.

26. **How is HCV transmitted? What are the possible courses of the disease?**
Blood transfusions, shared and contaminated needles among IV drug abusers, intranasal drugs, high-risk sexual behavior, tattoos, and vertical transmission from infected mothers to unborn children (accounts for 3–6%). Before 1992, when widespread screening of blood donors began in the United States, HCV was also commonly spread through blood transfusions and organ transplants. Nearly 30% of persons infected with HCV have no known risk exposure. Detection of HCV-RNA by polymerase chain reaction is the definitive test for active HCV. Chronic infection developed in at least 55–85% of affected persons. Five percent to 20% of persons infected will develop cirrhosis over a period of 20–25 years, and they are at risk for the development of HCC.

27. **How can HCV transmission be prevented? How is HCV infection treated?**
Risk modification to minimize exposure is the only means of prevention. No vaccine is available for HCV. Treatment is recommended for all HCV infected patients, unless life expectancy is limited. HCV treatment regimens have dramatically changed in the last 5 years. Direct-acting antiviral (DAA) drugs have revolutionized HCV treatment, and now treatment regimens using DAA drugs have superseded the use

of pegylated interferon and ribavirin alone. Choice of treatment regimen and length of treatment depend on the HCV genotype and whether cirrhosis is present or absent. Cure rates (measured as sustained virologic response) have improved from 50–80% to greater than 90% with the advent of DAA drugs.

American Association for the Study of Liver Diseases and the Infectious Diseases Society of America. HCV guidance: recommendations for testing, managing, and treating hepatitis C, Available at: www.hcvguidelines.org. Accessed January 19, 2018.

28. **How is hepatitis D virus (HDV) or delta virus transmitted?**
Through contact with the blood or other body fluids of an infected person. HDV is a very small RNA virus that contains a defective genome and requires HBsAg to become pathogenic. Infection may occur under two circumstances:
- In conjunction with simultaneous infection with HBV in a previously unexposed patient (coinfection).
- In the chronic carrier of HBsAg (superinfection).

29. **What is hepatitis E virus (HEV)?**
A small RNA virus that is transmitted via fecal-oral route due to fecal contamination of drinking water. HEV is endemic to Southeast and Central Asia, Africa, and Mexico and is responsible for large epidemics of acute hepatitis in these areas but is rare in the United States. HEV may be transmitted from animal contact in areas where animal hosts are abundant, including pig farming areas in the United States. HEV illness is particularly severe in pregnant women with mortality rates from acute liver failure approaching 20%.

30. **What conditions require hospitalization for a patient with acute viral hepatitis?**
- Older age
- Underlying systemic illnesses
- Encephalopathy
- Ascites
- Bilirubin > 15 mg/dL
- Hypoglycemia
- Pregnancy
- Underlying chronic hepatitis of another cause
- Volume depletion or inability to hold down fluids
- PT > 15 seconds; INR > 1.4
- Albumin < 3 mg/dL
- Social problems that may result in loss to follow-up

31. **What blood tests predict fulminant hepatic failure?**
Worsening PT/INR or bilirubin with improving transaminases.

32. **What three conditions result in very high transaminases (>1000 U/L)?**
- Ischemia
- Viral hepatitis
- Drug-induced hepatitis

33. **What causes chronic liver disease?**
- Viral HBV and HCV
- Wilson disease
- Alcoholism
- Drug-induced disease
- Autoimmune hepatitis
- Alpha$_1$-antitrypsin deficiency (AATD)
- Hemochromatosis
- Nonalcoholic fatty liver disease (NAFLD)

34. **Discuss the significant features of fulminant hepatic failure.**
Fulminant hepatic failure usually occurs in a previously healthy patient who develops acute and progressive liver failure. Early symptoms include malaise, anorexia, and low-grade fever with progression to signs and symptoms of liver failure (e.g., jaundice, encephalopathy). The mortality rate is approximately 80% if untreated. The most common cause of death in fulminant hepatic failure is either brain edema due to increased intracranial pressure or sepsis. The most definitive therapy is liver transplantation.

35. List the common causes of fulminant hepatic failure.
    - **Drugs:** Acetaminophen (most common cause of acute liver failure in the United States), amiodarone, ecstasy (illicit drug), isoniazid, ketoconazole, NSAIDs, rifampin, phenytoin, propylthiouracil, sulfonamides, tetracycline, tricyclic antidepressants, and troglitazone
    - **Indeterminate:** Second most common cause of acute liver failure in the United States
    - **Viral:** HAV, HBV (most common viral cause of fulminant hepatic failure), HCV, HDV, and HEV
    - **Herbal medications:** Jin bu huan, comfrey, germander
    - **Toxins:** *Amanita phalloides*, carbon tetrachloride, trichloroethylene
    - **Vascular:** Budd-Chiari syndrome, veno-occlusive disease, ischemia or hypoxia, portal vein thrombosis
    - **Miscellaneous:** Malignant infiltration, Wilson disease, acute fatty liver of pregnancy, Reye syndrome, heatstroke, autoimmune hepatitis

36. What is Budd-Chiari syndrome?
    Partial or complete obstruction of blood flow out of the liver, usually involving the hepatic veins. The patient characteristically presents with hepatomegaly, ascites, and abdominal pain. Underlying causes include myeloproliferative disorders (~50%), malignancy, infections of the liver, oral contraceptive pills, pregnancy, collagen vascular diseases, and hypercoagulable states.

37. What is Wilson disease?
    An autosomal recessive genetic disorder characterized by an accumulation of copper in the liver, basal ganglia, and cornea with resulting Kayser-Fleischer rings. The Wilson gene is *ATP7B*, which is either absent or markedly diminished in Wilson disease. The lack of the gene results in diminished synthesis of ceruloplasmin or defective transport of hepatocellular copper into bile for excretion. The diagnosis of Wilson disease is suspected in patients with low serum ceruloplasmin, increased copper in the liver on biopsy, and increased urinary copper excretion.

38. What is AATD?
    An autosomal codominant disorder (meaning two different versions of the gene can be active or expressed) resulting from a defect in the *SERPINA1* gene. The disorder is characterized by hepatic disease including cirrhosis and HCC, pulmonary emphysema mainly involving the lung bases, panniculitis, vascular disease including arterial aneurysms and fibromuscular dysplasia, and glomerulonephritis. The actual degree of organ involvement depends on the phenotype of the patient.

39. What is hereditary hemochromatosis (HH)?
    An autosomal recessive disorder resulting from the mutations in the *HFE* gene that lead to increased intestinal iron absorption. Patients with HH have increased iron deposition in their vital organs resulting in liver disease, skin pigmentation, diabetes mellitus, arthropathy, impotence, and cardiac enlargement with heart failure or conduction defects. (Remember "bronze diabetes" for iron accumulation in skin causing bronze color and in pancreas causing diabetes.)

NUTRITION

40. Name six common vitamins and trace minerals and the clinical manifestations of their respective deficiency states in adults.
    - **Thiamine (vitamin B_1):** Beriberi, muscle weakness, tachycardia, heart failure, Wernicke-Korsakoff syndrome
    - **Niacin (vitamin B_3):** Pellagra, glossitis
    - **Vitamin A:** Xerophthalmia, hyperkeratosis of skin
    - **Vitamin E:** Cerebellar ataxia, areflexia
    - **Zinc:** Hypogeusia, acrodermatitis, diarrhea
    - **Chromium:** Glucose intolerance primarily in diabetics

41. What disorders lead to major and minor folate deficiency?
    Major disorders
    - Chronic alcoholism
    - Celiac sprue
    - Tropical sprue
    - Blind loop syndrome

Minor disorders
- Crohn disease
- Following partial gastrectomy
  Because folate is mainly absorbed in the upper small intestine, malabsorption is worse in disorders that affect the upper gut; however, any intestinal disorder accompanied by a decrease in dietary folate intake or rapid transport may result in folate deficiency.

42. An elderly man presents with profound peripheral neuropathy and a markedly low serum level of vitamin B_{12}. Physical examination reveals an abdominal scar consistent with previous laparotomy, but the patient does not remember what kind of surgery was done. What two operations may result in vitamin B_{12} deficiency? Why?
    Gastrectomy and terminal ileum resection. Vitamin B_{12} absorption starts in the acid environment of stomach, where it binds R proteins. In the duodenum, the R proteins are hydrolyzed off the vitamin B_{12} in the presence of an alkaline environment, which then allows for further binding of vitamin B_{12} with intrinsic factor (produced in the stomach). Vitamin B_{12} cannot be absorbed unless it is bound to intrinsic factor. If the patient's stomach was completely or partially removed, he would have insufficient intrinsic factor. This patient may also have had resection of a large portion (>100 cm) of terminal ileum, the site of absorption of the vitamin B_{12}–intrinsic factor complex.

43. How are vitamin B_{12} deficiencies related to surgery treated?
    With IM cyanocobalamin (vitamin B_{12}) injections.

44. What is the most common disorder of carbohydrate digestion in humans?
    Lactase deficiency. Lactase-deficient adults retain 10–30% of intestinal lactose activity and develop symptoms (diarrhea, bloating, and gas) only when they ingest sufficient lactose. Symptoms result from the colonic bacteria metabolizing lactose to methane, carbon dioxide, and short-chain fatty acids. Lactase deficiency is highest among African Americans, Hispanic Americans, Asian Americans, and Native Americans.

45. After avoiding dairy products, the patient's GI symptoms have disappeared. Does this confirm the diagnosis of lactose deficiency?
    No. The diagnosis cannot be made simply by symptom improvement after the patient avoids dairy products for 2 weeks. Many patients who respond to these manipulations are actually not lactase-deficient. The diagnostic test to be used is the lactose hydrogen breath test.

46. Which patients may need total parenteral nutrition (TPN)?
    - Any patient in whom enteral feedings are either impossible or contraindicated
    - Burn victims
    - Cancer patients
    - Patients undergoing bone marrow transplants
    - Critically ill patients
    - Perioperative management of severely malnourished patients

47. What are the most common complications of TPN?
    Infections as well as venous thrombosis, nonthrombotic occlusion, and other mechanical complications during line placement. Catheter-related complications can be minimized by maintaining strict and reproducible technique as well as meticulous line care.

48. What long-term complications may arise?
    Liver dysfunction, bone disease, and gallstones. In prolonged TPN, especially when excessive carbohydrate calories are given, patients frequently develop liver tenderness and transaminase elevations. The increased liver values are thought to reflect hepatic steatosis. AST/SGOT and ALT/SGPT abnormalities usually return to normal when TPN is discontinued. If TPN is continued, one should decrease the dextrose infusion and increase the amount of fat calories provided. Metabolic bone disease similar to osteomalacia and osteoporosis can occur. The addition of acetate or phosphate may offset the urinary calcium losses and restore positive calcium balance in these patients. Cholelithiasis and cholecystitis are related to gallbladder stasis.

49. What is body mass index (BMI)?
    BMI = Body Weight in kilograms (kg)/Height in meters squared (m^2).

BMI is the first step in determining the degree of obesity in overweight individuals. BMI provides a better estimate of total body fat rather than body weight alone.

National Heart, Lung, and Blood Institute. Calculate your body mass index. Available at: www .nhlbi.nih.gov/guidelines/obesity/BMI/bmicalc.htm. Accessed November 15, 2016.

50. **Summarize the standards of weight and obesity according to BMI.**
Weight categories:

BMI	Category
<18.5 kg/m^2	Underweight
18.5–24.9 kg/m^2	Normal
25.0–29.9 kg/m^2	Overweight
>30 kg/m^2	Obese

The "obese" category is further categorized as:

BMI	Class
30.0–34.9 kg/m^2	Class I
35.0–39.9 kg/m^2	Class II
≥40 kg/m^2	Class III (extreme or massive obesity)

51. **What is the rationale for routinely screening for obesity in the U.S. adult population?**
Obesity is a chronic disease that is considered to be a global epidemic. Obesity is associated with a significant increase in overall mortality rate and increases the risk of many disorders. Health care expenditures are significantly higher for overweight and obese individuals. Without screening, many high-risk patients may not receive counseling about health risks, lifestyle changes, obesity treatment options, and risk factor reduction.

52. **What comorbid diseases are directly attributable to obesity?**
- Type 2 diabetes mellitus
- Hypertension
- Coronary artery disease
- Cerebrovascular accident
- Cancer (colon, esophageal, gastric, gallbladder, liver, breast, uterine, leukemia, and prostate)
- Osteoarthritis
- Gallstones
- NAFLD
- Gout
- Gastroesophageal reflux disease (GERD)
- Infection
- Depression

53. **What GI disorders are associated with obesity?**
- **Esophagus:** GERD symptoms, erosive esophagitis, Barrett esophagitis, esophageal adenocarcinoma (EAC)
- **Gallbladder:** gallstones and cancer
- **Pancreas:** cancer, worsened acute pancreatitis
- **Colon:** adenoma and cancer
- **Liver:** NAFLD, advanced HCV-related disease, cirrhosis, and HCC
- **Stomach:** nonspecific abdominal pain, bloating, diarrhea, cancer

CANCER

54. **At what age should screening for colorectal cancer (CRC) begin?**
Age 50 in asymptomatic people without increased risk of CRC. Several studies increasingly support screening beginning at age 45 for African-American women. Routine screening ends at age 75; screening is performed on an individual basis for patients age 76 to 85.

55. What are commonly used methods for colon cancer screening?

Test	Frequency
Fecal immunochemical testing (FIT)	Annually
Flexible sigmoidoscopy with insertion to the splenic flexure	Every 5 years
Air-contrast barium enema (ACBE)	Every 5 years
Computed tomographic colonography (CTC)	Every 5 years
Colonoscopy	Every 10 years

The U.S. Preventive Services Task Force (USPSTF) currently recommends the following:
- The guidelines support the following screening options:
  - Stool-based tests: Guaiac studies (gFOBT [fecal occult blood test]), FIT, FIT-DNA
  - Direct visualization: Flexible sigmoidoscopy ± FIT, colonoscopy, computed tomography (CT) colonography
  - Serologic test: *SETP9* DNA test
- USPSTF found no head-to-head studies proving that any one of these tests was superior to the others.
   U.S. Preventive Services Task Force, Bibbins-Domingo K, Grossman DC, Curry SJ. Screening for colorectal cancer: US Preventive Services Task Force Recommendation Statement. *JAMA.* 2016;315(23):2564–2575.

56. List the risk factors for CRC.
- Colon cancer in a first-degree relative < 60 years old
- Chronic ulcerative colitis with involvement beyond left colon
- Familial adenomatous polyposis
- Hereditary nonpolyposis colon cancer (HNPCC)
- Personal history of uterine, endometrial, or breast cancer
- Lynch syndrome (HNPCC)
- Personal history of CRC or adenomatous polyp > 1 cm
- Family cancer syndrome
- Advanced age > 80 years

57. What is the significance of an adenomatous polyp?
Malignant potential. Nearly all colonic carcinomas arise from adenomatous polyps. These polyps are most often in the colon, giving rise to symptoms only when they become large, and are frequently detected incidentally on colonoscopic examination or barium enema. About 75% of adenomatous polyps are tubular adenomas, 15% are tubulovillous adenomas, and the rest are villous adenomas.

58. What factors increase the likelihood that a polyp is malignant?
Villous tumors are more likely to be malignant than tubular adenomatous polyps. Other factors that relate to malignant potential include tumor size > 1 cm, degree of cellular atypia, and number of polyps present.

59. How are adenomatous polyps managed?
Through endoscopic polypectomy. Patients with polyps should undergo colonoscopy at routine intervals so that additional polyps may be removed before they progress to malignancy.

60. Summarize the guidelines for repeat surveillance time intervals of patients after polypectomy.
- Hyperplastic polyps that should be considered "normal": 10 years
- One or two adenomatous polyps < 1 cm, and negative family history of CRC: 10 years
- Two adenomatous polyps or adenomatous polyp > 1 cm: 5 years
- Villous appearance or high-grade dysplasia: 3 years
- Family history of CRC: 3 years
- Large, sessile, or numerous adenomatous polyps: 3–5 years, based on clinical judgment that should be individualized for each patient
- Dirty preparation: Variable based on clinical judgment with acknowledgment that patient had suboptimal examination and, therefore, lesions may have been missed
- Piecemeal resection of > 2 cm sessile adenoma: 2–6 months to exclude dysplasia of the flat mucosa then subsequent follow-up based on clinical judgment
- Negative follow-up for new polyps: every 5 years

61. **Summarize the guidelines for surveillance of patients after CRC resection.**
Colonoscopy should be performed in the perioperative period to clear the colon of any synchronous lesions. The next colonoscopy following clearing should be 3 years postoperatively *or* according to postpolypectomy surveillance guidelines if a polyp is detected in the perioperative colonoscopy. In the patient with a history of HNPCC, follow-up should be every 1–2 years. In patients with rectal cancer, a flexible sigmoidoscopy or rectal endoscopic ultrasound (US) should be performed every 3–6 months for 2 years because rectal cancer has a greater tendency to recur locally.

62. **Name the most common malignant neoplasms of the small intestine.**
- Adenocarcinoma (45%)
- Carcinoid (34%)
- Leiomyosarcoma (18%)
- Lymphoma (3%)

63. **List the most common benign neoplasms of the small intestine in order of frequency.**
Leiomyoma > lipoma > adenoma > hemangioma.

64. **What is the most common primary cancer of the liver?**
HCC ranks fourth in the annual mortality cancer rate in the United States. HCC often coexists with cirrhosis, but it can also occur in noncirrhotic patients, including those with HBV infection.

65. **What are the risk factors for HCC?**
Major risk factors
- Chronic HBV and HCV
- Dietary exposure to aflatoxin B1
- Cirrhosis

Minor risk factors
- Cigarette smoking
- Oral contraceptives
- HH
- Wilson disease
- AATD

66. **How is HCC diagnosed?**
According to the American Association for the Study of Liver Diseases (AASLD), the diagnosis of HCC is guided by the nodule size and characteristic features on imaging studies.
- For nodule < 1 cm: No initial diagnosis of HCC but surveillance with US every 3–6 months.
- For nodule 1–2 cm in a cirrhotic liver: The diagnosis of HCC is made when the lesion has an appearance typical of HCC on two dynamic studies (CT scan, contrast US, or magnetic resonance imaging [MRI] with contrast).
- For nodule > 2 cm: The diagnosis of HCC is made when there are typical features of HCC on one dynamic imaging technique or an alpha-fetoprotein (AFP) value > 200 ng/mL.
- Biopsy is recommended for nodules > 1 cm when the diagnosis is not clear on dynamic imaging studies or AFP.

67. **What are the GI endocrine tumors and their associated findings and symptoms?**
- **Gastrinoma (Zollinger-Ellison syndrome [ZES]):** Peptic ulcer disease, diarrhea, and gastric acid hypersecretion; frequently associated with multiple endocrine neoplasia type I (MEN I)
- **Insulinoma:** Hypoglycemia
- **VIPoma (vasoactive intestinal peptide):** Watery diarrhea, hypokalemia, and achlorhydria known as *WDHA syndrome* or *Verner-Morrison syndrome*
- **Glucagonoma:** Dermatitis, glucose intolerance, weight loss, and anemia
- **Somatostatinomas:** Abdominal pain, weight loss

INFLAMMATORY BOWEL DISEASE

68. **How do Crohn disease (CD) and ulcerative colitis (UC) differ?**
See Table 7.2.

Table 7.2. Distinguishing Features of Crohn Disease and Ulcerative Colitis

	CROHN DISEASE	ULCERATIVE COLITIS
Symptoms	Pain is more common; bleeding is uncommon	Diarrhea with a bloody-mucosal discharge, cramping
Location	Can affect GI tract from mouth to anus	Limited to colon
Pattern of colonic involvement	Skip lesions	Continuous involvement
Histology	Transmural inflammation, granulomas, focal ulceration	Mucosal inflammation, crypt abscesses, crypt distortion
Radiologic	Terminal ileal involvement, deep ulcerations, normal haustra between involved areas, strictures, fistulas	Rectum involved, shortened colon, absence of haustra (lead-pipe sign)
Complications	Obstruction, fistulas, abscesses, kidney stones, gallstones, vitamin B_{12} deficiency	Bleeding, toxic megacolon, colon cancer

GI, gastrointestinal.

69. **What are the pathologic gold standards for differentiating between CD and UC?**
The finding of a granuloma = CD. The finding of crypt abscesses = UC. These findings are documented in fewer than one third of patients, but when found, they are considered pathognomonic for these diseases.

70. **What are the extraintestinal manifestations of IBD?**
- **Musculoskeletal:** arthritis, ankylosing spondylitis, sacroiliitis, osteoporosis
- **Mucocutaneous:** erythema nodosum, pyoderma gangrenosum, aphthous ulcers
- **Ocular:** iritis, uveitis, episcleritis
- **Hepatobiliary:** fatty liver, gallstones, primary sclerosing cholangitis, cholangiocarcinoma
- **Renal:** kidney stones
- **Miscellaneous:** venous thrombosis, weight loss, hypoalbuminemia, anemia, vitamin and electrolyte disturbances

71. **What is the goal of treatment for IBD?**
To induce and maintain remission, which will ultimately help with patient's symptoms and improve quality of life. When choosing a treatment, careful consideration of the adverse effects of short- and long-term therapy is essential.

72. **What are the classes of medications available to treat CD and UC?**
- **5-Aminosalicylates (5-ASA):** include sulfasalazine, mesalamine, olsalazine
- **Antibiotics:** such as ciprofloxacin and metronidazole
- **Glucocorticoids**
- **Immunomodulators:** such as 6-mercaptopurine and azathioprine, methotrexate, cyclosporine
- **Biologic agents:** include anti-tumor necrosis factor (TNF) modulators (i.e., infliximab, adalimumab, certolizumab) and anti-alpha-4 integrin agents (i.e., natilizumab and vedolizumab)

73. **If medical therapy fails, what are the surgical options for IBD?**
In CD, fibrostenotic structuring disease does not respond well to medical therapy and can lead to bowel obstruction that requires limited small bowel or ileocolonic resection. In UC, medically refractory disease is treated with curative total proctocolectomy with either end-ileostomy or ileal pouch anal anastomosis (for this a neorectum is made from a segement of ileum and connected to the anus to maintain continence).

74. **Name the side effects associated with each IBD medication.**
- **Sulfasalazine:** agranulocytosis, headache, rash, reversible male infertility
- **Mesalamine:** pancreatitis, hepatitis, pericarditis, pleuritis
- **Azathioprine:** pancreatitis, bone marrow suppression, hepatitis

- **Glucocorticoids:** sleep and mood disorders, acne, adrenal suppression, infections, glucose intolerance, cataracts, bone loss, impaired wound healing
- **Anti-TNF agents:** infections, lymphoma, nonmelanoma skin cancer, psoriatic lesions, heart failure
- **Methotrexate:** hepatotoxicity, hypersensitivity pneumonitis, megaloblastic anemia, teratogenic
- **Natalizumab:** progressive multifocal leukoencephalopathy

ULCERS

75. **What are the two major functions of acid secretion in the stomach?**
    - Activation of the enzyme pepsin by converting pepsinogen to pepsin, initiating the first stages of protein digestion
    - Antibacterial barrier that protects the stomach from colonization

76. **List the factors that lead to recurrent ulcer after ulcer surgery.**
    - Untreated *H. pylori* infection
    - NSAID use
    - Incomplete vagotomy
    - Adjacent nonabsorbable suture that acts as an irritant
    - "Retained antrum" syndrome, in which antral tissue left behind at surgery produces a continued source of gastric acid production
    - Antral G-cell hyperplasia (uncommon)
    - ZES (gastrinoma)
    - Gastric cancer
      Other factors that may contribute to recurrent ulcers but have not necessarily been implicated as primary causes include smoking, enterogastric reflex (bile acid reflux), primary hyperparathyroidism, and gastric bezoar.

77. **List the most common causes of peptic ulcer disease in order of frequency.**
    - *H. pylori* infection (duodenal >> gastric)
    - NSAIDs (gastric >> duodenal)
    - Hyperacidity states (e.g., ZES)

78. **How common is *H. pylori* infection?**
    Approximately 1 in 10 persons worldwide are infected, and *H. pylori* infection is the most infectious disease worldwide. This microaerophilic spiral bacterium that inhabits the mucous layer of the stomach is associated with the development of peptic ulcer disease and occurs in > 90% of patients with duodenal ulcers. Although millions are infected, only about 10% develop peptic ulcer disease.

79. **Which diseases are strongly associated with *H. pylori* infection?**
    - Peptic ulcer disease (duodenal >> gastric)
    - Chronic active gastritis
    - MALToma (mucosa-associated lymphoid tissue)
    - Gastric carcinoma

80. **How is *H. pylori* infection treated?**
    Over 60 treatment regimens for *H. pylori* have been used. Triple therapy (two antibiotics plus a PPI) is the most widely used regimen, resulting in eradication of *H. pylori* in approximately 80% of patients. At present, no regimen results in 100% cure. Knowledge of the antibiotic resistance patterns in the community assists in antibiotic selection. A typical oral treatment regimen with an eradication rate of 70–80% includes:
    - Clarithromycin, 500 mg twice daily
    - Amoxicillin, 1000 mg twice daily
    - PPI, maximum dose twice daily

81. **What are the diagnostic tests for *H. pylori*?**
    - **Noninvasive tests:** Do not require sampling of the gastric mucosa
    - **Serologic testing:** IgG antibody, useful for initial diagnosis but not useful to confirm eradication after treatment
    - **Urea breath tests:** Useful for initial diagnosis and to confirm eradication

- **Stool antigen tests:** For *H. pylori,* useful for initial diagnosis and to confirm eradication
- **Invasive tests:** Require sampling of the gastric mucosa
- **Histologic examination:** Excellent sensitivity and specificity but expensive
- **Polymerase chain reaction:** Excellent sensitivity and specificity but not widely available
- **Culture:** Excellent specificity but expensive, difficult to perform, and not widely available
- **Rapid urease testing:** Inexpensive, provides rapid results

82. **What is the clinical triad of ZES?**
Remember the mnemonic PIG:

P = Peptic ulcer disease
I = Islet cell tumor of nonbeta cells of pancreas
G = Gastric acid hypersecretion

83. **What are other diagnostic features of ZES?**
In addition to symptoms of peptic ulcer disease (abdominal pain, heartburn, GI bleeding, and weight loss), diarrhea is common and may be present for many years before diagnosis. ZES should be suspected in patients with a compatible clinical history and gastric acid hypersecretion or a personal/family history of MEN type I.

84. **How is the diagnosis of ZES made?**
- Serum fasting gastrin concentration > 1000 pg/mL
- Secretin stimulation test with an increased serum gastrin level of ≥ 200 pg/mL
- Localization studies: octreotide scan, endoscopic ultrasonography, CT of the abdomen

PANCREATITIS

85. **What are the most common causes of acute pancreatitis in the United States?**
Choledocholithiasis, ethanol abuse, and idiopathic causes account for > 90% of cases of acute pancreatitis in the United States. Most patients previously classified with idiopathic pancreatitis have subsequently been found to have diminutive gallstones (microlithiasis). In the private hospital setting, 50% of patients with acute pancreatitis have gallstones (gallstone pancreatitis). In public hospitals, up to 66% of first episodes are caused by excessive alcohol consumption. Other causes include hypertriglyceridemia, autoimmune disorders, and malignancy.

86. **Which drugs have the strongest association with acute pancreatitis?**
- Asparaginase
- Azathioprine
- 6-Mercaptopurine
- Dideoxyinosine
- Pentamidine
- Vinca alkaloids
- Didanosine
- Valproic acid
- Mesalamine
- Estrogen preparations
- Opiates
- Tetracycline
- Corticosteroids
- Trimethoprim/sulfamethoxazole
- Sulfasalazine
- Furosemide

87. **List other drugs that may be associated with acute pancreatitis.**
- **Analgesics:** Acetaminophen, piroxicam, NSAIDs, morphine
- **Diuretics:** Thiazides, metolazone
- **Antibiotics:** Sulfonamides, erythromycin, ceftriaxone
- **Anti-inflammatory agents:** Salicylates, 5-ASA products, cyclosporine
- **Toxins:** Ethanol, methanol

- **Hormones:** Oral contraceptive pills
- **Others:** Octreotide, cimetidine, valproic acid, ergotamine, methyldopa, propofol, alpha interferons, zalcitabine, isotretinoin, ritonavir, ranitidine

88. **List Ranson criteria for the prognosis in acute pancreatitis.**
See Table 7.3.

Table 7.3. Ranson Criteria for Prognosis in Acute Pancreatitis

ON ADMISSION	IN INITIAL 48 HOURS
Age > 55 yr	Hematocrit decrease of > 10%
WBC count > 16,000/mm^3	BUN rise of > 5 mg/dL
Serum LDH > 350 IU/L	Serum calcium < 8 mg/dL
Blood glucose > 200 mg/dL	Pao$_2$ < 60 mm Hg
SGOT/AST > 250 IU/L	Base deficit > 4 mEq/L Estimated fluid sequestration > 6 L

BUN, blood urea nitrogen; LDH, lactate dehydrogenase; PaO$_2$, arterial oxygen partial pressure; SGOT/AST, aspartate aminotransferase; WBC, white blood cell.
From Ranson JH. Etiologic and prognostic factors in human acute pancreatitis: a review. *Am J Gastroenterol.* 1982;77:633–638.

89. **How are Ranson criteria used to make a prognosis?**
By calculating the number of criteria present. When there are fewer than three positive signs, the patient has mild disease and an excellent prognosis. The mortality rate is 10–20% with three to five signs and > 50% with six or more signs.

90. **What components are used in the bedside index of severity in acute pancreatitis (BISAP)?**
- Blood urea nitrogen (BUN) > 25 mg/dL
- Impaired mental status
- >2 SIRS (systemic inflammatory response syndrome) criteria
- Age > 60
- Presence of pleural effusion
Common themes in these scores include increased inflammation and third spacing/decreased fluid in vascular space.

91. **How is BISAP used to calculate prognosis?**
A score of 0 indicates low mortality rate (<2%). Mortality rate increases greatly with a score of 3 or more.

92. **When are antibiotics indicated in pancreatitis?**
When > 30% pancreatic necrosis and suspicion of infection are present.

93. **What conditions other than acute pancreatitis may cause an increase in serum amylase?**
- Macroamylasemia
- Renal failure
- Mesenteric infarction
- Parotitis
- Burns
- Cholecystitis
- Post–endoscopic retrograde cholangiopancreatography
- Perforated peptic ulcer disease
- Ruptured ectopic pregnancy
- Diabetic ketoacidosis
- Peritonitis

- Tumors of pancreas, salivary glands, ovary, lung, prostate
- Pancreatitis complications (pseudocyst, abscess, ascites)
- Medications

94. **What features of a pancreatic pseudocyst suggest that surgery or percutaneous drainage is indicated?**
    - Persistence for > 6 weeks
    - Development of symptoms, including abdominal pain, nausea, emesis, obstruction (intestinal, biliary), and weight loss
    - Increasing size of pseudocyst
    - Onset of complications (infection)
    - Possible malignancy

95. **What may be a serious vascular complication of pancreatitis?**
    Splenic vein thrombosis, which is associated with pancreatic or peripancreatic inflammation and tumors. Splenic vein thrombosis classically results in gastric varices without accompanying esophageal varices. The definitive therapy is surgical splenectomy.

96. **What is chronic pancreatitis?**
    Irreversible damage to the pancreas resulting in inflammation, fibrosis, and destruction of exocrine and endocrine tissue.

97. **What are the causes of chronic pancreatitis?**
    - **Alcohol:** Most common cause
    - **Genetic:** Mutations in cationic trypsinogen gene (*PRSS1* mutation), cystic fibrosis transmembrane conductance regulator gene (*CFTR*), and pancreatic secretory trypsin inhibitor gene (*SPINK1*)
    - **Metabolic:** Hypercalcemia and hyperlipidemia
    - **Other:** Autoimmune, tropical calcific pancreatitis, and pancreatic duct obstruction

VASCULAR DISEASE

98. **What is dysphagia lusoria?**
    Vascular compression of the esophagus by an aberrant right subclavian artery that leads to difficulty swallowing. The right subclavian artery in dysphagia lusoria arises from the left side of the aortic arch and compresses the esophagus as it courses from the lower left to the upper right side posterior to the esophagus.

99. **What is intestinal angina?**
    Symptoms of pain after eating that occur when all three of the major intestinal arteries (celiac axis, superior mesenteric, and inferior mesenteric) (Fig. 7.2) to the bowel are obstructed by atherosclerosis. Patients with intestinal angina usually have the triad of crampy, epigastric discomfort (postprandial pain), nausea, and occasional diarrhea. The discomfort is similar to that of cardiac angina (substernal chest pressure with exercise), hence the term *intestinal angina*. Patients lose weight simply by avoiding meals secondary to a fear of recurrent symptoms. The pain is usually out of proportion to tenderness on physical examination.

100. **How is chronic mesenteric ischemia diagnosed and treated?**
    By noninvasive US and Doppler evaluation of the mesenteric arteries. CT and MR angiography can be used in patients when a diagnosis cannot be made by US because of obesity or overlying bowel gas. If the noninvasive tests are suggestive of significant disease, a more invasive angiogram is performed to verify findings. Treatment for severe stenoses is balloon angioplasty and stenting of *both* the celiac axis and the superior mesenteric artery. If occlusions are noted, surgical bypass or endarterectomy is the more accepted therapy.

101. **Which two colonic segments are most commonly involved in ischemic colitis? Why?**
    The splenic flexure, which lies between the inferior and the superior mesenteric arteries, and the rectosigmoid junction, which lies between the inferior mesenteric and the interior iliac arteries. Ischemic colitis most commonly occurs in the regions lying in the "watershed" areas between two adjacent arterial supplies.

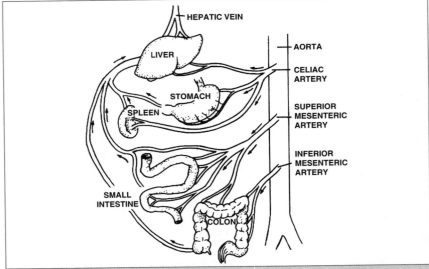

Fig. 7.2. Major splanchnic organs and vessels. *(From McNally PR, editor.* GI/Liver Secrets. *Philadelphia: Hanley & Belfus; 1996.)*

102. Describe the presentation of hepatic hemangioma.

A benign blood vessel tumor that is most commonly found incidentally on imaging examinations of the liver. Hemangiomas are usually single, asymptomatic, and < 5 cm. The incidence is thought to range from 0.4% to 20%.

103. Define *superior mesenteric artery syndrome.*

A narrowing of the aortomesenteric angle that may lead to compression of the duodenum and may be caused by weight loss, immobilization, scleroderma, neuropathies that reduce duodenal peristalsis (e.g., diabetes), and use of narcotics. Because of its anatomic position anterior to the aorta and posterior to the superior mesenteric vessels, the third portion of the duodenum is prone to luminal compression by these vessels.

DIARRHEA

104. What are the four pathophysiologic mechanisms of diarrhea?
- **Osmotic:** Due to the presence of an osmotically active agent in the intestinal lumen that cannot be absorbed and, therefore, draws fluid in the intestinal lumen
- **Exudative:** Due to infection, food allergy, celiac sprue, IBD, collagenous colitis, and graft-versus-host disease
- **Secretory:** Due to mucosal stimulation of active chlorine ion secretion associated with *Escherichia coli*, *Vibrio cholerae*, hormone-producing tumors, bile acids, and long-chain fatty acids
- **Altered intestinal transit**

105. What causes osmotic diarrhea?

The ingestion of excessive amounts of a poorly absorbable but osmotically active solute. Substances such as mannitol or sorbitol (seen in patients chewing large quantities of sugar-free gum), magnesium sulfate (Epsom salt), and some magnesium-containing antacids can cause osmotic diarrhea. Carbohydrate malabsorption also may cause osmotic diarrhea through the action of unabsorbed sugars (lactulose). Clinically, osmotic diarrhea stops when the patient fasts (or stops ingesting the poorly absorbable solute).

106. Name three characteristics of secretory diarrhea?
   - Stool volumes > 1 L/day
   - Occurs both day and night
   - Persists even with fasting
     See Table 7.4.

Table 7.4. Secretory Versus Osmotic Diarrhea

	SECRETORY	OSMOTIC
Stool osmolar gap	<50 mOsm/kg	>50 mOsm/kg
Effect of fasting	None	Ceases
Presence of WBCs, RBCs, fat	None	May be present

RBCs, red blood cells; WBCs, white blood cells.

107. How do you calculate the stool osmotic gap, and what is its purpose?
   The osmotic gap is determined by subtracting the sum of the stool sodium and potassium concentration multiplied by a factor of 2 from 290 mOsm/kg to account for unmeasured anions (i.e., $290 - 2([Na^+] + [K^+])$. An osmotic gap of > 125 mOsm/kg suggests an osmotic diarrhea, whereas a gap of < 50 mOsm/kg suggests a secretory diarrhea.

108. What are common causes of bloody diarrhea in adults?
   Shigella, nontyphoidal *Salmonella* (rare), *Campylobacter,* and enteroinvasive or enterohemorrhagic *E. coli. Shigella* is the most common cause of acute bloody diarrhea.

109. A 50-year-old woman complains of six to eight loose stools per day for 1 month. The cause is not immediately evident after a careful history and physical examination. What diagnostic tests should be performed at this stage?
   - **Blood tests:** CBC, serum chemistry profile, urinalysis
   - **Stool studies:** Bacterial culture and sensitivity, Sudan stain for fat, Wright stain, white blood cells (WBCs), occult blood testing, phenolphthalein test for the presence of laxative ingestion, and calculation of stool osmotic gap

110. Discuss the role of flexible sigmoidoscopy in the diagnosis of diarrhea.
   Flexible sigmoidoscopy is a very important part of the examination in most patients with chronic and recurrent diarrhea. In patients aged ≥ 50 years, this should be expanded to a full colonoscopy to allow screening for polyps. Examination of the rectal mucosa may reveal pseudomembranes seen with antibiotic-associated diarrhea, discrete ulceration typical of amebiasis, or a diffusely inflamed granular mucosa seen in UC. Biopsy specimens can be obtained through the scope for histologic examination, and fresh stool samples can be collected for cultures.

111. What is the most common cause of antibiotic-associated colitis?
   Clostridium difficile. Patients usually have a history of antibiotic use, especially cephalosporins, pencillins, clindamycin, or one of the fluoroquinolone antibiotics, or recent hospitalization. The diagnosis is usually based on a history of recent antibiotic use, detection of *C. difficile* toxin A or B in stool sample, PCR stool testing for *TCDB* gene, or sigmoidoscopy revealing colonic pseudomembranes.

112. What are the risk factors for *C. difficile*–associated diarrhea (CDAD) infection?
   - Antibiotics (most widely recognized cause)
   - Hospitalization
   - Advanced age
   - Severe illness
   - Gastric acid suppression
   - Use of an NG tube
   - GI surgery
   - Cancer chemotherapy
   - Obesity
     Of note, CDAD can occur in the absence of any risk factors.

113. **What is traveler's diarrhea?**

A common term given to the onset of diarrhea in patients who have traveled to other countries, usually in the Third World, where the enteric flora are different. Eighty percent of cases are caused by bacteria that can be transmitted via a fecal-oral route. Viruses account for 10% of cases, and parasites cause 2–3%. In the remainder of cases, the cause is unknown. Unfortunately > 50% travelers who visit these underdeveloped countries may develop *traveler's diarrhea.*

114. **How can traveler's diarrhea be prevented?**
- Eat only foods that are recently cooked and served hot.
- Avoid nonbottled water, ice, and cold beverages diluted with nonbottled liquids (e.g., fruit juices).
- Drink only bottled, sealed, carbonated, or boiled beverages.
- Avoid fresh, unpeeled fruits and vegetables that are washed in nonbottled water.

115. **What are the most common organisms implicated in traveler's diarrhea?**

Bacteria	*Virus*	*Parasites*
E. coli	Rotavirus	Giardia lamblia
Campylobacter jejuni	Norovirus	Cryptosporidium parvum
Salmonella	Enteric adenovirus	Cyclospora cayetanensis
Shigella		Microsporidium
Vibrio parahaemolyticus		Cystoisospora belli
Aeromonas hydrophila		Entamoeba histolytica (rare)
Plesiomonas shigelloides		
Yersinia enterocolitica		

116. **What prophylactic regimens are recommended for traveler's diarrhea?**

Nonantimicrobial agent
- Bismuth subsalicylate (Pepto-Bismol), 2 tablets four times a day

Antimicrobial agents
- Rifaximin, 200 mg once or twice daily
- Ciprofloxacin, 500 mg once daily
- Norfloxacin, 400 mg once daily *(not available in United States)*

The U.S. Centers for Disease Control and Prevention (CDC) currently recommends antibiotic prophylaxis only for short-term travelers with high-risk conditions such as immunosuppression, cardiac or renal disease, human immunodeficiency virus (HIV) status, previous organ transplantation; or those taking critical trips when acute diarrhea may significantly impede the trip's purpose.

Cooper B. Travelers' diarrhea. In: Brunette GW, ed. *The Yellow Book.* New York: Oxford University Press; 2016. Available at: wwwnc.cdc.gov/travel/page/yellowbook-home. [Accessed 24.09.16].

117. **How does the time of onset of illness relate to the possible causes of food poisoning?**

See Table 7.5.

NONHEPATITIS LIVER DISEASE

118. **Explain the Child-Pugh system for staging cirrhosis.**

See Table 7.6.

119. **What is a model for end-stage diseases (MELD) score?**

A validated chronic liver disease severity scoring system that uses a patient's serum bilirubin, serum creatinine, and the INR or PT to predict survival. The MELD score is mainly used to allocate donor organs for liver transplantation.

United Network for Organ Sharing. MELD/PELD calculator documentation. Available at: www.unos.org/wp-content/uploads/unos/MDLE_PELD_Calculator_Documentation.pdf. Accessed September 24, 2016.

120. **Summarize the clinical manifestations of liver disease and their pathogenic basis.**

See Table 7.7.

Table 7.5. Causes of Food Poisoning

ONSET	SYMPTOMS AND SIGNS	AGENTS
1 hr	Nausea, vomiting, abdominal cramps	Heavy metal poisoning (copper, zinc, tin, cadmium)
1 hr	Paresthesias	Scrombroid poisoning, shellfish poisoning, Chinese restaurant syndrome (MSG), niacin poisoning
1–6 hr	Nausea and vomiting	Preformed toxins of *Staphylococcus aureus* and *Bacillus cereus*
2 hr	Delirium, parasympathetic hyperactivity, hallucinations, disulfiram reaction, or gastroenteritis	Toxic mushroom ingestion
8–16 hr	Abdominal cramps, diarrhea	In vivo production of enterotoxins by *Clostridium perfringens* and *B. cereus*
6–24 hr	Abdominal cramps, diarrhea, followed by hepatorenal failure	Toxic mushroom ingestion (*Amanita* spp.)
16–48 hr	Fever, abdominal cramps, diarrhea	*Salmonella, Shigella, Clostridium jejuni*, invasive *Escherichia coli, Yersinia enterocolitica, Vibrio parahaemolyticus*
16–72 hr	Abdominal cramps, diarrhea	Norwalk agent and related viruses, enterotoxins produced by *Vibrio* spp., *E. coli*, and occasionally *Salmonella, Shigella*, and *C. jejuni*
18–36 hr	Nausea, vomiting, diarrhea, paralysis	Food-borne botulism
72–100 hr	Bloody diarrhea without fever	Enterotoxigenic *E. coli*, most frequently serotype O157:H7
1–3 wk	Chronic diarrhea	Raw milk ingestion

MSG, monosodium glutamate.
From Mandell GL, Bennett JE, Dolin R, et al, editors. *Principles and Practice of Infectious Diseases.* 4th ed. New York: Churchill Livingstone; 1995.

Table 7.6. Child-Pugh Staging of Cirrhosis

PARAMETER	SCORE 1	SCORE 2	SCORE 3
Albumin (g/dL)	>3.5	3.0–3.5	<3.0
Bilirubin (mg/dL)	<2.0	2.0–3.0	>3.0
Prolongation of PT	<4 sec	4–6 sec	>6 sec
Ascites	None	Moderate	Massive
Encephalopathy	None	Moderate	Severe
Child score:	A = 5–6	B = 7–9	C = >9

PT, prothrombin time.

Table 7.7. Clinical Manifestations of Liver Disease

SIGN/SYMPTOM	PATHOGENESIS	LIVER DISEASE
Constitutional		
Fatigue, anorexia, malaise, weight loss	Liver failure	Severe acute or chronic hepatitis Cirrhosis
Fever	Hepatic inflammation or infection	Liver abscess Alcoholic hepatitis Viral hepatitis
Fetor hepaticus	Abnormal methionine metabolism	Acute or chronic liver failure
Cutaneous		
Spider telangiectasias, palmar erythema	Altered estrogen and androgen metabolism	Cirrhosis
Jaundice	Diminished bilirubin excretion	Biliary obstruction Severe liver disease
Pruritus		Biliary obstruction
Xanthomas and xanthelasma	Increased serum lipids	Biliary obstruction/cholestasis
Endocrine		
Gynecomastia, testicular atrophy, diminished libido	Altered estrogen and androgen metabolism	Cirrhosis
Hypoglycemia	Decreased glycogen stores and gluconeogenesis	Liver failure
Gastrointestinal		
RUQ abdominal pain	Liver swelling, infection	Acute hepatitis Hepatocellular carcinoma Liver congestion (heart failure) Acute cholecystitis Liver abscess
Abdominal swelling	Ascites	Cirrhosis, portal hypertension
GI bleeding	Esophageal varices	Portal hypertension
Hematologic		
Decreased RBCs, WBCs, platelets	Hypersplenism	Cirrhosis, portal hypertension
Ecchymoses	Decreased synthesis of clotting factors	Liver failure
Neurologic		
Altered sleep pattern, subtle behavioral changes, somnolence, confusion, ataxia, asterixis, obtundation	Hepatic encephalopathy	Liver failure, portosystemic shunting of blood

GI, gastrointestinal; RBCs, red blood cells; RUQ, right upper quadrant; WBCs, white blood cells.
From Andreoli TE, Cecil RL, editors. *Cecil Essentials of Medicine*. 2nd ed. Philadelphia: WB Saunders; 1990, p 312.

121. A patient with known cirrhosis of the liver presents with massive swelling of the abdomen. A fluid wave can be elicited on examination of the abdomen by striking one flank and feeling the transmitted wave on the opposite flank. What is the appropriate diagnostic procedure at this point?
Abdominal paracentesis. After the diagnosis of new-onset ascites on physical examination, all patients should undergo abdominal paracentesis with ascitic fluid analysis. A small amount of fluid is aspirated from the midline of the abdomen between the umbilicus and the pubis with a small-gauge needle. The most important tests to order are the serum albumin value and ascitic fluid cell count and albumin.

122. **Explain the significance of the serum–to–ascitic fluid albumin gradient.**
The serum albumin value should be measured within a few hours of the abdominal paracentesis to ensure accuracy. Ascitic fluid with a serum–to–ascitic fluid albumin gradient (S-A AG) > 1.1 g/dL is designated as high-gradient ascites. Fluids with values < 1.1 g/dL are designated as low-gradient ascites. The terms *high-albumin gradient* and *low-albumin gradient* should replace the terms *transudative* and *exudative* in the description of ascites.

123. **Which diseases are associated with high-gradient ascites?**
    - Portal hypertension (i.e., cirrhosis)
    - Constrictive pericarditis
    - Hypoalbuminemia
    - Myxedema
    - Nephrotic syndrome (occasionally)
    - Congestive heart failure
    - Inferior vena cava obstruction
    - Meigs syndrome
    - Fulminant hepatic failure
    - Mixed ascites

124. **Which diseases are associated with low-gradient ascites?**
    - Peritoneal neoplasms
    - Tuberculosis
    - Bowel obstruction or infarction
    - Pancreatic ascites
    - Nephrotic syndrome
    - Connective tissue diseases

125. **Explain the significance of the ascitic fluid cell count.**
A large number of RBCs in the fluid or grossly bloody ascites suggests neoplasm. An ascitic fluid neutrophil count of > 250/mL is strongly suggestive of a peritoneal infection or an inflammatory process.

126. **What other ascitic fluid tests should be considered in the diagnosis of ascites?**
Cytologic tests; lactic dehydrogenase (LDH); specific tumor markers; glucose; cultures for bacteria, mycobacteria, and fungi; and adenosine deaminase.

127. **List the benign primary hepatic lesions.**
    - Cavernous hemangioma (most common benign tumor of the liver)
    - Focal nodular hyperplasia (composed of nodules of benign hyperplastic hepatocytes)
    - Hepatic adenoma (associated with the use of oral contraceptive steroids)
    - Bile duct adenoma
    - Bile duct hamartoma
    - Biliary cyst
    - Focal fat

128. **List the malignant primary hepatic lesions.**
    - HCC: Most common primary malignant tumor of the liver
    - Hepatoblastoma: Most common malignant tumor of the liver in children
    - Intrahepatic cholangiocarcinoma: Originates from small intrahepatic bile ducts
    - Angiosarcoma: Most common malignant mesenchymal tumor of the liver
    - Biliary crystadenoma or carcinoma
    - Sarcoma

129. **How is acetaminophen toxic to the liver?**
Through the accumulation of the toxic metabolite of acetaminophen, *N*-acetyl-*p*-benzoquinone. When the dosage of acetaminophen is excessive or the protective detoxifying pathway in the liver is overwhelmed, the metabolite accumulates and hepatocytes die. Acetaminophen is the second most common cause of death from poisoning in the United States.

130. **At what doses does acetaminophen become toxic to the liver?**
>7.5 g in nonalcoholic patients. A potentially lethal effect is seen with ingestion of >140 mg/kg (10 g in a 70-kg man). Chronic alcoholics are at greater risk of acetaminophen injury owing to alcohol induction of the cytochrome P450 system and attendant malnutrition and low levels of glutathione. Glutathione is an intracellular protectant naturally found in the hepatocyte.

131. **What are contraindications to liver transplantation?**
    - Malignancy: extrahepatic malignancy, HCC with metastatic spread
    - Hemangiosarcoma
    - Acquired immunodeficiency syndrome (AIDS)
    - Active/ongoing substance abuse
    - Uncontrolled systemic infection
    - Inability to comply with the posttransplant immunosuppression regimen
    - Advanced cardiopulmonary disease
    - MELD score < 15
    - Anatomic abnormality that precludes liver transplantation
    - Fulminant hepatic failure with sustained intracranial pressure > 50 mm Hg
    - Lack of adequate social support system

132. **What is the most prevalent liver disease in the United States?**
    Nonalcoholic steatohepatitis (NASH), also known as nonalcoholic fatty liver disease (NAFLD). This disease is present in approximately 20% of the American population and perhaps as high as 30–80% of people who are obese. NAFLD is clinically silent except for abnormal liver tests and is most often discovered incidentally, but it can be progressive and result in end-stage liver disease. Imaging studies usually show steatosis of the liver.

ESOPHAGEAL DISEASE

133. **Describe the approach to treatment of GERD.**
    See Table 7.8.
    - Dietary and lifestyle changes
        - Elevation of head of bed 6–8 inches
        - Avoid meals 2–3 hours prior to bedtime
        - Limit intake of trigger foods that may reduce lower esophageal sphincter (LES) pressure: spicy foods, caffeine, chocolate, citrus, carbonated beverages
        - Avoid tight-fitting garments around the abdomen
    - Medications
        - PPI: Most potent single agent for treating GERD; acts by increasing gastric pH

Table 7.8. Treatment of Gastroesophageal Reflux Disease

Dietary and Lifestyle Changes
Postural therapy: elevate head of bed 6–8 inches; avoid lying down after eating; remain upright at least 2 hr after eating (most important lifestyle change)
Limit intake of foods and drink that reduce LES pressure: fatty foods, peppermint, acidic foods, onions, chocolate, caffeine, alcohol
Avoid medications that reduce LES pressure: theophylline, nitrates, tranquilizers, progesterone, calcium blockers, anticholinergic agents, beta-adrenergic agonists
Stop smoking
Decrease the size of meals
Weight reduction if obese (BMI > 30)
Avoid tight-fitting garments around abdomen
Proton Pump Inhibitor
Most potent single agent for treating severe reflux esophagitis (e.g., omeprazole, lansoprazole, rabeprazole, pantoprazole, and esomeprazole)
Acts to increase the pH of gastric contents and heal erosive esophagitis
Endoscopic Therapy
To increase LES pressure
Surgery (Endoscopic or Open)
Aimed at restoring LES competence or preventing reflux

BMI, body mass index; LES, lower esophageal sphincter.

- PPI therapy for 8 weeks is therapy of choice for symptom relief and healing of erosive esophagitis
- PPI should be taken 30 minutes prior to meal
- Surgical therapy
  - Includes laparoscopic or open Nissen fundoplication (restores LES competence)
  - As effective as medical therapy for treatment of GERD
  - Rule of thumb: Surgery not recommended for patients who do not respond to PPI

134. What are the extraesophageal signs and symptoms of GERD?
- **Cardiac:** Atypical chest pain or tightness
- **Ear, nose, and throat:** Hoarseness, cough, sore throat, laryngitis/pharyngitis, otitis media, granuloma, ulcers, interarytenoid changes
- **Respiratory:** Chronic or recurrent cough, adult-onset asthma, recurrent bronchitis, aspiration or chronic interstitial pneumonia, irreversible airway disease, pulmonary fibrosis, sleep apnea
- **Oral:** Burning mouth syndrome, dental erosions
- **Other:** Sudden infant death syndrome

135. How is extraesophageal GERD treated?
If a patient has typical symptoms of GERD (heartburn or acid regurgitation) in addition to extraesophageal symptoms, then trial of PPI therapy for 8 weeks is recommended. If patient only has extraesophageal symptoms, then reflux monitoring to confirm the presence of GERD is recommended prior to a PPI trial.

136. What is Barrett esophagus?
A complication that develops in patients with longstanding reflux that represents a unique reparative process in which the original squamous epithelial cell lining of the esophagus is replaced by a metaplastic columnar-type epithelium. In most adults, this epithelium resembles intestinal mucosa, complete with goblet cells.

137. Summarize the clinical significance of Barrett esophagus.
The risk of EAC is increased 30 to 40 times among patients with Barrett esophagus compared with those without this condition. The actual incidence of EAC in Barrett esophagus patients is unknown, but the average range is 0.2–7%. Currently, adenocarcinoma of the junction, which primarily arises from Barrett epithelium, is the fastest growing GI cancer among white men in the United States.

138. How is Barrett esophagus managed?
By acid suppression with PPIs to control symptoms and heal esophageal damage. Although the inflammatory changes associated with Barrett epithelium can be healed, once Barrett epithelium has developed, the process cannot be reversed by any form of antireflux therapy. If Barrett esophagus has dysplastic cells (low grade or high grade), then endoscopic ablation therapy is recommended.

139. Is routine surveillance for esophageal cancer necessary in patients with Barrett esophagus?
Probably. Although there are no prospective clinical trials that demonstrate a benefit of endoscopic surveillance, the heterogeneity of the available studies makes it prudent to continue to perform endoscopic surveillance of Barrett esophagus patients. The interval for surveillance depends on the degree of dysplasia (no dysplasia, low-grade dysplasia, or high-grade dysplasia).

140. Name the two types of dysphagia.
- **Oropharyngeal:** Occurs when there is difficulty moving the food bolus from the oral cavity to the cervical esophagus
- **Esophageal:** Occurs when there is difficulty with the passage of solid or liquid material through the esophagus, specifically the region between the upper and lower esophageal sphincters. It results from either abnormal motility of this segment of the esophagus or physical impairment to passage (obstruction) due to intrinsic lesions blocking the esophagus (e.g., peptic strictures, cancer) or extrinsic lesions (e.g., mediastinal tumors) compressing the esophagus.

141. Describe the typical history of a patient with oropharyngeal dysphagia.
Symptoms relate to difficulty in the initiation or initial transport of a solid or liquid food bolus. Patients frequently describe choking sensation, aspiration, or sensation of food getting stuck in oral cavity or neck region. Typically seen in patients with neuromuscular disorders such as myasthenia gravis, amyotrophic lateral sclerosis, or stroke.

142. What is the typical history of a patient with esophageal dysphagia related to abnormal motility?

Difficulty in swallowing both liquids and solids. Symptoms may be sensation of food getting stuck in midchest, regurgitation of food/liquids, chest pain. Dysphagia that worsens on ingesting cold liquids and improves with warm liquids suggests a motility disorder.

143. How does esophageal dysphagia related to obstruction typically present?

Difficulty in swallowing solids primarily (this may progress to difficulty with liquids too if obstruction is severe). Patients usually give a history of eating only soft foods, chewing foods longer, and avoiding steak, apples, and fresh bread. Solid-food dysphagia associated with a long history of heartburn and regurgitation suggests a peptic stricture. For patients with ongoing weight loss and progressive dysphagia to solids, an esophageal malignancy must be ruled out.

144. What is the initial diagnostic step for obstructive dysphagia after a thorough history and examination?

An upper GI endoscopy is the standard for diagnosis and any therapeutic intervention.

145. Define *achalasia*.

A disorder of unknown cause with lack of peristalsis in the lower esophagus and failure of the LES to relax. Achalasia is the best-known motor disorder of the esophagus and usually occurs in patients aged 25–60 years, with an equal frequency between the sexes. Symptoms include dysphagia with solids and liquids, regurgitation of undigested foods, heartburn, and chest pain.

146. How is achalasia diagnosed?

By esophageal manometry, which yields the following characteristic findings:
- Loss of peristalsis (absolute requirement)
- Failure of the LES to relax
    Note: increased LES pressure is seen in 60% of cases, but this finding is not required for diagnosis.

147. Define *pseudoachalasia*.

Conditions that mimic the clinical and x-ray findings of achalasia. Distal esophageal obstruction by tumor, stricture, or surgical manipulation may result in pseudoachalasia.

148. How is 24-hour pH monitoring endoscopy used to assess patients with suspected esophageal disease?

Specific variables measured include the number of reflux episodes in 24 hours, esophageal exposure to acid, and symptom index (which measures if patient symptoms correlate temporally with reflux episodes); 24-hour pH monitoring is the gold standard for documenting or excluding GERD and determining whether atypical GERD symptoms are a result of acid reflux.

149. Summarize the role of esophageal manometry in the assessment of esophageal disease.

Esophageal manometry measures the function of the LES and the muscles of the esophagus and is primarily used to evaluate patients with suspected esophageal motility disorders (i.e., patients with noncardiac chest pain or dysphagia to both solids and liquids). Esophageal manometry is also required prior to surgery for GERD to rule out an esophageal motility disorder such as achalasia, which may be a contraindication to surgery.

150. Why is endoscopy useful in assessing esophageal disorders?

Because it provides a direct view of the esophageal mucosa and allows directed biopsy when necessary. Endoscopy and biopsy are necessary to make a definitive diagnosis of many esophageal diseases (e.g., malignancy). The benefits of endoscopy include the ability to perform therapeutic intervention such as biopsy, cytologic tests, brushing, dilatations, and stent placement.

MALABSORPTION

151. What causes Whipple disease?

Tropheryma whipplei, a bacterium. Whipple disease is a systemic disease that may affect almost any organ system of the body, but in most cases, it involves the small intestine. Patients present with intestinal malabsorption, weight loss, diarrhea, abdominal pain, fever, anemia, lymphadenopathy, and arthralgias. Nervous system symptoms, pericarditis, or endocarditis may also be present.

152. How is Whipple disease diagnosed?

By small intestinal biopsy. Whipple disease is confirmed if the biopsy shows infiltration of involved tissues with large glycoprotein-containing macrophages that stain strongly positive with a periodic acid–Schiff stain. One can also see characteristic rod-shaped, gram-positive bacilli that are not acid-fast.

153. How is Whipple disease treated?

With oral double-strength trimethoprim/sulfamethoxazole given for a minimum of 1 year. Repeat intestinal biopsy should document the disappearance of the Whipple bacillus before therapy is discontinued. Relapses are common and are re-treated for a minimum of 6–12 months. Patients allergic to sulfonamides should receive parenteral penicillin.

154. In a small bowel biopsy, the mucosa shows flat villi with markedly hyperplastic crypts. What is the diagnosis?

Celiac sprue, also called *gluten-sensitive enteropathy*. Celiac sprue is an allergic disease character-ized by malabsorption of nutrients secondary to the damaged small intestinal mucosa. The respon-sible antigen is gluten, a water-insoluble protein found in cereal grains such as wheat, barley, and rye. Withdrawal of gluten from the diet results in complete remission of both the clinical symptoms and the mucosal lesions.

155. What tests are used to diagnose celiac disease?

Serologic tests include anti-tissue transglutaminase and, if positive, anti-endomysial antibody. The combination is > 90% sensitive for celiac disease. Causes for false-negative results include IgA deficiency, age < 2 years old, and mild enteropathy. Small bowel biopsy is considered the "gold standard" and should always be performed if celiac disease is suspected.

156. What is dermatitis herpetiformis?

A pruritic skin condition that may be reversed with gluten restriction and is characterized by papulovesicular lesions in a symmetrical distribution on the elbows, knees, buttocks, face, scalp, neck, and trunk.

157. How does dermatitis herpetiformis relate to celiac sprue?

Patients with dermatitis herpetiformis usually have the spruelike mucosal lesion in the small bowel, although most patients with celiac sprue do not develop skin lesions of dermatitis herpetiformis. The two diseases appear to be distinct entities that respond to the same dietary restrictions. Unlike the intestinal disease, the skin lesions can be treated with the antibiotic dapsone, with a clinical response within 1–2 weeks.

158. What is the blind-loop syndrome?

A constellation of symptoms and laboratory abnormalities that include malabsorption of vitamin B_{12}, steatorrhea, hypoproteinemia, weight loss, and diarrhea attributed to overgrowth of bacteria within the small intestine. Bacterial overgrowth is associated with a number of diseases and surgical abnormalities. The common link between these conditions is abnormal motility of a segment of small intestine, resulting in stasis. The aim of therapy is to reduce the bacterial overgrowth and consists of antibiotics and, when feasible, correction of the small intestinal abnormality that led to the condition.

159. Describe the process of normal fat absorption.

Normal fat absorption requires all phases of digestion to be intact. The process begins in the small intestine with secretion of pancreatic lipase and colipase. These enzymes are activated intraluminally and require an optimal pH of 6–8. Both enzymes are necessary for triglyceride hydrolysis in the duodenum. The products of triglyceride hydrolysis (i.e., fatty acids and monoglycerides) then must be solubilized by bile salts to form micelles, which are subsequently absorbed by the small intestinal epithelium.

160. What mechanisms may lead to fat malabsorption?

- Deficiencies of pancreatic enzyme secretion
- Presence of an acidic intraluminal environment in the small bowel
- Interruption of the enterohepatic circulation or secretion of bile salts may impair micelle formation
- Diseased intestinal epithelial cells leading to impairment of monoglyceride absorption and processing into chylomicrons for transport
- Diseased intestinal lymphatics with impaired chylomicron transport

161. **Which diseases can affect fat absorption?**
   - Chronic pancreatitis
   - Cystic fibrosis
   - Pancreatic carcinoma
   - Postgastrectomy syndrome
   - Biliary tract obstruction: Stones, tumors
   - Terminal ileal resection or disease
   - Cholestatic liver disease
   - Intestinal epithelial disease: Whipple disease, sprue, eosinophilic gastroenteritis
   - Lymphatic disease: Abetalipoproteinemia, intestinal lymphangiectasia, lymphoma, tuberculous adenitis
   - Small bowel bacterial overgrowth: Bile salts are deconjugated and inactivated by bacteria
   - ZES: Low intraluminal pH

162. **What type of kidney stones is most often seen in a person with fat malabsorption?**
   Calcium oxalate stones. Fat malabsorption leads to excess free fatty acids in the intestine, which then bind to luminal calcium, decreasing the calcium available to bind and clear oxalate. The increased luminal oxalate is absorbed, resulting in hyperoxaluria, which leads to calcium oxalate stone formation in the kidneys.

163. **Summarize the pathologic mechanism of small bowel bacteria overgrowth. How is it diagnosed?**
   Any abnormality of the small intestine that results in local stasis or recirculation of intestinal contents is likely to be associated with marked proliferation of intraluminal bacteria. The gold standard for diagnosing bacterial overgrowth is a culture of aspirate from the upper small bowel showing > 100,000 colony-forming units (CFUs)/mL. However, this test is technically difficult to perform. Small intestinal bacterial overgrowth leads to malabsorption of carbohydrates and fat.

164. **What disorders are associated with small bowel bacteria overgrowth?**
   - **Hypochlorhydric or achlorhydric states:** Lead to gastric proliferation of bacteria particularly when in combination with motor or anatomic disturbances
   - **Small intestinal stagnation:** Associated with anatomic alterations following surgery, such as afferent loop syndrome after a Billroth II procedure
   - **Duodenal and jejunal diverticulosis:** Particularly as seen in scleroderma
   - **Surgically created blind loops:** End-to-side anastomoses
   - **Chronic low-grade obstruction:** Secondary to small intestinal strictures, adhesions, inflammation, or carcinoma
   - **Motor disturbances of the small intestine:** Scleroderma, idiopathic pseudo-obstruction, diabetic neuropathy
   - **Abnormal communication between the proximal small intestine and the distal intestinal tract:** Seen in gastrocolic or jejunocolic fistulas or resection of the ileocecal valve
   - **Immunodeficiency syndromes:** AIDS, primary immunodeficiency states, malnutrition

165. **How does bacterial overgrowth of the small bowel result in fat malabsorption?**
   Through the excess production of enzymes that deconjugate intraluminal bile salts to free bile acids. Free bile acids are reabsorbed in the jejunum and are, therefore, unable to solubilize monoglycerides and free fatty acids into micelles for absorption by the intestinal epithelial cells. The result is impaired absorption of fat and fat-soluble vitamins.

166. **What constitutes a normal fecal fat concentration? What is steatorrhea?**
   Normal concentration is 4–6 g/day, ranging to an upper limit of normal of approximately 7 g/day. The typical U.S. diet consists of 100–150 g of fat/day. Fat absorption is extremely efficient, and most of the ingested fat is absorbed with very little excretion into the stool. Patients with steatorrhea, or increased excretion of fecal fat, may have up to 10 times this amount in the stool.

167. **How is steatorrhea detected?**
   Through a 72-hour stool sample collected while the patient is on a defined dietary fat intake of > 100 g/day. Chemical analysis of the stool collection measures the amount of fat present. This test is highly reliable but neither specific nor sensitive in determining the cause of steatorrhea.

OBSTRUCTION

168. **Name the four most common causes of mechanical small bowel obstruction in adults.**
    - Adhesions (~74%)
    - Hernias (8%)
    - Malignancies of the small bowel (8%)
    - IBD with stricture formation

169. **Define *small bowel ileus*.**
    Distention due to intestinal muscle paralysis. Paralytic ileus is a relatively common disorder and occurs when neural, humoral, and metabolic factors combine to stimulate reflexes that inhibit intestinal motility.

170. **What seven entities may cause small bowel ileus?**
    - Abdominal surgery
    - Peritonitis
    - Generalized sepsis
    - Electrolyte imbalance (especially hypokalemia and hypomagnesemia)
    - Retroperitoneal hemorrhage
    - Spinal fractures
    - Pelvic fractures

171. **What role do drugs play in small bowel ileus?**
    Drugs such as anticholinergics and narcotics inhibit small bowel motility and also may contribute to paralysis.

172. **How is small bowel ileus treated?**
    With NG suction to relieve distention and IV fluids to replace fluid losses, followed by correction of the underlying disorder.

173. **What conditions may aggravate or be associated with colonic pseudo-obstruction?**
    See Table 7.9.

Table 7.9. Conditions Associated With Colonic Pseudo-Obstruction
1. Trauma (nonoperative) and surgery (gynecologic, orthopedic, urologic)
2. Inflammatory processes (pancreatitis, cholecystitis)
3. Infections
4. Malignancy
5. Radiation therapy
6. Drugs (narcotics, antidepressants, clonidine, anticholinergics)
7. Cardiovascular disease
8. Neurologic disease
9. Respiratory failure
10. Metabolic disease (diabetes, hypothyroidism, electrolyte imbalance, uremia)
11. Alcoholism

174. **What are bezoars?**
    Clusters of food or foreign matter that have undergone partial digestion in the stomach, then failed to pass through the pylorus into the small bowel, forming a mass in the stomach. Substances typically composing bezoars include hair (trichobezoars) and, more commonly, plant matter (phytobezoars).

175. **How do patients with bezoars present?**
    With abdominal mass, gastric outlet obstruction, attacks of nausea and vomiting, and peptic ulceration when bezoars become large. Factors important in the formation of bezoars include the

amount of indigestible materials in the diet (pulpy, fibrous fruit or vegetables such as oranges), the quality of the chewing mechanism, and loss of pyloric function, which limits the size of food particles that may enter the duodenum.

BILIARY TRACT DISEASE

176. **Which U.S. ethnic groups have the highest prevalence of cholesterol gallstone formation?**
American Indians and Mexican Americans.

177. **List the types of gallstones.**
- **Cholesterol** (70–80% of all stones in Western countries): Risk factors are female gender, obesity, age > 40 years, and multiparity.
- **Pigmented** (20–30%).
- **Black calcium bilirubinate:** Risk factors are cirrhosis, chronic hemolytic syndromes.
- **Brown calcium salts:** Can form de novo in bile ducts; risk factors are infections of the biliary system.

178. **What is Charcot triad?**
Right upper quadrant pain, jaundice, and fever. Charcot triad is present in approximately 50% of patients with bacterial cholangitis.

179. **What is Reynold pentad?**
Charcot triad (right upper quadrant pain, jaundice, and fever), plus hypotension and altered mental status.

180. **Which tests are used in the initial diagnostic evaluation of a patient with suspected obstructive jaundice?**
Clinical history, physical examination, and routine laboratory tests (serum total and unconjugated or indirect bilirubin, ALP, PT, ALT, AST, and albumin). The only special study that is routinely useful in the early evaluation of obstructive jaundice is an US study of the gallbladder, bile ducts, and liver. US is fairly specific for detecting gallstones and ductal dilatation (the latter signifying ductal obstruction). However, a negative US finding does not prove the absence of stones or obstruction, because the sensitivity of US in detecting obstruction is only about 90%.

181. **What are the advantages of endoscopic ultrasound (EUS)?**
- Noninvasive
- Images the entire pancreaticobiliary system
- Detects presence of tumors, stones, and strictures
- Can be used with fine-needle aspiration for biopsy or tissue samples

182. **Discuss the role of CT in the evaluation of obstructive jaundice.**
Abdominal CT is fairly sensitive for detecting ductal dilatation and can be useful in localizing the site of ductal obstruction. A CT scan is less able to detect stones of the gallbladder and common bile duct than US, but it is better able to image mass lesions and to evaluate the pancreas. Generally, US is considered first line if considering stone disease, and CT is considered if suspicion of tumor is high.

183. **Is magnetic retrograde cholangiopancreatography (MRCP) useful in the evaluation of obstructive jaundice?**
Yes. MRCP is a useful diagnostic tool in the evaluation of jaundice. MRCP can reveal the size of the ducts and document presence of stones and other masses. In many centers, MRCP has supplanted diagnostic endoscopic retrograde pancreatography (ERCP) as a primary screening modality.

184. **Are liver scans helpful in the evaluation of jaundice?**
No. Liver scan in the patient with extrahepatic ductal obstruction is not routinely useful. It may reveal evidence of cholestasis and cholangitis but will not help to determine the cause. A liver scan using technetium sulfur colloid is of very little value in the jaundiced patient.

185. **What causes air in the biliary system?**
- Previous surgery or endoscopy procedures (most common)
- Penetrating ulcers
- Erosion of gallstone into the bowel lumen

- Traumatic fistula
- Neoplasms
- Bowel obstruction

IRRITABLE BOWEL SYNDROME

186. What is irritable bowel syndrome (IBS)?
A functional bowel disorder. The Rome IV criteria characterize the symptoms as abdominal pain occurring generally once a week during the past 3 months and associated with at least two of the following symptoms:
- Relief with defecation
- Onset associated with a change in frequency of stool
- Onset associated with a change in form or appearance of stool

187. What findings suggest organic disease instead of IBS?
- New onset of symptoms in an elderly patient
- Pain that interferes with normal sleep patterns
- Weight loss
- Anemia
- Blood in the stools
- Pain on awakening from sleep
- Diarrhea that awakens the patient
- Fever
- Steatorrhea
- Physical examination abnormalities

188. What is the differential diagnosis of IBS?
- Psychiatric disorders (depression, anxiety, somatization)
- Diabetes
- Scleroderma
- IBD
- Chronic pancreatitis
- Postgastrectomy syndromes
- Side effects of medications
- Hypothryoidism
- Lactose malabsorption
- Endocrine disorders
- Celiac sprue
- Infectious diarrhea

WEBSITE

1. UpToDate: www.uptodate.com

BIBLIOGRAPHY

1. Low V. *Case Review: Gastrointestinal Imaging.* Philadelphia: Elsevier; 2013.
2. Lichetenstein GR, Wu GD, eds. *The Requisites in Gastroenterology: vol 2: Small and Large Intestines.* St. Louis: Mosby; 2003.
3. Reddy KR, Long WB, eds. *The Requisites in Gastroenterology: Vol 3: Hepatobiliary Tract and Pancreas.* St. Louis: Mosby; 2003.
4. Rustgi AK, ed. *The Requisites in Gastroenterology: vol 1: Esophagus and Stomach.* St. Louis: Mosby; 2003.
5. Feldman M, Friedman LS, Brandt LJ. *Sleisenger and Fordtran's Gastrointestinal and Liver Disease: Pathophysiology, Diagnosis, and Management.* 10th ed. Philadelphia: Elsevier; 2016.
6. Tytgat GNJ, Classen M, Waye JD, et al. *Practice of Therapeutic Endoscopy.* 2nd ed. London: WB Saunders; 2000.

CHAPTER 8

NEPHROLOGY

Sharma S. Prabhakar, MD, MBA, FACP, FASN

He [Dr. Richard Bright] is rightfully regarded as one of the founding fathers of nephrology, with his name immortalized in the eponym Bright's disease.

Jay V: Richard Bright: physician extraordinaire,
Arch Pathol Lab Med. 2000;124:1262

ASSESSMENT OF RENAL FUNCTION

1. **What is the glomerular filtration rate (GFR)?**
   The ultrafiltrate of plasma that exits the glomerular capillary tuft and enters the Bowman capsule to begin the journey along the tubule of the nephron. The GFR is the initial step in the formation of urine and is usually expressed in milliliters per minute.

2. **How is the GFR measured clinically?**
   The GFR is measured indirectly with a marker substance contained in glomerular filtrate, which is then excreted in the urine. The amount of this substance leaving the kidney (urinary mass excretion) must equal the amount of marker substance entering the kidney as glomerular filtrate; it must not be reabsorbed, secreted, or metabolized after entering the kidney tubule. The marker substance is chosen so that its concentration in the glomerular filtrate is equal to its concentration in the plasma (i.e., the substance is freely filterable across the glomerular capillary). Therefore, the amount of substance X entering the kidney equals the GFR multiplied by the plasma concentration of the substance (P_x). Likewise, the amount of the substance leaving the kidney in the urine equals the urinary concentration of the substance (U_x) multiplied by the urine flow in mL/min (V). Therefore, the formula for calculating GFR using our marker substance X becomes:

   $$GFR \times P_x = U_x V \text{ or } GFR = U_x V / P_x$$

   A stable plasma concentration of the substance (steady-state situation) is required to make the preceding equation useful.

3. **Why is creatinine used as a marker substance for GFR determinations in clinical settings?**
   Because creatinine is an endogenous substance, derived from the metabolism of creatine in skeletal muscle, and fulfills almost all of the requirements for a marker substance: it is freely filterable, not metabolized, and not reabsorbed once filtered. A small amount of tubular secretion makes the creatinine clearance a slight overestimate of the GFR, but this overestimate becomes quantitatively important only at low levels of GFR. Creatinine is released from muscle at a constant rate, resulting in a stable plasma concentration. The creatinine clearance is commonly determined from a 24-hour collection of urine. This time period is used to average out the sometimes variable creatinine excretion that may occur from hour to hour. Creatinine is easily measured, making it a nearly ideal marker for GFR determination.

4. **Is any other substance used as a marker of GFR in laboratory settings?**
   The polysaccharide **inulin** is often used in laboratory determinations of GFR. However, it requires constant intravenous (IV) infusion, making it somewhat impractical for routine clinical use in patients. In clinical practice, clearance of endogenous creatinine is used as a surrogate for GFR. More recently serum cystatin C levels have been shown to be a better marker of GFR than serum creatinine. It is not affected by age, sex, race, and muscle mass as much as serum creatinine, but cystatin levels are affected by thyroid dysfunction and presence of cancer.

5. **Can the completeness of a 24-hour urine collection be judged?**
   Yes, by knowing the estimated creatinine excretion value. Because total creatinine excretion in the steady state is dependent on muscle mass, day-to-day creatinine excretion remains fairly constant for an individual and is related to lean body weight. In general, men excrete 20–25 mg creatinine/kg body weight/day, whereas women excrete 15–20 mg/kg/day. Therefore, a 70-kg man excretes approximately 1400 mg creatinine/day. Creatinine excretion levels measured on a 24-hour urine collection that are substantially less than the estimated value suggest an incomplete collection.

6. **What is the relationship between the plasma creatinine concentration (P_{Cr}) and GFR?**
   Because creatinine production and excretion remain constant and equal, the amount of creatinine entering and leaving the kidney remains constant. Thus:

   $$GFR \times P_{Cr} = U_{Cr} \times V = \text{constant or } GFR = (1/P_{Cr}) \times \text{constant}$$

   Creatinine excretion remains constant as GFR declines until the GFR reaches very low levels. Therefore, the GFR is a function of the reciprocal of the P_{Cr}.

7. **Does a given P_{Cr} reflect the same level of renal function in different patients?**
   Not necessarily. Remember that creatinine production is directly proportional to muscle mass and that the P_{Cr} is determined in part by creatinine production. Examination of the creatinine clearance (C_{Cr}) for an 80-kg man compared with that of a 40-kg woman, assuming both individuals have P_{Cr} of 1.0 mg/dL (0.01 mg/mL), shows the following:
   For the 80-kg man, creatinine excretion should be:

   $$80 \text{ kg} \times 20 \text{ mg/kg/day} = 1600 \text{ mg/day} = 1.11 \text{ mg/min}$$

   $$GFR = (1.11 \text{ mg/min}) / (0.11 \text{ mg/mL}) = 111 \text{ mL/min}$$

   For the 40-kg woman, creatinine excretion should be:

   $$40 \text{ kg} \times 15 \text{ mg/kg/day} = 600 \text{ mg/day} = 0.42 \text{ mg/min}$$

   $$GFR = (0.42 \text{ mg/min}) / (0.01 \text{ mg/mL}) = 42 \text{ mL/min}$$

   This example demonstrates that the same P_{Cr} can represent markedly different GFRs in different individuals.

8. **What formulas are used to estimate GFR when a measured C_{Cr} is not immediately available?**
   The following formula was first devised to provide a rough estimate of the GFR when a measured C_{Cr} is not immediately available:

   $$C_{Cr} \text{ (mL/min)} = \frac{(140 - \text{age in years}) \times \text{lean body wt in kg}}{(P_{Cr} \times 72)} \times (0.85 \text{ if female})$$

   This is the Cockcroft-Gault formula, which gives creatinine clearance in mL/min. These estimates are in the range of those determined previously and serve to illustrate the relative differences in the GFR calculated for two individuals with the same P_{Cr}. Recognizing this fact and using this formula to estimate GFR could prevent a serious error when selecting the dose of a drug that is excreted by the kidneys.
   The modification of diet in renal disease (MDRD) formula is now the most widely used method (and has replaced the use of the Cockcroft-Gault formula in many instances) to estimate the GFR (eGFR) in the context of chronic kidney disease (CKD).

   eGFR =
   $$170 \times S_{Cr}^{-1.154} \times \text{age}^{-0.203} \times [1.21 \text{ if black}] \times [0.74 \text{ if female}] \times BUN^{-0.170} \times \text{albumin}^{+0.138}$$

   where the serum creatinine (S_{Cr}) and blood urea nitrogen (BUN) concentrations are both in mg/dL. The albumin concentration is in g/dL. The GFR is expressed in mL/min/1.73 m^2. However, this formula underestimates the GFR in healthy people with GFR over 60 mL/min.

The Chronic Kidney Disease Epidemiology Collaboration (CKD-EPI) formula was developed recently (May 2009) to circumvent this problem:

eGFR =
$$141 \times \min(S_{Cr}/K,1)^a \times \max(S_{Cr}/K,1)^{-1.209} \times 0.093^{age} \times (1.108 \text{ if female}) \text{ or} \times (1.159 \text{ if black})$$

where k is 0.7 for females and 0.9 for males, a is −0.329 for females and −0.411 for males, min indicates the minimum of S_{Cr}/k or 1, and max indicates the maximum of S_{Cr}/k or 1.
This formula is slowly replacing the MDRD formula to estimate C_{Cr}.
Levey AS, Stevens LA, Schmid CH, et al. A new equation to estimate glomerular filtration rate. *Ann Intern Med.* 2009;50:604–612.

9. **How does BUN relate to the GFR?**
BUN is excreted primarily by glomerular filtration, and the plasma level tends to vary inversely with GFR. BUN, however, is a much less ideal marker of GFR than is creatinine. The production of urea is not constant and varies with protein intake, liver function, and catabolic rate. In addition, urea can be reabsorbed once filtered into the kidney, and this reabsorption increases in conditions with low urine flow, such as volume depletion. Volume depletion is one cause of a high (>15:1) BUN-to-creatinine ratio in plasma. Thus, creatinine is the better marker for GFR. The plasma level of BUN can be used along with the C_{Cr} to indicate the presence of certain states, such as volume depletion.

10. **What is the difference between urinary excretion and clearance?**
Urinary **excretion** of a substance is simply the total amount of a substance excreted per unit of time, usually expressed in mg/min. **Clearance** expresses the efficiency with which the kidney removes a substance from the plasma. The volume of plasma that must be completely cleared of a substance per unit of time accounts for the amount of that substance appearing in the urine per unit of time. Clearance is expressed in volume per unit of time, usually mL/min.

11. **Give an example of clearance.**
Substance (X) with a plasma concentration (P_x) of 1.0 mg/mL, urine concentration (U_x) of 10 mg/mL, and urine flow (V) of 1.0 mL/min have the following clearance:

$$Cl_x = (U_x/P_x) \times V = (10 \text{ mg/mL} \times 1 \text{ mL/min}) / 1.0 \text{ mg/min} = 10 \text{ mL/min}$$

The calculated clearance of 10 mL/min indicates that the amount of substance X appearing in the urine is the same as if 10 mL of plasma were completely cleared of the substance and excreted in the urine each minute. The urinary excretion of X is 10 mg/min, but this measurement does not indicate the efficiency with which the substance is removed from the plasma.

12. **How does measurement of urinary protein excretion help in the evaluation of renal disease?**
Normal urinary protein excretion <150 mg/day, with albumin constituting <50% of this protein. Failure of the tubules to reabsorb the normally filtered small-molecular-weight proteins leads to **tubular proteinuria.** This occurs in diseases that affect tubular function, and the proteins are almost entirely of smaller molecular weight rather than albumin. **Glomerular proteinuria** occurs when the normal glomerular barrier to the passage of plasma proteins is disrupted. This results in variable quantities of albumin and sometimes larger molecular weight proteins spilling into the urine. Quantitatively, tubular proteinuria is usually <1 g/24 hours, and glomerular proteinuria is usually >1 g/24 hours. When the proteinuria is >3.5 g/1.73 m^2 body surface area, it is said to be in the **nephrotic range**. Significant degrees of proteinuria (>150 mg/day) could indicate intrinsic renal disease. Quantification and characterization of the proteinuria are useful in detecting the presence of renal disease and in determining involvement of the tubule, glomerulus, or both.

13. **What information can be gained from examining urine sediment?**
Urine sediment is normally almost cell free, is usually crystal free, and contains a very low concentration of protein (<1+ by dipstick). Examination of this sediment is an important part of the work-up of any patient with renal disease. The examination should be performed by the physician before diagnostic or therapeutic decisions are made. The information must be correlated with all other aspects of the patient's history, physical examination, and laboratory database. The examination can provide evidence of many conditions, including renal inflammation (cells, protein), infection (white blood cells [WBCs], bacteria), stone disease (crystals), and systemic diseases (e.g., bilirubin, myoglobin, and hemoglobin).

14. Define *oliguria*.

A urine volume that is inadequate for the normal excretion of the body's metabolic waste products. Because the daily load of metabolic products amounts to approximately 600 mOsm and the maximal urine concentrating ability of the human kidney is about 1200 mOsm/kg H_2O, there is a minimal obligate urine volume of 500 mL/day for most people. Therefore, a 24-hour urine volume **< 500 mL/ day** is said to represent oliguria. When associated with acute kidney injury (AKI), oliguria portends a poorer prognosis than does nonoliguric AKI.

15. Define *anuria*.

A 24-hour urine volume < 100 mL. Anuria denotes a severe reduction in urine volume that is commonly associated with obstruction, renal cortical necrosis, or severe acute tubular necrosis (ATN). It is important to make the distinction between oliguria and anuria so that these diagnostic entities will be considered and appropriate therapy planned.

PROTEINURIA, NEPHROTIC SYNDROME, AND NEPHRITIC SYNDROME

16. List the four general mechanisms by which abnormally increased urinary protein excretion (>150 mg/day) occurs.
   - Glomerular
   - Tubular
   - Overflow
   - Secretory

17. What causes glomerular proteinuria?

Damage to the glomerular filtration barrier (in glomerulonephritis), leading to leakage of plasma proteins into the glomerular ultrafiltrate.

18. Describe the mechanism behind tubular proteinuria.

Suboptimal reabsorption of the normally filtered protein as a result of tubular disease. This recovery of the small amount of normally filtered protein (usually ~2 g/day) allows for the normal excretion of <150 mg/day of protein.

19. Explain overflow proteinuria.

Proteinuria resulting from disease states that leads to excessive levels of plasma proteins (e.g., in multiple myeloma). The proteins are filtered and overload the reabsorptive capacity of the renal tubules.

20. What is secretory proteinuria?

Proteinuria that occurs because of the addition of protein to the urine after glomerular filtration. The protein may come from the renal tubules (e.g., Tamm-Horsfall protein from the ascending limb of the loop of Henle) or from the lower genitourinary (GU) tract.

21. What conditions are associated with heavy proteinuria despite severely reduced GFR?

Usually glomerular disease. In most glomerular diseases, proteinuria tends to decrease with diminishing GFR as the filtration of proteins also tends to decrease. However, in certain conditions, such as diabetic nephropathy, amyloidosis, focal glomerulosclerosis, and probably reflex nephropathy, proteinuria (often in the nephrotic range) persists despite severely diminished GFR.

22. Define *nephrotic syndrome*.

A symptom complex resulting from various causes and characterized by heavy proteinuria (usually >3.5 g/day), generalized edema, and lipiduria with hyperlipidemia. Because all the other features are a consequence of marked proteinuria, some authorities restrict the definition of "nephrosis" to heavy proteinuria alone.

23. What are the common causes of nephrotic syndrome in adults and children?

In **adults,** the most common cause is diabetes nephropathy, which is a secondary cause of nephritic syndrome. Membranous nephropathy is the most common primary glomerulopathy in adults. In **children,** the most common cause of nephrotic syndrome is minimal change disease, also called "lipoid nephrosis" or "nil disease." Other causes of nephrotic syndrome include focal and segmental glomerulosclerosis and amyloidosis.

24. **When evaluating patients with nephrotic syndrome, which diseases must you rule out before considering the syndrome to be due to a primary renal disease?**
    - Drugs that may result in excessive urinary protein excretion (gold and penicillamine)
    - Systemic infections (hepatitis B and C, human immunodeficiency virus [HIV], malaria)
    - Neoplasia (lymphomas)
    - Multisystem collagen vascular diseases (systemic lupus erythematosus [SLE])
    - Diabetes mellitus (DM)
    - Heredofamilial diseases (Alport syndrome)

25. **Why is it important to distinguish primary renal disease from these conditions?**
    The distinction between these causes and primary renal disease is important for a number of reasons. Diagnostically, identification of some of these processes may help to identify the renal lesion without the need for a renal biopsy (as in DM). Treatment of such disorders may involve simple discontinuation of the offending agent (e.g., a drug). Management may need to be directed at a systemic disease (infection) rather than at the renal lesion itself.

26. **Name the common complications of the nephrotic syndrome.**
    - Edema and anasarca.
    - Hypovolemia with acute prerenal or parenchymal renal disease or both. In the nephrotic syndrome, decreased effective arterial blood volume can lead to various degrees of renal underperfusion, resulting in renal failure in severe cases.
    - Protein malnutrition due to massive protein losses in excess of dietary replacement.
    - Hyperlipidemia, which raises the risk of atherosclerotic cardiovascular disease.
    - Increased susceptibility to bacterial infection often involving the lungs, meninges (meningitis), and peritoneum. Common organisms include *Streptococcus* (including *Streptococcus pneumoniae*), *Haemophilus influenzae*, and *Klebsiella* spp.
    - Proximal tubular dysfunction leading to Fanconi syndrome with urinary wasting of glucose, phosphate, amino acids, uric acid, potassium, and bicarbonate.
    - Hypercoagulable state manifested by an increased incidence of venous thrombosis, particularly in the renal vein, which may be due to urinary loss of antithrombotic factors.

27. **Define *nephritic syndrome*.**
    A renal disorder resulting from diffuse glomerular inflammation characterized by the sudden onset of gross or microscopic hematuria, decreased GFR, oliguria, hypertension (HTN), and edema. Nephritic syndrome results from many different causes but is traditionally represented by postinfectious glomerulonephritis following infections with certain strains of group A beta-hemolytic streptococci.

28. **What are the various causes of an acute nephritic syndrome?**
    - **Postinfectious glomerulonephritis:** bacterial (pneumococci, *Klebsiella* spp., staphylococci, gram-negative rods, and meningococci), viral (varicella, infectious mononucleosis, mumps, measles, hepatitis B, and coxsackievirus), rickettsial (Rocky Mountain spotted fever and typhus), and parasitic (*Plasmodium falciparum* malaria, toxoplasmosis, and trichinosis)
    - **Idiopathic glomerular diseases:** membranoproliferative glomerulonephritis, mesangial proliferative glomerulonephritis, and immunoglobulin A (IgA) nephropathy
    - **Multisystem diseases:** SLE, Henoch-Schönlein purpura, essential mixed cryoglobulinemia, and infective endocarditis
    - **Miscellaneous:** Guillain-Barré syndrome and postirradiation of renal tumors

29. **Are the syndromes of nephritis and nephrosis mutually exclusive?**
    No. Some forms of glomerular diseases are characteristically nephrotic in their presentation, whereas some aggressive forms of proliferative glomerulopathies present as nephritic syndrome. Some others manifest mixed features (Table 8.1).

30. **A 62-year-old man with nephrotic syndrome is found to have no systemic cause. What is the differential diagnosis?**
    As opposed to a minimal lesion in children, a minimal lesion on renal biopsy in an elderly patient warrants an extensive search to rule out underlying malignancy, especially lymphomas (both Hodgkin and non-Hodgkin) and other solid tumors (e.g., renal cell carcinoma). One third of elderly patients with membranous nephropathy have underlying malignancy (colon, stomach, or breast).

Table 8.1. Interrelationship of Morphologic and Clinical Manifestations of Glomerular Injury

	NEPHROSIS	NEPHRITIS
Minimal change glomerulopathy	+ + + +	
Membranous glomerulopathy	+ + +	
Focal glomerulosclerosis	+ +	+
Mesangioproliferative glomerulopathy	+ +	+ +
Membranoproliferative glomerulopathy	+ +	+ + +
Proliferative glomerulonephritis	+	+ + +
Acute diffuse proliferate glomerulonephritis	+	+ + + +
Crescentic glomerulonephritis		+ + + +

From Mandal AK, et al. *Diagnosis and Management of Renal Disease and Hypertension*. Philadelphia: Lea & Febiger; 1988, p. 248.

GLOMERULAR DISORDERS

31. Define *primary glomerulopathy.*
    A heterogeneous group of kidney diseases in which the glomeruli are predominantly involved. Extrarenal involvement, if present, is usually secondary to consequences of the glomerular insult. Most of these disorders are idiopathic. The cardinal manifestations of the primary glomerular disorders or glomerulopathy are proteinuria, hematuria, alterations in GFR, and salt retention leading to edema, HTN, and pulmonary congestion.

32. What are the characteristics of the clinical syndromes that are manifested by the primary glomerulopathies?
    - **Acute glomerulonephritis:** Acute onset of variable degrees of hematuria, proteinuria, decreased GFR, and fluid and salt retention that is usually associated with an infectious agent and tends to resolve spontaneously.
    - **Nephrotic syndrome:** Insidious onset characterized primarily by heavy proteinuria of usually >3.5 g/day in an adult and usually associated with hypoalbuminemia, lipidemia, and anasarca.
    - **Chronic glomerulonephritis:** Insidious onset of vague symptoms with progressive renal insufficiency and a protracted downhill course of 5–10 years' duration. Varying degrees of proteinuria, hematuria, and HTN are present.
    - **Rapidly progressive glomerulonephritis (RPGN):** Subacute onset of symptoms but with rapid progression to renal failure and no tendency toward spontaneous recovery. Patients are usually hypertensive, hematuric, and oliguric.
    - **Asymptomatic urinary abnormalities:** No clinical symptoms but microscopic hematuria or proteinuria (usually <3 g/day).

33. How does routine urinalysis help in the evaluation of a primary glomerular disease?
    In glomerular disease, the urinary sediment usually conforms to one of three different forms:

Nephrotic	*Nephritic*	*Chronic*
Heavy proteinuria	Red blood cells	Less proteinuria and hematuria
Free fat droplets	Red blood cell casts	Broad, waxy casts
Oval fat bodies	Variable proteinuria	Pigmented granular casts
Fatty casts	Frequent white blood cell and granular cells	
Variable hematuria		

Schreiner GE. The identification and clinical significance of casts. *Arch Intern Med.* 1957;99:356–369.

34. **Which strains of streptococci cause poststreptococcal glomerulonephritis (PSGN)?**

    Only certain serotypes of group A (beta-hemolytic) streptococci are nephritogenic. Type 12 is the most common type, but types 1, 2, 3, 18, 25, 49, 55, 57, and 60 are also nephritogenic. In contrast, all strains of streptococci can cause acute rheumatic fever, which is why the incidence of nephritis differs from that of rheumatic fever in outbreaks of streptococcal infection. The M-protein in streptococci is poorly linked to nephritogenicity. Recent evidence indicates that nephritogenicity is more closely related to endostreptosin, a cell membrane antigen. Other streptococcal cytoplasmic antigens and autologous antigens also have been implicated.

35. **What abnormalities are seen in patients with PSGN?**

    The urinalysis in PSGN is characterized by a nephritic sediment, high specific gravity, and nonselective proteinuria. The proteinuria is <3 g/day in >75% of patients, although proteinuria in the nephrotic range is occasionally seen. Pyuria is often noted, indicating glomerulitis. Hematuria is almost always present in either gross (smoky urine) or microscopic form. Red blood cell (RBC) casts, if present, are very diagnostic. Dysmorphic erythrocytes are found in abundance. However, a benign urinary sediment does not rule out acute PSGN if clinical features are suggestive. In some cases, biopsy studies have confirmed PSGN.

36. **What is the prognosis in acute PSGN? What are the poor prognostic signs?**

    In **children,** the immediate and late prognoses are quite favorable in both epidemic and sporadic cases. A diuresis occurs in 1 week, and S_{Cr} returns to normal in 3–4 weeks. The mortality rate in acute cases is <1%, and chronic sequelae are uncommon. Microscopic hematuria may last 6 months, and proteinuria may persist for as long as 3 years in 15% of patients. In **adults**, the prognosis is good in epidemic forms but less predictable in sporadic cases.

37. **What are the poor prognostic signs in PSGN?**

    In **adults,** severe impairment of renal function at the onset, persistent proteinuria, elderly age, and crescent formation on biopsy are poor prognostic factors. In **children,** the factors indicating a poor prognosis include persistent heavy proteinuria, extensive crescents or atypical humps in initial biopsy, and severe disease in the acute phase requiring hospitalization.

38. **A 31-year-old black man is referred to the renal clinic for increasing swelling of feet and elevated serum creatinine. He was diagnosed with HTN about 7 years ago. He admits using heroin for the past 13 years. Urinalysis is positive for blood and protein (4+) and an occasional RBC cast. His eGFR is 26 mL/min. What would a renal biopsy most likely show?**

    Focal and segmental glomerulosclerosis. Chronic heroin abuse has been associated with the development of focal and segmental glomerulosclerosis.

39. **What are the biopsy findings of RPGN?**

    Extensive glomerular crescent formation, in most cases involving over 75% of glomeruli. The cells of the crescents are thought to be derived from blood-borne monocytes.

40. **Is RPGN synonymous with crescentic nephritis?**

    No. RPGN is strictly a clinical expression, whereas crescentic nephritis denotes the histologic picture in such patients. Several primary glomerulopathies demonstrate variable degrees of crescent formation, but they do not progress as rapidly as in RPGN.

41. **Define *fibrillary* and *immunotactoid glomerulonephritis* (GN).**

    These two related yet distinct glomerular diseases are characterized by deposition of Congo red–negative fibrils and by a variety of light microscopic features and a progressive clinical course. **Fibrillary GN** is defined as Congo red–negative fibrils <30 nm in diameter, whereas **immunotactoid GN** is defined by glomerular deposition of hollow stacked microtubules >30 nm in diameter. Both entities are relatively uncommon, accounting for less than 1% of native renal biopsies. Recurrence of these diseases is common after transplantation.

    Rosenstock JL, Markowitz GS, Valeri AM, et al. Fibrillary and immunotactoid glomerulonephritis: distinct entities with different clinical and pathologic features. *Kidney Int.* 2003;63:1450–1461.

42. **What are the renal manifestations of infective endocarditis?**

    Initially, microscopic or gross hematuria and proteinuria. Renal failure is usually mild or absent. The histologic examination in these cases reveals focal proliferative glomerulonephritis. Rarely, a rapidly progressive renal failure with extensive crescent formation is reported. Nephrotic syndrome is rare. Serum IgG and C3 levels are often decreased, and immunofluorescence often demonstrates IgG, IgM, and subendothelial and subepithelial deposits, suggesting an immune-complex cause.

43. **What are the current strategies for treatment of lupus nephritis?**
Active treatment of HTN, especially with angiotensin-converting enzyme (ACE) inhibitors, delays the progression of all classes of lupus nephritis. In general, classes II and V lesions are amenable to therapy and are associated with better prognosis. A combination of cyclophosphamide (oral or IV) with oral low-dose steroids is effective in improving the prognosis of classes III and IV lupus nephritis. IV pulse cyclophosphamide has become popular in view of fewer gonadal and bladder toxicities. Azathioprine and mycophenolate mofetil are used as alternates to cyclophosphamide. Treatment is generally ineffective in class VI lesions. See Chapter 10, Rheumatology, for description of nephritis classification.
      Berden JHM. Lupus nephritis. *Kidney Int.* 1997;52:538–558.

44. **A 36-year-old Caucasian woman is seen in the clinic for dark-colored urine with symptoms of progressive weakness, generalized arthralgias, and intermittent fever. Her blood pressure (BP) is 153/96 mm Hg, and she has an erythematous rash on her face and forearms. Her blood tests show BUN 38 mg/dL, serum creatinine 1.9 mg/dL, weakly positive antinuclear antibody (ANA), high titer positive anti-DNA, low complement levels, and negative rheumatoid factor (RF). Urinalysis is positive for protein and blood. What is your next diagnostic test?**
Order a renal biopsy. This young woman with fever, hematuria, modest HTN, and renal failure has features suggestive of lupus nephritis. Before initiating the appropriate therapy, which often includes immunosuppressive therapy, it is necessary to establish the histologic class, which only can be provided by a renal biopsy. Steroids or ACE inhibitors can be started as initial therapy, but if she has severe renal disease she may be need more aggressive therapy.

45. **What are the main causes of recurrent isolated glomerular hematuria?**
    • Berger disease (IgA nephropathy)
    • Thin basement membrane nephropathy
    • Idiopathic hypercalciuria
      Berger disease and thin basement membrane nephropathy may require biopsy for confirmation.

46. **A 39-year-old Hispanic woman has undergone renal biopsy for heavy proteinuria. The renal biopsy shows diffuse thickening of glomerular basement membrane with subepithelial deposits. What systemic conditions are associated with this finding?**
Hepatitis B, SLE, and solid organ tumors. Subepithelial deposits are characteristic of membranous nephropathy, which may be found with these conditions.

47. **What are the signs and symptoms of Berger disease?**
Recurrent episodes of painless hematuria, often gross, and presence of RBC casts in urine. HTN and proteinuria are often minimal or modest. Only 25% of patients progress to end-stage renal disease (ESRD). The symptoms are often exacerbated during an upper respiratory infection (not 2–3 weeks later as in PSGN) and hence the term *synpharyngitic nephritis* to describe Berger disease. Episodes of gross hematuria may often be associated with worsening of renal function. Berger disease is the most common primary glomerulopathy worldwide.

DIABETIC RENAL DISEASE

See also Chapter 14, Endocrinology.

48. **What is the incidence of renal involvement in DM?**
Among type 1 diabetics, 30–40% develop CKD between 10 and 30 years after onset of DM. Although about one third of type 2 diabetics develop proteinuria, only 4% develop nephrotic syndrome and 6% develop ESRD. The fraction of patients with diabetic nephropathy progressing to ESRD has decreased over the past decade, owing primarily to the widespread use of renin angiotensin system (RAS) inhibitors and probably better diabetic control. However, due to the large number of type 2 diabetics, they constitute the majority of diabetics on dialysis. DM contributes up to 40% of all cases of ESRD in the United States.

49. **What is the earliest evidence of renal involvement in DM?**

An increase in GFR of 25–50% (hyperfiltration) and a slight enlargement of the kidney (hypertrophy) that persists for 5–10 years. At this stage, there may be a slight increase in albumin excretion rate (microalbuminuria), but the total protein excretion remains in the normal range. Studies indicate that patients with this "microalbuminuria" (>20 µg/min of albumin) are more likely to develop overt diabetic nephropathy than those who do not exhibit microalbuminuria. The clinical phase starts with the appearance of proteinuria on urine dipstick (corresponding to >300 mg/day).

50. **Why is diabetic nephropathy associated with large kidneys?**

Elevated levels of growth hormone, often seen with uncontrolled hyperglycemia, are incriminated in this renal hypertrophy; however, the exact cause remains unknown. Renal size is increased early in the course of diabetic renal disease and involves hypertrophy and hyperplasia.

51. **What interventions are used for renal protection in diabetic nephropathy?**

Control of BP, blood sugar levels, and dietary protein restriction have been shown to decrease proteinuria and retard the progression of renal failure. The hyperfiltration and hypertrophy seen early in the course of diabetic nephropathy can be corrected with insulin treatment. Strict glycemic control can reverse the elevated GFR and renal hypertrophy and also can decrease the spontaneous or exercise-induced microalbuminuria seen in the preclinical phase. Renin-angiotensin system inhibitors are also renoprotective and have contributed to significant improvement in slowing the progression to ESRD.

52. **What are the goals of glucose and BP control in diabetic patients?**

Maintenance of a blood glucose level within or close to the normal range while avoiding hypoglycemic attacks and maintaining a hemoglobin $A_{1c} < 7\%$. However, once overt nephropathy begins and progressive renal insufficiency ensues, the benefit of tight glycemic control is still observed, although it is less pronounced than in the preclinical phase. HTN control significantly slows the progression of diabetic nephropathy. The BP target level is <130/80 mm Hg for patients without proteinuria and <125/75 mm Hg for patients with significant proteinuria. ACE inhibitors have been shown to slow diabetic nephropathy progression, as do angiotensin receptor blockers (ARBs). The more recent Action to Control Cardiovascular Risk in Diabetes (ACCORD) and Action in Diabetes and Vascular Disease: Preterax and Diamicron Modified Release Controlled Evaluation (ADVANCE) trials, though, suggest that a lower hemoglobin A_{1c} may be associated with an increased cardiovascular mortality rate, although these data continue to be analyzed carefully. At this time, most experts continue to recommend modification of all cardiovascular risk factors, including control of blood glucose and HTN.

See also Chapter 4, Cardiology.

Boyko EJ. ACCORD glycemia results continue to puzzle. *Diabetes Care.* 2010;33:1149–1150.

Diabetes Control and Complications Trial Research Group. The effect of intensive treatment of diabetes on the development and progression of long-term complications in insulin-dependent diabetes mellitus. *N Engl J Med.* 1993;329:977–986.

The Action to Control Cardiovascular Risk in Diabetes Study Group, Gerstein HC, Miller ME, Byington RP, et al. Effects of intensive glucose lowering in type 2 diabetes. *N Engl J Med.* 2008;358:2545–2559.

The ADVANCE Collaborative Group, Patel A, MacMahon S, Chalmers J, et al. Intensive blood glucose control and vascular outcomes in patients with type 2 diabetes. *N Engl J Med.* 2008;358:2560–2572.

53. **How do inhibitors of the renin-angiotensin-aldosterone system (RAAS) slow the renal disease in diabetic nephropathy?**

Activation of RAAS occurs early in diabetic nephropathy and contributes to glomerular HTN by causing efferent arteriolar constriction. The resulting hyperfiltration leads to microalbuminuria, which predisposes to overt proteinuria. In addition, angiotensin II directly leads to oxidative stress. Other intracellular mediators result in functional and structural demise of the kidney in DM. By inhibiting angiotensin II production and action, the inhibitors of RAAS such as ACE inhibitors and ARBs slow down the progression of renal damage in diabetic nephropathy.

54. **Why are ACE inhibitors preferred in diabetic kidney disease?**

Because ACE inhibitors reduce intraglomerular HTN and thereby reduce proteinuria by decreasing the tone of efferent arterioles. Sufficient data now exist to support the use of ACE inhibitors, especially in diabetic patients with clinical or subclinical renal involvement, to retard the progression of diabetic nephropathy (in terms of both proteinuria as well as renal failure). A recent, large-scale, multicenter, prospective study concluded that captopril treatment was associated with a 50% reduction in the risk of death, dialysis, or transplantation in diabetics. This renal protective effect was independent of BP control. Patients with insulin-dependent DM with microalbuminuria (30–300 mg/day in at least two out of three measurements) or overt albuminuria (>300 mg/day) should receive an ACE inhibitor even in the absence of HTN or renal failure. ACE inhibitors should be the first-line agents in therapy for HTN in DM. Shortly after ACE inhibitors are started, S_{Cr} and potassium should be monitored to detect patients who develop hyperkalemia or an abrupt reduction in GFR. If no adverse effects are seen for at least 2 weeks, ACE inhibitors can be safely continued. ARBs can be used in place of ACE inhibitors when the latter are not tolerated.

Lewis EJ, Hunsicker LG, Bain RP, et al. The effect of angiotensin-converting enzyme inhibition on diabetic nephropathy. *N Engl J Med.* 1993;329:1456–1462.

55. **What other agents may be considered for BP control in diabetes?**
ARBs such as losartan and valsartan are also effective and renoprotective. Direct renin inhibitors (aliskiren) can effectively control HTN in the context of diabetes. But the combination of ACE inhibitors with ARB or ACE inhibitors or ARB with direct renin inhibitors is contraindicated because of increased adverse effects and poor outcomes. Although effective in controlling BP in renal failure, calcium channel blockers may not be as effective as ACE inhibitors in slowing the renal damage from DM. Nondihydropyridine calcium channel blockers (diltiazem and verapamil) have some renoprotective and antiproteinuric effects, whereas dihydropyridine calcium channel blockers (nifedipine and amlodipine) have no such benefits. Beta blockers may be effective, but their effects on the lipid profile and need for dose modification in renal failure and dialysis make them less desirable.

Parving HH, Brenner BM, McMurray JJ, et al. Cardiorenal end points in a trial of aliskiren for type 2 diabetes. *N Engl J Med.* 2012;367:2204–2213.

Parving HH, Smidt UM, Hommel E, et al. Effective antihypertensive treatment postpones renal insufficiency in diabetic nephropathy. *Am J Kidney Dis.* 1993;22:188–195.

56. **A 64-year-old white woman is being evaluated in the renal clinic for declining renal function. She has longstanding history of tobacco abuse, type 2 diabetes, osteoarthritis, and recently worsening HTN. Her BP is now 155/103 mm Hg. HbA$_{1c}$ is 9.2%, S_{Cr} is 2.8 mg/dL, and proteinuria is 6.3 g/day. What would you prescribe to this patient to slow down her renal disease?**
- Optimize antidiabetic medication for better glycemic control
- ACE inhibitors/ARB to be part of antihypertensive regimen
- Avoid nonsteroidal anti-inflammatory drugs (NSAIDs)
- Discontinue smoking

This patient has a profile that fits well with advanced diabetic nephropathy with uncontrolled diabetes, HTN, and history of arthritis and chronic smoking. The proven strategies to prevent progression of diabetic nephropathy include optimal control of diabetes, altering HTN regimen, discontinuation of NSAIDs, and tobacco cessation.

57. **Do diabetics with renal failure tolerate dialysis as well as nondiabetics?**
No. Previously, diabetics were not considered good candidates for dialytic therapy because about 80% of diabetics with ESRD who were placed on hemodialysis died in the first year. Results have since improved significantly. One report indicates a 1-year survival rate of 85% and a 3-year survival rate of 60% in diabetics on hemodialysis. However, even today, diabetics tend to do poorly compared with nondiabetics. Their 3-year survival rate is 20–30% less, and their mortality rate is 2.25 times higher than that of nondiabetics. Atherosclerotic cardiac disease is the most common cause of death, with infections a close second.

ACUTE KIDNEY INJURY

58. **What is AKI?**
AKI, a syndrome of many causes, is characterized by a sudden decrease in renal function leading to a compromise in the kidney's ability to regulate normal homeostasis. The kidney is unable to maintain the content and volume of the extracellular fluid or perform its routine endocrine functions. In most cases, AKI is a potentially reversible process. The clinical manifestations of AKI are generally more severe than those associated with chronic renal failure (CKD) because of the rapidity of development

of symptoms. Unlike CKD, a cause for AKI can usually be identified and must be addressed to prevent further kidney or other organ damage. AKI is a potentially reversible disorder if the causative factor or factors are identified and corrected, and appropriate supportive care must be given to optimize the chances for recovery of renal function. The cause of AKI is frequently multifactorial.

59. **What is the RIFLE classification of AKI?**
A stratified definition of AKI using five groups proposed by the Acute Dialysis Quality Initiative that improves consistency across studies and allows greater ability to compare clinical results (Table 8.2).

Table 8.2. RIFLE Classification

	GFR CRITERIA	URINE OUTPUT CRITERIA
Risk	S_{Cr} > 1.5 times baseline or GFR decrease > 25%	<0.5 mL/kg/hr × 6 hr
Injury	S_{Cr} > 2.0 times baseline or GFR decrease > 50%	<0.5 mL/kg/hr × 12 hr
Failure	S_{Cr} > 3.0 times baseline or GFR decrease > 75%; or S_{Cr} > 4.0 mg/dL	<0.5 mL/kg/hr × 24 hr
Loss	Persistent AKI = complete loss of renal function for >4 wk	
ESRD	End-stage kidney failure >3 mo	

AKI, acute kidney injury; ESRD, end-stage renal disease; GFR, glomerular filtration rate; RIFLE, risk, injury, failure, loss, ESRD; S_{Cr}, serum creatinine.
From Ricci Z, Cruz D, Ronco C. The RIFLE criteria and mortality in acute kidney injury: a systematic review. *Kidney Int.* 2008;73:538–546.

60. **How are the causes of AKI classified?**
Prerenal, renal, or postrenal.

61. **What is meant by prerenal failure?**
A decrease in renal function resulting from a decrease in renal perfusion. The decrease in renal perfusion leads to functional changes within the kidney, which in turn compromise the kidney's ability to perform its homeostatic functions. This disorder is potentially correctable by addressing the factors leading to renal hypoperfusion. In some cases, renal hypoperfusion can be severe and prolonged enough to result in structural damage and, hence, can lead to the "renal" category of AKI. Therefore, it is important that the prerenal syndrome be identified and corrected promptly.

62. **List the common prerenal causes of AKI in the United States.**
   • True volume depletion: as seen with gastrointestinal (GI) losses (vomiting, diarrhea, and bleeding), renal losses (diuretics, osmotic diuresis [glucose], hypoaldosteronism, salt-wasting nephropathy, and diabetes insipidus), skin or respiratory losses (insensible losses, sweat, and burns), and third-space sequestration (intestinal obstruction, crush injury or skeletal fracture, and acute pancreatitis)
   • Hypotension: shock
   • Edematous states: heart failure, hepatic cirrhosis, and nephrosis
   • Selective renal ischemia: hepatorenal syndrome, NSAIDs, bilateral renal artery stenosis, and calcium channel blockers

63. **List the typical findings in the urine of patients with prerenal azotemia.**
   • Low urinary sodium concentration: <20 mEq/L
   • Low fractional excretion of sodium: <1.0%
   • Low free-water excretion: high urine osmolality > 500 mOsm/L and urine specific gravity > 1.015

64. **What are the renal causes of AKI?**
   • **Ischemia:** all causes of severe prerenal disease, particularly hypotension.
   • **Nephrotoxins:** drugs and exogenous toxins. Common examples include aminoglycoside antibiotics, radiocontrast media, cisplatin, and NSAIDs. Rare examples include cephalosporins, rifampin, amphotericin B, polymyxin B, methoxyflurane, acetaminophen overdose, heavy metals (mercury, arsenic, and uranium), carbon tetrachloride, ethylenediamine tetraacetic acid, and tetracyclines. In addition, heme pigments may lead to rhabdomyolysis (myoglobinuria) and intravascular hemolysis (hemoglobinuria).

65. Define *acute tubular necrosis*.

A syndrome characterized by structural and functional damage of the renal tubules and a functional decrease of glomerular function. If the patient survives, ATN is self-limited, with most patients recovering renal function within 8 weeks. It is most commonly caused by ischemia, but there are a multitude of other causes.

66. How can the use of urinary indices help to distinguish prerenal failure from ATN?

Patients with prerenal azotemia have intact tubular function. The kidney, in this setting, is attempting to minimize solute and water excretion in an effort to preserve extracellular fluid volume, and this will be reflected in the urinary excretion of sodium and water. By contrast, the tubules of patients with ATN do not properly recover solutes and water that have been filtered into the kidney.

67. What are the urinary indices of patients with ATN?

- Urinary Na > 40 mEq/L
- Fractional Na excretion > 3.0%
- Urine osmolality < 350 mOsm/L
- Urine specific gravity < 1.010

The urinary indices of patients with ATN reveal the kidney's relative inability to reabsorb sodium and to reabsorb water. Remember that there is considerable crossover between renal and prerenal failure with regard to these indices, and hence, no value absolutely indicates one or the other diagnosis. The indices should be used along with other data (i.e., history and physical examination) to arrive at a clinical impression.

68. How is the FE_{Na}^+ calculated?

$$FE_{Na}^+ = \left(U_{Na}^+ \times P_{Cr} \times 100\right) / \left(P_{Na}^+ \times U_{Cr}\right)$$

where U_{Na}^+ is urinary plasma sodium (mEq/L); P_{Na}^+ is plasma sodium (mEq/L); U_{Cr} is urinary creatinine (mg/dL); and P_{Cr} is plasma creatinine (mg/dL).

69. What is the relevance of FE_{Na}^+ to the diagnosis of AKI?

An FE_{Na}^+ value <1% favors prerenal states, whereas a value >1% indicates intrarenal states or ATN. The test is more accurate than urinary Na measurement in this differentiation. However, it should be noted that FE_{Na}^+ < 1% is occasionally reported for various causes of AKI other than prerenal states. In addition, an intact sodium reabsorptive capacity is necessary for the use of this test. Thus, in conditions such as underlying chronic renal disease, hypoaldosteronism, diuretic therapy, or metabolic alkalosis with bicarbonaturia, the FE_{Na}^+ will be inappropriately high despite the presence of volume depletion.

70. What are the postrenal causes of AKI?

- Obstruction due to strictures
- Stones
- Malignancies
- Prostatic enlargement

71. What is renal-dose dopamine?

A widespread practice to use a low-dose dopamine IV infusion in critically ill patients with oliguria to prevent or treat AKI. This practice is based on the belief that dopamine increases the urine output through direct tubular effects and may also help to increase the tubular delivery of diuretics and renal blood flow. However, in low doses, dopamine may cause tachycardia and myocardial ischemia. In extreme cases, dopamine may also predispose to digital and bowel ischemia. Low-dose dopamine infusion is not without risk.

Chertow GM, Sayegh MH, Lazarus JM. Is dopamine administration associated with adverse or favorable outcomes in AKI? *Am J Med.* 1996;101:49–53.

72. List the indications for dialysis in patients with AKI.

- Uncontrolled hyperkalemia
- Acute pulmonary edema
- Uremic pericarditis
- Uremic encephalopathy (coma)
- Bleeding diathesis due to uremia

- Refractory metabolic acidosis (HCO_3^- < 10 mEq/L)
- Severe azotemia (BUN >100 mg/dL, S_{Cr} > 10 mg/dL)

73. What are CRRTs? What is their role in AKI?
Continuous renal replacement therapies, which are now increasingly used for treatment of AKI. These therapies are slow forms of dialytic treatments that are performed continuously. They are particularly beneficial in patients with hemodynamic instability that may preclude the use of conventional hemodialysis and are specifically advantageous when fluid removal is an important aspect of therapy.

74. What is the mortality rate of AKI?
Approximately 40–60% despite the availability of dialysis. The mortality rate is worse in the subcategory of patients with a history of surgery or trauma. The prognosis is better in the absence of respiratory failure, bleeding, and infection and in patients with nonoliguric ATN. AKI in the obstetric setting also has a better prognosis, with only a 10–20% mortality rate.

75. In which situations do ACE inhibitors lead to AKI?
Bilateral renal artery stenosis and renal artery stenosis of a single kidney or transplant kidney. AKI under these conditions may be mediated by ACE inhibitor–induced poststenotic dilatation of efferent arterioles and consequent reduction of glomerular hydrostatic pressure. In normal persons, this effect is offset by dilatation of afferent sites and maintenance of GFR. There have been reports of reversible renal failure in patients with chronic essential HTN treated with ACE inhibitors. In patients with severe nephrosclerosis, GFR depends on angiotensin-induced efferent arteriolar constriction. In patients with decreased effective renal blood flow, as in congestive heart failure, cirrhosis, or nephrosis, systemic hypotension and effective arteriolar dilatation caused by ACE inhibitors result in AKI.

Toto RD, Mitchell HC, Lee HC, et al. Reversible renal insufficiency due to angiotensin-converting enzyme inhibitors in hypertensive nephrosclerosis. *Ann Intern Med.* 1991;115:513–519.

76. Name the important risk factors for contrast-induced AKI.
Azotemia (Cr > 1.5 mg/dL)
Albuminuria > 2+
HTN
Age > 60 years
Dehydration
Uric acid > 8.0 mg/dL
Multiple radiologic studies
Solitary kidney
Contrast medium > 2 mL/kg
Multiple myeloma with renal insufficiency

Berns AS. Nephrotoxicity of contrast media. *Kidney Int.* 1989;36:730–740.

KEY POINTS: NEPHROLOGY

1. Reduce the frequency of contrast-induced renal failure by maintaining adequate hydration, minimizing the dose of contrast medium, and routinely using *N*-acetylcysteine.
2. Early detection of AKI is important because half of these patients may regain normal renal function with prompt intervention. Without intervention, mortality rate is high.
3. Renal replacement therapy in the form of hemodialysis, CAPD, or renal transplantation should be considered once creatinine clearance drops to 10 mL/min (15 mL/min in diabetics).
4. Diabetic patients with microalbuminuria or overt proteinuria should be treated with ACE inhibitors or ARBs even if BP is not elevated.
5. Reduction of proteinuria is critical in the management and prognosis of diabetic and nondiabetic glomerulopathies because proteinuria not only affects the progression of renal disease but is an independent risk factor for cardiovascular complications.

ACE, angiotensin-converting enzyme; AKI, acute kidney injury; ARBs, angiotensin receptor blockers; BP, blood pressure; CAPD, chronic ambulatory peritoneal dialysis.

CHRONIC KIDNEY DISEASE

77. **List the five stages of CKD.**
    - **Stage 1:** Kidney damage with normal renal reserve (GFR > 90 mL/min)
    - **Stage 2:** Mild renal insufficiency (GFR 60–89 mL/min)
    - **Stage 3:** Moderate renal failure (GFR 30–59 mL/min)
    - **Stage 4:** Severe renal failure or uremic syndrome (GFR 15–29 mL/min)
    - **Stage 5:** ESRD (GFR < 15 mL/min)

78. **Summarize the evolution of CKD through the five stages.**
    Patients with normal renal function have nephron mass in excess of that necessary to maintain a normal GFR. With progressive loss of renal mass, the **renal reserve** is initially lost, and subsequently, there is not a rise of BUN and creatinine or a disturbance of homeostasis. If the progression continues, mild **renal insufficiency** occurs, associated with mild elevation of BUN and creatinine and very mild symptoms, such as nocturia and easy fatigability. With further progression, moderate **renal failure** ensues. Abnormalities of renal excretory function become apparent, including disturbances in water, electrolyte, and acid-base metabolism. Continued worsening of renal function is followed by the stage of severe renal failure with **uremic syndrome,** which includes multiple dysfunction of major organ systems in addition to the abnormalities of excretory function described. Finally, **ESRD** appears, at which time renal replacement therapy (dialysis or transplantation) is required to sustain life.

79. **How do the remaining intact nephrons adapt in the diseased kidney?**
    By increasing the GFR and excretion of salt and water to maintain the same excretory function performed by the normal kidney. The increased excretory function is accomplished by reducing reabsorption of filtered salt and water, often resulting in polyuria and nocturia.

80. **What happens to the adaptation process in patients with chronic renal insufficiency?**
    The ability to respond to changes in intake with appropriate changes in excretory function is reduced. The remaining functioning nephrons of persons with decreased GFR are chronically excreting a higher salt load and are thus much closer to their maximum salt-excreting ability. Hence, these patients are less able to adjust to an increased salt intake by increasing salt excretion. At the opposite extreme, the remaining nephrons of the patient with a decreased GFR are less able to reduce their high salt excretion to compensate for a reduction in salt intake. These patients are more at risk of becoming salt-depleted in response to salt restriction than are patients with normal renal function.

81. **Why is the renal potassium excretory ability usually well maintained down to very low (10–15 mL/min) levels of GFR in patients with progressive CKD?**
    As is the case for salt excretion, the remaining intact nephrons increase potassium excretion, and the level of excretion per nephron is much higher than when there was a full contingent of nephrons, allowing for a total renal K^+ excretion that is nearly normal. In addition, there is evidence that the extrarenal K^+ excretion, especially by the colon, is increased in patients with CKD. By these mechanisms, patients with a significant decrease in GFR are unlikely to be hyperkalemic purely as a result of chronic renal insufficiency. In this clinical situation, if hyperkalemia is seen, consideration should be given to acute rather than chronic renal insufficiency, hormonal disorders (i.e., hyporeninemic hypoaldosteronism), or tubular disorders (i.e., obstructive uropathy).

82. **Name the common causes of CKD and their frequency of occurrence.**
    - **DM:** 38%
    - **HTN:** 25%
    - **Glomerulonephritis:** 16%
    - **Obstructive uropathy:** 2%
    - **Polycystic kidney disease and other interstitial diseases:** 3%
    - **Others:** 10%
      United States Renal Data System. 2015 USRDS annual data report: Epidemiology of kidney disease in the United States. Bethesda, MD: National Institutes of Health, National Institute of Diabetes and Digestive and Kidney Diseases; 2015. Available at: www.usrds.org.

83. About half a million patients in the United States are receiving renal replacement therapy for ESRD. What are the most common causes of ESRD?

Diabetic nephropathy, hypertensive nephrosclerosis, glomerulonephritides, cystic diseases, and interstitial nephritides. With the global epidemic of diabetes, the number of patients developing nephropathy from this single condition has become the leading cause of ESRD in not only the United States but also most parts of the world. As per the United States Renal Data System (USRDS), a federal agency that tracks the ESRD patient population in the United States, diabetic nephropathy has accounted consistently for over 35–40% of all ESRD for the past 2 decades, which is higher than any other condition that causes ESRD.

84. A 56-year-old obese white man is followed in your clinic for 4 years for a 12-year history of HTN, a 7-year history of gout, and a 6-year history of type 2 diabetes. His renal function has been deteriorating for the past 5 years. His current laboratory values are blood glucose 145 mg/dL (fasting), BUN 92 mg/dL, serum creatinine 6.8 mg/dL, and hemoglobin 8.7 g/dL. What is the cause of his anemia?

Likely a combination of iron deficiency, bleeding diathesis and blood losses, uremic toxins, and erythropoietin deficiency. Anemia occurs very commonly in CKD. Although diminished synthesis of erythropoietin in the kidney is the most common and dominant cause of anemia in CKD, it is truly multifactorial. Iron deficiency is very common in progressive renal failure. In fact correction of iron deficiency not only corrects anemia at least partially but also decreases the need for erythropoietin therapy. Other contributory factors for renal anemia include bleeding diathesis of uremia, blood losses due to GI bleeding and blood sampling, and bone marrow suppression by uremic toxins.

85. Discuss the new developments in the treatment of anemia of CKD.

The most important development is the use of recombinant human erythropoietin. Studies have documented the efficacy of this agent in improving the anemia and minimizing the need for blood transfusion. More important, the significance of correcting the iron deficiency in these patients by not only restoring the iron stores but also decreasing the requirements of the more expensive erythropoietin has been recognized.

Eschbach JW, Abdulhadi MH, Browne JK, et al. Recombinant human erythropoietin in anemic patients with end stage renal disease. *Ann Intern Med.* 1989;111:992–1000.

86. What are ESAs?

Erythropoietin-stimulating agents. These agents are human recombinant erythropoietin preparations that have been approved for the treatment of anemia in CKD and ESRD. These agents include erythropoietin alpha and darbepoietin.

87. Is it safe to normalize hemoglobin in CKD and dialysis patients?

No. The target hemoglobin in CKD and dialysis subjects who need ESAs is usually 11–12 g/dL. The Correction of Hemoglobin Outcomes in Renal Insufficiency (CHOIR) study showed that such higher hemoglobin levels of 13–15 g/dL are associated with increased cardiovascular morbidity and mortality rates.

Singh AK, Szczech L, Barnhart H, et al. Correction of anemia with epoetin alfa in chronic kidney disease. *N Engl J Med.* 2006;355:2085–2098.

88. A 67-year-old African-American man is being followed for chronic progressive renal insufficiency from focal sclerosis and is currently in stage IV CKD. The patient has no signs of uremia except pedal edema and modest anemia. His latest eGFR from MDRD is 23 mL/min, and intact parathyroid hormone (iPTH) is 478 IU. What is the most likely contributing factor for high iPTH level in advanced CKD?

Multiple factors including hypocalemia, decreased renal synthesis of 1,25(OH)D3, and hyperphosphatemia. Although hypocalcemia has been known for many decades to stimulate PTH secretion, observations in the past 2 decades have established the role of decreased renal synthesis of 1,25-dihydroxycholecalciferol and elevated phosphorus in independently increasing PTH levels.

DIALYSIS

89. What are the indications for dialysis in a patient with CKD?

When conservative management fails to maintain the patient in reasonable comfort. Usually, dialysis is required when the GFR drops to 5–10 mL/min, but it is both unnecessary and risky to adhere to strict biochemical indications. Broadly speaking, the development of uremic encephalopathy, neuropathy, pericarditis, and bleeding diathesis is an indication to start dialysis immediately. Fluid overload, congestive heart failure, hyperkalemia, metabolic acidosis, and HTN uncontrolled by conservative measures are also indications for starting patients on dialysis therapy.

90. **What are the contraindications for dialysis?**
The presence of potentially reversible abnormalities is a major contraindication for dialysis. These abnormalities include volume depletion, urinary tract infection (UTI), urinary obstruction, hypercatabolic state, uncontrolled HTN, hypercalcemia, nephrotoxic drugs, and low cardiac output state.

91. **Which clinical manifestations of uremia (CKD) can be improved with dialysis? Which ones persist or worsen?**

Improve	Persist	Develop or Worsen
Uremic encephalopathy	Renal osteodystrophy	Dialysis dementia
Seizures	Hypertriglyceridemia	Nephrogenic ascites
Pericarditis	Amenorrhea and infertility	Dialysis pericarditis
Fluid overload	Peripheral neuropathy	Dialysis bone disease
Electrolyte imbalances	Pruritus	Accelerated atherosclerosis
GI symptoms	Anemia	Carpal tunnel syndrome (amyloid-related)
Metabolic acidosis	Risk of hepatitis	

92. **Which poisons and toxins are dialyzable?**
   - Alcohols: ethanol, methanol, ethylene glycol
   - Salicylates
   - Heavy metals: mercury, arsenic, and lead
   - Halides
     In addition, hemoperfusion successfully removes barbiturates, sedatives (meprobamate, methaqualone, and glutethimide), acetaminophen, digoxin, procainamide, quinidine, and theophylline.

93. **What is chronic ambulatory peritoneal dialysis (CAPD)?**
A manual form of peritoneal dialysis, usually performed by the patient, in which 1–2 L of dialysate fluid are infused into the peritoneal space through a Tenckhoff catheter and then drained after a dwell time of 4–6 hours. The exchanges are repeated four to five times a day. CAPD is indicated in any patient with ESRD.

94. **What are the indications and contraindications for CAPD?**
CAPD is the treatment of choice for diabetics with severe peripheral vascular disease because hemodialysis is not a viable option for such patients. This method provides more independence and mobility, and it should be offered to all young patients leading active lives. The contraindications include blindness, severe disabling arthritis, presence of colostomy, poor patient motivation, and quadriplegia.

95. **What are the common mechanical complications of CAPD?**
Pain, bleeding, leakage, inadequate drainage, intraperitoneal catheter loss, abdominal wall edema, scrotal edema, incisional hernia, other hernia, intestinal hematoma, and intestinal perforation.

96. **What are the common metabolic complications of CAPD?**
Hyperglycemia, hyperosmolar nonketotic coma, postdialysis hypoglycemia, hyperkalemia, hypokalemia, hypernatremia, hyponatremia, metabolic alkalosis, protein depletion, hyperlipidemia, and obesity.

97. **List other potential complications of CAPD.**
   - **Infections and inflammation:** bacterial or fungal peritonitis, tunnel infection, exit-site infection, diverticulitis, sterile peritonitis, eosinophilic peritonitis, sclerosing peritonitis, and pancreatitis
   - **Cardiovascular:** acute pulmonary edema, fluid overload, hypotension, arrhythmia, cardiac arrest, and HTN
   - **Pulmonary:** basal atelectasis, aspiration pneumonia, hydrothorax, respiratory arrest, and decreased forced vital capacity (FVC)

98. What are the causes of peritonitis in a patient on peritoneal dialysis?
    - *Staphylococcus epidermidis* and *Staphylococcus aureus*: 70%
    - Gram-negative organisms: 20%
    - Fungi and mycobacteria: 5%
    The frequency of infection has decreased considerably since this dialysis method was first introduced, to about one episode every 18–24 patient-months. This decrease is mainly due to the addition of a Luer-Lok adapter between the catheter and the tubing and the institution of monthly tubing changes.

RENAL CANCER

99. A 59-year-old Hispanic man with history of diabetes and HTN has been on dialysis for the past 6 years. His past medical history is remarkable for angina, PVD, and a recent stroke. What is the most likely cause of death for this patient?
    Cardiovascular diseases. Although accidental falls, trauma, and renal causes are a true risk and account for significant morbidity in ESRD, with the huge cardiovascular disease burden and risk, cardiovascular events remain the most common cause of death in these patients, followed by infectious complications.

100. What is dialysis-associated amyloidosis?
    The accumulation and deposition of amyloid fibrils containing beta$_2$ microglobulin associated with long-term dialytic therapy. Amyloidosis is usually manifested after 5–7 years of chronic dialytic therapy and is seen in most patients after 10 years of dialysis. Clinical findings include asymptomatic lytic bone lesions, carpal tunnel syndrome (often bilateral), tenosynovitis, scapulohumeral periarthritis, and destructive arthropathy. No satisfactory preventive measures are available.
    Koch KM. Dialysis related amyloidosis. *Kidney Int.* 1992;41:1416–1429.

NEPHROLITHIASIS

101. What three mechanisms are important in the development of nephrolithiasis?
    - Precipitation of a substance from supersaturated solutions to form stones that is related to many factors, including solubility and concentration of the substance and urine characteristics (e.g., pH).
    - Reduced concentration of normal constituents of urine that inhibit stone formation including citrate, pyrophosphate, and magnesium.
    - Contribution of the protein matrix to the formation, growth, and aggregation of stones. This matrix derives in part from renal tubular epithelial cells and from the uroepithelium.

102. What are the common constituents of urinary stones in the United States, and what is their frequency?
    - Calcium oxalate: 35%
    - Calcium apatite: 35%
    - Magnesium ammonium phosphate (struvite): 18%
    - Uric acid: 6%
    - Cystine: 3%

103. Summarize the conditions that favor the formation of each kind of stone.
    In general, an alkaline urine pH favors precipitation of inorganic stone such as calcium phosphate that undergoes rearrangement into hydroxyapatite. Alkaline urine pH and high concentrations of urinary ammonia lead to supersaturation of magnesium ammonium phosphate (struvite). This environment is created by the presence of urea-splitting bacteria (commonly *Proteus*, *Pseudomonas*, *Klebsiella*, and *Staphylococcus*), which contain the enzyme urease and convert urea to ammonia and CO_2. An acid pH favors precipitation of organic stone such as uric acid and cystine. Urine pH has little effect on calcium oxalate solubility and, therefore, little influence on the formation of these stones.

104. List common metabolic conditions that predispose to the formation of urinary stones.
    - **Idiopathic hypercalciuria** (50%): may be related to increased GI absorption, bone resorption, and renal loses of calcium
    - **Low urinary citrate excretion** (50%): frequently occurs with other conditions

- **Hyperuricosuria** (30%): occurs with and without gout and may contribute to calcium stone formation
- **Hyperoxaluria** (15%): due to various causes

105. **What are the less common causes of urinary stones?**
   - Chronic UTI
   - Primary hyperparathyroidism
   - Cystinuria
   - Distal renal tubular acidosis (RTA)

   Typically, more than one of these conditions are present in a stone-forming patient.

106. **What are the symptoms of urinary obstruction by a stone?**
   Usually severe, colicky pain that radiates toward the lower abdomen and genital area. The ureteropelvic junction, the midureter as it crosses the iliac artery, and the ureterovesical junction are the common sites for urinary obstruction by stones. In women who have children, the pain is often described as more severe than the pain of labor. The increased pressure inside the collecting system decreases the net pressure for glomerular filtration, resulting in a decreased GFR. The resulting urinary stasis predisposes to infection.

107. **Do the consequences of acute urinary obstruction have permanent effects?**
   No. The GFR corrects toward normal if the stone passes or is removed from the urinary tract within a few days. If the obstruction becomes chronic, permanent renal injury can ensue, with an irreversible reduction in GFR and chronic dilatation of the collection system. This dilated collecting system is less efficient in delivering urine to the bladder (because of compromised peristalsis), predisposing to urinary stasis and infection.

108. **How should you manage the patient with acute urinary obstruction due to a stone?**
   Initially with supportive management with analgesics and oral fluids because most stones spontaneously pass in a few hours to days. Serum chemistries should be done to document the degree of renal dysfunction (if any) and an imaging procedure (renal ultrasound [US], noncontrast helical computed tomography [CT]) is performed to locate the stone and estimate its size in order to help determine the possible need for surgical intervention.

109. **What should you do once the acute phase of obstruction ends?**
   Evaluate the patient for underlying conditions that led to the formation of the stone, which will lead to a protocol for long-term management. A reasonable percentage of patients recover stone material from their urine. However, laboratory analysis is usually not readily available, and the approach to further management is more often empirical than based on analysis of recovered stones.

110. **Describe the general approach to avoidance of recurrent stones.**
   Maintenance of a dilute urine through high intake of hypotonic fluids. More specific management depends on the predisposing condition.

111. **What measures are appropriate for patients with absorptive or renal hypercalciuria?**
   Absorptive hypercalciuria can be managed by reducing dietary calcium (type 2 only), reducing intestinal calcium absorption by using cellulose sodium phosphate (type 1), or a thiazide diuretic, which promotes renal calcium reabsorption. **Renal** hypercalciuria can also be treated with thiazides.

112. **How is primary hyperparathyroidism treated?**
   With parathyroidectomy in selected patients. (See also Chapter 16, Endocrinology.)

113. **Summarize the management of uricosuric states.**
   Uricosuric states result from the overproduction of uric acid and can be treated with allopurinol or with potassium citrate if patients have hyperuricosuria associated with calcium oxalate stones.

114. **Describe the treatment of patients with excessive intestinal oxalate absorption.**
   With a low-oxalate diet and use of magnesium or calcium salts, which bind oxalate and inhibit its reabsorption.

115. **How is cystinuria treated?**
With conservative management and maintenance of a dilute or alkaline urine or with penicillamine, which increases the solubility of cysteine if the conservative measures are ineffective.

116. **How should you manage patients with struvite stones?**
Treat UTIs with antibiotics, and use the urease inhibitor acetohydroxamic acid, if needed.

117. **What is lithotripsy?**
Litho (stone or calculus) *tripsy* (crushing) is a way of breaking up stones by use of shock waves or US and may serve as an alternative to operation or cystoscopy for the removal of stones in the kidney and urinary tract.

118. **What are the three forms now available for lithotripsy?**
- Extracorporeal shock-wave lithotripsy
- Percutaneous ultrasonic lithotripsy
- Endoscopic ultrasonic lithotripsy

URINARY TRACT OBSTRUCTION

119. **List the common causes of ureteric obstruction in adults.**
- Renal stones
- Prostatic, bladder, or pelvic malignancy
- Retroperitoneal lymphoma, metastasis, or fibrosis
- Accidental surgical ligation
- Blood clot
- Pregnancy
- Stricture

120. **How do unilateral and bilateral obstructions differ in their effects on the GFR?**
Unilateral obstruction does not necessarily lead to a clinically measurable decrease in GFR in patients with normal renal function, but bilateral obstruction quite often leads to a decreased GFR in patients with both normal and abnormal renal function.

121. **Describe in detail how unilateral obstruction affects the GFR.**
In patients with normal renal function, unilateral obstruction with complete obliteration of ipsilateral function forces recruitment of the nephron reserve of the unaffected, contralateral kidney, resulting in no changes or only small changes in total GFR. Relatively large reductions in functioning nephron mass (~40%) are necessary to elicit an appreciable rise in the P_{Cr} concentrations when baseline renal function is normal (P_{Cr} 0.8–1.2 mg/dL). The relatively small change in GFR in patients with normal baseline renal function who are subjected to unilateral obstruction probably will not be reflected by a rise in P_{Cr}. The response is different for patients with baseline renal insufficiency. Such patients have already lost their reserve nephron mass and are likely using compensatory mechanisms to maintain their GFR. Unilateral obstruction in such patients may result in a significant fall in GFR and is more likely to be associated with a rise in P_{Cr}.

122. **Describe the differences in clinical presentation between acute and chronic obstruction of the urinary tract.**
Partial or complete obstruction of the urinary tract compromises urine passage whether it is acute or chronic. Nevertheless, the urinary findings and clinical consequences differ depending on the duration of the obstruction. After release of an **acute (>24-hour) obstruction**, there is commonly a decrease in excretion of sodium, potassium, and water. This results in excretion of a urine low in sodium and with increased osmolarity, a situation also seen with volume depletion. In contrast, release of **chronic obstruction** commonly results in increased excretion of sodium and water and decreased excretion of acid (with urinary loss of bicarbonate) and potassium. These abnormalities can lead to volume depletion, free-water deficit (reflected by hypernatremia), and hyperkalemic non–anion gap metabolic acidosis.

123. **What abnormalities of tubular function can occur with chronic obstruction?**
Chronic obstruction affects primarily distal rather than proximal nephron functions, including reabsorption of sodium and water and secretion of acid and potassium. The decreased **water** reabsorption results from decreased responsiveness of the collecting tubule to antidiuretic hormone,

yielding a form of nephrogenic diabetes insipidus. The **acid** secretory defect results in incomplete bicarbonate recovery from the urine and a non–anion gap metabolic acidosis. The **potassium** secretory defect results in potassium retention and hyperkalemia. Therefore, obstructive nephropathy is a common cause of hyperkalemic, hyperchloremic, non–anion gap metabolic acidosis. These abnormalities usually resolve after correction of the obstruction but may require weeks or months to do so. In addition to the decrease in GFR and the potential tubular abnormalities, the resulting urinary stasis can predispose to infection, renal stones, and papillary necrosis. The salt and water retention can lead to HTN.

124. **Which components of polyuria (postobstructive diuresis) are seen immediately after correction of chronic obstruction?**
The patient with obstruction and compromised renal function accumulates solute and water that are ordinarily excreted by the normally functioning kidney. Correction of the obstruction results in appropriate excretion of the accumulated urea, NaCl, and water in an effort to return the volume and content of the extracellular fluid to normal. This polyuria is physiologic. However, a minority of such patients have a pathologic polyuria, resulting from poor salt and water reabsorption. These abnormalities commonly resolve within a few hours but may last for days. Usually, the polyuria is physiologic, but the patient must be observed. Pathologic polyuria may occur because of either salt or water loss (or both). Pathologic salt loss is reflected by continued excretion of a large amount of urinary sodium in the setting of volume depletion. Pathologic water loss is reflected by excretion of large volumes of dilute urine in spite of rising serum osmolality.

125. **Should the polyuria after correction of obstruction be treated?**
In pathologic polyuria, appropriate fluid replacement therapy should be instituted. If replacement is instituted during the physiologic polyuria, one will "chase" the patient's volume status so that polyuria continues as a result of the fluids that are administered.

126. **Explain "functional" obstruction of the urinary tract.**
Abnormalities that compromise the exit of urine from the kidney in the absence of anatomic obstruction of the outflow tract. Two examples are an atonic bladder and vesicoureteral reflux.

127. **What is an atonic bladder?**
A bladder that is unable to empty itself completely and hence contains urine, continuously yielding a higher than normal hydrostatic pressure. This high bladder pressure is transmitted via the ureters and may cause the abnormalities described earlier.

128. **What causes vesicoureteral reflux?**
Retrograde flow of urine into the ureter or kidney or both during voiding due to an incompetent vesicoureteral valve. The transmitted pressure is felt to contribute to the renal abnormalities. Both of these conditions also predispose to infection.

129. **How is the diagnosis of lower urinary tract obstruction (LTO) made?**
By history, clinical setting, and the laboratory findings. A palpable urinary bladder on examination is strong evidence for LTO or an atonic bladder. A postvoid residual urine volume of >100 mL on Foley catheter insertion is supportive of LTO. Imaging studies help confirm the diagnosis.

130. **Which imaging studies are helpful in the diagnosis of LTO?**
   - Plain abdominal radiographs: can show distended bladder as well as large kidney
   - Renal US: can detect hydronephrosis
   - Abdominal CT scan: if further imaging is needed
   - Retrograde pyelography (selective catheterization and insertion of contrast dye into both ureters via cystoscopy): may be necessary if LTO is suspected but not found by x-ray, US, or CT examinations
   - Radionuclide renal scans: suggest LTO when there is prompt uptake of the dye with prolonged excretion

   IV pyelograms should be avoided owing to the risk of additional renal injury from the contrast dye.

131. **How does imaging help determine the prognosis of LTO?**
Development of hydronephrosis usually up to 48 hours; therefore, the absence of hydronephrosis does not rule out LTO. The chances of recovery of renal function in LTO can be predicted based on the extent and duration of parenchymal injury. The US studies will reflect this by the degree of cortical thinning and echogenicity of the renal parenchyma.

RENAL BONE DISEASE

132. **What is the Bricker "trade-off" hypothesis?**
The theory propounded by Neil Bricker to explain the secondary hyperparathyroidism seen in renal failure.

133. **Explain the trade-off hypothesis.**
Early in the course of renal failure, the kidney fails to excrete phosphorus, leading to a transient and often undetectable rise in serum phosphorus. This tends to lower the serum level of ionized calcium temporarily, leading to stimulation of PTH secretion. The increased levels of PTH reduce tubular reabsorption of phosphate, leading to phosphate excretion and thereby tending to normalize the serum calcium and phosphorus levels. However, this process occurs at the expense of an elevated PTH level. With further declines in renal function, the serum phosphorus tends to rise, and the whole cycle is repeated. With advancing renal failure, these changes tend to keep serum calcium and phosphorus levels below normal at the expense of increasing serum PTH levels. The serum level of PTH is increased in an attempt to normalize serum phosphate and calcium levels, but the "trade-off" is the bone disease (osteitis fibrosa cystica) caused by the elevated PTH levels.

134. **List the three major bone histologic subtypes found in renal osteodystrophy.**
Osteitis fibrosa cystica, which is a result of high bone turnover (bone changes due to secondary hyperparathyroidism), **osteomalacia,** and occasionally, **osteosclerosis.** With better management of patients with ESRD, the long-term course of renal bone disease and its clinical features have changed, and newer entities have emerged. Adynamic or aplastic bone disease or low bone turnover has become a fairly common bone disease. Aluminum accumulation causes osteomalacia, which is one cause of adynamic bone disease. Decreased vitamin D, DM, and iron accumulation are other factors associated with adynamic bone disease.

135. **Why do patients with CKD and marked hypocalcemia often fail to manifest tetany?**
Because of the acidemia seen in CKD, ionized calcium is usually not reduced enough to cause tetany. Tetany is the result of decreased ionized calcium, which is decreased in the presence of alkemia. Tetany is usually only manifested in the presence of an alkaline pH. However, if the acidosis of CKD is excessively treated with alkalizing agents, tetany may become manifest.

136. **How do you manage secondary hyperparathyroidism in patients with CKD?**
By reducing the serum PTH levels with vitamin D analogs. However, vitamin D therapy should not be attempted before the serum phosphorus level is normalized or the product of calcium and phosphorus is lowered to <70. The most commonly used vitamin D preparation is calcitriol (1,25-dihydroxycholecalciferol) in either oral or IV form. More recently, other analogs of vitamin D such as 19-nor-cholecalciferol and 1-alpha-calcidiol have been successfully used and may cause less hypercalcemia.

137. **Does bone disease improve with dialysis?**
No. Renal osteodystrophy does not always improve with dialytic therapy. Indeed, the symptoms may worsen or progress because a number of additional factors are introduced that either directly or indirectly influence the severity of renal bone disease, including the aluminum content of dialysate, heparin administration, and administration of large amounts of acetate.

Sherrard DJ, Hercz G, Pei Y, et al. The spectrum of bone disease in end stage renal failure—an evolving disorder. *Kidney Int.* 1993;43:436–442.

138. **Does renal transplantation improve bone disease?**
Yes. In patients who undergo renal transplantation, the uremic bone disease improves to a great extent. Increased osteoclastic and osteoblastic activities are noted within a few weeks after transplantation. However, in some patients, osteoporosis and the effects of secondary hyperparathyroidism may persist for as long as 1–2 years. In addition, steroid therapy may be responsible for osteoporosis and osteonecrosis that complicate the later phases of the posttransplant period. Another abnormality that may develop in the posttransplant phase is a renal phosphate leak, which, if severe, may contribute to osseous abnormalities.

RENAL TRANSPLANTATION

139. **Who is a potential candidate for renal transplantation?**
All patients with ESRD who need some form of renal replacement therapy.

140. What are the absolute contraindications to renal transplantation?
- Reversible renal disease
- Active infection
- Recent malignant disease
- Active glomerulonephritis
- Presensitization to donor class I major transplantation antigens
- Acquired immunodeficiency syndrome (AIDS)

141. List the relative contraindications to renal transplantation.
- Fabry disease (an inherited lysosomal storage disease)
- Oxalosis
- Advanced age
- Psychiatric problems
- Presence of anatomic urologic abnormality
- Iliofemoral occlusion
- Chronic active hepatitis

142. A 45-year-old school teacher with longstanding history of type 2 diabetes and HTN is seen for progressive fatigue, fluid retention, nausea, and pruritus. His current laboratory values are serum creatinine 5.9 mg/dL, BUN 88 mg/dL, hemoglobin 9.1 g/dL, phosphorus 7.2 mg/dL, calcium 8.2 mg/dL, iPTH 365 IU. After explaining that he will need renal replacement therapy, what would you recommend as the option with the best outcomes?

Renal transplantation. This patient with near end-stage renal failure has azotemia, hypocalcemia, hyperphosphatemia, and high PTH levels. He clearly needs initiation of renal replacement therapy. Although all modalities extend patient survival significantly, renal transplantation offers the best outcomes in terms of survival and quality of life parameters. Considering the relatively young age of this patient, renal transplantation is the best option for him.

143. What are the donor-selection criteria for living-related transplantation?

Normal physical examination, age < 65 years, and the same ABO blood group as the recipient or type O. An angiogram is necessary to exclude the presence of multiple or abnormal renal arteries, because such abnormalities make the surgery prolonged and difficult. In general, the left kidney is preferred because of the longer renal vein. Some relative contraindications for kidney donation include severe HTN, DM, HIV positivity, active medical illness, urologic abnormalities, persistently abnormal urinalyses, and family history of nephritis, polycystic kidney disease, or other renal disease.

144. What factors are considered important in evaluating suitability of a cadaver kidney?

No history of neoplastic or infectious disease, preferably age < 60 years, and good urine output and a normal S_{Cr} before death. Urinalyses should be normal, and urine cultures should be negative. The kidney should be transplanted as early after harvesting as possible. The graft function tends to be worse 24 hours after harvesting. The donor should be free of infection with hepatitis B virus and HIV.

145. Give the current survival figures for renal transplant recipients in the United States.

The 1-year patient survival rate for living-related renal transplantation is now around 95–100% and for cadaveric transplantation approximately 90%. With cyclosporine therapy, graft survival rates are 90% and 80%, respectively, for living and cadaveric kidney transplants.

146. What are the common immunosuppressive agents used in renal transplantation?
- **Induction therapy (perioperatively):** corticosteroids (IV methylprednisolone at engraftment followed by oral prednisone tapered over the first 3 months) and possibly monoclonal antibodies such as basiliximab or daclizumab that block interleukin 2 (IL-2) receptors
- **Maintenance therapy (during the life of the kidney):** oral corticosteroids, antimetabolites (mycophenolate mofetil), and calcineurin inhibitors (cyclosporine and tacrolimus)

147. **What is acute rejection, and how is it treated?**
An acute deterioration in renal allograft function associated with specific pathologic changes in the graft. Acute rejection can occur at any time but most often occurs in the first 6 months after transplant. As a result of better immunosuppressive regimens, the incidence of acute rejection is declining and is currently <20% in the first year in many transplant centers. Acute rejection could be acute cellular or acute humoral rejection. The treatment of acute cellular rejection usually includes high-dose IV corticosteroids, polyclonal antibodies such as antithymocyte globulins, or monoclonal antibodies such as OKT3 and rituximab. Acute humoral rejection can also be treated with plasmapheresis, steroids, and IV immunoglobulin (IVIG).

MISCELLANEOUS RENAL DISORDERS

148. **How is a patient with recurrent hematuria evaluated?**
Initially with renal imaging and urinary instrumentation to exclude urinary stones and other structural lesions such as tumors of the upper and lower urinary tract. The presence of dysmorphic erythrocytes or RBC casts helps to distinguish glomerular bleeding from lower tract bleeding. Glomerular bleeding accounts for recurrent hematuria in over a quarter of patients younger than age 40 years.

149. **What are the risk factors associated with aminoglycoside nephrotoxicity?**
    - Dose and duration of drug therapy
    - Recent aminoglycoside therapy
    - Preexisting renal or liver failure
    - Older age
    - Volume depletion
    - Concurrent nephrotoxin administration
    - Potassium or magnesium depletion or both

    Fumes D. Aminoglycoside nephrotoxicity. *Kidney Int.* 1988;33:900–911.

150. **How should antibiotic doses be adjusted in patients with renal failure?**
Several antibiotics need dosage modification in the presence of renal failure, notably aminoglycosides, most cephalosporins, many penicillins, most fluoroquinolones, and vancomycin. The adjustments can be made by maintaining the usual dose and varying the dosing interval, maintaining the dosing interval and varying the dose, or a combination of the two. The objective is to obtain a therapeutic drug concentration–time profile that is therapeutic and not toxic. For most commonly used antibiotics, dosing guidelines are established and readily accessible. No adjustment is needed for erythromycin, doxycycline, rifampin, and oral vancomycin. Tetracyclines, nitrofurantoin, nalidixic acid, and bacitracin should be totally avoided in renal failure.

    Brier ME, Aronoff GR, Burns JS, et al. *Drug Prescribing in Renal Failure.* 5th ed. Philadelphia: American College of Physicians; 2007, pp 45–75.

151. **How do drugs interfere with assessment of renal function?**
Cimetidine, trimethoprim, and acetylsalicylic acid increase S_{Cr} by interfering with the tubular creatinine secretion, whereas methyldopa and cefoxitin interfere with creatinine assay, artificially elevating the S_{Cr} level. Tolbutamide, penicillins, cephalosporins, sulfonamides, and contrast media can cause a false-positive reaction for protein in the urine.

152. **How do antacids interact with other drugs in cases of renal failure?**
Antacids impair the gastric absorption of **beta blockers** and **ferrous sulfate.** These drugs should be given 1–2 hours apart.

153. **With what drug may Scholl solution interact in patients with renal failure?**
Aluminun hydroxide. Scholl solution contains sodium citrate, and citrate increases aluminum absorption so that aluminum toxicity may result. The combination has to be avoided.

154. **Explain the interaction between azathioprine and allopurinol.**
Azathioprine levels in the blood are elevated when used in conjunction with allopurinol owing to decreased xanthine oxidase metabolism of azathioprine. The azathioprine dose, therefore, has to be decreased and leukocyte counts followed.

155. **Which drugs alter cyclosporine levels in the plasma?**
Phenytoin, phenobarbital, and **rifampin** increase cyclosporine clearance by the liver, and higher doses may be needed. Conversely, **erythromycin, amphotericin B,** and **ketoconazole** decrease cyclosporine clearance by the liver; thus, the dose needs to be decreased.

156. **How does pregnancy affect healthy kidneys?**
Owing to increased blood volume and hyperdynamic circulation in pregnancy, renal hemodynamics are altered. Most important, clearances of urea, creatinine, and uric acid are increased, leading to a decrease in the serum concentrations of these compounds. Urine protein excretion rates are increased. There is some dilatation of the collecting system, including the ureters, partially due to the pressure from the gravid uterus but mainly due to the effect of progestational hormones on the muscular tone of the ureters. All of these changes revert to normalcy once the patient delivers.

157. **How does pregnancy affect diseased kidneys?**
Most renal diseases with proteinuria demonstrate increases in proteinuria during pregnancy. In diabetics with no renal disease, pregnancy does not adversely affect the renal function. However, there are no data about effects of pregnancy on renal function in patients with advanced diabetic nephropathy. Lupus nephritis is associated with an increased rate of spontaneous abortion and increased fetal loss. However, there is no evidence that pregnancy affects the long-term prognosis of lupus nephritis.

158. **Describe a simple renal cyst.**
Simple cysts represent 60–70% of renal masses. They are common after age 50, most often asymptomatic, and usually detected as incidental findings in radiologic procedures done for other reasons.

159. **How is a simple renal cyst distinguished from a malignant cyst?**
On sonography, a simple cyst has smooth, sharply delineated margins, no echoes within the mass, and a strong posterior wall echo indicating good transmission through the cyst. These features generally exclude the possibility of malignancy. However, if there is any further suspicion, a CT scan should be done. CT findings consistent with a simple cyst include fluid that is homogeneous with a density of 0–20 Hounsfield units and no enhancement of the cyst fluid following the administration of radiocontrast medium. Characteristics of renal cysts are summarized in Table 8.3.

160. **You evaluate a 53-year-old man admitted to the hospital with fever, chills, right flank pain, and dysuria. Two years ago when he was evaluated for newly detected HTN, he was noted to have polycystic kidney disease. Urinalysis shows 15–20 RBCs, plenty of WBCs, and 3+ bacteria. An abdominal US examination is unremarkable except for bilateral polycystic kidneys, showing one of the renal cysts in the right kidney filled with highly echogenic material. What should be done first?**
Start IV ciprofloxacin. One does not need to wait for urine culture results, but empiric therapy should be started. An antibiotic such as ampicillin would not penetrate the cyst wall (demonstrated on US as infected) and reach adequate concentration to clear the infection. Surgical drainage is needed only in cases resistant to IV antibiotics.

161. **What are the renal manifestations of HIV disease?**
The most common chronic renal disease from HIV infection is a type of focal glomerulosclerosis, the so-called HIV nephropathy. Typically, nephrotic proteinuria, large echogenic kidneys, minimal or modest HTN, and rapidly progressive renal failure characterize the disease. Dialysis is well tolerated; however, the mean survival time is less than 1 year in patients with full-blown AIDS. The other renal manifestations include hyponatremia, hyperkalemia (often secondary to adrenal disease or hyporenin hypoaldosteronism), hypouricemia, and AKI, often due to anti-HIV medications. (See also Chapter 13, AIDS and HIV Infection.)

162. **Describe the major differences between fibromuscular dysplasia (FMD) and atherosclerotic renal artery stenosis.**
See Table 8.4.

Table 8.3. Characteristics of Renal Cystic Disorders

FEATURE	CYSTS	ADPKD	ARPKD	ACKD	MCD	MSK
Inheritance pattern	None	Autosomal dominant	Autosomal recessive	None	Often present, variable pattern	None
Incidence or prevalence	Common, increasing with age	1/200–1/1000	Rare	40% in patients on dialysis	Rare	Common
Age of onset	Adult	Usually adults	Neonates, children	Older adults	Adolescents, young adults	Adults
Presenting symptom	Incidental finding, hematuria	Pain, hematuria, infection, family screening	Abdominal mass, renal failure, failure to thrive	Hematuria	Polyuria, polydipsia, enuresis, renal failure, failure to thrive	Incidental, UTIs, hematuria, renal calculi
Hematuria	Occurs	Common	Occurs	Occurs	Rare	Common
Recurrent infections	Rare	Common	Occurs	No	Rare	Common
Renal calculi	No	Common	No	No	No	Common
Hypertension	Rare	Common	Common	Present from underlying disease	Rare	No
Diagnosis	Ultrasound	Ultrasound, gene linkage analysis	Ultrasound	CT scan	None reliable	Excretory urogram
Renal size	Normal	Normal to very large	Large initially	Small to normal, occ. large	Small	Normal

ACKD, acquired cystic kidney disease; ADPKD, autosomal dominant polycystic kidney disease; ARPKD, autosomal recessive polycystic kidney disease; CT, computed tomography; MCD, medullary cystic disease; MSK, medullary sponge kidney; UTIs, urinary tract infections.
Adapted from Grantham JJ. Cystic diseases of kidney. In: Goldman L, Bennett JC, eds. *Cecil Textbook of Medicine.* 21st ed. Philadelphia: WB Saunders; 2000.

Table 8.4. Fibromuscular Dysplasia Versus Therosclerotic Renal Artery Stenosis

	FMD	**ATHEROSCLEROSIS**
Age at onset	<40 yr	>45 yr
Gender	80% female	Primarily male
Distribution of lesion	Distal main renal artery	Aortic orifice and proximal main renal artery and intrarenal branches
Progression	Uncommon	Common; may progress to complete occlusion

FMD, fibromuscular dysplasia.

163. **When should you consider renovascular HTN?**
When the onset of HTN occurs before age 20 or after age 50. Similarly, the development of a refractory phase in a previously stable hypertensive patient, the presence of spontaneous hypokalemia, and the presence of an abdominal bruit are also suggestive.

164. **What laboratory tests are useful in screening for renovascular HTN?**
Imaging techniques have largely replaced laboratory tests now in diagnosing renovascular HTN, but previously, a **high plasma renin** profile was found in 80% of patients with renovascular HTN. Another previously used screening is the **captopril test.** The administration of oral captopril causes a reactive rise of renin that is greater in patients with renovascular as opposed to essential HTN. The overall sensitivity is 74% and specificity is 89%.

165. **What imaging techniques are useful in screening for renovascular HTN?**
Duplex renal sonography, CT angiography, and magnetic resonance (MR) angiography are the most useful screening tests for renal artery stenosis. The gold standard test for confirmation of renal artery stenosis is renal angiography.
Hirsch AT, Haskal ZJ, Hertzer NR, et al. ACC/AHA 2005 practice guidelines for the management of patients with peripheral arterial disease (lower extremity, renal, mesenteric, and abdominal aortic). *Circulation.* 2006;113:1474–1547.

166. **What are ANCAs?**
Antineutrophil cytoplasmic antibodies that are autoantibodies directed against intracellular antigens in neutrophils. ANCAs have two immunofluorescence patterns: cytoplasmic (c-ANCA) and perinuclear (p-ANCA) staining. c-ANCAs are directed toward proteinase 3 (PR3), and p-ANCAs are specific for myeloperoxidase (MPO). (See also Chapter 10, Rheumatology.)

167. **How do ANCAs help in distinguishing glomerular disorders?**
ANCAs are often positive in pauci-immune vasculitides. Approximately 85–90% of patients with Wegener granulomatosis are positive for c-ANCA, and 50–80% with microscopic polyarteritis are positive for p-ANCA. However, many other autoimmune disorders with small vessel vasculitis, such as SLE, rheumatoid arthritis, and Sjögren syndrome, are also positive for p-ANCA. It is highly recommended to obtain tissue biopsy in ANCA-positive vasculitis before immunosuppressive therapy is begun.
Jeaneete JC, Falk RJ. Small vessel vasculitis. *N Engl J Med.* 1997;337:1512–1523.

168. **A 29-year-old man is admitted with severe generalized weakness, dark-colored urine, and shortness of breath. Examination reveals severe fluid overload, pulmonary edema, pallor, and HTN. His laboratory results show a hemoglobin of 9.6 g/dL, serum creatinine of 7.6 mg/dL, BUN 93 mg/dL, negative ANA, normal complement profile, and strongly positive ANCA PR3. Two months ago his renal function was normal. What lesion is likely on renal biopsy?**
Cresentic nephritis. This young male patient with rapidly progressive renal failure has a pulmonary renal syndrome associated with ANCA; therefore, his renal biopsy would show crescentic nephritis or RPGN.

169. **What causes AKI secondary to rhabdomyolysis?**
Frequently ATN. Rhabdomyolysis occurs in various clinical conditions, including trauma, ischemic tissue damage after a drug overdose, alcoholism, seizures, and heat stroke (especially in untrained subjects or those with sickle cell trait). Hypokalemia and severe hypophosphatemia can also precipitate rhabdomyolysis, which is the most common cause of AKI in patients abusing illicit IV drugs.

170. **Summarize the signs and symptoms of AKI secondary to rhabdomyolysis.**
Typical patients have pigmented granular casts in urine sediment, a positive orthotolidine test in the urine supernatant (indicating the presence of heme), and markedly elevated plasma creatine kinase and other muscle enzymes, owing to their release from damaged muscle tissue. Other characteristics of AKI due to rhabdomyolysis include hyperphosphatemia, hyperkalemia, and a disproportionate increase in P_{Cr} (all of these being due to release of cellular constituents). A high–anion gap metabolic acidosis and severe hyperuricemia are also characteristic, and oliguria or anuria is common.

171. **What is the mechanism of renal failure in rhabdomyolysis?**
The mechanism of renal failure is not completely understood. Although myoglobin is not directly nephrotoxic, concurrent vasoconstriction or volume depletion decreases the renal perfusion and rate of urine flow in tubules, thereby promoting the precipitation of these pigment casts.

BIBLIOGRAPHY

1. Skoredi K, Cherkow GM, eds. *Brenner & Rector's The Kidney.* 10th ed. Philadelphia: Elsevier; 2012.
2. Goldman L, Schafer A, eds. *Goldman-Cecil Textbook of Medicine.* 25th ed. Philadelphia: Saunders; 2015.
3. Gilbert SJ, Weiner DA, eds. *National Kidney Foundation's Primer on Kidney Disease.* 6th ed. Philadelphia: Elsevier; 2014.
4. Rose BD, Post TW. *Clinical Physiology of Acid-Base and Electrolyte Disorders.* 5th ed. New York: McGraw-Hill; 2001.
5. Schrier RW, Coffman TM, Falk RI, et al. *Diseases of the Kidney.* 9th ed. Philadelphia: Lippincott Williams & Wilkins; 2007.
6. Schrier RW, ed. *Renal and Electrolyte Disorders.* 7th ed. Philadelphia: Lippincott Williams & Wilkins; 2010.
7. Singh A, ed. *Educational Review Manual in Nephrology.* 2nd ed. New York: CCGM; 2008.

CHAPTER 9

ACID-BASE AND ELECTROLYTE DISORDERS

Sharma S. Prabhakar, MD, MBA, FACP, FASN

In all things you shall find everywhere the Acid and the Alcaly.

Otto Tachenius (1670)
Hyppocrates Chymacus, Chapter 21

Hence if too much salt is used in food, the pulse hardens.

Huang Ti (The Yellow Emperor) (2697–2597 BCE)
Nei Chung Su Wen, Bk. 3, Sect. 10, trans. by Ilza Veith,
in *The Yellow Emperor's Classic of Internal Medicine*

REGULATION OF SODIUM, WATER, AND VOLUME STATUS

1. **List the osmolality and electrolyte concentrations of serum and commonly used intravenous (IV) solutions.**
   See Table 9.1.

2. **How do you estimate a patient's serum osmolality?**
   A close estimate can be derived from measurements of the serum sodium concentration ([Na⁺]), glucose, and blood urea nitrogen (BUN), using the following equation:

   $$Osmolality = 1.86 \times \left[Na^+\right] + \frac{Glucose}{18} + \frac{BUN}{2.8} + 9$$

3. **What percentage of the adult human body consists of water? What percentage of the water content is intracellular versus extracellular?**
   Approximately 60% of the adult man and 50% of the adult woman is water. About two thirds of this volume is intracellular, and one third is extracellular. About 20% of the extracellular fluid (ECF) volume is plasma water.

4. **What are the sources and daily amounts of water gain and loss?**
   The average adult male gains and loses 2600 mL of water each day. The gains occur from direct fluid ingestion (1400 mL/day), from the fluid content of ingested food (850 mL/day), and as a product of water produced by oxidation reactions (350 mL/day). Water losses occur through urine (1500 mL/day), perspiration (500 mL/day), respiration (400 mL/day), and feces (200 mL/day).

5. **List the factors necessary to allow the kidney to excrete free water.**
   • A filtrate must be formed to allow renal excretion of free water.
   • Glomerular filtrate must escape reabsorption in the proximal tubule to reach the diluting segment (ascending loop of Henle), where free water is created.
   • An adequately functioning diluting segment must be present.
   • The free water formed by the diluting segment must leave the nephron without being reabsorbed by the collecting tubule. This nephron segment is intrinsically impermeable to water but is made permeable by antidiuretic hormone (ADH).

6. **Summarize the relationship between glomerular filtration rate (GFR) and excretion of free water.**
   The lower the GFR, the lower the kidney's ability to respond rapidly to a free-water challenge with excretion of free water.

Table 9.1. Osmolality and Electrolyte Concentrations of Commonly Used Intravenous Solutions

SERUM AND SOLUTIONS	OSMOLALITY (mOsm/KG)	GLUCOSE (g/L)	SODIUM (mEq/L)	CHLORIDE (mEq/L)
Serum	285–295	65–110	135–145	97–110
5% D/W	252	50	0	0
10% D/W	505	100	0	0
50% D/W	2520	500	0	0
½ NS (0.45% NaCl)	154	0	77	77
NS (0.9% NaCl)	308	0	154	154
3% NS	1026	0	513	513
Ringer lactate*	272	0	130	109

*Ringer lactate also contains 28 mEq/L lactate, 4 mEq/L K^+, and 4.5 mEq/L Ca^{2+}.
D/W, dextrose in water; NS, normal saline.

7. **What pathologic states can affect fluid reabsorption in the proximal tubule?**
   True volume depletion and states of decreased effective arterial blood volume, such as congestive heart failure, cirrhosis, and nephrotic syndrome. These states involve vigorous fluid reabsorption in the proximal tubule and are associated with a compromised ability to excrete free water.

8. **What pathologic states can affect functioning of the diluting segment?**
   Intrinsic disorders of function of the diluting segment are unusual. Endogenous prostaglandin E_2 and loop diuretics inhibit NaCl transport in this segment and can thereby limit formation of free water.

9. **Explain the meaning of serum sodium concentration with respect to sodium balance and water balance.**
   [Na^+], measured in mEq/L, reflects the concentration of this cation in ECF. Because its units are measured as mass per unit volume, [Na^+] indicates the relationship between Na^+ and water in the body. It is not indicative of total body Na^+ content but is more an indication of the water status (hydration) of the body. [Na^+] may be low, normal, or increased with any given perturbation of total body Na^+ content. Alterations of the [Na^+] reflect alterations in free-water balance. Therefore, a true low [Na^+] indicates a free-water excess compared with Na^+ content, and a high [Na^+] indicates a relative free-water deficit.

10. **Why is normal saline (with 154 mEq/L of Na^+) isotonic with plasma, which has a sodium concentration of 145 mEq/L?**
    The plasma sodium concentration reflects the concentration of sodium per liter of water in the plasma. Because the plasma has other solid components, the sodium concentration per liter of just water in the blood compartment is 154 mEq/L and, hence, the sodium concentration in normal saline.

11. **What is meant by a state of decreased effective arterial blood volume?**
    The extracellular space is dynamic, with an ongoing balance between its capacity and its actual volume. Both parameters are biologically monitored and normally coordinated to maintain optimal tissue perfusion. A state of decreased effective arterial blood volume occurs when a large capacity is combined with a smaller volume, as seen most commonly with congestive heart failure, cirrhosis, and nephrotic syndrome. Isotonic fluid losses, such as hemorrhage, cause a decrease in ECF volume with no change in [Na^+]. If, however, these losses are replaced with hypotonic fluids, dilutional hyponatremia results.

12. **Why does Na^+ have an effective distribution in total body water (TBW) despite being confined largely to the extracellular space?**
    Na^+ is the major determinant of serum osmolality, and changes in its concentration lead to water shifts between the extracellular and the intracellular compartments. This osmotic shift of water gives Na^+ an effective distribution greater than its chemical distribution and equivalent to that for TBW.

13. **What is the initial step in evaluating a patient with hyponatremia?**
    Determining the serum osmolality (both measured and calculated) (Fig. 9.1).

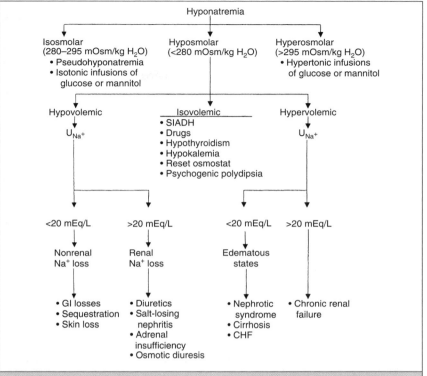

Fig. 9.1. Classification of hyponatremia. CHF, congestive heart failure; GI, gastrointestinal; SIADH, syndrome of inappropriate antidiuretic hormone secretion.

14. **What is hyperosmolar hyponatremia?**
Serum osmolarity > 295 mOsm/kg H_2O, usually resulting from administration of hypertonic solutions of dextrose or mannitol.

15. **Define *isotonic hyponatremia*.**
Serum osmolality of 280–295 mOsm/kg H_2O, seen with administration of isotonic solutions of dextrose and mannitol.

16. **What is hyposmolar hyponatremia?**
Serum osmolality < 280 mOsm/kg H_2O that can be associated with low, normal, or increased volume status. Diuretic administration, salt-losing renal conditions, syndrome of inappropriate antidiuretic hormone secretion (SIADH), chronic kidney disease (CKD), and a wide range of other causes can lead to hyposmolar hyponatremia.

17. **How can patients with hyposmolar hyponatremia be categorized according to history and physical findings?**
As hypovolemic, hypervolemic, or euvolemic.

18. **What findings suggest a hypovolemic state?**
A history of volume loss or decreased intake and orthostatic blood pressure changes on examination.

19. **How is the hypovolemia treated?**
By replacing the lost volume to turn off the factors that limit the kidney's ability to excrete free water.

20. How do you recognize the hypervolemic patient?

By a history of a condition with decreased effective arterial blood volume and an examination showing edema.

21. Describe the treatment of the hypervolemia.

Therapeutic attention must be directed to the underlying disorder. If the hyponatremia is mild and asymptomatic, free-water restriction, in addition to specific treatment of the underlying disorder, is the suggested initial therapeutic approach. If the hyponatremia is severe and symptomatic, more aggressive treatment with hypertonic saline and furosemide may be required.

22. Summarize the approach to euvolemic hyposmolar hyponatremia.

In patients with hyposmolar hyponatremia and apparently normal volume status or euvolemia, a wide variety of pathologic processes must be considered in the diagnostic evaluation, including SIADH and drugs that can limit free-water excretion (e.g., chlorpropamide).

23. Define *pseudohyponatremia*.

Pseudohyponatremia occurs when a quantitative $[Na^+]$ measurement is performed on a given volume of plasma that contains a greater-than-normal amount of water-excluding particles, such as lipid or protein. In this setting, plasma water (which contains the Na^+) composes a smaller fraction of the plasma volume, leading to a factitiously low serum $[Na^+]$ (when expressed in mEq/L). The $[Na^+]$ in plasma water is normal, and therefore, patients are asymptomatic. Attention should be directed to hyperlipidemia or hyperproteinemia.

24. How is spurious hyponatremia different from pseudohyponatremia?

Spurious hyponatremia results from hyperosmolality of the serum (i.e., from hyperglycemia), resulting in movement of intracellular water to the extracellular space and subsequent dilution of the Na^+ in the ECF. These patients are not symptomatic from hyposmolality (unlike patients with true hyponatremia). If they are symptomatic at all, it is due to their hyperosmolar state. Attention should be directed to correcting the hyperosmolar state. It is important to distinguish these two categories of hyponatremia from true hyponatremia associated with hyposmolality because the diagnostic work-up and therapeutic management are different.

25. How do you correct the $[Na^+]$ for a given level of hyperglycemia?

Hyperglycemia, one of the causes of spurious hyponatremia, causes a decrease in the measured $[Na^+]$. For each increase in serum glucose of 100 mg/dL up to 600 mg/dL (an increase of 500, or $5 \times$ 100 mg/dL), the $[Na^+]$ decreases by 8.0 mEq/L (5×1.6 mEq/L). However, recent studies suggested that the relationship is not linear, especially with plasma glucose levels of more than 400 mg/dL, and a factor of 2.4 mEq/L may be a more accurate correction factor.

Hillier TA, Abbott RD, Barrett EJ. Hyponatremia: evaluating the correction factor for hyperglycemia. *Am J Med*. 1999; 106(4):399–403.

26. Define *essential hyponatremia*.

Hyponatremia in the absence of a water diuresis defect. One hypothesis is that the osmoreceptor cells in the hypothalamus are reset so that they maintain a lower plasma osmolality. This is seen in several conditions, such as congestive heart failure, cirrhosis, and pulmonary tuberculosis, and is diagnosed by demonstrating normal urinary Na^+ concentration and dilution in the face of hyponatremia. Generally, this entity does not require treatment and is sometimes called "sick cell syndrome."

27. What are the signs and symptoms of hyponatremia?

The manifestations are mainly attributable to central nervous system (CNS) edema, which is usually not seen until the $[Na^+]$ falls to ≤ 120 mEq/L. Symptoms range from mild lethargy to seizure, coma, and death. The signs and symptoms of hyponatremia are more a function of the rapidity of the drop in $[Na^+]$ than the absolute level. In patients with chronic hyponatremia, there has been time for solute equilibration, resulting in less CNS edema and less severe manifestations. In acute hyponatremia, there is no time for equilibration, and so smaller changes in $[Na^+]$ are accompanied by larger degrees of CNS edema and more severe manifestations.

28. Why is hyponatremia often seen after transurethral resection of the prostate (TURP)?

Because large volumes of solutions containing mannitol, glycerol, or sorbitol are used to irrigate the prostate. A variable fraction of these fluids is absorbed into the systemic circulation, producing hyponatremia.

29. **How do you manage hyponatremia in edematous states?**

    Treatment depends on the underlying cause, any symptoms, and the rapidity of the drop in [Na$^+$]. In general, patients with edematous states such as the nephrotic syndrome, who have ECF expansion, have some degree of hyponatremia if they are not water-restricted. Generally, this condition is asymptomatic and requires no treatment. Treatment is required only if the hyponatremia is severe (<125 mEq/L), and especially if there are symptoms such as lethargy, confusion, stupor, and coma.

30. **A 41-year-old black man is hospitalized with acute bacterial meningitis. His chemistry profile shows BUN and creatinine levels of 11 mg/dL and 1.2 mg/dL, respectively, but his [Na$^+$] is 127 mEq/L. What is the likely cause of his hyponatremia?**

    SIADH. Hyponatremia in the setting of bacterial meningitis (or any pathologic CNS process) is usually due to SIADH. SIADH is a form of hyponatremia involving sustained or spiking levels of ADH that are inappropriate for the osmotic or volume stimuli that normally affect ADH secretion.

31. **List the essential points in the diagnosis of SIADH.**
    - Presence of hypotonic hyponatremia
    - Inappropriate antidiuresis (urine osmolality higher than expected for the degree of hyponatremia)
    - Significant Na$^+$ excretion when the patient is normovolemic
    - Normal renal, thyroid, and adrenal function
    - Absence of other causes of hyponatremia, volume depletion, or edema

32. **Describe the work-up for the patient with suspected SIADH.**

    Measurement of serum and urine Na$^+$ concentration and osmolality. In most cases, urinary osmolality exceeds plasma osmolality, often by >100 mOsm/L. Urinary Na$^+$ excretion exceeds 20 mEq/L unless the patient is wasting, and it improves with fluid restriction. In most cases, restriction of fluids to 1000–1200 mL/day is all that is needed. Occasionally, patients with symptomatic and marked hyponatremia may require demeclocycline therapy or hypertonic saline.

33. **What is cerebral salt-wasting?**

    A syndrome that mimics SIADH in all aspects including hypouricemia except that in cerebral salt-wasting, patients are volume depleted. In SIADH, patients are euvolemic. Owing to impaired renal water excretion, this condition is associated with hyposmolar hyponatremia in patients with cerebral trauma or disease. The high urinary Na$^+$ despite hypovolemia reflects renal salt-wasting. The cause of this salt-wasting is unknown, although increased secretion of cerebral natriuretic factors is one likely explanation. A circulating factor that impairs renal tubular Na$^+$ reabsorption is another likely possibility.

    Al-Mufti H, Arieff AI. Cerebral salt wasting syndrome: combined cerebral and distal tubular lesion. *Am J Med.* 1984;77:740–746.

34. **How do you estimate the free-water deficit in a patient with hypernatremia?**

    It can be assumed that the patient has lost free water without salt, and thus the patient has reduced TBW but maintains the same total body Na$^+$ content. This change results in an increase in the [Na$^+$] that is proportional to the decrease in TBW. In other words, the ratio of the initial [Na$^+$] (which is assumed to be normal) to the current [Na$^+$] (which is higher than normal) is equal to the ratio of the present TBW (which is less than normal) to the initial TBW (which is assumed to have been normal).

    $$\text{Current TBW} \div \text{Initial TBW} = \text{Initial } \left[Na^+\right] \div \text{Current } \left[Na^+\right]$$

    This relationship can be used to calculate the current TBW. Subtracting this value from the initial (normal) TBW yields the estimated free-water deficit. This calculated free-water deficit must be replaced with fluids.

35. **What are the manifestations of hypernatremia?**

    Basically they are similar to the symptoms manifested by other causes of hyperosmolality, such as hyperglycemia. These changes are produced mainly by fluid shifts from the CNS and increased CNS osmolality, resulting in "shrinking" of the brain. The symptoms range from lethargy to seizures, coma, and death. The severity of the symptoms depends on the severity of the hyperosmolality and the speed with which it develops.

36. **What are some common causes of hypernatremia?**
Diabetes insipidus, severe dehydration due to extrarenal fluid losses (e.g., burns, excessive sweating), and hypothalamic disorders (e.g., tumors, granulomas, cerebrovascular accidents) leading to defective thirst and vasopressin regulation.

37. **How do you correct hypernatremia?**
By replacement of the water. In mild cases, this can be accomplished by simply having the patient drink, or if IV fluids are used, dextrose in water can be given. If salt-containing fluids are deemed necessary, the equivalent free-water volume must be given. For example, if half-normal saline is used (1 L of which contains 500 mL of normal saline and 500 mL of free water), then twice the amount of the estimated free-water deficit is needed to correct the free-water deficit. This volume deficit should be replaced slowly. The first half is given over 24 hours. If the patient is hemodynamically unstable, with signs of severe ECF volume depletion, therapy with 0.9% normal saline is warranted before dextrose infusion is started.

POTASSIUM BALANCE

38. **How is potassium (K^+) distributed between the intracellular fluid (ICF) and the ECF compartments?**
A 70-kg man contains approximately 3500 mEq of K^+ (~50 mEq/kg body weight). The vast majority of this (98%) is in the ICF space. Therefore, the amount in the ECF compartment (the portion that we routinely measure) represents only a small percentage of the total body K^+.

39. **How is the large chemical gradient between intracellular and extracellular K^+ concentration maintained?**
The Na^+-K^+ adenosine triphosphate (ATP) pump actively extrudes Na^+ from the cell and pumps K^+ into the cell. This pump is present in all cells of the body. In addition, the cell is electrically negative compared with the exterior, which serves to keep K^+ inside the cell.

40. **Because the extracellular K^+ concentration is relatively small compared with the intracellular concentration of K^+, why are some electrical processes (cardiac conduction, skeletal and smooth muscle contraction) sensitive to changes in the ECF K^+ concentration?**
Because the ratio of the ECF to the ICF K^+ concentration is more significant than the absolute level of either in determining the sensitivity of these electrical processes. Because the ECF concentration of K^+ is small compared with the ICF concentration, a small absolute change in ECF K^+ concentration results in a large change in the ECF-to-ICF K^+ ratio.

41. **What factors commonly influence the movement of K^+ between the intracellular and the extracellular compartments?**
   - **Acid-base changes:** Acidemia (increased concentration of H^+ in serum) leads to intracellular buffering of H^+, with subsequent extrusion of K^+ into the ECF, increasing the concentration of K^+ in this compartment. Similarly, alkalemia leads to hypokalemia.
   - **Hormones:** Insulin, epinephrine, growth hormone, and androgens all promote net movement of K^+ into cells.
   - **Cellular metabolism:** Synthesis of protein and glycogen is associated with intracellular K^+ binding.
   - **Extracellular concentration:** All other things being equal, K^+ tends to enter the cell when its extracellular concentration is high and vice versa.

42. **How is K^+ handled by the kidney?**
Through reabsorption in the proximal tubule, and there is net secretion or net resorption in the distal nephron, depending on the body's K^+ needs. Under most conditions, we are in K^+ excess, and the kidney must excrete K^+ to maintain whole body K^+ balance. K^+ restriction leads to renal K^+ conservation, but this process is neither as rapid nor as efficient as the process for Na^+.

43. **How does aldosterone influence K^+ metabolism?**
By promoting Na^+ resorption and K^+ secretion in the distal nephron, gut, and sweat glands. Aldosterone is the main regulatory hormone for K^+ metabolism. Quantitatively, its greatest effect is in the kidney. Its secretion is increased by an increasing K^+ concentration in the ECF and is decreased by low K^+ concentrations.

44. **How does hypoaldosteronism affect K^+ and Na^+ levels?**
    Asymptomatic hyperkalemia is a common presentation of patients with mineralocorticoid deficiency. Na^+ deficiency and volume depletion are not seen unless there is concomitant glucocorticoid deficiency. Na^+ balance is maintained by other factors, such as angiotensin II and catecholamines, although the ability to conserve Na^+ maximally is generally lost. Thus, urine $Na^+ < 10$ mEq/L is unusual in primary hypoaldosteronism.

45. **How is hypoaldosteronism diagnosed?**
    First by excluding drug-induced hyperkalemia (such as caused by angiotensin-converting enzyme [ACE] inhibitors, beta blockers, nonsteroidal anti-inflammatory drugs [NSAIDs], heparin, or K^+-sparing diuretics). The next step is to obtain morning samples of plasma for renin, aldosterone, and cortisol measurements. Administration of furosemide (20–40 mg) at 6 pm and 6 am before samples are drawn enhances the utility of the test by stimulating plasma renin activity in normal persons but not in those with hypoaldosteronism.

46. **What is meant by transtubular K^+ gradient (TTKG)?**
    An indirect method of evaluating the effect of aldosterone on the kidney. The principle is to measure K^+ at the end of the cortical collecting tube after all the distal K^+ secretion has taken place:

    $$TTKG = \frac{U_{K^+} / (U_{osm}/P_{osm})}{P_{K^+}}$$

    where P_{K^+} is plasma K^+ concentration. It is assumed that urine osmolality (U_{osm}) at the end of the cortical collecting tube is the same as that of plasma (P_{osm}) because the interstitium here is iso-osmotic. It is also assumed that no further K^+ secretion or resorption takes place. But because ADH-mediated water permeability continues in the medullary collecting tubule, the K^+ concentration in this duct rises. This formula is applicable as long as the urine Na^+ concentration is 25 mEq/L, because Na^+ delivery should not be a limiting factor.

47. **What is the TTKG value in normal and hyperkalemic subjects?**
    The TTKG in normal subjects is 8–10 on a normal diet. On a high K^+ diet, TTKG > 11 because of increased K^+ secretion. Thus, in a hyperkalemic subject, a TTKG < 5 indicates impaired tubular K^+ secretion and is highly suggestive of hypoaldosteronism.
    Ethier JH, Kamel KS, Magner PO, et al. The trans-tubular potassium gradient in patients with hypokalemia and hyperkalemia. *Am J Kidney Dis*. 1990;15:309–315.

48. **List conditions that can lead to increased renal K^+ excretion.**
    - Increased dietary K^+ intake
    - Increased aldosterone secretion (as in volume depletion)
    - Alkalosis
    - Increased flow rate in the distal tubule
    - Increased Na^+ delivery to the distal nephron
    - Decreased chloride concentration in tubular fluid in the distal nephron
    - Natriuretic agents

49. **How does increased sodium delivery promote renal excretion of K^+?**
    Increased Na^+ delivery to the distal nephron promotes Na^+ resorption in exchange for K^+ secretion. The process is accelerated in the presence of aldosterone.

50. **Explain how decreased chloride concentration leads to an increased renal excretion of K^+.**
    Decreased chloride concentration in tubular fluid in the distal nephron allows Na^+ to be resorbed with a less permeable ion (e.g., bicarbonate or sulfate) that increases the negativity of the tubular lumen in the distal nephron. The increased negativity of the tubular lumen promotes K^+ secretion.

51. **How do natriuretic agents increase renal excretion of K^+?**
    Natriuretic agents, such as loop diuretics, thiazides, and acetazolamide, lead to increased Na^+ delivery to the distal nephron, volume depletion with increased aldosterone secretion, and subsequent increased renal K^+ excretion.

52. **In addition to the kidney, what is the other major route of K^+ loss?**
The gastrointestinal (GI) tract. Fluids in the lower GI tract, particularly those of the small bowel, are high in K^+. Therefore, diarrhea can result in significant losses of K^+. However, upper GI losses, such as vomiting or nasogastric suction, cause renal K^+ loss. This renal K^+ loss is multifactorial and includes the following:
   - Alkalosis
   - Volume depletion, which leads to increased aldosterone secretion
   - Chloride depletion from the loss of HCl in gastric fluid, which leads to a high tubular concentration of HCO_3^- anion

53. **What causes a spuriously elevated serum K^+ determination?**
   - **Hemolysis,** with the release of intraerythrocytic K^+.
   - **Pseudohyperkalemia,** seen in marked thrombocytosis or leukocytosis due to the disproportionately increased amounts of the normally released K^+ that occurs with clotting. This condition can be corrected by inhibiting clotting and measuring the plasma K^+ concentration.

54. **List the four common mechanisms by which hyperkalemia develops.**
   - Inadequate excretion of K^+
   - Excessive intake of K^+
   - Shift of potassium from tissues
   - Pseudohyperkalemia (due to thrombocytosis, leukocytosis, poor venipuncture technique, in vitro hemolysis)
     Singer GG, Brenner BM. Fluids and electrolytes. In: Fauci A, Braunwald E, Kaspar DL, et al, eds. *Harrison's Principles of Internal Medicine.* 17th ed. New York: McGraw-Hill; 2008.

55. **What factors lead to inadequate potassium excretion?**
   - Renal disorders (acute renal failure, severe CKD, tubular disorders)
   - Hypoaldosteronism
   - Adrenal disorders
   - Hyporeninemia (as with tubulointerstitial diseases, drugs such as NSAIDs, ACE inhibitors, and beta blockers)
   - Diuretics that inhibit potassium secretion (spironoloactone, triamterene, amiloride)

56. **Is there a difference in the risk for hyperkalemia between ACE inhibitors and angiotensin receptor blockers (ARBs)?**
The risk of hyperkalemia caused by ARBs is similar to that of ACE inhibitors, although in many large-scale clinical studies, the frequency was found to be less with ARBs than with ACE inhibitors. Although the exact reason is unclear, it may depend partly on the differential degree of inhibition of aldosterone with these two classes of agents.

57. **What factors lead to a shift of potassium from tissues?**
   - Tissue damage (muscle crush, hemolysis, and internal bleeding)
   - Drugs (succinylcholine, arginine, digitalis poisoning, and beta blockers)
   - Acidosis
   - Hyperosmolality
   - Insulin deficiency
   - Hyperkalemic periodic paralysis

58. **What is the first step in the diagnostic approach to patients with disturbances in serum K^+ concentration?**
Determine whether the disturbance results from:
   - Abnormal K^+ intake or metabolism (excessive catabolism or anabolism)
   - Intra- and extracellular compartmental shifts
   - Disturbances in renal excretion or extrarenal loss

59. **What should you do next?**
After the patient is placed in one of these three categories, it is possible to narrow the differential diagnosis, order appropriate diagnostic tests, and decide on the appropriate management. Disturbances of intake can be investigated by history and physical examination. The possibility of cellular shifts can be investigated by looking for any of the disturbances that result in compartmental movement of this cation. Determination of the urinary K^+ concentration can help in distinguishing

renal from nonrenal causes. High urinary K^+ excretion in the setting of hypokalemia is compatible with a renal cause for K^+ deficiency. In contrast, an appropriately low urinary K^+ excretion in the setting of hypokalemia suggests extrarenal (possibly GI) losses.

60. **How does hypokalemia present clinically?**
Usually with neuromuscular symptoms. When K^+ falls to 2.0–2.5 mEq/L, muscular weakness and lethargy are seen. With further decreases, the patient manifests paralysis with eventual respiratory muscle involvement and death. Hypokalemia also can cause rhabdomyolysis, myoglobinuria, and paralytic ileus. Prolonged hypokalemia can lead to renal tubular damage (called "hypokalemic nephropathy").

61. **How do you manage a patient with hypokalemia?**
First with correction of the disturbance causing the abnormal K^+ concentration. If hypokalemia is associated with alkalosis, then the alkalosis should be corrected in addition to providing K^+ supplements. In general, patients with K^+ depletion should be given supplements slowly to replace the deficit. The oral route is preferred because of its safety as well as its efficacy. Some instances require more rapid repletion with IV supplements, but this should not exceed 20 mEq/hour. Cardiac monitoring should accompany infusions of > 10 mEq/hour.

62. **What are the manifestations of hyperkalemia besides electrocardiogram (ECG) changes?**
The most important manifestation is the increased excitability of cardiac muscle. With severe elevations in K^+, a patient can suffer diastolic cardiac arrest. Skeletal muscle paralysis also can be seen. Again, the symptoms produced by hyperkalemia are dependent on the rapidity of the change. Patients with chronically elevated serum K levels can tolerate higher levels with fewer symptoms than patients with acute hyperkalemia. (See also Chapter 4, Cardiology.)

63. **How is chronic hyperkalemia generally managed?**
Treatment depends on the extent of the hyperkalemia and the clinical setting. Mild levels of hyper-kalemia (5.0–5.5 mEq/L) associated with the hyporenin-hypoaldosterone syndrome are tolerated well and usually require no treatment. Higher levels not associated with ECG changes may require treatment with a synthetic mineralocorticoid.

64. **Describe the management of hyperkalemia as a medical emergency.**
    - IV calcium must be administered to immediately counteract the effect of hyperkalemia on the conduction system.
    - Calcium administration must be followed by maneuvers to shift K^+ into cells, thereby decreasing the ratio of extracellular to intracellular K^+. This goal can be accomplished by administering glucose with insulin and bicarbonate to increase serum pH.
    - Finally, a maneuver to remove K^+ from the body must be instituted, such as a cation-exchange resin (Kayexalate) and hemodialysis or peritoneal dialysis.

65. **A 61-year-old woman with end-stage renal disease missed her dialysis twice and presents to the emergency department with a serum K^+ of 6.4 mEq/L. How should you manage this patient?**
The severity of hyperkalemia is assessed by both the serum K^+ level and ECG changes. If the ECG shows only tall T waves and the serum K^+ < 6.5 mEq/L, the hyperkalemia is mild, whereas K^+ levels of 6.5–8.0 mEq/L are associated with more severe ECG changes, including absent P waves and wide QRS complexes. At higher K^+ levels, ventricular arrhythmias tend to appear, and the prognosis is grave unless proper treatment is given.

66. **If the ECG shows only tall T waves, which agents should you administer? Why?**
    - **Hypertonic glucose infusion,** along with 10 units of insulin (e.g., 10 units of insulin with 200–500 mL of 10% glucose in 30 minutes followed by 1 L of the same in the next 4–6 hours)
    - **Sodium bicarbonate,** 50–150 mEq given by IV (if the patient is not in fluid overload)
    Both of these agents shift K^+ into cells and start acting within an hour. Total body K^+ can be decreased by using cation-exchange resins, such as sodium polysterone sulfonate; usually 20 g with 20 mL of 70% sorbitol solution is started every 4–6 hours.

67. **If the ECG shows the more severe changes, what should you do?**
Give 10% calcium gluconate (10–30 mL IV) with cardiac monitoring. Arrangements must be made to dialyze the patient as soon as possible to correct the hyperkalemia.

68. **A 71-year-old diabetic with a nonhealing foot ulcer is on tobramycin and piperacillin. This patient has a resistant hypokalemia. How do you approach this problem?**
Aminoglycosides and penicillins are both known to deplete serum K^+. The former do this by defective proximal tubular K^+ resorption and the latter by increased renal K^+ excretion induced by the poorly resorbable anion (penicillin). With aminoglycosides, magnesium-wasting is another complication. Hence, in addition to K^+ repletion, correction of hypomagnesemia is important, because hypokalemia is often resistant to correction unless the magnesium deficit is also corrected.

69. **A 67-year-old man with congestive heart failure treated with furosemide has a serum K^+ of 2.4 mEq/L. How would you correct his K^+ deficit?**
Hypokalemia is an important complication of diuretic therapy (except with K^+-sparing diuretics). It is important to monitor serum K^+ periodically in these patients, especially those with cardiac illnesses who are likely to be on digoxin because hypokalemia can exacerbate digitalis toxicity. The K^+ deficit requires replacement (except in patients who are on minimal doses of diuretics), particularly if serum $K^+ < 3$ mEq/L. The serum K^+ level is not an exact indicator of the total body deficit, but severe hypokalemia with serum $K^+ < 3$ mEq/L is usually associated with a deficit of approximately 300 mEq. KCl elixir or tablets are the treatment of choice. Enteric-coated K^+ supplements are known to cause gastric ulceration.

70. **What is the primary defect in Bartter syndrome?**
Impaired NaCl reabsorption in the thick ascending loop of Henle or distal tubule. Recent genetic studies indicate the defect involves a mutation of Na^+-K^+-2Cl cotransporter or K^+ channel in the thick ascending limb of Henle. The diagnosis is often made by exclusion. Surreptitious use of diuretics and vomiting (urine Cl^- is often low!) can mimic most of the findings of this syndrome.
Rodríguez-Soriano, J. Pediatr Nephrol. 1998;12:315. https://doi.org/10.1007/s004670050461

71. **Describe the treatment of Bartter syndrome.**
A K^+-sparing diuretic (such as amiloride in doses of 10–40 mg) and NSAIDs to raise the plasma K^+ by reversing the physiologic abnormalities.

72. **A 55-year-old man with a history of congestive heart failure and chronic obstructive pulmonary disease (COPD) presents with extreme weakness and fatigue. His medications include digoxin 0.25 mg/day, furosemide 40 mg/day, and albuterol inhalations for his asthma. The patient reports a few days of exacerbation of COPD symptoms, forcing him to use the inhaler more frequently. What is the likely cause of his weakness?**
Severe hypokalemia resulting from overuse of beta agonists such as albuterol especially in the presence of potassium-losing diuretics, because both effects could be additive. The hypokalemic effects of inhaled beta agonists are often so potent that they are used to treat patients with hyperkalemia acutely.

ACID-BASE REGULATION

73. **What is the Henderson-Hasselbalch equation?**
An acid-base disorder is suspected on clinical grounds and confirmed by arterial blood gas (ABG) analysis of the pH, arterial carbon dioxide pressure ($Paco_2$), or HCO_3^- concentration.
   The Henderson-Hasselbalch equation is used to test whether a given set of parameters is mutually compatible:

$$pH = pK_a + \log \frac{HCO_3^-}{\alpha CO_2 \times Paco_2} = 6.1 + \log \frac{HCO_3^-}{0.03 \times Paco_2}$$

   The value of pK_a, the negative log of the equilibrium constant K, and the CO_2 solubility coefficient (αCO_2) are constant at any given set of temperature and osmolality. In plasma, at 37° C, the $pK_a = 6.1$ and the $\alpha CO_2 = 0.03$.

74. **Explain the significance of the Henderson-Hasselbalch equation.**
The Henderson-Hasselbalch equation shows that pH is dependent on the ratio of $[HCO_3^-]$ to $Paco_2$ and not on the absolute individual values alone. A primary change in one of the values usually leads to a compensatory change in the other value. This serves to limit the degree of the resulting acidosis or alkalosis.

75. **The integrated action of which three organs is involved in acid-base homeostasis?**
    Liver, lungs, and **kidneys.** The **liver** metabolizes proteins contained in the standard American diet such that net acid (protons) is produced. Hepatic metabolism of organic acids (lactate) can consume acid, which is the equivalent of producing bicarbonate. Acid released into the ECF titrates HCO_3^- to H_2O and CO_2. The **lungs** excrete this CO_2 and the CO_2 produced from cellular metabolism. The **kidney** reclaims the filtered HCO_3^- and excretes the accumulated net acid.

76. **What is the fate of a load of nonvolatile acid administered to the body?**
    Initially, buffering by extracellular (40%) and intracellular (60%) buffers and eventual excretion by the kidneys. The buffers minimize the decrease in pH that otherwise would occur. The major ECF buffer is the HCO_3^- system, and most intracellular buffering is provided by histidine-containing proteins. The administered acid reduces ECF HCO_3^-, and new HCO_3^- is then regenerated by the kidney during the process of proton (acid) secretion.

77. **How does the kidney excrete acid to maintain the acid-base balance?**
    The kidney must **reclaim** the filtered HCO_3^- and **regenerate** the HCO_3^- lost by acid titration. This latter process is equivalent to acid excretion. Reclamation of HCO_3^- is quantitatively a more important process than regeneration (4500 mEq/day vs. 70 mEq/day). Nevertheless, without regeneration of new HCO_3^- (excretion of acid), the plasma HCO_3^- concentration could not be maintained, and net acid retention would result. Two principal urinary buffers allow net acid excretion (new HCO_3^- regeneration): dibasic phosphate and ammonia. By accepting a proton, they become monobasic phosphate and ammonium ions, respectively, and are excreted in the urine. The phosphate is measured as titratable acid, and the ammonium is measured directly. Urinary excretion of these two substances minus urinary HCO_3^- excretion constitutes net acid excretion.

78. **List the four primary acid-base disturbances.**
    - Metabolic acidosis
    - Metabolic alkalosis
    - Respiratory acidosis
    - Respiratory alkalosis

79. **Explain what is meant by *acidosis* and *alkalosis*.**
    Acidosis refers to an imbalance in the steady-state acid-base balance that leads to a net increase in $[H^+]$. **Alkalosis** refers to an imbalance that leads to a net decrease in $[H^+]$. In the maintenance of normal acid-base balance, the addition of H^+ to the body fluids is balanced by their excretion, such that the H^+ concentration of the ECF remains relatively constant at 40 nM (40×10^{-9} M, or pH = 7.40).

80. **What is meant by *metabolic* and *respiratory* in referring to acid-base disturbances?**
    Metabolic and *respiratory* are terms used to describe how the imbalance occurred. Describing a disorder as **metabolic** implies that the imbalance leading to the change in H^+ occurred either because of the addition of nonvolatile acid or base or because of a gain or loss of available buffer (HCO_3^-). HCO_3^- as a buffer reduces the concentration of free H^+ in solution. Referring to an acid-base disorder as **respiratory** implies that the net change in $[H^+]$ occurred secondary to a disturbance in ventilation that resulted in either a net increase or decrease in CO_2 gas in the ECF.

81. **Define *metabolic acidosis*.**
    A net increase in $[H^+]$ as a result of a net gain in nonvolatile acid or from a net loss of HCO_3^- buffer.

82. **Define *respiratory acidosis*.**
    A net increase in $[H^+]$ as a result of decreased ventilation, leading to CO_2 retention.

83. **Define *metabolic alkalosis*.**
    A net decrease in $[H^+]$ as a result of gain of HCO_3^- or loss of acid.

84. **Define *respiratory alkalosis*.**
    A net decrease in $[H^+]$ because of increased ventilation leading to decreased CO_2.

85. **What important points should be kept in mind about these four disorders?**
These disorders refer to the imbalance that leads to the directional change in $[H^+]$ and do not denote what the final $[H^+]$, Pco_2, and $[HCO_3^-]$ will be. Two important facts should be kept in mind:
1. Compensatory changes occur in response to these disorders.
2. More than one acid-base disturbance may occur simultaneously; the final parameters measured depend not only on the algebraic sum of the different disorders but also on their respective compensatory responses.

86. **How are the four primary acid-base disorders diagnosed?**
See Table 9.2.

Table 9.2. Relationships Between Bicarbonate and Arterial Carbon Dioxide Pressure in Simple Acid-Base Disorders

CONDITION	pH	HCO$_3^-$	Paco$_2$	PREDICTED RESPONSE
Metabolic acidosis	↓	↓	↓	$\Delta\Delta Paco_2$ (↓) = 1–1.4 ΔHCO_3^-*
Metabolic alkalosis	↑	↑	↑	$\Delta Paco_2$ (↑) = 0.4–0.9 ΔHCO_3^-*
Respiratory acidosis	↓	↑	↑	Acute: ΔHCO_3^- (↑) = 0.1 $\Delta Paco_2$ Chronic: ΔHCO_3^- (↑) = 0.25–0.55 $Paco_2$
Respiratory alkalosis	↑	↓	↓	Acute: ΔHCO_3^- (↓) = 0.2–0.25 $\Delta Paco_2$ Chronic: ΔHCO_3^- (↓) = 0.4–0.5 $\Delta Paco_2$

*After at least 12–24 hours.
From Hamm L. Mixed acid-base disorders. In: Kokko JP, Tannen KL, editors. *Fluids and Electrolytes*. 3rd ed. Philadelphia: WB Saunders; 1996, p 487.
HCO$_3^-$, bicarbonate; Paco$_2$, arterial carbon dioxide pressure.

87. **What are secondary acid-base disturbances?**
Compensatory physiologic responses to the cardinal acid-base disturbances. The phrase *secondary acid-base disturbance* is actually a misnomer. They usually alleviate the change in H^+ concentration and, therefore, the pH change that otherwise would occur.

88. **What equation helps explain the compensatory physiologic responses to acid-base disturbances?**
The mass-action equation, derived from the more familiar Henderson-Hasselbalch equation, defines the relationship of H^+, HCO_3^-, and the $Paco_2$:

$$[H^+] = \frac{Paco_2 \times 24}{(HCO_3^-)}$$

One can see that in the setting of metabolic acidosis, with a primary decrease in $[HCO_3^-]$, the $[H^+]$ increases. It is also evident that the increase in $[H^+]$ in this setting can be alleviated by concomitantly decreasing the $Paco_2$, which is exactly what occurs as a result of a **physiologic** increase in ventilation. This situation is properly described as metabolic acidosis with a directionally appropriate respiratory response. It is incorrect to describe the condition as primary metabolic acidosis with secondary respiratory alkalosis. To say that a patient has respiratory alkalosis is to say that a patient has **pathologic** hypoventilation, which is not the case in this situation. Tables and formulas can be used to calculate the expected respiratory response to a given degree of metabolic acidosis.

89. **What is a mixed acid-base disorder?**
If the decrease in $Paco_2$ in response to the degree of metabolic acidosis is exactly what we would have predicted from the formulas, the patient is said to have one acid-base disorder: metabolic acidosis. In contrast, if the measured decrease in $Paco_2$ is more than that predicted for the degree of metabolic acidosis, then the patient has an additional (not secondary) acid-base disorder: respiratory

alkalosis in addition to metabolic acidosis. In other words, the patient has a mixed disorder, which is actually very common. If the measured $Paco_2$ is higher than predicted, then the patient has an additional respiratory acidosis.

90. **What causes respiratory acidosis?**
Alveolar hypoventilation that leads to a drop in the pH. The alveolar hypoventilation leads to a rate of excretion of CO_2 that is less than its metabolic production. This net gain in CO_2 causes a rise in the $Paco_2$. The lungs may be subject to diffuse hypoventilation (global alveolar hypoventilation), or only parts of the lungs may be involved (regional alveolar hypoventilation). As can be seen in the Henderson-Hasselbalch equation, any increase in the $Paco_2$, if not accompanied by an increase in $[HCO_3^-]$, leads to a measurable drop in the pH.

91. **Describe the treatment of respiratory acidosis.**
Correction of the cause of the hypoventilation. This goal may involve the treatment of airway obstruction or, in respiratory failure, even mechanical ventilation.

92. **What causes respiratory alkalosis?**
Alveolar hyperventilation that leads to a rise in pH. Alveolar hyperventilation, in turn, leads to an increase in the excretion of CO_2 and a drop in the $Paco_2$. The causes of respiratory alkalosis include:
   - CNS stimulation of ventilation: physiologic (voluntary, anxiety, fear, fever, and pregnancy) or pathologic (intracranial hemorrhage, stroke, tumors, brainstem lesions, and salicylates)
   - Peripheral stimulation of ventilation: reflex hyperventilation due to abnormal lung or chest wall mechanics (pulmonary emboli, myopathies, and interstitial lung diseases), arterial hypoxemia, high altitudes, pain, congestive heart failure, shock of any cause, and hypothermia
   - Hyperventilation with mechanical ventilation
   - Others: severe liver disease and uremia

93. **Are the plasma electrolytes alone (Na^+, K^+, Cl^-, and HCO_3^-) sufficient to determine a patient's acid-base status?**
No. Remember that the regulatory systems of the body work to maintain the pH (or $[H^+]$) and that pH is a function of the ratio of $Paco_2$ to $[HCO_3^-]$. The pH is not determined by the absolute value of $Paco_2$ or $[HCO_3^-]$ alone. Thus, a set of plasma electrolytes demonstrating a normal $[HCO_3^-]$ does not necessarily indicate a normal acid-base status.

94. **Give two interpretations of a low $[HCO_3^-]$ and high $[Cl^-]$.**
Either a metabolic acidosis (probably a non–anion gap [AG] acidosis) or a chronic respiratory alkalosis with an appropriate metabolic response (renal lowering of $[HCO_3^-]$ as a response to the chronically low $Paco_2$). This is an attempt to maintain a more normal pH.

95. **Give two interpretations of a high $[HCO_3^-]$ and low $[Cl^-]$.**
A metabolic alkalosis or a chronic respiratory acidosis with an appropriate metabolic response (renal increase in $[HCO_3^-]$ in response to chronically high $Paco_2$) in an attempt to maintain a more normal pH. Note that without an accompanying pH and $Paco_2$, one cannot tell whether an abnormal $[HCO_3^-]$ is due to a metabolic cause (a metabolic acidosis or alkalosis) or to a metabolic response to a primary respiratory disorder. This illustrates the importance of obtaining ABGs (with a pH and $Paco_2$) in addition to an $[HCO_3^-]$ to properly assess a patient's acid-base status.

96. **What is meant by the anion gap (AG)?**
The difference between the routinely measured cations and anions in the plasma. It is usually calculated as follows:

$$AG = [Na^+] - [Cl^- + HCO_3^-]$$

97. **Is the AG really a gap?**
No. Because electroneutrality is always maintained in solution, there is no actual anion "gap." The calculated gap is composed predominantly of negatively charged proteins in plasma and averages 12 ± 3 mEq/L. An increase is most commonly caused by addition of an acid salt (H^+A), which reduces plasma HCO_3^- concentration and leads to an increased AG. Note that the AG would not change if the added acid were HCl. Other circumstances that can increase the AG include increased protein concentration and alkalemia, which increase the net negative charge on plasma proteins. The presence of a large quantity of cationic (positively charged) proteins, as with multiple myeloma, can reduce the AG.

98. **What is the conceptual difference between an AG and a non-AG metabolic acidosis?**

An AG acidosis is caused by the addition of a nonvolatile acid to the ECF. Examples include diabetic ketoacidosis, lactic acidosis, and uremic acidosis. A non-AG acidosis commonly (but not exclusively) represents a loss of HCO_3^-. Examples include lower GI losses from diarrhea and urinary losses due to renal tubular acidosis (RTA). Therefore, when approaching a patient with an AG acidosis, one should look for the source and identity of the acid gained. By contrast, when evaluating a patient with a non-AG acidosis, one should begin by looking for the source of the HCO_3^- loss.

99. **What are the causes of AG metabolic acidosis?**

The mnemonic KUSMAL can be used to remember the differential diagnosis of AG metabolic acidosis.

K = **K**etones (diabetic, alcohol, starvation)
U = **U**remia
S = **S**alicylates
M = **M**ethyl alcohol
A = **A**cid poisoning (ethylene glycol, paraldehyde)
L = **L**actate (circulatory/respiratory failure, sepsis, liver disease, tumors, toxins)

Morganroth ML. An analytical approach in the diagnosis of acid-base disorders. *J Crit Illness.* 1990;5:138–150.

100. **What is the significance of the plasma osmolal gap? How does it help in the evaluation of a patient with metabolic acidosis?**

The difference between the measured and the calculated plasma osmolality. A plasma osmolal gap of 0.25 mOsm/kg suggests, in a patient with AG metabolic acidosis, the possibility of ingestion of methanol or ethylene glycol. Isopropyl alcohol and ethanol increase the osmolal gap but not the AG, because acetone is not an anion.

101. **What are the common causes of a non-AG metabolic acidosis?**

Associated with K⁺ Loss	*Drugs*
Diarrhea	Acetazolamide
Renal tubular acidosis (proximal or distal)	Amphotericin B
Interstitial nephritis	Amiloride
Early renal failure	Spironolactone
Urinary tract obstruction	Toluene ingestion
Posthypocapnia	Urethral diversions
Infusions of HCl (HCl, arginine HCl, lysine HCl)	Ureterosigmoidostomy
	Dual bladder
	Ileal ureter

Toto RD. Metabolic acid-base disorders. In: Kokko JP, Tannen RL, eds. *Fluids and Electrolytes.* 3rd ed. Philadelphia: WB Saunders; 1996.

102. **How does the serum protein level affect the interpretation of AG?**

The AG is significantly influenced by serum albumin level. If the concentration of serum albumin falls to 2 g/dL (which is approximately half the normal level), the expected normal AG should be reduced to half. The paraproteins that accumulate in multiple myeloma are usually positively charged because they are rich in lysine and arginine. If there is a significant accumulation of these positively charged particles, the measured cations remain in the normal range. But because these "unmeasured" cations are associated with Cl⁻ (which is measured), the calculated AG will be reduced proportionately and may even become negative.

103. **Why is ammoniagenesis reduced in renal failure?**

Because in renal failure, the renal mass is reduced and there is a decrease in the ATP stores. Consequently, less ATP can be used to oxidize glutamine to ammonia. Ammonia then combines with H⁺ to form ammonium, which is then excreted in the urine. Renal ammoniagenesis is an important mechanism for removal of acid and H⁺ from the body.

104. **How is the urine AG useful in the evaluation of metabolic acidosis?**
     For the evaluation of some cases of hyperchloremic metabolic acidosis.

$$\text{Urine AG} = \text{Unmeasured cations} - \text{unmeasured anions} = (Na^+ + K^+) - Cl^-$$

     In normal subjects excreting 20–40 mEq of NH_4^+/L, the urine AG is positive or near zero. Conversely, in metabolic acidosis, the NH_4^+ excretion increases if the renal acidification mechanisms are intact. Consequently, urinary Cl^- excretion also increases to maintain electroneutrality. Urinary Cl^- therefore exceeds cation $(K^+ + Na^+)$ excretion, and the urine AG is negative (often −20 to greater than −50 mEq/L). Conversely, in acidosis in which the renal acidification mechanisms are impaired (as in renal failure and RTA), the urine AG remains positive, as in normal subjects.
     Battle DC, Hizon M, Cohen E, et al. The use of the urine anion gap in the diagnosis of hyperchloremic metabolic acidosis. *N Engl J Med.* 1988;318:594–599.

105. **Why is K^+ factored in the calculation of urine AG and not in plasma AG?**
     Potassium is predominantly an intracellular cation with the plasma K^+ level being ~4 mEq/L under normal conditions. The cations in plasma, therefore, are almost entirely represented by Na^+, because Ca and Mg are also present in very small amounts. Conversely, the urine K^+ is usually much greater because most of the dietary K^+ is excreted daily in the urine with some being excreted in fecal route. Thus, K^+ is a major cation in the urine and used in the calculation of urine AG.

106. **In which two clinical situations should the urine AG not be used?**
     - In **ketoacidosis,** the excretion of ketoacids neutralize the increased excretion of NH_4^+ cations, decreasing the negativity of the AG.
     - In **hypovolemia,** the avid proximal Na^+ reabsorption causes decreased distal Na^+ delivery resulting in a defect in acidification. The Cl^- reabsorption that accompanies Na^+ prevents NH_4Cl excretion, and the urine AG remains positive.

107. **What causes a decreased AG?**
     An increase in **unmeasured cations** such as K^+, Ca^{2+}, or Mg^{2+}, the addition of **abnormal** cations (lithium), or an increase in **cationic immunoglobulins** (plasma cell dyscrasias). AG also can be decreased by loss of unmeasured anions such as albumin (serum hypoalbuminemia) or if the effective negative charge on albumin is decreased by acidosis.

108. **What is RTA?**
     A disorder of tubular function in which the kidney has a compromised ability to excrete acid or recover filtered HCO_3^- in the setting of higher than normal $[H^+]$ in the ECF. The laboratory presentation is that of a non-AG metabolic acidosis. There are four types of RTA.

109. **Describe type I RTA.**
     Type I RTA (distal or classic RTA) is characterized by reduced net proton secretion by the distal nephron in the setting of systemic acidemia. Because the distal nephron is largely responsible for net acid excretion, patients with this disorder have continuous net acid retention (less net acid excretion than net acid production) and are, therefore, not in net acid balance. The diagnosis is made by demonstrating an inappropriately alkaline urine (pH > 5.5) in the setting of an acidemic serum (pH < 7.36) and by excluding the presence of drugs that alkalinize the urine (acetazolamide) or urea-splitting bacteria in the urine that can increase the urinary pH.

110. **Describe type II RTA.**
     Type II RTA (proximal RTA) is characterized by a reduced capacity for HCO_3^- recovery by the proximal tubule but intact distal nephron function. These patients waste HCO_3^- in the urine until the ECF concentration of HCO_3^- is reduced to a level such that the reduced filtered load of HCO_3^- (GFR × plasma HCO_3^-) can now be more completely resorbed and the urine becomes nearly bicarbonate-free. The reduction in plasma HCO_3^- concentration results in an increase in $[H^+]$. However, in the steady-state condition of low plasma HCO_3^-, these patients can excrete an appropriately acid urine (pH < 5.5) because distal nephron function is intact, and they are thus in acid balance (amount of acid excreted equals amount of acid produced), unlike the situation described for type I.

111. What is type III RTA?

Type III RTA represents a variant of type I, and the term is rarely used.

112. Describe type IV RTA.

Type IV RTA is characterized by a reduced aldosterone effect on the renal tubules, which may result in insufficient secretion of acid necessary to maintain normal acid-base status. These patients nevertheless can excrete an appropriately acidic urine in the face of acidemic stress. Unlike the other types of RTA, type IV RTA is commonly associated with hyperkalemia due to a coexisting reduction in K^+ secretion. This disorder is commonly seen in patients with hyporenin-hypoaldosteronism but also in isolated aldosterone deficiency and resistance.

KEY POINTS: RENAL TUBULAR ACIDOSIS

1. Type IV is the most common type of RTA seen in clinical practice.
2. Type IV RTA is often secondary to diabetic or nondiabetic renal disease (e.g., obstructive uropathy, aldosterone deficiency).
3. Drugs (e.g., triamterene and trimethoprim) are another common cause of RTA.

RTA, renal tubular acidosis.

113. How is type I (distal) RTA managed?

Alkali is given in amounts necessary (usually 1–2 mEq/kg/day) to correct the acidosis and to buffer the acid being retained. K^+ supplements are commonly required at the initiation of treatment but usually not in the steady-state treatment once the acidosis has been corrected.

114. How is type II (proximal) RTA managed?

Alkali is not usually required in adults because they do not have net acid retention and have only mild acidemia. But because the chronic acidemia inhibits bone growth in children, they must be treated with large amounts of alkali (10–20 mEq/kg/day) as well as large K^+ supplements (the increased urinary HCO_3^- losses are accompanied by accelerated urinary K^+ losses).

115. How is type IV RTA managed?

The clinically mild degrees of acidemia rarely require alkali treatment. Hyperkalemia is more commonly a clinical concern and dictates whether mineralocorticoid replacements with synthetic steroids are required.

116. What is lactic acidosis?

The accumulation of lactic acid, the end product of glycolysis. This accumulation leads to a depletion of the body's buffers and a drop in pH. Lactate, being an unmeasured anion, is one of the causes of an increased AG acidosis.

117. List the causes of lactic acidosis.

- Cellular hypoxia
- Decreased hepatic utilization of lactic acid (seen in advanced hepatocellular insufficiency of any cause)
- Cyanide poisoning
- Alcohol consumption
- Neoplasms with a large tumor burden
- Diabetic ketoacidosis (even in the absence of shock or other causes)
- Lactic acidosis X (severe lactic acidosis without obvious cause)
- Factitious lactic acidosis

118. How does cellular hypoxia cause lactic acidosis?

Oxygen is required for the oxidative phosphorylation of the lactic acid produced by glycolysis. Anything interfering with the available cellular supply of O_2 or its utilization will lead to the accumulation of lactic acid. This category includes respiratory failure, circulatory failure, and CO poisoning. This also can be seen in thiamine deficiency and has been reported in patients on long-term total parenteral nutrition without supplementation with thiamine.

KEY POINTS: LACTIC ACIDOSIS

1. In patients with lactic acidosis, bicarbonate administration is useful only when the pH < 7.15.
2. Alkali may cause paradoxical increase in lactate production in patients with milder acidosis.
3. The most common causes of lactic acidosis are cellular hypoxia, decreased hepatic utilization of lactic acid, alcohol consumption, neoplasms with a large tumor burden, and diabetic ketoacidosis.
4. "Lactic acidosis X" refers to severe lactic acidosis without obvious cause.

119. **How does cyanide poisoning cause lactic acidosis?**
By blocking oxidative phosphorylation, leading to increased glycolysis, decreased utilization of lactic acid, and therefore lactic acid accumulation.

120. **Explain how alcohol consumption may lead to lactic acidosis.**
Alcohol causes a modest increase in lactic acid production. In association with caloric depletion, the lactic acidosis can be severe.

121. **How does large tumor burden lead to lactic acidosis?**
By the increased rates of glycolysis in tumor cells compared to normal cells. This occurs even with sufficient O_2.

122. **What causes factitious lactic acidosis?**
Storage of blood for prolonged periods of time. The red and white blood cells generate lactic acid in the tube as it is stored; factitious lactic acidosis is most commonly seen in patients with high white blood cell counts.

123. **What is D-lactic acidosis, and how is it treated?**
An uncommon condition seen in patients with short bowel syndrome, as in patients with a history of small bowel resection, jejunoileal bypass, and other conditions. In these patients, glucose is rapidly transported into the large bowel and is metabolized by lactobacilli into D-lactate. The D-lactate is then rapidly absorbed into plasma and cannot be metabolized, because humans lack the D-lactate dehydrogenase (the enzyme in the human body is L-lactate specific). This results in the accumulation of D-lactate and leads to D-lactic acidosis. Clinically, patients present with ataxia, confusion, neurologic deficits, and speech and memory defects, typically after a large meal containing carbohydrates. The condition is diagnosed by measuring lactate using D-lactate dehydrogenase. The treatment usually consists of oral antibiotics to kill lactate-producing bacilli, low-carbohydrate diets using starch polymers rather than glucose, and of course, bicarbonate therapy.

124. **What causes metabolic alkalosis?**
The addition of excess HCO_3^- or alkali or loss of acid. Note that a low Cl^- and a high HCO_3^- concentration can result from both metabolic alkalosis as well as from a metabolic response to a respiratory acidosis. However, the pH and $Paco_2$ help to differentiate these two disorders.

125. **What are the two categories of metabolic alkalosis?**
Chloride-responsive (urine Cl^- < 10 mEq/L) and **chloride-resistant** (urine Cl^- > 20 mEq/L). Forms of alkalosis responsive to chloride salt administration are generally associated with ECF volume depletion and low urinary Cl^- concentration in spot urine tests, whereas the Cl^--unresponsive alkaloses are associated with ECF volume expansion and urine Cl^- > 20 mEq/L.

126. **What conditions are associated with chloride-responsive metabolic alkalosis?**
- Gastric fluid loss
- Postdiuretic therapy
- Posthypercapnia
- Congenital chloride diarrhea

127. **List the conditions associated with chloride-resistant metabolic alkalosis.**
- Primary aldosteronism
- Primary reninism
- Hyperglucocorticoidism

- Hypercalcemia
- Potassium depletion
- Liddle syndrome (an autosomal dominant disorder with increased Na^+ reabsorption in the collecting tubules and, usually, K^+ secretion)
- Bartter syndrome (an autosomal recessive disorder with impaired Na^+ in the loop of Henle)
- Chloruretic diuretics

128. **Which is the most common acid-base disturbance seen in cirrhosis?**
Primary respiratory alkalosis due to centrally mediated hyperventilation, especially with superimposed encephalopathy. The exact cause is unclear but may be related to the hormonal imbalance associated with liver failure. Estrogens and progesterone have been implicated, a situation somewhat similar to that seen in pregnancy.

129. **How do you treat a patient with metabolic alkalosis and edema?**
Frequently with NaCl with or without potassium. But in patients with edematous conditions presenting with metabolic alkalosis, using saline may be risky. In such patients, acetazolamide (a carbonic hydrase inhibitor and a diuretic) may be useful. It increases renal Na HCO_3^- excretion and ameliorates edema and alkalosis. In patients resistant to acetazolamide, isotonic HCl may be given cautiously in a period of 8–24 hours (the amount needed is TBW $\times$ 0.5 $\times$ ΔHCO_3^-. If all measures fail, dialysis can be performed to ameliorate alkalosis.

130. **How do you diagnose a mixed acid-base disorder?**
    1. Define the primary disturbance and the compensatory process involved. The primary disturbance is identified by the direction of the changes in pH, HCO_3^-, and $Paco_2$ levels.
    2. Determine whether the pulmonary or renal compensation is appropriate (see Table 9.2). Two facts must be kept in mind while making these interpretations. First, adequate compensation takes 12–24 hours to occur, and second, "overcompensation" never occurs in primary acid-base disturbances.
    3. Consider the patient's history and clinical presentation to formulate a differential diagnosis. In general, the underlying clinical condition gives clues to the possible mixed acid-base disturbance, which is then defined using the nomograms of expected compensation.
    Narins R, Emmett M. Simple and mixed acid-base disorders: a practical approach. *Medicine.* 1980;59:161–187.

131. **What findings suggest a combined metabolic and respiratory acidosis?**
A distinctly lower pH, even though the HCO_3^- and $Paco_2$ may not be changed.

132. **What findings suggest combined metabolic acidosis and metabolic alkalosis?**
In combined metabolic acidosis and metabolic alkalosis, the pH and HCO_3^- can be lower, normal, or higher, but an elevated AG with a high or normal HCO_3^- suggests the diagnosis.

133. **What findings suggest combined metabolic alkalosis and respiratory acidosis?**
Combined metabolic alkalosis and respiratory acidosis (which can be seen in patients with acute respiratory distress syndrome [ARDS] or COPD who are vomiting) causes HCO_3^- levels of higher-than-predicted compensation for a given high $Paco_2$.

134. **A 34-year-old woman is admitted to the hospital because of nausea and vomiting for the past 2 days. She admits to having taken several aspirin pills to alleviate her joint pains before she noticed epigastric pain and vomiting. Her ABG analysis reveals the following: pH 7.64, $Paco_2$ 32 mm Hg, and plasma bicarbonate 33 mEq/L. What kind of acid-base disorder is present in this patient?**
The patient has an alkalotic state because the pH is higher than the normal range. Because the patient presented with significant emesis, it is logical to think that the primary disturbance is metabolic alkalosis, which is supported by the fact that plasma bicarbonate is significantly elevated. The expected respiratory compensatory response is to increase $Paco_2$ by 6–7 mm Hg for every 10-mEq/L increase in plasma bicarbonate. However, in this patient, the $Paco_2$ is actually lower than normal, indicating a primary respiratory alkalosis. Thus, this patient has a mixed acid-base disorder. The combined metabolic and respiratory alkalosis explains why the pH is so disproportionately high.

135. **In what situations are potentially fatal mixed acid-base disorders encountered?**
In general, combined respiratory and metabolic acidosis or metabolic and respiratory alkalosis can result in pH changes that are fatal. Common examples include:
- An alcoholic with ketoacidosis (metabolic acidosis) may have superimposed vomiting from gastritis (metabolic alkalosis) and hyperventilation associated with withdrawal (respiratory alkalosis).
- A combination of metabolic acidosis and respiratory alkalosis is seen typically in patients with sepsis, salicylate intoxication, and severe liver disease.
- Metabolic acidosis can coexist with metabolic alkalosis in patients with renal failure or with alcoholic or diabetic ketoacidosis (acidosis) who are vomiting or having gastric suction (alkalosis).
- Vomiting in a pregnant woman or a patient with liver failure causes a mixture of respiratory and metabolic alkalosis.

CALCIUM, PHOSPHATE, AND MAGNESIUM METABOLISM

136. **How is calcium distributed in the body and in the serum?**
A 70-kg man has approximately 1000 g of calcium in his body. Of this amount, bone contains 99%, whereas the ECF and ICF contain only 1%. Furthermore, only about 1% of skeletal calcium is freely exchangeable with ECF calcium. The routine measurement for serum calcium (normal = 9–10 mg/mL = 4.5–5.0 mEq/L = 2.25–2.5 mM/L) measures total calcium. Approximately 40% is protein bound, 5–10% is complexed to other substances (e.g., phosphate, sulfate), and 50% is ionized.

137. **Explain the significance of the ionized fraction of calcium.**
The ionized fraction determines the activity of calcium in cellular and membrane function. The concentration of total calcium can vary without changing the ionized fraction by changing the protein concentration. It is also possible to vary the ionized fraction without changing the total calcium by changing serum pH. Increasing serum pH decreases the ionized fraction of calcium and vice versa.

138. **What are the major sites of calcium reabsorption in the nephron?**
About 50% of the filtered calcium is reabsorbed in the proximal tubule, and most of the remainder (~40% of the total) is reabsorbed in the loop of Henle, primarily in the ascending limb. A small amount of calcium is reabsorbed in the distal convoluted tubule and an even smaller amount in the collecting tubule.

139. **What are the major hormones involved in calcium metabolism?**
Parathyroid hormone (PTH), vitamin D, and calcitonin.

KEY POINTS: ELECTROLYTE DISTURBANCES

1. Magnesium deficiency must be excluded in patients with resistant hypokalemia.
2. Hyperglycemia is the most common cause of nonhypotonic hyponatremia.
3. Although hypoalbuminemia results in reduction of total serum calcium, ionized calcium remains unchanged (physiologically more important fraction).

140. **Summarize the roles of these hormones in calcium metabolism.**
PTH is secreted in response to a decrease in serum calcium and promotes calcium resorption from bone because it enhances renal resorption of calcium and excretion of phosphate. Low serum calcium concentration stimulates 1-hydroxylation of 25-hydroxyvitamin D by the kidney to form 1,25-dihydroxyvitamin D (the active form of **vitamin D**). This hormone promotes calcium resorption from the gut and mineralization of bone. Increases in serum calcium lead to increased secretion of **calcitonin.** This hormone inhibits bone reabsorption and 1-hydroxylation of 25-hydroxyvitamin D and thereby ameliorates hypercalcemia.

141. **What factors affect renal calcium excretion?**
With some exceptions, renal calcium handling varies directly with renal Na^+ handling. Therefore, renal calcium excretion is increased by saline diuresis, loop diuretics, and volume expansion. In contrast, renal calcium excretion is decreased in volume depletion and other states associated with renal salt retention. One notable exception to this general rule is that the natriuresis associated with thiazide diuretics is accompanied by decreased, rather than increased, urinary calcium excretion.

142. Define *pseudohypocalcemia* and *pseudohypercalcemia*.

These terms refer to an alteration of the total calcium concentration in the setting of a normal ionized fraction. Because the ionized fraction is normal, such patients are asymptomatic. Abnormalities in the concentration of serum proteins are a common cause of these disorders. Hypoalbuminemia causes a decrease in the total serum calcium level without a change in the level of ionized calcium. For each decrease of 1.0 g/dL in serum albumin, one should expect a drop in the total serum calcium of approximately 0.8 mg/dL.

143. List the common causes of true hypocalcemia.

- Hypoparathyroidism (usually following thyroid or parathyroid surgery)
- Vitamin D deficiency
- Magnesium depletion (usually at levels <0.8 mEq/L)
- Liver disease (decreased synthesis of 25-hydroxyvitamin D)
- CKD (hyperphosphatemia and decreased synthesis of 1,25-dihydroxyvitamin D)
- Acute pancreatitis
- Tumor lysis syndrome
- Rhabdomyolysis

144. What are the signs and symptoms of hypocalcemia?

The symptoms depend on the magnitude of the decrease in serum calcium, the rate of the drop, and its duration. The symptoms of hypocalcemia are due to the resultant decrease in the excitation threshold of neural tissue, which causes an increase in excitability, repetitive responses to a single stimulus, reduced accommodation, or even continuous activity of neural tissue. Specific signs and symptoms include:

- Tetany and paresthesia
- Altered mental status (lethargy to coma)
- Seizures
- QT interval prolongation on the ECG
- Increased intracranial pressure
- Lenticular cataracts

145. What are Trousseau and Chvostek signs?

Both are indications of the latent tetany caused by hypocalcemia. Of the two signs, the Trousseau sign is more specific and reliable.

- **Trousseau sign:** A sphygmomanometer is placed on the arm and inflated to greater than systolic blood pressure and left in place for at least 2 minutes. A positive response is carpal spasm of the ipsilateral arm. Relaxation takes 5–10 seconds after the pressure is released.
- **Chvostek sign:** Tapping the facial nerve between the corner of the mouth and the zygomatic arch produces twitching of the ipsilateral facial muscle, especially the angle of the mouth. This sign may be seen in 10–25% of normal adult patients.

146. What causes hypercalcemia?

Primary hyperparathyroidism (~50% of cases), malignancy, use of thiazide diuretics, vitamin D excess, hyper- and hypothyroidism, granulomatous disorders, immobilization, and milk-alkali syndrome.

147. What are the signs and symptoms of hypercalcemia?

Weakness, constipation, nausea, anorexia, polyuria, polydipsia, and pruritus. Severe hypercalcemia may present with progressive CNS symptoms of lethargy, depression, obtundation, coma, and seizures. Rapid onset is more likely to be symptomatic than a slowly progressive level, regardless of the ultimate level at presentation.

148. Describe the appropriate treatment for hypercalcemia.

Treatment depends on the calcium level and symptoms of the patient. Acute symptomatic hypercalcemia should be treated aggressively, first with saline infusion to expedite calcium excretion. Most patients with hypercalcemia are significantly volume depleted as a result of the osmotic diuresis related to the hypercalciuria.

149. How is normal saline infused for aggressive treatment of hypercalcemia?

At a rapid rate, ≥300 mL/hour, with KCl and possibly magnesium added to the solution depending on measured blood values. After the patient is volume-repleted, furosemide may be given to promote calciuresis. Care must be taken to keep input equal to or greater than output to avoid making the patient hypovolemic again.

150. **How is calcitonin used in the treatment of hypercalcemia?**
Calcitonin is useful for decreasing serum calcium and has the added advantage of rapid onset of action. It may be given in the presence of renal insufficiency or thrombocytopenia or when mithramycin is contraindicated. Its disadvantage is that rapid resistance often develops, probably related to the development of antibodies. This resistance can sometimes be delayed by concomitant administration of prednisone.

151. **Describe the role of bisphosphonates in the treatment of hypercalcemia.**
Bisphosphonates inhibit osteoclast activity and are effective with those cancers in which this mechanism is present. They are given via IV infusion over 5 days or as oral tablets.

152. **What other agents are useful for treatment of less significant levels of hypercalcemia?**
Glucocorticoids (prednisone, 20–40 mg/day), phosphates (1–6 g/day), prostaglandin inhibitors (aspirin and NSAIDs), or oral bisphosphonates. All of these agents are less effective but may suffice for chronic maintenance.
Bilizekian JP. Management of acute hypercalcemia. *N Engl J Med.* 1992;326:1196–1203.

153. **What factors regulate phosphate metabolism in the body?**
Serum phosphate is lowered by insulin, glucose (by stimulating insulin secretion), and alkalosis, which cause transcellular translocation of phosphate from plasma. Phosphate is resorbed predominantly in the proximal tubule, with small amounts being absorbed in the distal tubule. Renal phosphate excretion is increased by PTH, alkalosis, saline diuresis, ketoacidosis, and increased dietary phosphate intake.

154. **In which clinical situations can hypophosphatemia develop?**
- Decreased intake of phosphorus
- Shifts of phosphorus from serum into cells
- Increased excretion of phosphorus into urine
- Spurious hypophosphatemia (mannitol infusion)

155. **What factors may lead to decreased intake of phosphorus?**
- Decreased dietary intake
- Alcoholism
- Decreased intestinal absorption due to vitamin D deficiency, malabsorption, steatorrhea, secretory diarrhea, vomiting, or phosphate binders

156. **What factors may cause shifts of phosphorus from serum into cells?**
- Respiratory alkalosis (e.g., sepsis, heat stroke, hepatic coma, salicylate poisoning, gout)
- Recovery from hypothermia
- Hormonal effects (e.g., insulin, glucagon, androgens)
- Recovery from diabetic ketoacidosis
- Carbohydrate administration (hyperalimentation, fructose or glucose infusions)

157. **List the factors that may lead to increased excretion of phosphorus in urine.**
- Hyperparathyroidism
- Renal tubule defects (as in aldosteronism, SIADH, mineralocorticoid administration, diuretics, corticosteroids)
- Hypomagnesemia

158. **What electrolyte disturbances are commonly seen in progressive renal disease?**
Patients with progressive renal disease develop hyperphosphatemia, hypocalcemia, and secondary hyperparathyroidism. They are also at risk of developing at least two kinds of bone diseases.

159. **What are the main disturbances thought to be responsible for the abnormalities of calcium and phosphate metabolism in progressive renal disease?**
- A rise in inorganic phosphate concentration in the serum due to poor renal excretion. This rise leads to a decrease in serum calcium concentration and stimulation of PTH secretion. The increased PTH secretion leads to increased bone resorption and osteitis fibrosa cystica.
- Resistance to the action of vitamin D. One function of this hormone is to promote calcium resorption from the gut. Decreased gut resorption of calcium exacerbates the hypocalcemia and reduces available calcium for bone mineralization.

- Defective synthesis of 1,25-dihydroxyvitamin D (the active form of this hormone). Reduced levels of 1,25-dihydroxyvitamin D result in defective bone mineralization (osteomalacia in adults, rickets in children).

160. **How does magnesium depletion affect calcium and phosphate metabolism?**
Magnesium depletion results in decreased secretion and end-organ responsiveness of PTH. This leads to functional hypoparathyroidism and the resultant effects on the serum level and urinary excretion of calcium and phosphate. This disorder can be corrected with magnesium repletion.

161. **What are some common causes of magnesium deficiency?**
Dietary insufficiency (decreased intake, protein-calorie malnutrition, prolonged IV feeding), intestinal malabsorption, chronic loss of GI fluids, loop diuretics (Mg^{2+} is reabsorbed predominantly in the thick ascending limb of the loop of Henle), other drugs (gentamicin, cisplatin, pentamidine, cyclosporine), alcoholism, hyperparathyroidism, and lactation.

162. **What is the milk-alkali syndrome?**
The presence of hypercalcemia, increased BUN and creatinine, increased serum phosphate, and metabolic alkalosis in a patient ingesting large quantities of milk and calcium carbonate–containing antacids. The patient usually presents with nausea, vomiting, anorexia, weakness, polydipsia, and polyuria. If it continues, metastatic calcification can occur, leading to mental status changes, nephrocalcinosis, band keratopathy, pruritus, and myalgias. The treatment is withdrawal of the milk and antacid.

163. **What electrolyte abnormalities are seen in human immunodeficiency virus (HIV) infection?**
In addition to the main proteinuric syndrome caused by focal sclerosis (so-called HIV nephropathy), a variety of electrolyte disorders are commonly seen in patients with HIV. Asymptomatic **hyperkalemia** is a common manifestation. The hyperkalemia may be due to many possible causes, including hyporenin-hypoaldosteronism, adrenal insufficiency, drugs such as pentamidine and trimethoprim-sulfamethoxazole, and even isolated hypoaldosteronism. **Hyponatremia** is frequently caused by hypovolemia, adrenal insufficiency, and SIADH due to associated pulmonary or cerebral diseases. Other electrolyte abnormalities include hypocalcemia, hypomagnesemia, and hypouricemia. Hypercalcemia is seen in association with lymphomas and cytomegalovirus infection.
Klotman ME, Klotman PE. AIDS and the kidney. *Semin Nephrol.* 1998;18:371–372.

164. **List the electrolyte disturbances associated with alcoholism.**
- Hypokalemia
- Hypophosphatemia
- Hypomagnesemia
- Hyponatremia

165. **How common is hypokalemia in alcoholics? Explain.**
Hypokalemia is seen in one half of hospitalized, withdrawing alcoholics. This does not necessarily mean a total body K^+ deficit. Respiratory alkalosis, inadequate dietary intake, and GI losses (vomiting, diarrhea) are the common etiologic factors for hypokalemia. Withdrawal as well as severe liver failure causes respiratory alkalosis.

166. **How common is hypophosphatemia in alcoholics? Explain.**
Hypophosphatemia (<2.5 mg/dL) is a common finding in hospitalized severe alcoholics, noted in more than half (50%) of patients in some series. The common predisposing factors are respiratory alkalosis, decreased dietary intake, transcellular shifts due to glucose administration, and rarely, associated proximal tubular injury leading to phosphate wasting.

167. **Explain the relationship between chronic alcoholism and hypomagnesemia.**
Chronic alcoholism is the most common cause of hypomagnesemia in the United States. It is seen in alcoholics who are withdrawing and more commonly in those who had withdrawal seizures. GI losses, cellular uptake, dietary deficiencies, and possibly lipolysis leading to fatty acid–magnesium precipitation are the possible causes.

168. **How may beer contribute to hyponatremia?**
Beer is virtually solute free, so when large quantities are ingested, this free-water volume exceeds the excretory capacity of the kidney, and hyponatremia results.

BIBLIOGRAPHY
1. Skoredi K, Cherkow GM, eds. *Brenner & Rector's The Kidney*. 10th ed. Philadelphia: Elsevier; 2010.
2. Goldman L, Ausiello D, eds. *Cecil Textbook of Medicine*. 23rd ed. Philadelphia: WB Saunders; 2007.
3. Rose BD, Post T, eds. *Clinical Physiology of Acid-Base and Electrolyte Disorders*. 5th ed. New York: McGraw-Hill; 2001.
4. Schrier RW, ed. *Renal and Electrolyte Disorders*. 7th ed. Philadelphia: Lippincott Williams & Wilkins; 2010.

CHAPTER 10

RHEUMATOLOGY

Roger Kornu, MD, FACR, Kathryn H. Dao, MD, FACP, FACR, Catalina Orozco, MD, and Rahul K. Patel, MD, FACP, FACR

The wolf, I'm afraid, is inside tearing up the place.

Letter from Flannery O'Connor (1925–1964)
Author afflicted with systemic lupus erythematosus

1. Give an operational definition of rheumatic diseases.
   Syndromes of pain or inflammation or both in articular or periarticular tissues.

2. How common are the rheumatic diseases?
   Fairly common: 52.5 million (22.7%) adults have self-reported doctor-diagnosed arthritis, including 49.7% of adults 65 years or older, according to data from the National Health Interview Survey (2010–2012). By the year 2030, 67 million (25% of the adult population) are projected to have physician-diagnosed arthritis. Overall, 2% of the general population has one form of inflammatory arthritis, and half of those have rheumatoid arthritis (RA).
   Centers for Disease Control and Prevention. *Arthritis.* 2016. Available at: http://www.cdc.gov/arthritis [accessed 05.06.16].

SIGNS AND SYMPTOMS

3. What are the key points in a rheumatic history?
   - Pain location
   - Symmetry of symptoms
   - Presence of morning stiffness (tends to be present in inflammatory disease patients)
   - Effect of exercise (tends to lead to improvement in inflammatory disease patients)
   - Additional constitutional symptoms (fatigue, low-grade fever, and weight loss)
   - Daily function
   - Family history (such as positive human leukocyte antigen [HLA-B27 in ankylosing spondylitis [AS])

4. What is the "squeeze test"?
   A physical examination maneuver to assess the possible presence of inflammatory arthritis. The metacarpophalangeal (MCP) squeeze test is performed by squeezing all four MCP joints together to elicit tenderness. The metatarsophalangeal (MTP) squeeze test elicits tenderness across the four MTP joints.

5. What is the Finkelstein test?
   A maneuver to demonstrate de Quervain tenosynovitis in which a fist is made around the thumb and the wrist is moved toward the ulnar side. In a positive test, a sharp pain is felt at the base of the thumb.

6. Define *Tinel sign*.
   The sensation of focal pain and electrical sensations occurring when a nerve is tapped at the site of entrapment.

7. How do you elicit the Phalen sign?
   Ask the patient to:
   - Raise both arms to shoulder level.
   - Press the back (dorsum) of the hands together.
   - Slightly drop the elbows, causing maximal flexion of the wrist, and maintain for 30–60 seconds.
   If the patient has carpal tunnel syndrome (CTS), the discomfort will be reproduced.

8. **What do the Speed's test and the Yergason maneuver detect?**
   Both check for bicipital tendinitis of the shoulder.
   - Speed's test: Pain in the bicipital groove when the forearm is supinated, elbow is extended, and there is resistance to forward flexion of shoulder
   - Yergason maneuver: Pain in the bicipital groove with resisted supination of the forearm and elbow is flexed 90 degrees and held at the patient's side.

9. **What condition does the Adson test elicit, and how is it done?**
   Thoracic outlet syndrome. With the Adson test, the radial pulse is lost when the patient's arm is abducted, extended, and externally rotated and the patient rotates the head on the ipsilateral side and inhales deeply. This suggests compression of the subclavian artery.

10. **What does the Schober test detect?**
    Limited forward flexion of the lumbar spine. The modified Schober test is useful in the diagnosis of a spondyloarthropathy by detecting limitation of the forward flexion of the lumbar spine. While the patient is standing, the examiner marks one point at the level of the posterior iliac spine and another point 10 cm above the midline. The patient then touches the toes while keeping the knees straight (maximal forward flexion). A measure distance < 5 cm suggests spine stiffness.

11. **Straight leg raising (SLR) is a useful diagnostic maneuver in what common condition?**
    Low back pain. If the pain is due to nerve root compression, the symptoms are reproduced with SLR. To perform the maneuver, lift the lower leg by the calcaneus with the knee remaining straight. The cross-table SLR test additionally brings the heel across the other leg and may increase the sensitivity of this maneuver.

12. **What distinguishes Bouchard nodes and Heberden nodes?**
    The location of the bony enlargement. Bouchard nodes involve the proximal interphalangeal (PIP) joints; Heberden nodes, the distal interphalangeal (DIP) joints. Both are associated with osteoarthritis (OA), and women are affected more frequently than men in a 10:1 ratio. Heredity plays a particularly strong role in mothers, daughters, and sisters.

13. **What is a Jaccoud deformity?**
    Changes of the hands secondary to chronic inflammation of the joint capsule, ligaments, and tendons. The deformities may mimic those of RA such as ulnar deviation of the fingers and MCP joint subluxation. Erosions are not present on x-ray study, although after several recurrences, notches may be seen radiographically on the ulnar side of the metacarpal heads. Although originally described in rheumatic fever, this disorder has been extended to include the arthropathy of other conditions, most commonly systemic lupus erythematosus (SLE).

14. **Name dermatologic findings associated with some rheumatic diseases.**
    See Table 10.1.

Table 10.1. Dermatologic Findings in Rheumatic Diseases

DERMATOLOGIC FINDING	DESCRIPTION	DISEASE
Malar rash	Butterfly appearance on face of rash that spares the nasolabial folds	Systemic lupus erythematosus
Palpable purpura	Slightly elevated purpuric rash over one or more areas of the skin	Vasculitis
Erythema nodosum	Reddish/violet subcutaneous nodules that tend to develop in a pretibial location	Sarcoidosis, inflammatory bowel disease, tuberculosis, streptococcal infection
Keratoderma blennorrhagicum	Hyperkeratotic skin lesions on soles and palms	Reactive arthritis
Heliotrope rash	Violaceous eruption on the upper eyelids	Dermatomyositis

(Continued)

Table 10.1. Dermatologic Findings in Rheumatic Diseases—cont'd

DERMATOLOGIC FINDING	DESCRIPTION	DISEASE
Gottron papules	Erythematous rash extensor on the regions of MCP and IP joints	Dermatomyositis
Erythema chronicum migrans	Reddish, central clearing known as a "target lesion"	Lyme disease
Morphea	Small area(s) of skin fibrosis	Systemic sclerosis
Linear scleroderma	Band-like lesion, which may expand across dermatomes	Systemic sclerosis
"En coup de sabre"	Specific curvilinear band that resembles a dueling scar that occurs across the face	Systemic sclerosis

IP, interphalangeal; MCP, metacarpophalangeal.

15. **Which rheumatic syndromes have been associated with uveitis?**
    - Spondyloarthopathies (ankylosing spondylitis, inflammatory bowel disease, psoriatic arthritis, reactive arthritis)
    - Juvenile idiopathic arthritis
    - Sjögren syndrome (SS)
    - Sarcoidosis
    - Behçet disease (BD)
    - Kawasaki disease (KD)
    - Relapsing polychondritis (RP)

16. **Describe the Raynaud phenomenon.**
    The presence of triphasic color changes (usually white, blue, then red) in the hands (or any distal part of the body) incited by exposure to cold or intense emotion.

17. **Distinguish between primary and secondary Raynaud phenomenon.**
    Primary Raynaud phenomenon occurs without association with another condition and is estimated to occur in 3–4% of the population, more commonly in females. Raynaud phenomenon occurring in association with another condition is usually termed *secondary Raynaud phenomenon.*

18. **Name some conditions that are typically associated with Raynaud phenomenon.**
    - Systemic rheumatologic diseases: systemic sclerosis (SSc), CREST syndrome (calcinosis, Raynaud's, esophageal dysmotility, sclerodactyly, and telangiectasia), SLE, polymyositis, SS, RA
    - Drugs: beta blockers, ergot alkaloids, stimulants (i.e., methylphenidate)
    - Hyperviscosity-related diseases: cryoglobulinemia, cold agglutinins
    - Other causes: carcinoid, complex regional pain syndrome, bacterial endocarditis

19. **What factors predict the development of a systemic autoimmune disease in a patient presenting with Raynaud phenomenon?**
    Positive antinuclear antibodies (ANAs) (positive predictive value 30%), abnormal nail bed capillaries (positive predictive value 47%), or abnormal pulmonary function studies. One study showed that 12.6% of patients presenting with Raynaud phenomenon went on to develop a rheumatic disease.

20. **What is erythromelalgia?**
    Intense burning pain with pronounced erythema and increased skin temperature often in response to mild thermal stimuli or exercise. Erythromelalgia is often thought of as the opposite to Raynaud phenomenon. The condition is believed to arise from vasomotor abnormalities resulting in abnormal blood flow to the extremities. Primary erythromelalgia can be idiopathic or genetic; secondary erythromelalgia most commonly is due to a myeloproliferative disorder or medications but can occur in the setting of infection and polycythemia vera or essential thrombocytosis.

LABORATORY AND IMAGING EVALUATION

21. **When is an arthrocentesis (joint aspiration) indicated?**
When joint infection is suspected. Synovial fluid analysis on patients with a mono- or polyarticular arthropathy of unclear etiology may be helpful in determining the cause.

22. **Which studies should generally be performed on synovial fluid after arthrocentesis?**
    - Gram stain and culture for aerobic and anaerobic bacteria
    - Total leukocyte count and differential white blood cell (WBC) count
    - Crystal evaluation by polarized light microscopy
    - Culture for mycobacteria or fungi, if suspected

23. **Describe the typical findings in synovial fluid analysis.**

Type of Fluid	Visual Appearance	WBC Count (cells/mm³)	PMNs (%)
Normal	Transparent, clear, viscous	0–200	<10
Noninflammatory	Transparent, yellow, viscous	0–2000	<25
Inflammatory	Translucent-opaque, yellow, not viscous	2000–50,000	25–75
Septic	Opaque, yellow-green, variable viscosity	50,000–100,000	>75
Hemorrhagic	Bloody, red, variable viscosity	200–2000	50–75

PMN, polymorphonuclear leukocyte; WBC, white blood cell.

24. **What are rice bodies?**
Aggregates of fibrin frequently found in the synovial fluid of patients with RA.

25. **What is the erythrocyte sedimentation rate (ESR)?**
A measurement of the distance in millimeters that red blood cells travel in a Westergen or Wintrobe tube over 1 hour that is an indirect measurement of acute-phase reactants in systemic inflammation.

26. **Describe the clinical utility of C-reactive protein (CRP). How does it compare to ESR?**
CRP can monitor disease progression and therapy response in inflammatory conditions. CRP is an acute-phase reactant protein that is synthesized in response to tissue injury, rising within 4–6 hours, peaking in 24–72 hours, and normalizing within 1 week. CRP rises more rapidly than ESR and rapidly falls back to normal reference range before ESR has returned to normal after an active disease process has subsided.

27. **What is a major difference between quantitative CRP, high-sensitivity CRP (hsCRP), and cardiac CRP (cCRP)?**
Quantitative or conventional CRP assays are clinically used for the evaluation of inflammatory disorders and infection. hsCRP can be used for conditions thought to be associated with inflammation in otherwise healthy individuals. cCRP is used to aid in the identification and stratification of risk for cardiovascular disease.

Callaghan, James V. Guidance for Industry and FDA Staff: Review criteria for assessment of CRP, hsCRP, and cCRP assays, 2005. Available at: http://www.fda.gov/downloads/MedicalDevices/DeviceRegulationandGuidance/GuidanceDocuments/ucm071017.pdf [accessed 28.11.16].

28. **What are rheumatoid factors (RFs)?**
Autoantibodies directed at the Fc portion of the immunoglobulin G (IgG) molecule. Although IgM RFs are the most common, all immunoglobulin isotypes have been reported. IgG RFs are associated with a greater likelihood of vasculitis.

29. **Name some causes of positive RFs.**
Remember the mnemonic CHRONIC:
CHronic disease: interstitial lung disease, primary biliary cirrhosis
Rheumatoid arthritis

Other rheumatologic diseases: SLE, SS, SSc, sarcoidosis
Neoplasm
Infections: hepatitis C, bacterial endocarditis, parvovirus B19 infection, tuberculosis
Cryoglobulinemia

30. **Do all patients with RA have circulating RFs?**
No. RFs may be detectable in 50% of RA patients in the first 6 months of diagnosis and in 85% in the first 2 years; however, up to 25% of patients with clinical RA have no circulating RFs. The titer has little prognostic value in an individual patient, and remeasurements provide little added information.

31. **What are anti-CCP antibodies?**
Anti-cyclic citrullinated peptide (anti-CCP) antibodies are directed against the citrullinated residue of certain molecules (such as filaggrin and fibrin). These autoantibodies are found in the sera of patients with RA.

32. **What are the sensitivity and specificity of RF and anti-CCP antibodies?**
   - **RF:** 66% sensitivity, 70% specificity
   - **Anti-CCP antibodies:** 82% sensitivity, 95% specificity
   Measurement of anti-CCP antibodies is superior in specificity compared with RF alone, but the diagnostic yields of both tests are very good in patients suspected with RA. High titers of either RF or anti-CCP antibodies correlate with more severe disease including erosive disease and extra-articular manifestations.

33. **What is the ANA?**
Any autoantibody that reacts to certain nuclear antigens (e.g., histones, ribonucleoproteins, DNA, or centromere). With the development of immunofluorescence microscopy techniques, different staining patterns were discovered, and it became clear that many different nuclear antigens can elicit an antibody response. Thus, many antibodies can be classified as ANA (Table 10.2). Testing for the presence of an ANA can be done by immunoassay or indirect fluorescent antibody (IFA). IFA is considered the gold standard.

Table 10.2. Antigens and Antinuclear Antibodies

ANTIGEN	ANTIBODY
Deoxyribose phosphate backbone of DNA	Anti-DNA (double-stranded or native)
Purine and pyrimidine bases	Anti–single-stranded DNA
H1, H2A, H2B, H3, H2A/H2B complex, H3/H4 complex	Antihistones
DNA topoisomerase I	Anti–SCL-70
Histidyl tRNA transferase	Anti–Jo-1
Kinetochore	Anticentromere
RNA polymerase I	Antinucleolar
Y1–Y5 RNA and protein	Anti-Ro
U1–6 RNA and protein	Anti-RNP (includes anti-Sm)

Adapted from von Mühlen CA, Tan EM. Autoantibodies in the diagnosis of systemic rheumatic diseases. *Semin Arthritis Rheum.* 1995;24:323–358.

34. **What is the significance of a positive ANA test in a patient who is otherwise healthy?**
Very little. ANA test positivity is common and may not carry any significance. In 1997, the ANA Subcommittee of the International Union of Immunological Societies (IUIS) Standardization Committee completed a multicenter study with the objective of identifying the range of ANA titers in normal individuals and in patients with certain rheumatic diseases. The study found that a positive ANA test can be found in 31.7% of healthy individuals at 1:40 serum dilution, 13.3% at 1:80, 5.0% at 1:160, and 3.3% at 1:320. Despite these high frequencies of occurrence, the ANA titer may be useful in determining the presence of disease. Setting a low cutoff of 1:40 (high sensitivity, low specificity)

could aid in diagnosis because it would classify most patients who have SLE, SSc, or SS. Conversely, setting a high cutoff at 1:160 serum dilution (high specificity, low sensitivity) could be useful to confirm the presence of disease and would likely exclude 95% of normal individuals.

Tan EM, Feltkamp TE, Smolen JS, et al. Range of antinuclear antibodies in "healthy" individuals. *Arthritis Rheum.* 1997;40:1601–1611.

35. **Do ANA staining patterns detect specific ANAs? What is their clinical relevance?**
No. The fluorescence test for ANA is performed by incubating the patient's serum with a fixed monolayer of human larynx epithelioma cancer (HEp-2) cell lines. If ANAs are present in the serum, they bind to the nuclear component of the substrate. Next, fluorescent anti-Ig is added, which binds to antibodies (if present) in the test serum. With the fluorescent tag, the ANA can be directly visualized under fluorescent light. Different patterns of staining occur, and although they may provide some information, they do not identify the specific antibody present, nor are they specific for a disease entity or clinically relevant. For example, the rim or peripheral pattern (usually associated with antibodies directed against nuclear membrane proteins) may be obscured if another autoantibody (staining a homogeneous pattern) is present.

36. **Why is it helpful to know which specific ANA is present in a given patient?**
To increase the diagnostic likelihood of a specific rheumatic diagnosis and provide a prognosis. Anti-double-stranded DNA antibody is associated with lupus and lupus nephritis; the anti-SSA and SSB antibodies are associated with SS and neonatal lupus.

37. **What rheumatic diseases are associated with specific ANAs?**
See Table 10.3.

Table 10.3. Specific Antinuclear Antibodies and Disease Association

ANTIBODY	ASSOCIATED DISEASES
Ro/SSA	SLE, neonatal lupus syndrome, subacute lupus, SS, RA
dsDNA	SLE (with nephritis)
Sm	SLE
Jo-1	Polymyositis (pulmonary involvement)
Centromere	CREST syndrome (limited scleroderma)
SCL-70	Systemic sclerosis
Histone	SLE, drug-induced lupus
RNP	SLE, MCTD
Ribosomal P	SLE (with psychosis)
Cardiolipin	SLE (with thromboembolic events), antiphospholipid syndrome

CREST, calcinosis cutis, Raynaud phenomenon, esophageal dysfunction, sclerodactyly, and telangiectasia; MCTD, mixed connective tissue disease; RA, rheumatoid arthritis; SLE, systemic lupus erythematosus; SS, Sjögren syndrome.

38. **What are antineutrophil cytoplasmic antibodies (ANCAs)?**
Antibodies directed against enzymes (proteinase 3 [PR3] and myeloperoxidase [MPO]) found in primary granules of neutrophils and lysosomes of monocytes. Immunofluorescence detects two principal staining patterns: (1) a fine granular cytoplasmic staining (c-ANCA) and (2) a perinuclear collection of antibody (p-ANCA).

39. **What is the association of HLA-B27 in rheumatic disease?**
HLA-B27 is encoded by an allele of the major histocompatibility complex (MHC) class I HLA-B, and its structure has been hypothesized to play a role in seronegative spondyloarthopathies such as AS, reactive arthritis, psoriasis, and psoriatic arthritis. HLA-B27 positivity cannot be the sole reason for pathogenesis, as HLA-B27 is present in over 90% of patients with AS, but only 5% of HLA-B27–positive people will ever develop a spondyloarthropathy.

40. Which diseases are associated with soft tissue calcification on plain radiographs?
    - Calcific tendinitis
    - Chondrocalcinosis
    - Dermatomyositis
    - Diabetes
    - Ehlers-Danlos syndrome
    - Neoplasia
    - Neuropathic arthropathy
    - Parathyroid disease
    - Renal osteodystrophy
    - Sarcoidosis
    - Scleroderma
    - Trauma

41. Describe typical radiographic features of inflammatory arthritis in early and progressive disease.
    Soft tissue swelling and juxta-articular osteoporosis in early disease and more diffuse osteoporosis with uniform loss of cartilage in chronic disease. Further inflammation will lead to synovial hypertrophy and erosions with marginal areas of the synovium.

42. List five classic radiographic findings of OA.
    - Subchondral cyst formation
    - New bone formation (osteophytes)
    - Bone sclerosis
    - Joint space narrowing
    - Lack of osteoporosis

43. Describe the role of magnetic resonance imaging (MRI) and peripheral ultrasound (US) in inflammatory arthritis.
    To detect subtle bony abnormalities that may not be seen on plain radiographs. MRI is able to detect early bony erosions. Peripheral US is also a sensitive test for detecting erosions. US is less expensive than MRI, but accurate results are operator dependent.

KEY POINTS: DIAGNOSING RHEUMATIC DISEASES

1. Inflammatory arthritis tends to involve small joints, has a morning stiffness component, and improves with activity.
2. Joint arthrocentesis is most useful in evaluating for joint infection.
3. RF and anti-CCP antibodies help improve sensitivity and specificity in diagnosing RA.
4. Although ANA positivity may occur in normal patients, its titer and its presence with other autoantibodies are useful in diagnosing connective tissue diseases.
5. The HLA-B27 association with arthritis is highest in ankylosing spondylitis and reactive arthritis but lower with the spondylitis associated with psoriasis and inflammatory bowel disease.
6. Imaging may be a useful tool in diagnosing rheumatologic disease and determining the severity of disease, especially in evaluation for bony erosions.

anti-CCP, anti-cyclic citrullinated peptide; ANA, antinuclear antibody; RA, rheumatoid arthritis; RF, rheumatoid factor.

RHEUMATOID ARTHRITIS

44. What is the basis for the revised RA classification criteria established in 2010 by the American College of Rheumatology (ACR) and European League Against Rheumatism (EULAR)?
    Definite RA is based on:
    - Presence of synovitis in at least one joint
    - Absence of an alternative diagnosis to explain the synovitis
    - Achievement of a total score ≥ 6 from individual scores from four domains:
        - Number and site of involved joints (score range 0–5)
            - 2–10 medium to large joints: 1 point
            - 1–3 small joints: 2 points

- 4–10 small joints (with or without large joint involvement): 3 points
- >10 joints (at least one small joint involved): 5 points
- Serologic abnormalities (score range 0–5)
  - Negative RF and negative anti-CCP antibodies: 0 points
  - Low positive RF or low positive anti-CCP antibodies (over three times the normal upper limit): 2 points
  - High positive RF or high positive anti-CCP antibodies (over three times the normal upper limit): 3 points
- Elevated acute-phase response (score range 0–1)
  - Normal CRP and normal ESR: 0 points
  - Abnormal CRP or abnormal ESR: 1 point
- Symptom duration (two levels; range 0–1)
  - <6 weeks: 0 points
  - >6 weeks: 1 point

Aletaha D, Neogi T, Silman AF, et al. 2010 Rheumatoid arthritis classification criteria: an American College of Rheumatology/European League Against Rheumatism Collaborative Initiative. *Arthritis Rheum.* 2010;62:2569–2581.

45. What is the advantage of these new criteria?
To identify patients with new symptoms of inflammatory synovitis who are likely to develop persistent or erosive joint disease.

46. What is the differential diagnosis of RA?
- Connective tissue disease (SLE, SS, Sjögren disease)
- Psoriatic arthritis
- Inflammatory bowel disease
- Polyarticular gout
- Lyme disease–related arthropathy
- Viral-induced arthropathies (i.e., parvovirus B19, hepatitis C)

47. Describe the epidemiology of RA.
RA occurs in up to 1% of the general population worldwide, with lower prevalence in parts of Africa (0.1%) and China (0.3%) and higher prevalence in Pima and Chippawa Indians (5%). Peak incidence is in the fourth and fifth decades of life, but almost any age can be affected.

48. What are the genetic associations in RA?
First-degree relatives of patients with RA have a 1.5-fold increased risk of developing RA compared with the general population. Monozygotic twin studies found a concordance rate for RA of 12–15%. An increased prevalence of RA is present in a subset of populations with the presence of HLA-DR4 (Western European descent) and HLA-DR1 or HLA-DR10 (Spanish, Basque, and Israeli descent). RA susceptibility is associated with the third hypervariable region of DR1β-chains from amino acids 70–74 referred to as the "shared epitope" (QKRAA, QRRAA, or RRRAA) and is associated with both susceptibility and severity of RA.

49. Explain the influence of gender in RA.
Females have a two to three times increased likelihood of developing RA compared with males. Estrogen has been shown to inhibit T suppressor cell function and enhance T helper function, leading to stimulatory effects on the immune system. In addition, nulliparity increases RA risk. The last trimester of pregnancy is associated with decreased RA disease activity. Men with RA tend to have lower testosterone levels than other men and later disease onset than women.

50. What are nongenetic risk factors for RA?
Smoking and infections (bacterial and viral). A 25-pack-year or more history of tobacco use is associated with more severe disease with greater seropositivity, nodules, and radiographic changes. Bacterial infections have been implicated in initiation of RA through activation of Toll-like receptors on mast cells and stimulation of innate immunity. Viruses have also been considered in the etiology of RA. Epstein-Barr virus (EBV), parvovirus B19, and retroviruses have similar amino acid sequences to the shared epitope and may trigger an autoimmune response leading to inflammation.

51. What is the synovium?
A 1- to 2-cell-thick lining of the joint made up of two types of synoviocytes: type A (macrophage-like cells probably derived from bone marrow) and type B (fibroblast-like cells that are probably of mesenchymal origin). The subsynovium constitutes the second layer of normal synovium.

52. **How does RA affect the synovium?**
By inducing intimal lining hyperplasia and subsynovial infiltration with mononuclear cells (especially CD4-negative T cells, macrophages, and B cells). Increased numbers of type A and type B synoviocytes are added to the synovial lining. The lining is the main source of the inflammatory cytokines and proteases thought to lead to the joint destruction in RA. Activated chondrocytes and osteoclasts may also be involved. In addition, other cell types including plasma cells, T and B lymphocytes, and dendritic cells may accumulate in RA synovium. Synovial fluid has elevated PMNs with lesser cell types including lymphocytes, macrophages, natural killer cells, and fibroblasts present.

53. **What is pannus?**
The area of proliferating synovium that can erode the adjacent cartilage and bone. (*Pannus* means cloth in Latin.) Angiogenesis allows the synovium to hypertrophy, leading to enlargement of pannus and an influx of inflammatory cells.

54. **How does pannus contribute to joint destruction in RA?**
By adhering to articular cartilage. The cells within the pannus produce proteinases that can destroy cartilage. The marginal erosions on radiographs are likely due to bone invasion by pannus. Synovial tissue analysis also reveals inflammatory mediators including cytokines, enzymes, adhesion molecules, and transcription factors. Notable examples include interleukin 1 (IL-1), tumor necrosis factor-alpha (TNF-alpha), IL-6, IL-8, IL-17, matrix metalloproteinases, cathepsins, and other proteases. Receptor activator for nuclear factor kappa-B ligand (RANK-L) production leads to osteoclast activation, which may be involved in the bone loss in RA.

55. **Which joints and distribution are most commonly involved in RA?**
Multiple diarthrodial joints (with free motion) in a symmetric distribution. In early disease, the MCP, PIP, wrist, and MTP joints are involved. Larger joints of the upper and lower extremities, such as the elbows, shoulders, ankles, and knees, are also commonly affected, although symptoms may appear later. Less common are cervical spine, temporomandibular, and sternoclavicular joint involvement. Joints that are very uncommon in RA include the DIP joints and thoracic and lumbar spine.

56. **Describe the typical late joint deformities in RA.**
Hands
- Swan neck deformity: typically resulting from inflammation and flexor contraction of the MCP joints, which causes flexion at the MCP and DIP joints with hyperextension of the PIP joints
- Boutonnière deformity: due to flexion contracture at the PIP joint with extension of the DIP joint caused by injury or weakening of the extrinsic extensor tendon
- Ulnar deviation: due to MCP joint subluxation
- "Piano key sign": characterized by softening of the ulnar styloid due to destruction of the ulnar collateral ligament

Feet
- Claw toes or hammer toes, which are due to subluxation of the metatarsal heads and occur late

57. **Describe cervical spine involvement in RA.**
Initial symptoms include pain with motion in the neck and occipital headache. Risk factors for cervical spine disease include high RF seropositivity, later onset RA, active synovitis, and rapid progression of erosive disease. Significant laxity at the atlantoaxial joint with subluxation makes patients prone to slowly progressive spastic quadriparesis. If this laxity is present, the hyperextension of the neck that occurs during intubation for general anesthesia can produce quadriplegia. Therefore, patients with neck pain or longstanding disease should undergo cervical spine evaluation before any surgical procedure.

58. **What are rheumatoid nodules?**
Firm, usually movable nodules ranging in size from a few millimeters to 2 cm found over pressure areas. The classic rheumatoid nodule has a central area of necrosis surrounded by a rim of palisading fibroblasts surrounded by a collagenous capsule with perivascular collections of chronic inflammatory cells. Rheumatoid nodules occur in 20–35% of patients with RA and can be found at the elbow, knuckles, wrist, soles, Achilles tendon, head, bridge of the nose (if pressure area from glasses), and sacrum. RF is usually positive, as are anti-CCP antibodies. Accelerated nodule formation has been described in patients receiving methotrexate treatment for RA, even when methotrexate shows efficacy at calming the arthritis and the patient has had no previous nodule formation. Nodulosis can go away when methotrexate is discontinued.

59. **What are typical laboratory findings in RA?**
    - Anemia of chronic disease (see also Chapter 14, Hematology)
    - Elevated ESR
    - Elevated CRP
    - Positive RF (70–80% sensitivity, >85% specificity)
    - Positive anti-CCP (50–60% sensitivity, 93–97% specificity)

60. **What are typical radiographic findings in RA?**
    In early disease, juxta-articular osteopenia. Later, more diffuse osteopenia and erosions at the margins of small joints may occur. Late findings include joint space narrowing and deformities.

61. **What factors suggest an aggressive disease course in RA?**
    - Acute onset of disease with involvement of multiple joints
    - High titers of RF and anti-CCP antibodies
    - Positive ANA test
    - Presence of rheumatoid nodules
    - Lower socioeconomic status

62. **List some extra-articular manifestations of RA.**
    See Table 10.4.

Table 10.4. Extra-articular Manifestations of Rheumatoid Arthritis

ORGAN SYSTEM	EXTRA-ARTICULAR MANIFESTATION
Constitutional	Fever, fatigue, weight loss
Skin	Rheumatoid nodules
Pulmonary	Pulmonary nodules, pleural thickening, pleural effusions, diffuse interstitial lung disease, BOOP
Ophthalmologic	Keratoconjunctivitis sicca, episcleritis, scleritis
Vascular	Small vessel vasculitis
Neurologic	Cervical spine subluxation causing cervical myelopathy, nerve entrapments
Cardiac	Pericarditis, coronary atherosclerosis
Muscular	Muscle atrophy
Hematologic	Anemia of chronic disease, thrombocytosis, lymphoma

BOOP, bronchiolitis obliterans with organizing pneumonia.

63. **Which patients with RA are at highest risk for extra-articular manifestations?**
    Those with:
    - High titers of RF or anti-CCP antibodies
    - HLA-DR4 positivity
    - Shared epitope (antigenic determinant); individuals with certain genetic sequence found in DR4, DR14, and DR1 beta-chains have higher chance for more severe disease
    - Male gender
    - 10 years or more of disease activity

64. **What is Felty syndrome?**
    The triad of RA, splenomegaly, and leukopenia. Felty syndrome occurs in 1% of RA patients with severe disease who typically have RF positivity, rheumatoid nodules, and other extra-articular manifestations. Leukopenia predominantly affects neutrophils with WBC count < 2000/mm^3. Patients are more susceptible to bacterial infections and have a higher risk of development of non-Hodgkin lymphoma. Around 30–40% of Felty syndrome patients may also develop large granular lymphocyte (LGL) syndrome with CD2, CD3, CD8, CD16, and CD57 markers and increased susceptibility to recurrent infections.

65. **What is Caplan syndrome?**
    The development of lung inflammation and scarring in patients with RA and pneumoconiosis from mining dust exposure. Multiple perihilar lung nodules with pathologic change similar to that of rheumatoid nodules are also found. These patients can develop massive fibrosis and are at increased risk of tuberculosis.

66. **Why is functional capacity so important in patients with RA?**
Because decreased functional status may be one of the best predictors of premature death.

67. **Why is early treatment of RA so important?**
Because the joints can be significantly damaged early in the disease if not treated. The structural damage produces mechanical derangements in the joint leading to deformity and profoundly impaired joint function.

68. **How does pregnancy affect RA?**
Usually with improvement. Signs and symptoms of RA subside in approximately 70% of women during pregnancy. No data suggest that RA has a detrimental effect on the fetus; however, arthritis should be assessed before pregnancy, if possible, because anesthesia and intubation (if needed) can be problematic and even dangerous when cervical spine disease is present. Delivery also can be difficult if arthritis limits hip motion. Postpartum flares of disease occur in approximately 90% of women who experience improvement during pregnancy.

69. **Describe the basic mechanism of action of nonsteroidal anti-inflammatory drugs (NSAIDs).**
Inhibition of production of prostaglandins (and other inflammatory cytokines) through competition with arachidonic acid for cyclooxygenase (COX) binding. There are two main subtypes of COX. COX-1 is often described as a "housekeeping" enzyme and has been associated with regulating normal cellular processes such as gastric cellular protection, platelet aggregation, and kidney function. COX-2 is expressed in the brain, kidney, bone, and possibly, the cardiovascular system. COX-2 seems to be involved more specifically in the synthesis of inflammatory mediators than COX-1. Without COX, there are fewer circulating prostaglandins and therefore less inflammation and pain.

70. **What is the advantage of selective COX-2 inhibition over nonselective COX inhibition?**
Decreased risk of gastrointestinal (GI) injury. COX-1 is known to be involved in gastric cellular protection, so selective inhibition of COX-2 would theoretically lead to less gastric and duodenal injury. Clinical studies do show this, but toxicity still may occur with COX-2 inhibition. Although improved GI tolerance has been shown, there has been no significant improvement in efficacy with selective COX-2 inhibition. Patients at risk of peptic ulcer disease (PUD) who use NSAIDs chronically should be evaluated for proton pump inhibitor (PPI) prophylaxis. (See Chapter 2, General Medicine and Ambulatory Care.)

71. **What are side effects of NSAIDs?**
- **Renal:** hypertension, acute renal failure, and papillary necrosis
- **Gastointestinal:** dyspepsia, peptic ulcer disease, gastric and duodenal mucosal damage
- **Hepatic:** elevated transaminases and rarely acute hepatic injury
- **Nervous system:** dizziness, headache, and cognitive dysfunction
- **Cardiovascular:** increased risk for myocardial infarction
Also see Chapter 2, General Medicine and Ambulatory Care.

72. **Describe two proposed mechanisms of cardiovascular risks associated with COX-2 inhibitors.**
One theory relates to the balance of COX-1 and COX-2. The inhibition of COX-2 leads to decreased prostacyclin, less vasodilation, and inhibition of platelet aggregation. If COX-1 is not opposed, there is continued thromboxane A_2 production, which would predispose to more atherogenesis and plaque formation. Another theory proposes that less COX-2 leads to decreased prostaglandins, which leads to decreased renal flow, lower glomerular filtration rate, increased aldosterone production, and eventual hypertension leading to cardiovascular events. Nonselective NSAIDs of COX-1 and COX-2 still increase cardiovascular risk by an unknown mechanism, but it may be due to differing COX-2 selectivity.
   Pirlamarla P, Bond R. FDA labeling of NSAIDs: review of nonsteroidal anti-inflammatory drugs in cardiovascular disease. *Trends Cardiovasc Med.* 2016:26(8):675–680. Epub April 29, 2016. Available at: https://doi.org/10.1016/j.tcm.2016.04.011.

73. **How do the effects of aspirin on platelets differ from those of other NSAIDs?**
Acetylated salicylates (such as aspirin) irreversibly destroy the COX enzyme that leads to decreased platelet aggregation. Other NSAIDs (including nonacetylated salicylates) allow the return of normal enzyme function once the drug level has decreased. Because COX-2 does not regulate platelet aggregation, newer COX-2 NSAIDs have little effect on platelet function.

74. **What is the role of glucocorticoids (GCs) in the management of RA?**
    Mainly for managing disease flares and bridging more targeted therapy. GCs reduce synthesis of enzymes involved in the production of prostaglandins and proinflammatory cytokins such as IL-1, IL-6, and TNF-alpha. Because of more specific, safer agents, GCs are currently used less often in the long-term management of RA. The relatively quick onset of action (hours to days) makes GCs a good agent for treating disease flare-ups. Low-dose GCs are also used as bridging therapy concurrently with disease-modifying antirheumatic drug (DMARD) therapy.

75. **What are common adverse side effects from long-term use of GCs?**
    - Osteoporosis (secondary)
    - Hyperglycemia
    - Increased incidence of cardiovascular disease
    - Cushing syndrome
    - Increased risk of cataracts
    - Increased risk of infection

76. **What mechanisms contribute to bone loss with the use of GCs?**
    Inhibition of osteoblast proliferation and stimulation of osteoblast and osteocyte apoptosis (physiologic cell death). Increased bone resorption also occurs by increasing osteoclast proliferation via stimulating production of receptor activator of nuclear factor kappa-B (RANK) leading to osteoclastogenesis. Corticosteroids have also been shown to decrease intestinal absorption of calcium and increase urinary calcium excretion, stimulating parathyroid hormone (PTH) production. The severity of bone loss parallels the dose and duration of treatment. Patients at doses of >7.5 mg/day will generally have some bone loss, usually in trabecular bone.
    Khosla S. Minireview: the OPG/RANKL/RANK system. *Endocrinology*. 2001;2:5050–5055.
    Sambrook PN, Jones G. Corticosteroid osteoporosis. *Br J Rheum*. 1995;34:8–12.

77. **What are DMARDs, and how are they used in the treatment of RA?**
    DMARDs are thought to alter the natural history of RA, lessening the likelihood of joint destruction and deformity. Conventional DMARDs are typically oral and have been used clinically for many years. Biologic DMARDs are structurally engineered versions of already natural molecules such as monoclonal antibodies and have more specific targets in the inflammatory cascade of disease.

78. **Name the most commonly used conventional DMARDs, list each mechanism of action, and name associated side effects.**
    See Table 10.5.

Table 10.5. Mechanism of Action and Side Effects of Nonbiologic Disease-Modifying Antirheumatic Drugs

NONBIOLOGIC DMARDS	MECHANISM OF ACTION	COMMON SIDE EFFECTS
Methotrexate	Inhibits dihydrofolate reductase, which leads to anti-inflammatory effects and downregulation of cytokines, although the exact mechanism is still unclear	Nausea, stomatitis, alopecia, fatigue, elevated liver transaminases, bone marrow suppression, pneumonitis
Sulfasalazine	Suppresses lymphocyte and leukocyte functions	Nausea, rash, leukopenia
Hydroxychloro-quine	Accumulation in lysosomes raises the intravesical pH and interferes with antigenic peptides	Nausea, rash, hyperpigmentation, retinopathy
Leflunomide	Inhibits pyrimidine synthesis, which inhibits T-cell function	Nausea, stomatitis, alopecia, fatigue, elevated liver transaminases, bone marrow suppression

DMARDs, disease-modifying antirheumatic drugs.

79. Name other less common conventional DMARDs.

Minocycline has shown efficacy in small clinical trials. Gold compounds were used more frequently in the past but much less frequently now because of high levels of toxicity. Cyclosporine, tacrolimus, and azathioprine have been shown to have efficacy as well.

80. Name current biologic DMARD therapies in RA, describe the mechanisms of action, and list common side effects.

See Table 10.6.

Table 10.6. Mechanism of Action and Side Effects of Biologic Disease-Modifying Antirheumatic Drugs

BIOLOGIC DMARDS	CLASS	MECHANISM OF ACTION AND ROUTE OF ADMINISTRATION	COMMON SIDE EFFECTS
Infliximab	TNF-α inhibitor	Chimeric monoclonal antibody that binds to both soluble and membrane-bound TNF-α; intravenous administration	Infection (including reactivation of TB and fungal infection), infusion reaction, lymphoma, demyelinating disorder, drug-induced lupus
Entanercept	TNF-α inhibitor	Soluble receptor fusion protein that binds to soluble TNF-α; subcutaneous administration	Infection (including reactivation of latent TB and fungal infection), injection site reaction, lymphoma, demyelinating disorder, drug-induced lupus
Adalimumab	TNF-α inhibitor	Fully humanized monoclonal antibody that binds to both soluble and membrane-bound TNF-α; subcutaneous administration	Infection (including reactivation of latent TB and fungal infection), injection site reaction, lymphoma, demyelinating disorder, drug-induced lupus
Golimumab	TNF-α inhibitor	Fully humanized monoclonal antibody that binds to both soluble and membrane-bound TNF-α; subcutaneous administration	Infection (including reactivation of latent TB and fungal infection), injection site reaction, lymphoma, demyelinating disorder, drug-induced lupus
Certolizumab pegol	TNF-α inhibitor	Pegylated humanized antibody Fab fragment chemically linked to polyethylene glycol and binds to soluble and membrane-bound TNF-α and does not contain an Fc portion unlike the other monoclonal antibodies to TNF-α; subcutanous administration	Infection (including reactivation of latent TB and fungal infection), injection site reaction, lymphoma, demyelinating disorder, drug-induced lupus, pancytopenia
Abatacept (CTLA-4Ig)	T-cell inhibitor	Recombinant fusion protein that binds to CD80/CD86 on the surface of APC and prevents binding onto CD28 on T cells (blocks T-cell second signals); intravenous administration	Infection, infusion reaction, malignancy, COPD exacerbations
Rituximab	B-cell inhibitor	Chimeric anti-CD20 monoclonal antibody that involves inhibition of T-cell activation through reduction of antigen presentation by B cells; intravenous administration	Infection, infusion reactions, headache, fever
Tocilizumab	IL-6 inhibitor	Humanized IL-6 receptor antibody; IL-6 has proinflammatory effects and activates T cells, B cells, and macrophages	Infection, infusion reaction, elevated hepatic function tests, elevated total cholesterol, neutropenia

APC, antigen-presenting cell; COPD, chronic obstructive pulmonary disease; DMARDs, disease-modifying antirheumatic drugs; IL, interleukin; TB, tuberculosis; TNF, tumor necrosis factor.

81. Describe the jakinibs (janus kinase inhibitors).

A novel class of oral DMARD therapies that inhibit janus kinase (JAK) and are a group of tyrosine kinases. JAK1, JAK2, JAK3, and tyrosine kinase (TYK2) are intracellular proteins that activate transcription factors known as signal transducers and activators of transcription (STATs). This activation results in phosphorylation and dimerization and translocation to the nucleus, where it directly modulates gene transcription. The jakinibs uncouple cytokine receptor signaling from downstream STAT transcription activation, which modulates immune responses in immune-mediated diseases. Tofacitinib is an inhibitor of JAK1 and JAK3. Baricitinib, currently in phase III development, inhibits JAK1 and JAK2. Safety has been similar to that for biologic DMARDs with the potential for increased infections (notably herpes zoster), neutropenia, anemia, hyperlipidemia, elevated liver function, and elevated creatine levels.

Schwartz DM, Bonelli M, Gadina M, et al. Type I/II cytokines, JAKs, and new strategies for treating autoimmune diseases. *Nat Rev Rheumatol*. 2016;12: 25–36.

82. What is a biosimilar?

A biologic medicine that is highly similar, but not identical, to another biologic medicine (known as a *reference product*) that is already approved for use. Biosimilars are not supposed to have clinically meaningful differences in efficacy or safety from the reference product. Minor differences in clinically inactive components are allowable in biosimilar products. The Food and Drug Administration (FDA) approved an infliximab biosimilar, CT-P13, in early 2016 for all infliximab indications except pediatric ulcerative colitis based on one trial for moderate to severe RA and one trial of AS. Many biosimilars are in current development, but there are still many outstanding issues that need to be explored such as the viability of extrapolating indications, antidrug antibody development, and long-term safety.

Dörner T, Kay J. Biosimilars in rheumatology: current perspectives and lessons learnt. *Nat Rev Rheumatol*. 2015;11:713–724.

KEY POINTS: TREATMENT OF INFLAMMATORY ARTHRITIS

1. COX-2 selective inhibits have fewer GI toxicities than traditional NSAIDs but are no more efficacious and may have a higher cardiovascular risk.
2. Patients taking chronic NSAIDs who are at risk of PUD may benefit from prophylactic treatment with PPIs to prevent PUD.
3. Disease-modifying medications including the biologic agents have improved clinical outcomes in rheumatoid arthritis.
4. Although glucocorticoid treatments are common in managing several rheumatic diseases, there are many untoward side effects including osteoporosis, increased risk of cardiovascular disease, elevated glucose levels, and increased risk of infection.

COX-2, cyclooxygenase-2; GI, gastrointestinal; NSAIDs, nonsteroidal anti-inflammatory drugs; PPIs, proton pump inhibitors; PUD, peptic ulcer disease.

SYSTEMIC LUPUS ERYTHEMATOSUS AND RELATED DISEASES

83. What is SLE?

An autoimmune inflammatory disease that can affect many organ systems with protean manifestations. The pathogenesis of lupus is largely unknown, but immunologic abnormalities can give rise to excessive autoantibody production that can cause tissue damage.

84. What are the classification criteria for SLE?

Two classification criteria for SLE are commonly used. The 1997 American College of Rheumatology (ACR) SLE criteria are frequently used in which patients are classified with lupus if they meet 4 out of 11 criteria. However, these criteria have undergone many criticisms. For example, they were never validated and did not include other clinical features of lupus that are commonly seen. In 2012, the Systemic Lupus International Collaboration Clinics (SLICC) developed new criteria, validating these and the ACR Criteria. Notably in the new criteria, patients can be classified as having lupus if they meet 4 out of 17 criteria with at least 1 clinical criterion and 1 immunologic criterion OR biopsy-proven lupus nephritis and positive ANA or anti-dsDNA antibody. In addition, the SLICC criteria removed photosensitivity as a criterion and acknowledged other cutaneous lupus lesions (tumid lupus, toxic epidermal necrolysis, bullous lupus, chilblain lupus), other neurologic manifestations (myelitis, mononeuritis multiplex, neuropathy), other antiphospholipid antibodies (beta-glycoprotein-1 antibodies), low complements (CH50, C3, C4), and the direct Coombs test. See Table 10.7.

Table 10.7. American College of Rheumatology Criteria for Classification of Systemic Lupus Erythematosus*

FINDING	DESCRIPTION
Malar rash	Fixed erythema, flat or raised, over the malar eminences, sparing the nasolabial folds
Discoid rash	Erythematous raised patches with adherent keratotic scaling and follicular plugging: atrophic scarring may occur in older lesions
Photosensitivity	Skin rash as a result of unusual reaction to sunlight, by patient history or physician observation
Oral ulcers	Oral or nasopharyngeal ulceration, usually painless, observed by physician
Nonerosive arthritis	Involving two or more peripheral joints, characterized by tenderness, swelling, or effusion
Pleuritis or pericarditis	a. Pleuritis: convincing history of pleuritic pain or rub heard by physician or evidence of pleural effusion or b. Pericarditis: documented by electrocardiogram or rub or evidence of pericardial effusion
Renal disorder	a. Persistent proteinuria > 0.5 g/day or > 3+ protein if quantitative analysis not performed or b. Cellular casts: may be red blood cell, hemoglobin, granular, tubular, or mixed
Seizures or psychosis	a. Seizures: in the absence of offending drugs or known metabolic derangement (e.g., uremia, ketoacidosis, electrolyte imbalance) b. Psychosis: in the absence of offending drugs or known metabolic derangement (e.g., uremia, ketoacidosis, electrolyte imbalance)
Hematologic disorder	a. Hemolytic anemia with reticulocytosis or b. Leukopenia: <4000/mm^3 on two occasions or c. Lymphopenia: <1500/mm^3 on two occasions or d. Thrombocytopenia: <100,000/mm^3 in the absence of offending drugs
Immunologic disorder	a. Anti-DNA: antibody to native DNA in abnormal titer or b. Anti-Sm: presence of antibody to Sm nuclear antigen or c. Positive findings of antiphospholipid antibodies based on: 1. An abnormal serum concentration of IgG or IgM anticardiolipin antibodies 2. A positive test for lupus anticoagulant using standard method or 3. A false-positive test for at least 6 mo and confirmed by *Treponema pallidum* immobilization fluorescent treponemal antibody absorption test
Positive ANA	An abnormal titer of ANA by immunofluorescence or an equivalent assay at any point in time in the absence of drug

*Four of these criteria must be present in order for the patient to enroll in an SLE research study.
ANA, antinuclear antibody; Ig, immunoglobulin; SLE, systemic lupus erythematosus.
Adapted from Hochberg MC. Updating the American College of Rheumatology revised criteria for the classification of systemic lupus erythematosus [letter]. *Arthritis Rheum.* 1997;40:1725.

85. **How are these criteria used for the diagnosis of SLE in an individual patient?**
    The ACR and SLICC classification criteria were proposed to identify SLE patients for enrollment into clinical trial, providing a uniform base for which studies can be conducted in lupus patients. They are intended to reflect the major clinical features of the disease (e.g., dermatologic, renal, neurologic, articular, hematologic, and immunologic findings). Although these criteria may be helpful in aiding the diagnosis of lupus, patients who do not fulfill the classification criteria may still have the disease. The diagnosis of SLE in clinical practice is based upon autoantibody analysis, symptoms, laboratory tests of involved organ systems, and physical examination findings.

    Petri M, Magder L. Classification criteria for systemic lupus erythematosus: a review. *Lupus*. 2004;1311:829–337.

    Petri M, Orbai AM, Alarcón GS. Derivation and validation of the Systemic Lupus International Collaborating Clinics classification criteria for systemic lupus erythematosus. *Arthritis Rheum*. 2012;648:2677–2868.

86. **What are common laboratory and clinical findings in SLE?**
    See Table 10.8.

Table 10.8. Frequencies of Various Manifestations of Systemic Lupus Erythematosus by Disease Stage

MANIFESTATION	EARLY DISEASE (%)	LATE DISEASE (%)
Arthritis	46–53	83–95
Rash	9–11	81–88
Fever	3–5	77
Mucosal ulcers	—	7–23
Alopecia	—	37–45
Serositis	5	63
Pulmonary inflammation	—	9
Liver function test abnormalities	1	—
Vasculitis	—	21–27
Myositis	—	5
Osteoporosis	—	High
Osteonecrosis	—	7–24
Leukopenia	41–66	41–66
Thrombocytopenia	2	19–45
Anemia	2	57–73
CNS abnormalities	3	55–59
Nephritis	6	31–53
Renal failure	<1	20

CNS, central nervous system.
From Lahita RG: The clinical presentation of systemic lupus erythematosus in adults. In: Lahita RG (ed): *Systemic Lupus Erythematosus*, 4th ed. San Diego: Academic Press; 2004, p 435.

87. **When is the peak incidence of SLE?**
    15–44 years of age, which is believed to be related to the hormonal changes that occur during puberty and the childbearing years. The incidence of SLE in prepubertal females is similar to that of postmenopausal females.

    Masi AT, Kaslow RA. Sex effects in systemic lupus erythematosus: a clue to pathogenesis. *Arthritis Rheum*. 1978;21:480–484.

88. **How can cutaneous lupus be categorized?**
    - Acute cutaneous lupus erythematosus (ACLE)
    - Subacute cutaneous lupus erythematosus (SCLE)
    - Chronic cutaneous lupus erythematosus (CCLE)

89. **Compare and contrast the typical rashes of ACLE with SCLE.**
    The prototypical lesion of ACLE is the malar or butterfly rash, which is an erythematous rash that can be flat or raised, spanning the bridge of the nose and extending over the malar eminences. Ultraviolet (UV) light may exacerbate the lesion; hence, the nasolabial folds are often spared because these regions receive fewer UV rays. The rash of SCLE is also photosensitive and is often located in the upper chest, shoulders, and neck. SCLE may start as erythematous, scaly papules or plaques, often progressing into larger papulosquamous or annular polycyclic lesions that can then coalesce to produce large confluent areas with central hypopigmentation. Neither ACLE nor SCLE results in dermal scarring.

90. **What are some examples of CCLE?**
    - Lupus tumidus
    - Lupus profundus
    - Chilblain lupus
    - Discoid lupus erythematosus (DLE)

91. **Describe DLE, and explain the relationship between SLE and DLE.**
    Discrete erythematous plaques covered by scales that extend into hair follicles, causing follicular plugging. The plaques can occur over the face, scalp, pinnae and conchae bowl of the ear, neck, and areas that may not be exposed to the UV rays. DLE can exist in patients with SLE or in isolation. About 10% of patients with discoid lesions will have SLE.
    Walling HW, Sontheimer RD. Cutaneous lupus erythematosus: issues in diagnosis and treatment. *Am J Clin Dermatol.* 2009;10:365–381.

92. **What are other cutaneous manifestations of lupus?**
    - Raynaud phenomenon
    - Periungual telangiectasia
    - Bullae
    - Livedo reticularis
    - Petechiae
    - Vasculitis
    - Alopecia

93. **List the differential diagnoses of a lupus patient who presents with musculoskeletal complaints.**
    - Synovitis
    - Fibromyalgia
    - Myositis
    - Osteonecrosis
    - Fractures
    - Myopathy
    - Septic arthritis
    - Adrenal insufficiency

    Some of these disorders are related to the disease itself, whereas others may be related to medication side effects or existing comorbid conditions.

94. **What is the prevalence of lupus nephritis, and how is nephritis categorized?**
    About 50%. The International Society of Nephrology/Renal Pathology Society (ISN/RPS) in 2003 revised the World Health Organization (WHO) classification of lupus nephritis by adding chronicity and activity scores. Classification is based on biopsy:
    - **Class I:** minimal mesangial lupus nephritis
    - **Class II:** mesangial proliferative lupus nephritis
    - **Class III:** focal lupus nephritis, subcategorized as proliferative with activity (class III [A]), proliferative and sclerosis with activity and chronicity (class III [A/C]), or sclerosing with chronicity (class III [C])
    - **Class IV:** diffuse lupus nephritis, subcategorized as segmental and active (class IV-S [A]), global proliferative and active (class IV-G [A]), segmental with activity and chronicity (class IV-S [A/C]), global proliferative with activity and chronicity (class IV-G [A/C]), segmental with chronicity (class IV-S [C]), or global proliferative with chronicity (class IV-G [C])

- **Class V:** membranous lupus nephritis
- **Class VI:** advanced sclerosis lupus nephritis
  Weening JJ, D'Agati VD, Schwartz MM, et al. The classification of glomerulonephritis in systemic lupus erythematosus revisited. *J Am Soc Nephrol.* 2004;15:241–250.

95. What happens to lupus activity in patients with renal failure?
    Often, lupus becomes quiescent with the onset of uremia and dialysis. Several studies note the ability to discontinue GCs without a return of extrarenal manifestations once dialysis has been initiated. Although there are reports of subsequent disease exacerbations, disease activity usually does not recur in transplanted kidneys.

96. How commonly does SLE affect the GI tract?
    Frequently. GI manifestations may be present in up to 50% of patients with SLE. Anorexia, nausea, and vomiting are among the most common symptoms. Oral ulcerations (most commonly painless buccal erosions) were identified in 40% of one group of patients. Esophageal involvement such as esophagitis, esophageal ulceration, or esophageal dysmotility seems to correlate with the presence of Raynaud phenomenon. Intestinal involvement results in abdominal pain, diarrhea, and occasionally hemorrhage. Intestinal ischemia may be present and may progress to infarction and perforation. Pneumatosis intestinalis in SLE is usually benign and transient but may represent an irreversible necrotizing enterocolitis. In addition, pancreatitis and abdominal serositis are well recognized. Abnormal liver function tests also occur. A vasculitic process has been implicated in the pathogenesis of GI manifestations.

97. What is the most common pathologic abnormality in patients with lupus central nervous system (CNS) disease?
    Small infarcts and hemorrhages. Vasculitis is suggested by such commonly used designations as "lupus cerebritis" and occurs in <15% of patients.
    Johnson RT, Richardson EP. The neurological manifestations of systemic lupus erythematosus. *Medicine.* 1968;47:337–369.

98. What are the neuropsychiatric manifestations of SLE?
    - Psychosis
    - Cranial, autonomic, and peripheral neuropathies
    - Migraine headaches
    - Seizure
    - Aseptic meningitis
    - Pseudotumor cerebri
    - Chorea
    - Cerebral infarction
    - Transverse myelitis (rare)
    - Posterior reversible encephalopathy syndrome (PRES)
    - Organic brain syndrome (delirium, mild memory loss, and impaired concentration)
      Because of the difficulty in establishing an unequivocal diagnosis, rates of CNS features in SLE cross a broad range. Neuropsychiatric manifestations of lupus may occur in approximately 70% of patients. The more subtle features of cognitive dysfunction may be the most common CNS finding. Abnormal single-photon emission computed tomography (SPECT) or positron emission tomography (PET) scanning and decreased intellectual function, as measured by a standard battery of neurocognitive function tests, are present. The cause for this problem is not known, but cytokines are believed to play an important role.

99. What is PRES?
    Posterior reversible encephalopathy syndrome, which is a rare neurologic manifestation in patients with SLE. PRES is often associated with acute hypertension and renal failure. Diagnosis is based on presenting symptoms of headaches, seizures, altered mental status, cortical blindness, focal neurologic deficits, and typical MRI findings of posterior cerebral edema.
    Leroux G, Sellam J, Costedoat-Chalumeau N, et al. Posterior reversible encephalopathy syndrome during systemic lupus erythematosus: four new cases and review of the literature. *Lupus.* 2008;17:139–147.

100. Describe the pulmonary manifestations of lupus.
     Pleurisy or pleural effusion is most common. Up to 60% of patients may have pleuritic pain over the course of their illness. Effusions can be either transudative or exudative, and in rare cases, effusions are the presenting feature. The so-called shrinking lung syndrome describes dyspnea associated with

diaphragmatic dysfunction, probably secondary to chronic pleural scarring. Pulmonary parenchymal involvement or lupus pneumonitis has been described, as have pulmonary hemorrhage, pulmonary emboli, and pulmonary hypertension. Emboli and hypertension are more common when antiphospholipid antibodies (APA) are also present.

101. **Which drugs are commonly associated with the development of a clinical syndrome of lupus and a positive ANA?**
   - Hydralazine
   - Procainamide
   - Quinidine
   - Diphenylhydantoin
   - Methyldopa
   - Minocycline
   - Isoniazid
   - Sulfasalazine
   - D-Penicillamine
   - Chlorpromazine
   - TNF-alpha inhibitors
   - Diltiazem

   So-called slow acetylators more commonly develop clinical symptoms, which typically include fever, rash, and arthritis. The clinical features usually regress fairly promptly, although the laboratory abnormality may persist (sometimes indefinitely) when the drug is discontinued. The clinical features commonly present in drug-induced lupus rarely, if ever, include CNS disease or nephritis. There are numerous published reports of many other drugs inducing lupus symptoms on a small number of patients.

102. **Which autoantibody is often touted to be diagnostic for drug-induced lupus?**
   Antihistone antibody. Although the antihistone antibody is present in as many as 90% of the cases of drug-induced lupus, it is also present in nearly 75% of patients with SLE; hence, it is not diagnostic for drug-induced lupus.

103. **Summarize the mortality rate associated with SLE.**
   Death rates from SLE declined significantly over the last half of the 20th century. The 5-year survival rate in the 1950s was only 50%, whereas it is now >90%. Survival in those with late-onset disease seems to be reduced compared with survival among those patients afflicted at an earlier age.

104. **List some factors that may contribute to the morbidity or mortality of patients with SLE.**
   - Nonadherence to medical advice and treatment
   - Presence of active disease
   - Medication toxicity
   - Infection
   - Cardiovascular events

   Death early in the course of disease is usually related to the disease itself. Nephritis and CNS disease are the most ominous prognostic factors. Of the causes of death not directly related to active disease, infection is most common, followed by myocardial infarction, stroke, and other atherosclerotic complications. Studies have shown the presence of accelerated atherosclerosis in SLE.

   Asanuma Y, Oeser A, Shintani AK, et al. Premature coronary-artery atherosclerosis in systemic lupus erythematosus. *N Engl J Med.* 2003;349:2407–2415.

   Roman MJ, Shanker BA, Davis A, et al. Prevalence and correlates of accelerated atherosclerosis in systemic lupus erythematosus. *N Engl J Med.* 2003;349:2399–2340.

105. **Discuss the interaction of pregnancy and SLE.**
   Recent studies documented that pregnancy rates in women with SLE are lower than in the general population. Impaired fertility may be related to (1) impaired hypothalamic pituitary ovarian function related to chronic inflammation, (2) reduced ovarian reserve and autoimmune oophoritis, and (3) prior exposure to gonadotoxic medications (cyclophosphamide). In addition, lupus pregnancies were twice as likely to end in fetal death.

   Dhar JP, Essenmacher LM, Ager JW, et al. Pregnancy outcomes before and after a diagnosis of systemic lupus erythematosus. *Am J Obstet Gynecol.* 2005;193:1444–1445.

Lawrenz B, Henes J, Henes M, et al. Impact of systemic lupus erythematosus on ovarian reserve in premenopausal women: evaluation by using anti-Müllerian hormone. *Lupus.* 2011;20:1193–1197.

Molokhhia M , Maconochie N, Patrick AL, et al. Cross-sectional analysis of adverse outcomes in 1,029 pregnancies of Afro-Caribbean women in Trinidad with and without systemic lupus erythematosus. *Arthritis Res Ther.* 2007;9:R124– R136.

106. **How does neonatal lupus occur?**
Through transplacental passage of maternal anti-SSA/Ro antibodies to the fetus. These antibodies have been linked to direct tissue injury. Babies born with neonatal lupus can exhibit cutaneous lesions as SCLE, hematologic aberrations, hepatic abnormalities, or congenital heart block (CHB), which potentially can be fatal.

107. **What is the incidence of CHB in neonatal lupus?**
1–2%, typically identified between 16 and 24 weeks of gestation. The risk for recurrence is 10 times higher in subsequent pregnancies.

Buyon JP, Hiebert R, Copel J, et al. Autoimmune-associated congenital heart block: demographics, mortality, morbidity and recurrence rates obtained from a national neonatal lupus registry. *J Am Coll Cardiol.* 1998;31:1658–1666.

108. **What drugs are approved by the FDA for the treatment of SLE?**
- Low-dose aspirin
- GCs
- Hydroxychloroquine
- Belimumab

109. **What is undifferentiated connective tissue disease (UCTD)?**
A syndrome with clinical and laboratory features that are suggestive of an autoimmune cause, but the diagnosis is unable to be confirmed. An exact diagnosis of a rheumatic disease is not always possible at initial presentation. The clinical manifestations of a given rheumatic disease may not develop all at once but may unfold over time, and many features are shared among different rheumatic diseases. Myositis, for example, can be found as a primary condition (polymyositis) or as part of other systemic diseases (dermatomyositis, SSc, and SLE). In addition to shared clinical features, rheumatic diseases may have shared serologic features. The most obvious example is ANA, which may be found in various diseases, including SLE, SSc, SS, inflammatory myopathies, Hashimoto thyroiditis, and IBD. When clinical and laboratory features suggest an autoimmune cause but clinical and serologic heterogeneity make the diagnosis uncertain, the designation UCTD may be used.

110. **How is UCTD different from mixed connective tissue disease (MCTD)?**
MCTD is defined by specific characteristics and was first described as a separate entity in 1972. MCTD is used specifically when features of SLE and SSc are present with high titers of antibody to U_1RNP (ribonucleoprotein).

111. **Describe the antiphospholipid antibody (APA) syndrome.**
A symptom complex that occurs in approximately 40% of SLE patients and includes one or more of the following: multiple miscarriages, arterial or venous thrombosis, and thrombocytopenia in association with a laboratory finding of APAs. These antibodies can be specific (such as anticardiolipin antibodies), or they may be identified by their effect on the clotting cascade (lupus anticoagulant). Common laboratory tests indicating the presence of antibodies to various phospholipids include prolonged partial thromboplastin time, false-positive Venereal Disease Research Laboratory (VDRL) test for syphilis, or positive anticardiolipin antibodies. A less common example is the dilute Russell viper venom clotting time. APA syndrome may occur by itself (primary APA syndrome) or in association with an underlying connective tissue syndrome, primarily lupus (secondary APA syndrome).

112. **What is Hughes syndrome?**
Antiphospholipid syndrome. Graham R. V. Hughes, a rheumatologist, originally described antiphospholipid syndrome in 1983.

113. **Describe catastrophic APA syndrome.**
Sudden overwhelming vascular occlusion mediated by APAs. Clinical features result from widespread thrombosis of small vessels and the systemic inflammatory response, which may include ischemic bowel, pulmonary emboli, acute respiratory distress syndrome (ARDS), infarctive skin lesions,

encephalopathy with altered consciousness, seizure, myocardial infarction, and cardiac valvular lesions. Renal involvement is present in the majority of cases.

114. What factors increase the risk of catastrophic APA syndrome?
- Presence of other diseases, such as SLE or BD, even if treated
- Infections
- Vaccination
- Flare of underlying disease
- Withdrawal of anticoagulation
The mortality rate is >50% even with prompt intervention.

115. How is catastrophic APA syndrome treated?
- Anticoagulation
- GCs
- Treatment of underlying conditions such as infection
- IV immunoglobulin
- Plasma exchange
- Cytotoxic agents

Petri M. Management of thrombosis in antiphospholipid antibody syndrome. *Rheum Dis Clin North Am.* 2001;27:633–641.

SJÖGREN SYNDROME

116. What is Sjögren syndrome (SS)?
An exocrinopathy manifested by sicca (dryness) symptoms. The lacrimal and salivary glands are primarily affected, but the urogenital and GI systems may be involved as well.

117. What are the revised ACR criteria for SS?
In 2012, the American College of Rheumatology published new criteria for SS that stated the terms *primary Sjögren syndrome* and *secondary Sjögren syndrome* are now obsolete. The diagnosis of SS should be given to all who fulfill two of the three following criteria:
- Positive serum anti-SSA and/or anti-SSB or (positive rheumatoid factor and ANA ≥ 1:320)
- Ocular staining score (OSS) ≥ 3
- Presence of focal lymphocytic sialadenitis (FLS) with focus score ≥ 1 focus/4 mm^2 in labial salivary gland biopsies
Interestingly, symptoms of dry eyes and mouth are not requirements with the new criteria. About 15% of patients who have SS do not have sicca symptoms. In addition, dry eyes/mouth symptoms did not show statistically significant association with the presence of FLS, serum anti-SSA/B, or an OSS ≥ 3.

Shiboski SC, Shiboski CH, Criswell L, et al. American College of Rheumatology classification criteria for Sjögren's syndrome: a data-driven, expert consensus approach in the Sjögren's International Collaborative Clinical Alliance cohort. *Arthritis Care Res.* 2012,64: 475–487.

118. How do you treat SS?
Primarily with symptom relief using ductal plugs, preservative-free artificial tears, cyclosporine ophthalmic drops, and cholinergic agonists or other secretagogues. Autologous serum ophthalmic drops have been proved useful in refractory cases of keratoconjunctivitis sicca. There is limited evidence to support the use of immunomodulatory agents in treating primary SS, but anecdotal published reports have reported that hydroxychloroquine may help with the musculoskeletal and dermatologic manifestations. Regular dental and ophthalmologic evaluations are extremely important to detect and treat damages from the sicca syndrome.

SYSTEMIC SCLEROSIS

119. What is scleroderma?
A connective tissue disease characterized by abnormal collagen deposition into the skin and other organs. The term *scleroderma* is derived from two Greek words: *skleros,* meaning hard, and *derma,* meaning skin. Disease pathogenesis is believed to occur as a consequence of aberrant immune activation causing endothelial damage, followed by fibroblast activation that results in obliterative vasculopathy and fibrosis. Of note, the disease is heralded by a vasculopathy, *not* vasculitis. The term *scleroderma* is being phased out and replaced by the term *systemic sclerosis (SSc)* with subcategories of localized sclerosis (morphea, linear scleroderma) and systemic sclerosis (diffuse SSc or limited SSc).

120. Describe CREST syndrome.

Calcinosis, **R**aynaud phenomenon, **e**sophageal dysmotility, **s**clerodactyly, and **t**elangiectasias. CREST is often found in patients with limited SSc but can be present in diffuse SSc.

121. Compare and contrast diffuse SSc and limited SSc.

Patients with diffuse SSc have truncal skin involvement, higher mortality rates, and greater risks of developing pulmonary fibrosis, tendon friction rubs, and scleroderma renal crisis than those with limited SSc. Anti-Scl-70 antibodies are more often found in diffuse SSc. Patients with limited SSc have a higher incidence of pulmonary hypertension and anticentromere antibodies.

122. Summarize the genetic component of SSc.

Family members of SSc patients have a significantly greater risk of developing scleroderma than someone with no family history. One likely culprit is an abnormality in the fibrillin gene. This has been elegantly shown in a population study of Choctaw indians, in whom a genetic defect has been traced to a single common ancestor.

Tan FK, Arnett FC. Genetic factors in the etiology of systemic sclerosis and Raynaud's phenomenon. *Curr Opin Rheumatol.* 2000;12:511–519.

123. List the noncutaneous features of SSc.
- Arthralgia
- Inflammatory muscle disease
- GI dysmotility with malabsorption
- Pulmonary interstitial fibrosis with or without pulmonary hypertension
- Scleroderma renal crisis

124. Do specific autoantibodies help predict the form of SSc a patient may develop?

Yes. Although >80% of patients with SSC have a positive ANA test, this test adds little specificity. Antitopoisomerase 1 (anti-Scl-70) has a positive predictive value of 70% for developing scleroderma. Centromere antibodies have a positive predictive value of 88% for the development of CREST.

Spencer-Green G. Tests performed in systemic sclerosis: anticentromere antibody and anti Scl-70 antibody. *Am J Med.* 1997;103:242–248.

125. What is scleroderma renal crisis?

A life-threatening aspect of diffuse SSc manifested by sudden onset of malignant hypertension, hemolytic anemia, hyperreninemia, and renal failure. Angiotensin-converting enzyme inhibition therapy has been shown to improve clinical outcomes.

126. What are the risk factors for scleroderma renal crisis?
- Diffuse skin involvement
- Rapid progression of skin thickening
- Disease duration < 4 years
- Anti-RNA-polymerase III antibodies
- New-onset anemia
- New-onset cardiac involvement
- High-dose corticosteroid therapy
- Pregnancy

Steen VD, Medsger Jr TA, Osial Jr TA, et al. Factors predicting development of renal involvement in progressive systemic sclerosis. *Am J Med.* 1984;1976:779–786.

127. What part of the GI tract can SSc affect?

Anywhere from mouth to anus. Patients may have small oral aperture, dry mucosal membranes with periodontal disease, esophageal dysmotility, reflux, esophagitis, stricture, dysphagia, delayed stomach emptying, pseudo-obstruction of the small intestines, bacterial overgrowth, malabsorption, wide mouth diverticuli, and fecal incontinence due to rectal sphincter fibrosis.

128. What abnormalities on pulmonary function testing can be seen with SSc?
- Decreased diffusing capacity for carbon monoxide (D_{LCO}) (earliest marker of pulmonary hypertension)
- Increased A-a gradient with exercise activity
- Decreased vital capacity and increased forced expiratory volume in 1 second/forced vital capacity (FEV_1/FVC) ratio (restrictive pattern)

129. **How does SSc affect the heart?**
    - Myocardial fibrosis
    - Dilated cardiomyopathy
    - Cor pulmonale
    - Arrhythmias
    - Pericarditis
    - Myocarditis
    - Heart failure with preserved ejection fraction (diastolic heart failure)
    - Myocardial infarction

130. **Are scleredema and scleromyxedema related to SSc?**
    No. Scleredema is a dermatosis of unknown cause characterized by symmetric truncal skin induration and thickening, sometimes with erythema. A high proportion of cases are associated with diabetes, malignancies, and infections. Skin biopsy of a patient with scleredema may reveal thickened dermal collagen with a mild infiltration of mucin in the deeper regions of the dermis. Scleromyxedema (also called *papular mucinosis*) is characterized by raised pale waxy papules that result from excessive mucin deposition distributed over the face, fingers, arms, and legs. This condition is associated with paraproteins, particularly IgG lambda. Cases of scleromyxedema have been described in patients with multiple myeloma, amyloidosis, and human immunodeficiency virus (HIV) infection. Patients with scleredema and scleromyxedema do not typically exhibit Raynaud phenomenon and positive autoantibodies, as would be found in SSc.

IDIOPATHIC INFLAMMATORY MYOPATHIES

131. **What are the idiopathic inflammatory myopathies (IIMs)?**
    Polymyositis, dermatomyositis, and inclusion body myositis (IBM).

132. **What are the diagnostic criteria for polymyositis and dermatomyositis?**
    - Symmetric proximal weakness
    - Elevated muscle enzymes (creatine phosphokinase [CPK], aldolase, aspartate aminotransferase [AST], alanine aminotransferase [ALT], lactate dehydrogenase [LDH])
    - Myopathic electromyography (EMG) abnormalities
    - Typical changes on muscle biopsy
    - Typical dermatologic features (Gottron sign, heliotropic rash)
    To make a definite diagnosis of dermatomyositis, three of four criteria plus the rash must be present. For a definite diagnosis of polymyositis, four criteria must be present without the rash. Note that the criteria do not distinguish polymyositis from inclusion body myositis (IBM).
    Bohan A, Peter JB. Polymyositis and dermatomyositis. *N Engl J Med.* 1975;292:344–347.

133. **Compare and contrast polymyositis with dermatomyositis.**
    Both polymyositis and dermatomyositis are characterized by muscle weakness and abnormal muscle findings, but the disorders differ significantly. In dermatomyositis, the inflammation is perivascular (e.g., surrounding the fascicles) with a predominance of CD4+ cells; whereas in polymyositis, CD8+ lymphocytes invade the muscle fiber (e.g., endomysial infiltration). Dermatomyositis can be associated with cancer and may overlap with SSc or mixed connective tissue disease (MCTD). Sclerotic thickening of the dermis, contractures, esophageal hypomotility, microangiopathy, and calcium deposits may be present in dermatomyositis but typically are not seen with polymyositis.
    Dalakas MC, Hohlfeld R. Polymyositis and dermatomyositis. *Lancet.* 2003;362:971–982.

134. **What is Gottron sign?**
    An erythematous rash that is frequently scaly and occurs over the MCP and IP joints in a symmetric pattern.

135. **Where does the term *heliotropic* rash come from?**
    A South American plant with clusters of rich purple flowers, whose scent is similar to cherry pie, named *heliotrope*. The heliotropic rash refers to the violaceous coloration similar to that of the plant seen along the eyelids of a patient with dermatomyositis.

136. **List some of the characteristic features of IBM.**
    - Usually occurs in older people
    - Insidious onset

- Incidence greater in men than women
- Muscle involvement may be focal or diffuse with asymmetry
- Involves both proximal and distal muscles (in contrast to polymyositis in which proximal muscles are affected and distal muscles are usually unaffected)
- CPK normal (25%) or only low to moderate elevation
- Light microscopy shows ragged red fibers, atrophic fibers, and intracellular rimmed vacuoles
- Electron microscopy shows intracytoplasmic, intranuclear tubular or filamentous inclusions that are amyloid

137. **What percentage of patients who have an IIM have normal muscle enzymes?**
≤33%.

138. **Give examples of myositis-associated/myositis-specific antibodies.**
Anti-Jo-1 is found in patients with IIM who can present with arthritis, interstitial lung disease, and Raynaud phenomenon. IIM patients with anti-U1RNP may have myositis overlap with MCTD. Anti-SRP is typically found in patients with polymyositis, and its presence portends a poor prognosis. Anti-Mi-2 is found in patients with classic dermatomyositis; these patients have good prognoses and will respond well to treatment.

139. **What is the antisynthetase syndrome?**
A subcategory of the IIM defined by the presence of autoantibodies to aminoacyl-tRNA synthetases. Specific clinical manifestations include myositis, interstitial lung disease, arthritis, Raynaud phenomenon, fever, and mechanics hands. Antibodies to Jo-1, PL-12, OJ, EJ, PL-7, KS, and Zo have been reported.

140. **What further evaluation for an occult malignancy should be undertaken in an adult diagnosed with dermatomyositis?**
Because of the increased risk of malignancy in patients with myositis, particularly dermatomyositis, age-appropriate cancer screening should be pursued. (See Chapter 2, General Medicine and Ambulatory Care.)

SPONDYLOARTHROPATHIES

141. **What is a spondyloarthropathy?**
A group of inflammatory diseases of uncertain etiology that affect the spine and sacroiliac joints characterized by the absence of RF autoantibodies and a high association with class 1 major histocompatibility antigen, HLA-B27. Other unifying features include peripheral oligoarthropathy, enthesopathy, and extra-articular foci of inflammation such as uveitis. Diseases classified as spondyloarthropathies include:
- Ankylosing spondylitis (AS)
- Reactive arthritis
- Juvenile spondyloarthritis
- SAPPHO (**s**ynovitis, severe **a**cne, **p**almoplantar **p**ustulosis, **h**yperostosis, and **o**steitis)
- Psoriatic arthritis
- Enteropathic arthritis
- Arthritis associated with Whipple disease

142. **What mechanisms may explain the association of HLA-B27 with spondyloarthropathy?**
Although the exact mechanism is unknown, one hypothesis suggests that B27 presents an arthritogenic peptide or alters immune repertoire through its antigen presentation role. Another possibility is that the B27 peptide itself may be prone to misfolding, forming homodimers that subsequently trigger an inflammatory response. Last, B27 may serve as a surface ligand for other immunomodulatory receptor families, such as KIRs (killer cell immunoglobulin receptors). In addition, we know that individuals who are homozygous for B27 are three times more likely to develop AS than heterozygotes, suggesting a gene dosage effect. However, evidence also suggests various other HLA and non-HLA genetic factors in association with spondyloarthropathy risk.

Melis L, Elewaut D. Progress in spondylarthritis. Immunopathogenesis of spondyloarthritis: which cells drive disease? *Arthritis Res Ther.* 2009;11:233–238.

143. **Describe the principal clinical features of ankylosing spondylitis.**
    - Occurs more often in men than in women in a 3:1 ratio
    - Begins in later adolescence
    - Presents with inflammatory low back pain and stiffness
    - Has inflammatory back pain pattern that improves with activity and worsens with rest
    - Has predominantly lower limb peripheral joint involvement (hips, knees, ankles), often asymmetric

144. **Name extra-articular features of ankylosing spondylitis.**
    - Anterior uveitis (occurring in ~25%)
    - Aortitis (often progressing to aortic valve insufficiency)
    - Cardiac conduction defects
    - Pulmonary fibrosis (<1%)

145. **What is the difference between a syndesmophyte and an osteophyte?**
    Syndesmophytes represent ossification of the outer layers of the annulus fibrosus (Sharpey fibers), creating an osseous bridge across vertebrae at the discovertebral junction. The syndesmophyte is a characteristic radiographic finding in AS, though it may be seen in any of the spondyloarthropathies. Spinal **osteophytes** are triangular ossifications, continuous with the vertebral bodies, forming at either the margins of a vertebral body or a few millimeters from the margin of the discovertebral junction. Osteophytes are often associated with degenerative disk disease.
    Brower AC. The "phytes" of the spine. In: Brower AC, Flemming DJ, eds. *Arthritis in Black and White*. 2nd ed. Philadelphia: WB Saunders; 1997: 175–191.

146. **Describe reactive arthritis.**
    An inflammatory arthritis that typically presents days or weeks after an infection of the genitourinary or enteric tract that involves mucocutaneous surface, usually presenting an asymmetric oligoarthritis of the larger joints and is often HLA-B27 related. One type has a classic triad of conjunctivitis, nongonococcal urethritis, and arthritis. Most patients are between the ages of 20 and 40; the most common infectious agents associated with reactive arthritis include *Chlamydia*, *Salmonella*, *Shigella*, and *Yersinia*.

147. **Describe the mucocutaneous manifestations of reactive arthritis.**
    - Small painless areas of **desquamation on the tongue** that may be unnoticed by the patient
    - **Circinate balanitis,** usually affecting the glans penis, that can range from small erythematous macules to large areas of dry, flaking skin
    - **Keratoderma blennorrhagica,** a thickening and keratinization of the skin that generally involves the feet, hands, and nails that resemble psoriasis clinically and on histopathologic examination

148. **Describe the relationship between psoriasis and psoriatic arthritis.**
    About 25% of psoriasis patients will develop psoriatic arthritis sometime in their lifetime. In the majority of patients, psoriasis will precede psoriatic arthritis by an average of 8–10 years. The extent of skin involvement does not necessarily correlate with joint involvement. Nail dystrophy and dactylitis are characteristic features of psoriatic arthritis.

149. **List the five patterns of joint involvement found in psoriatic arthritis and their relative frequencies.**
    - DIP joints of hands or feet: 8%
    - Peripheral asymmetric oligoarthropathy: 8%
    - Symmetric polyarthritis resembling RA: 18%
    - Arthritis mutilans ("opera glass hands"): 2%
    - Sacroilitis with or without higher levels of spinal involvement: 24%
    Arnett FC. Seronegative spondyloarthropathies. *Bull Rheum Dis.* 1987;37:1–12.

150. **What are the treatment options for ankylosing spondylitis (AS) and psoriatic arthritis (PsA)?**
    NSAIDs, either nonselective or selective COX-2 inhibitors, may be considered initially for arthritis in both conditions. Anti-TNF treatment such as etanercept, infliximab, adalimumab, or golimumab may be considered for those with persistent disease activity. Unlike RA, conventional DMARDs such as methotrexate and sulfasalazine do not have any demonstrable effect on axial disease, though they may have some benefit for peripheral arthritis, as well as methotrexate in particular for psoriatic skin disease. Anti-IL-17 inhibitor, secukinumab, may be an option for patients with radiographic axial disease in AS and skin disease and arthritis in PsA. In addition, the phosphodiesterase-4 inhibitor,

apremilast, may be another treatment option for active PsA. Nonpharmacologic treatment, including patient education and exercise programs, should also be part of the treatment approach.

Gossec L, Smolen JS, Ramiro S, et al. EULAR recommendations for the management of psoriatic arthritis with pharmacological therapies: 2015 update. *Ann Rheum Dis.* 2016;75:499–510.

Sieper J, Poddubnyy D. New evidence on the management of spondyloarthritis. *Nat Rev Rheumatol.* 2016;12:285–295.

Zochling J, van der Heijde D, Burgos-Vargas R, et al. ASAS/EULAR recommendations for the management of ankylosing spondylitis. *Ann Rheum Dis.* 2006;65:442–452.

VASCULITIS

151. **What is vasculitis?**
A varied group of disorders that share a common underlying pathology of inflammation of a single blood vessel or blood vessels. Vasculitis occurs as a primary disorder or secondary to a variety of diseases or drugs.

152. **How are noninfectious vasculitides classified?**
By the predominant sizes of the involved blood vessels (large, medium, and small).

153. **What are the possible immune-pathogenic mechanisms of vasculitis?**
- Deposition of circulating antigen-antibody complexes or in situ formation of immune complexes within the vessel wall
- Cell-mediated hypersensitivity
- Granulomatous tissue reaction

154. **What is polymyalgia rheumatica (PMR)?**
An inflammatory condition that causes pain or stiffness, usually in the neck, shoulder, and hip girdle with sudden onset and occurrence in patients older than 50 years. Patients typically have elevated ESR or CRP or both, which suggests a systemic inflammatory process.

155. **What are the types of large vessel vasculitis?**
Giant cell arteritis (GCA) and Takayasu arteritis (TAK).

156. **What is the association between PMR and GCA?**
Approximately 15% of patients with PMR develop GCA, and approximately 50% of patients with GCA have associated PMR.

157. **How does the distribution of blood vessels involved in GCA affect the symptoms?**
If the *extracranial* branches of the aorta (with sparing of the intracranial vessels) are involved, the classic manifestations of blindness, headache, scalp tenderness, and jaw claudication are seen. Vasculitis of the vertebral arteries can impair the posterior cerebral circulation and cause stroke, transient ischemic attacks, vertigo, and dizziness. Involvement of the subclavian, axillary, and proximal brachial arteries leads to the aortic arch syndrome of claudication of the arms and absent or asymmetric pulses.

158. **What is TAK?**
A large vessel vasculitis, often granulomatous, that predominantly affects the aorta and its major branches. TAK usually occurs before age 50. High-risk populations include adolescent or young adult women from Japan, Southeast Asia, India, and Mexico. Clinical manifestations range from asymptomatic disease with nonpalpable pulses to catastrophic neurologic impairment (stroke, postural dizziness, seizures, and amaurosis).

159. **What are the medium vessel vasculitides?**
- Polyarteritis nodosa (PAN)
- Kawasaki disease (KD)

160. **What is PAN?**
Necrotizing vasculitis of medium or small arteries, typically ANCA negative. PAN may present with polyvisceral involvement, single organ involvement, or isolated cutaneous disease but typically spares the lungs.

161. **What are the characteristics of KD?**
Fever, bilateral nonexudative conjunctivitis, erythema of the lips and oral mucosa, rash, extremity changes, and lymphadenopathy. The most serious complication is severe coronary aneurysmal dilations. KD is one of the most common vasculitides of childhood and usually occurs in children <5 years old.

162. **Compare the common clinical presentations and laboratory findings of GCA, TAK, KD, and PAN.**
See Table 10.9.

Table 10.9. Characteristics of Giant Cell Arteritis, Takayasu Disease, Kawasaki Disease, and Polyarteritis Nodosa

DISEASE	VESSELS AFFECTED	CLINICAL MANIFESTATIONS	LABORATORY DATA
GCA	Large extracranial vessels	Visual changes, headache, scalp tenderness, and jaw claudication	Elevated ESR and CRP
TAK	Large blood vessels with elastic lamina	From asymptomatic to severe neurologic impairment	Elevated ESR
KD	Medium vessel vasculitis	Fever, rash, conjunctivitis, erythema (lips/mucosa), LAD	Elevated ESR
PAN	Predominantly medium-sized venules	Systemic symptoms, HTN, renal insufficiency, abdominal pain, neurologic dysfunction	Possible hepatitis B, aneurysms on angiography

CRP, C-reactive protein; ESR, erythrocyte sedimentation rate; GCA, giant cell arteritis; HTN, hypertension; KD, Kawasaki disease; LAD, lymphadenopathy; PAN, polyarteritis nodosa; TAK, Takayasu disease.

163. **With which diseases are ANCAs associated?**
    - Granulomatosis with polyangiitis (GPA)
    - Microscopic polyangiitis (MPA)
    - Single-organ ANCA-associated vasculitis
    - Eosinophilic granulomatosis with polyangiitis (EGPA)
    - Drug-induced vasculitis: propylthiouracil, hydralazine, minocycline, and other drugs
    - Inflammatory rheumatic disease: RA, SLE, SS, SSc, inflammatory myopathies, and APA syndrome
    - Autoimmune gastrointestinal disorders: ulcerative colitis and primary sclerosing cholangitis

164. **What is GPA?**
Systemic necrotizing granulomatous vasculitis that affects small to medium-sized vessels. It typically affects the upper respiratory tract, lungs, and kidneys and is associated with c-ANCA. Over 80–90% of GPA patients have PR3 antibody positivity.

165. **Which organs are primarily affected in GPA?**
Respiratory tract (upper and lower) and kidneys. Respiratory tract involvement can manifest as recurrent sinusitis, otitis media, tracheobronchial inflammation and erosions, lung nodules, or pneumonitis with cavitation. Renal involvement occurs in the form of a pauci-immune glomerulonephritis.

166. **What are other symptoms in GPA?**
    - Arthritis
    - Neurologic symptoms including polyneuritis, meningitis, and mononeuritis multiplex
    - Skin ulcerations in the distal portions of arms or legs
    - Eye inflammation due to contiguous granulomatous sinus disease (nasolacrimal duct obstruction, proptosis, and ocular muscle or optic nerve involvement) or due to focal vasculitis (conjunctivitis, episcleritis, scleritis, corneoscleral ulceration, uveitis, and granulomatous vasculitis of the retina and optic nerve)

167. **What is EGPA?**
Eosinophilic granulomatosis with polyangiitis that often involves the respiratory tract. Nasal polyps, severe asthma, and eosinophilia are common. Other organs involved include GI tract, kidney, heart, and skin. p-ANCA with positive MPO antibodies is common in patients with glomerulonephritis.

168. **How is MPA characterized?**
By pauci-immune necrotizing small vessel vasculitis of the lungs and kidneys without evidence of necrotizing granulomatous inflammation. MPA is the most common pulmonary-renal syndrome. Other organs involved include the skin, musculoskeletal system, and GI tract. Over 80% of patients with MPA are ANCA-positive, most often p-ANCA (MPO positive).

169. **What is cryoglobulinemic vasculitis (CV)?**
Small vessel vasculitis caused by the deposit serum cryoglobulins in the vessel walls. The most frequent manifestations are purpura, arthralgia, and nephritis. Mixed cryoglobulins and RF are often positive. Most patients have an associated hepatitis C virus infection.

170. **Define IgA vasculitis.**
Small vessel vasculitis characterized by vascular deposition of IgA-dominant immune complexes. This is also known as Henoch-Schönlein purpura (HSP). Purpura, arthralgia, and colicky abdominal pain are the most frequent manifestations. Approximately half the patients have hematuria and proteinuria, but only 10–20% have renal insufficiency. HSP is the most common vasculitis in childhood and has an excellent prognosis.

171. **Compare the common clinical presentations and laboratory findings of MPA, GPA, EGPA, CV, and IgA vasculitis.**
See Table 10.10.

Table 10.10. Characteristics of Microscopic Polyangiitis, Granulomatosis wtih Polyangiitis, Eosinophilic Granulomatosis with Angiitis, Cryoglobulinemis Vasculitis, and IgA Vasculitis

DISEASE	VESSEL SIZE AFFECTED	CLINICAL FEATURES	FREQUENCY (%)	LABORATORY FINDINGS
MPA	Small to medium-sized vessels	Glomerulonephritis Pulmonary and skin Neurologic, GI	>90 50 Less common	Usually p-ANCA (anti-MPO)
GPA	Small to medium-sized vessels	Pulmonary, ENT Glomerulonephritis Neurologic, GI, and skin	90 80 50	Usually c-ANCA (anti-PR3)
EGPA	Small to medium-sized vessels	Pulmonary and peripheral nerve Skin, ENT, GI, renal, and musculoskeletal	70–80 50	Eosinophilia Usually p-ANCA (anti-MPO)
CV	Small vessels	Skin Musculoskeletal Renal Neurologic, GI	90 70 55 30–40	Cryoglobulins, RF
IgA vasculitis	Small vessels	Skin Musculoskeletal GI	90 75 60	IgA deposition

c-ANCA, cytoplasmic antineutrophil cytoplasmic antibody; EGPA, eosinophilic granulomatosis with angiitis; CV, cryoglobulinemic vasculitis; ENT, ear, nose, and throat; EGPA, eosinophilic granulomatosis with polyangiitis; GI, gastrointestinal; GPA, granulomatosis with polyangiitis; MPA, microscopic polyangiitis; MPO, myeloperoxidase; p-ANCA, perinuclear antineutrophil cytoplasmic antibody; PR3, proteinase 3; RF, rheumatoid factor.

172. **What is Behçet disease (BD)?**
A systemic vasculitis of unknown cause, characterized by relapsing episodes of oral aphthous ulcers, genital ulcers, skin lesions, and ocular lesions (retinal vasculitis, anterior and posterior uveitis). Other symptoms include arthralgia/arthritis, CNS vasculitis, meningitis, thrombosis, and GI ulcerations. BD affects blood vessels of all sizes and is most common along the "Old Silk Route," which spans the region from Japan and China in the Far East to the Mediterranean Sea, including the countries of Turkey and Iran.

173. What are the skin lesions of BD?
    - Folliculitis
    - Acneiform lesions
    - Erythema nodosum lesions that may ulcerate
    - Pathergy (pustular reaction to skin injury)
    - Palpable purpura
    - Pyoderma gangrenosum–type lesions

174. What are the ocular findings associated with BD?
    - Retinal vasculitis
    - Anterior and posterior uveitis
    - Hypopyon (severe anterior uveitis with purulent material in the anterior chamber)
    - Cataracts
    - Glaucoma
    - Neovascularization
    - Conjunctival ulceration

175. What treatments are available for the management of vasculitis?
    Corticosteroids and immunosuppressive medications. The treatment choices for vasculitis will be determined by the type and severity of the manifestations of the disease. Some commonly used immunosuppressants include cyclophosphamide, rituximab, azathioprine, and methotrexate. For more severe disease, plasma exchange and intravenous gamma globulin (IVIG) are also commonly used.

KEY POINTS: SPECIFIC RHEUMATIC DISEASES

1. Rheumatoid arthritis is a chronic, symmetric inflammatory disease that will lead to joint damage and destruction. Early diagnosis and early initiation of disease-modifying treatment lead to better outcomes.
2. SLE is a heterogeneous, autoimmune disease more common in premenopausal females and is associated with ANA autoantibodies.
3. UTCD is a description commonly applied to a patient with signs and symptoms definitive enough to be clearly autoimmune and inflammatory in nature but not sufficient to render a more exact diagnosis.
4. Spondyloarthropathies are characterized by inflammatory symptoms of the axial skeleton and have associated symptoms of enthesopathy and uveitis.
5. The vasculitides are a group of disorders that share a common underlying pathology of inflammation of one or more blood vessels. Nomenclature and presentation differ on the size of vessel involvement (small, medium, large vessel).

ANA, antinuclear antibody; SLE, systemic lupus erythematosus; UTCD, undifferentiated connective tissue disease.

OSTEOARTHRITIS

176. Is OA a genetic disease?
    Yes, in that there is a hereditary component. Perhaps the most recognized inherited feature is the presence of Heberden nodes in mothers and sisters of affected patients. Studies have uncovered a mutation in a type II collagen gene (Arg519 to Cys) that predisposes to early OA.
    Pun YL, Moskowitz RW, Lie S, et al. Clinical correlations of osteoarthritis associated with a single-base mutation (arginine 519 to cysteine) in type II procollagen gene: a newly defined pathogenesis. *Arthritis Rheum.* 1994;37:264–269.

177. Compare the biochemical changes of the aged joint with the osteoarthritic joint.
    See Table 10.11.

Table 10.11. Biochemical Differences Between the Aging Joint and Osteoarthritis

	AGING JOINT	OSTEOARTHRITIS
Bone	Osteoporosis	Thickened cortices, osteophytes, subchondral cysts, remodeling
Chondrocyte activity	Normal	Increased
Collagen	Increased cross-linking of fibrils	Irregular weave Smaller fibrils
Water	Slight decrease	Significant increase
Proteoglycan	Normal total content Decreased chondroitins Increased keratin Normal aggregation	Decreased total proteoglycan component Increased chondroitins Decreased keratin Decreased aggregation

From Brandt KD, Fife RS. Aging in relation to the pathogenesis of osteoarthritis. *Clin Rheum Dis.* 1986;12: 117–130.

178. **What is spinal stenosis syndrome?**
The progressive narrowing of the spinal canal, most commonly from OA of the lumbar or cervical spine. With cervical disease, patients typically present with pain and limitation of motion. Hyperreflexia is common. Other signs may include muscle weakness, spastic gait, and Babinski sign. In the lumbar region, the clinical manifestations are mostly those of neurogenic claudication and compression of the cauda equina when severe.

179. **What is diffuse idiopathic skeletal hyperostosis (DISH)?**
A form of degenerative arthritis characterized by extensive ossification of tendinous and ligamentous attachments to the bone. Spine involvement with flowing calcification over the anterior longitudinal ligament is among the most common findings. DISH has been associated with obesity, increased waist circumference, hypertension, dyslipidemia, diabetes mellitus, hyperuricemia, metabolic syndrome, and an increased risk for cardiovascular diseases.

180. **What radiographic features help to distinguish DISH from AS, degenerative spine disease, and spondylosis deformans?**
   - Flowing calcification along the anterolateral aspect of at least four contiguous vertebral bodies
   - Relative preservation of intervertebral disk height in the involved vertebral segment and absence of extensive radiographic changes of "degenerative" disk disease (disk space narrowing with vacuum phenomena, vertebral body marginal sclerosis)
   - Absence of apophyseal joint ankylosis and sacroiliac joint erosion, sclerosis, and intra-articular osseous fusion

181. **What is the vacuum phenomenon?**
A radiographic finding seen in degeneration of the intervertebral disk that has the appearance of a radiolucent stripe in an intervertebral disk. Radiolucencies represent gas or nitrogen that appears at the site of negative pressure produced by abnormal spaces of clefts.

INFECTIOUS ARTHRITIS

182. **What is the mechanism for acute rheumatic fever?**
Following antibody formation to group A streptococcus after pharyngeal infection, the antibodies cross-react with human antigens (molecular mimicry), leading to a persistent autoimmune reaction, tissue destruction, and development of immune complexes. Arthritis is one of the earliest manifestations of rheumatic fever and has a migratory pattern.

183. **What is St. Vitus dance?**
A neurologic disorder consisting of abrupt, purposeless involuntary movements that disappear during sleep. The disorder is found in patients with rheumatic fever and is also called *Syndenham's chorea* or *chorea minor.*

184. **What viral illnesses may be associated with arthropathy?**
   - Hepatitis A, B, and C
   - Parvovirus B19
   - Epstein-Barr virus (EBV)
   - Cytomegalovirus (CMV)
   - Enteroviruses (ECHO [enteropathic cytopathogenic human orphan] virus, coxsackievirus)
   - HIV
   - Mumps
   - Rubella
   - Smallpox (vaccinia)
   - Varicella
   - Flavivirus (Zika virus, dengue)
   - Group A arboviruses (Ross River, chikungunya, o'nyong-nyong, sindbis, Mayaro virus)

185. **What rheumatologic condition is associated with chronic hepatitis B infection?**
   Polyarteritis nodosa, likely associated with persistent circulating hepatitis B antigen.

186. **What are the articular manifestations of hepatitis C infection?**
   - Arthropathy
   - Nondestructive RA-like arthritis
   - Monoarthritis
   - Oligoarthritis
   Hepatitis C can also be part of the mixed cryoglobulinemia syndrome. Chronic hepatitis C infection may also lead to low positive autoantibodies like ANA and RF. Anti-CCP antibodies are usually negative.

187. **What arthropathy is associated with active parvovirus infection?**
   Nondestructive RA-like picture with positive RF. The arthropathy clears with no chronic or destructive sequelae.

188. **Summarize the association of rubella infection with arthropathy.**
   Joint symptoms usually begin within 1 week of the onset of the rash of rubella and include arthralgia and arthritis, especially in adult women. In the past, arthritis and arthralgia often were seen after rubella vaccination, but they are less common because a less arthrogenic strain of virus is used for the vaccine.

189. **What are the common articular problems experienced by patients infected with HIV?**
   - Arthralgia
   - Reactive arthritis associated with HLA-B27 (but axial disease and sacroiliitis are unusual)
   - Psoriatic arthritis with asymmetric polyarticular inflammatory arthritis that may be more severe than in non-HIV patients
   - "Painful articular syndrome" describing an exquisitely painful, asymmetric, minimally inflammatory arthritis involving the large joints of the lower extremities
   - Septic arthritis, typically *Staphylococcus aureus* but also with *Streptococcus, Salmonella,* atypical *Mycobacteria,* and other opportunistic infections
   Solomon G, Brancato L, Winchester R. An approach to the human immunodeficiency virus–positive patient with a spondyloarthropathic disease. *Rheum Dis Clin North Am.* 1991;17:43–58.

190. **What are the specific muscle problems encountered by patients infected with HIV?**
   - Inflammatory muscle disease (polymyositis and dermatomyositis)
   - Nemaline rod myopathy with findings of nemaline rods without inflammation on muscle biopsy
   - Noninflammatory myopathy associated with severe muscle wasting
   - Pyomyositis or direct muscle infection with small muscle abscesses frequently caused by *S. aureus, Mycobacterium avium,* cryptococci, *Microsporidium,* and other organisms
   - Medication-associated myopathy seen with zidovudine (AZT) and other nucleoside and nucleotide reverse transcriptase inhibitors (NRTIs)

191. **What is DILS?**
   Diffuse infiltrative lymphocytosis syndrome. DILS is a condition occurring in 3–8% of HIV-infected patients and causes massive salivary gland involvement and sicca symptoms due to CD8 infiltration. In addition to salivary glands, other organs may be involved in DILS, resulting in neuropathy, interstitial pneumonitis, interstitial nephritis, and hepatitis.

192. **Is DILS the same as SS?**
No. DILS is a distinct entity with different immunogenetics and pathophysiology from SS. DILS is a predominantly CD8 disease, whereas SS is a CD4 disease. In addition, African-American DILS sufferers show a high incidence of HLA-DR8, whereas DR6 and DR7 are more prevalent in Caucasians. By contrast, in patients with SS, HLA-DR2 and HLA-DR3 predominate.

193. **Which bacterial pathogens are most commonly responsible for septic arthritis?**
- *Neisseria gonorrhoeae*
- *Staphylococcus* spp.
- *Streptococcus* spp.
- Gram-negative bacilli

194. **What are the common clinical manifestations of gonococcal arthritis?**
Migratory tenosynovitis and macular or papular rash (keratoderma blennorrhagica) on a distal extremity. Gonococcal arthritis occurs in approximately 0.1–0.5% of patients with gonorrhea. Synovial fluid cultures are positive in <50% of cases.

195. **What are the clinical manifestations of Lyme disease and the time of their occurrence in the untreated disease course?**
Early localized
- Erythema chronicum migrans (ECM)
- Flu-like illness
Early disseminated
- Neurologic findings (meningitis, cranial neuropathies such as Bell palsy, peripheral neuropathy)
- Cardiac findings (atrioventricular block, myopericarditis)
Late
- Inflammatory arthritis with predilection for large joints

196. **What is the classic skin manifestation of Lyme disease?**
ECM, an expanding erythematous ring (often asymptomatic) with central clearing beginning at the site of the tick bite. The *Borrelia* organism can be cultured from the margin of the lesion. In endemic regions, ECM is the most common presenting feature of early Lyme disease. Other skin manifestations include benign lymphocytoma and acrodermatitis chronica atrophicans.

197. **Is chronic arthritis of Lyme disease produced by active joint infection?**
Likely not. Live spirochetes have rarely been documented. In addition, spirochetal DNA has not been reliably discovered after amplification with polymerase chain reaction (PCR) technology.

CRYSTAL ARTHROPATHY

198. **What three principal crystals are associated with joint inflammation?**
- Urate (gout)
- Calcium pyrophosphate (CPP; "pseudogout")
- Hydroxyapatite
Dieppe P, Calvert P. *Crystals and Joint Disease*. London: Chapman & Hall; 1983.

199. **What conditions have been associated with calcium pyrophosphate dihydrate (CPPD) disease?**
- Hemochromatosis
- Hypothyroidism
- Aging
- Hyperparathyroidism
- Gene mutations (*ANKH*)
- Hypophosphatasia
- Amyloidosis (likely)
- Trauma, including surgery
- OA (likely)
- Hypomagnesemia
- Gout

200. **Why is the polarizing microscope important in the diagnosis of rheumatic diseases?**
To analyze synovial fluid and identify the specific causes of inflammatory arthritis, in particular crystal-induced arthritis. The microscopy operates on the relatively simple observation that some crystals refract light into fast and slow rays (i.e., they are birefringent). Polarized light passing through a crystal is no longer parallel to light not passing through the crystal. If a second polarizer is added so that its axis is rotated 90 degrees (extinction) to the light as it emerges from the first polarizer but after some light is bent (rotated) by the crystal in between the polarizers, the only light reaching the observer's eye is the light that the crystal has rotated. Monosodium urate crystals have a strongly negative birefringent appearance on polarized light microscopy and appear yellow when oriented parallel to the axis of the compensator. Calcium pyrophosphate crystals are weakly positively birefringent and appear blue when oriented parallel to the axis of the compensator. Polarized microscopy requires operator expertise for accuracy.
     Rosenthal AK, Mandel N. Identification of crystals in synovial fluids and joint tissues. *Curr Rheumatol Rep.* 2011;3:11–16.

201. **Where is chondrocalcinosis commonly demonstrated roentgenographically?**
In the joint cartilages. The cartilages appear punctate or stippled, with linear densities within the articular hyaline or fibrocartilage in knee menisci, radiocarpal joints, annulus fibrosus of intervertebral disks, and symphysis pubis. When present in peripheral joints, the findings are usually bilateral. The prevalence in the general population (as assessed by multiple radiologic studies) is 10–15% in people aged 65–75 years but rises above 40% in people older than 80 years.

202. **What are the four stages of gout?**
   - **Stage 1:** asymptomatic hyperuricemia
   - **Stage 2:** acute gouty arthritis
   - **Stage 3:** intercritical gout (the period between attacks)
   - **Stage 4:** chronic tophaceous gout

203. **Describe stage 1 gout.**
Elevated serum urate levels in the absence of symptomatic articular disease or nephrolithiasis. Not all patients with asymptomatic hyperuricemia progress to gout, but the higher the serum level, the greater the likelihood of developing articular disease. With serum urate > 9 mg/dL, the annual incidence of gout is 4.9%, with 5-year incidence of 22%. In most cases, 20–30 years of sustained hyperuricemia pass before an attack of nephrolithiasis or arthropathy.
     Campion EW, Glynn RJ, DeLabry LO. Asymptomatic hyperuricemia. Risks and consequences in the Normative Aging Study. *Am J Med.* 1987;82:421–426.

204. **Describe the characteristics of the first attack of acute gouty arthritis (stage 2).**
Exquisite pain usually occurring in a single joint (monoarticular). Fever, swelling, erythema, and skin sloughing may be associated findings, suggesting cellulitis. Fifty percent of initial attacks occur as podagra (involving the great toe or MTP joint), and 90% of patients with gout have podagra at some stage of disease without treatment. Typical sites of acute gout attacks include foot (first MTP joint), ankle, knee, and less commonly, upper extremity joints such as elbow, wrist, and finger joint.

205. **What are the symptoms of stage 3 gout?**
None. Stage 3 gout refers to the asymptomatic period between attacks. However, 62% of patients have a second attack of articular disease within 1 year of the first attack, 16% within 1–2 years, 11% within 2–5 years, 4% after 5–10 years, and 7% after >10 years.

206. **What is chronic tophaceous gout (stage 4)?**
Chronic arthritis with extra-articular tissue deposition of urate. Gout flares in this stage are often polyarticular, with longer duration and severity. In some cases, chronic tophaceous gout may have an appearance mimicking RA (pseudo-rheumatoid pattern), with chronic, nearly symmetric arthritis with nodules (tophi in gout). The principal determinant of the rate of urate deposition is the serum urate concentration. Tophi are often observed on finger pads, olecranon bursae, pinnae of the ear, and pressure points.
     Teng GG, Nair R, Saag KG. Pathophysiology, clinical presentation and treatment of gout. *Drugs.* 2006;66:1547–1563.

207. **What are the treatment options for acute gout flares?**
NSAIDs, colchicine, and corticosteroids, either oral or intra-articular. Ideally, acute gout flares are treated within 12 hours of symptom onset to reduce the severity. Oral NSAIDs can be given at high dose for 2–3 days, then tapered off within 5–7 days. NSAIDs have potential GI and renal toxicities, especially in elderly

patients and those with comorbid conditions such as congestive heart failure or anticoagulation use. Oral colchicine at lower doses (1.2 mg initially, followed by 0.6 mg 1 hour later) was shown in a recent randomized study to have equal efficacy but better tolerability than traditional higher dose colchicine (1.2 mg initially, then 0.6 mg every hour for 6 hours) for acute gout flares. Severe diarrhea, nausea, and vomiting are among the common side effects of colchicine, especially with a higher dose regimen.

Terkeltaub R. Update on gout: new therapeutic strategies and options. *Nat Rev Rheumatol.* 2010;6:30–38.

208. **What are the treatment options for chronic gout?**
Allopurinol, probenecid, febuxostat, and lesinurad. New evidence-based guidelines focus on treating chronic gout to a target uric acid level < 6 mg/dL. Allopurinol is commonly used in uric acid overproducers and undersecreters. Uricosuric agents similar to probenecid are limited to undersecreters with normal renal function. Allopurinol can be initiated at a dose of 100 mg daily, titrating higher to a maximum approved dose of 800 mg/day. Allopurinol dosing should be more cautious in patients with renal insufficiency (creatinine clearance < 50 mL/min) or elderly patients. Febuxostat, a nonpurine inhibitor of xanthine oxidase, could be used for treatment in those patients with allopurinol hypersensitivity, intolerance, or treatment failure. Febuxostat is dosed at 40 mg daily, or 80 mg daily for those who do not attain adequate uric acid suppression at the lower dose. Lesinurad, a URAT1 inhibitor, is another urate-lowering option, dosed at 200 mg daily and for use in combination with xanthine oxidase inhibitors. Chronic urate-lowering therapy should not be started during acute gout flares but can be continued through acute flares in those already taking urate-lowering treatment. Also, it is not uncommon for patients starting chronic urate-lowering therapy to have more frequent acute gout flares owing to mobilization and destabilization of urate deposits in tissues and joints. These patients should receive acute gout prophylaxis with low-dose daily colchicine (0.6 mg daily or twice daily) or NSAIDs for the first 6 months of therapy.

Dalbeth N, Merriman TR, Stamp LK. Gout. *Lancet.* 2016;388:2039–2052. Epub April 21, 2016. Available at: https://doi.org/10.1016/S0140-6736(16)00346-9.

Teng GG, Nair R, Saag KG. Pathophysiology, clinical presentation and treatment of gout. *Drugs.* 2006;66:1547–1563.

Terkeltaub R. Update on gout: new therapeutic strategies and options. *Nat Rev Rheumatol.* 2010;6:30–38.

SOFT TISSUE RHEUMATISM

209. **What is fibromyalgia (FM)?**
A chronic syndrome characterized by fatigue, generalized pain, sleep disturbance (sometimes termed *nonrestorative* sleep), cognitive problems, and somatic symptoms. The old ACR classification criteria considered the diagnosis of fibromyalgia if a patient had 11 out of 18 tender points. In 2010, the ACR developed new diagnostic criteria, which indicate the presence of fibromyalgia if the patient has symptomatic widespread pain over a certain threshold lasting more than 3 months without other causes for pain. Note that patients may have FM alone or in association with other diseases such as RA, OA, Lyme disease, and sleep apnea. The disease is often mimicked by hypothyroidism.

Wolfe F, Smythe HA, Yunus MB, et al. The American College of Rheumatology 1990 criteria for the classification of fibromyalgia: Report of the Multicenter Criteria Committee. *Arthritis Rheum.* 1990;33:160–172.

Wolfe F, Clauw DJ, Fitzcharles MA, et al. The American College of Rheumatology preliminary diagnostic criteria for fibromyalgia and measurement of symptom severity. *Arthritis Care Res.* 2010;62:600–610.

210. **What other symptoms and syndromes may be associated with FM?**
- Irritable bowel syndrome (IBS)
- Tension headaches
- Irritable bladder (interstitial cystitis, daytime urinary frequency, nocturia, dysuria, urgency, urge incontinence)
- Chronic fatigue syndrome

211. **How is FM treated?**
Recent guidelines indicated treatment for FM should be with pharmacologic therapies (pregabalin, duloxetine, milnacipran, other antidepressants), muscle reconditioning (aerobic exercise), restoration of more normal sleep patterns, and pain control with tramadol. Avoid narcotics to manage FM pain as these are ineffective and increase the risk for dependency and addiction to these drugs.

212. **Define the following disorders named after occupations.**
    - **Housemaid's knee:** prepatellar bursitis
    - **Tailor's seat** (also called "weaver's bottom"): inflammation of the ischial bursa (the bursa that separates the gluteus maximus from the ischial tuberosity)

213. **Define the following disorders named after specific sports and activities.**
    - **Little Leaguer's shoulder:** separation of the proximal humeral epiphysis, probably secondary to the repetitive motion associated with pitching
    - **Tennis elbow:** lateral epicondylitis
    - **Golfer's elbow:** medial epicondylitis
    - **Jumper's knee:** Sinding-Larsen-Johannson (SLJ) syndrome or patellar tendinopathy usually seen in basketball and volleyball athletes but also in ballet dancers

214. **What is de Quervain tenosynovitis?**
    Inflammation of the synovial lining and subsequent narrowing of the membrane (stenosing tenosynovitis) of the abductor pollicis longus and extensor pollicis brevis tendons at the radial styloid.

215. **What is patellofemoral syndrome (PFS)?**
    Knee pain that worsens with activity, while descending stairs and after long periods of inactivity. PFS occurs when the patella does not move or "track" in a correct fashion when the knee is being bent and straightened. This movement can lead to damage of the surrounding tissues, such as the cartilage on the underside of the patella itself, which can lead to pain in the region. This injury is quite common in people who play sports, in particular adolescent girls.

OTHER RHEUMATIC CONDITIONS

216. **What is pyoderma gangrenosum?**
    Skin lesions that begin as pustules or erythematous nodules and break down to form spreading ulcers with necrotic, undermined edges. Pyoderma gangrenosum is frequently associated with inflammatory bowel disease (IBD) but also occurs in chronic active hepatitis, seropositive RA (without evidence of vasculopathy), leukemia, and polycythemia vera. Differential diagnoses of the lesions include necrotizing vasculitis, bacterial infection, and spider bites.

217. **What diseases are associated with complement deficiencies?**
    See Table 10.12.

Table 10.12. Clinical Manifestations of Complement Component Deficiency

DEFICIENT COMPONENT	CLINICAL SYNDROME*
Classic Pathway	
C1q	SLE, infections
C1r/C1s	SLE, infections
C4	SLE, infections
C2	SLE, infections
Lectin Pathway	
MBL	Infections
Central component	
C3	Severe infections, GN, SLE
Membrane attack component	
C5, C6, C7, C8, or C9	*Neisseria* infections
Alternative Pathway	
Properdin, factor D	*Neisseria* infections

*With early component deficiencies of the classic pathway (C1, C4, or C2), infections are caused by the commonly encountered pyogenic organisms. With a late component (C5–C9) or an alternative pathway component deficiency, *Neisseria* infections predominate, especially meningococcal infections.
GN, glomerulonephritis; MBL, mannan-binding lectin; SLE, systemic lupus erythematosus.
From Atkinson JD. Complement system. In: Firestein GS, Budd RS, Harris ED, et al, ed, *Kelley's Textbook of Rheumatology.* 8th ed. Philadelphia: WB Saunders; 2008.

218. Describe Still disease.

A syndrome characterized by high spiking fevers (usually ≤104° F), polyarthritis, evanescent rash typically on the trunk, leukocytosis, and elevated inflammatory markers including ferritin that occurs in children and adults. Fevers may occur only once or twice a day, and patients typically have negative RF and ANA antibody tests.

219. What are familial autoinflammatory syndromes?

Familial autoinflammatory syndromes (FAS) are a set of genetic syndromes characterized by recurrent episodes of inflammation that are not autoantibody or infection driven. Patients tend to have fever, rash, inflammatory arthritis, ocular inflammation, and elevated acute phase reactants.

220. What is the most common familial autoinflammatory syndrome?

Familial Mediterranean fever (FMF). It is one of the periodic fever syndromes. Around 90% of patients present younger than 20 years old and have eastern Mediterranean ancestry (Jewish, Arab, Italian, or Armenian). Fever can last 1–3 days with serositis (pleurisy/pleural effusion and abdominal pain), inflammatory arthritis (may be nonerosive, monoarticular mimics septic arthritis), and rash. Renal amyloidosis is a more serious complication. Attacks may recur every 2–4 weeks. Patients have a mutation in the Mediterranean fever (*MEFV*) gene, which encodes pyrin. Colchicine is effective during attacks, and IL-1 inhibitors such as anakinra have been shown to be effective in colchicine nonresponders.

221. What is Ehlers-Danlos syndrome?

A group of true connective tissue disorders characterized by hyperextensibility of skin and hypermobility of joints, predisposing to early development of OA.

222. Distinguish between Legg-Calvé-Perthes disease and Osgood-Schlatter disease.
   - **Legg-Calvé-Perthes disease:** idiopathic osteonecrosis of the femoral capital epiphysis usually in boys ages 3–8 that may result in a large flat femoral head
   - **Osgood-Schlatter disease** (also called *tibial tubercle apophysitis*): inflammation at the site where the patellar tendon inserts onto the tibial tubercle that is probably due to a repetitive motion injury, usually occurring in adolescents

223. Describe RS3PE syndrome.

Remitting **s**eronegative **s**ymmetric **s**ynovitis with **p**itting **e**dema (RS3PE). Mostly affecting men older than 70 years, this syndrome is characterized by an acute onset of severe synovitis of the small joints with pitting edema of the dorsal aspect of the hand. Symptoms respond to low-dose prednisone, and the syndrome can mimic such conditions as RA and PMR.

224. What is relapsing polychondritis (RP)?

RP is a relatively rare autoimmune disease that involves inflammation and destruction of cartilaginous tissues. The most common feature is unilateral or bilateral external ear inflammation leading to "cauliflower ear." Hearing loss, tinnitus, and vertigo have been known to occur. Patients may get nasal and tracheal involvement. Ocular involvement includes episcleritis, scleritis, and uveitis.

225. Define *Cogan syndrome*.

An unusual vasculopathy associated with interstitial keratitis, sensorineural hearing loss, tinnitus, and vertigo. Systemic features such as fever, weight loss, and fatigue are present in about one half of patients.

226. What is pigment villonodular synovitis (PVNS)?

A proliferative disorder of unknown cause characterized by inflammation and hemosiderin of the synovium. The knee is most commonly affected, and clinically, the patient presents with monoarticular joint swelling. MRI is the diagnostic modality of choice because it may detect the hemosiderin that will show nodular foci.

227. Describe Paget disease of bone.

A chronic disorder of bone remodeling in which there is increased osteoclast-mediated bone resorption leading to increased bone formation; however, this reorganization leads to a disorganized bone matrix and mechanical weakness of the bone. Patients are older than 40 years with a 2:1 incidence in men compared with women. Most patients are asymptomatic, but bone pain and joint pain at night tends to occur. Paget disease is typically found through serendipitous testing such as an elevated alkaline phosphatase or noted on radiographs ordered for other reasons. Radionuclide bone scan can show the extent of disease.

228. **What conditions are associated with avascular necrosis of bone?**
- Trauma (femoral head fracture)
- Gaucher disease
- Hemoglobinopathies
- Pregnancy
- Exogenous or endogenous overproduction of glucocorticoids
- SLE
- Alcoholism
- Lymphoproliferative diseases
- HIV infection
- Anticardiolipin antibody
- Kidney transplantation

229. **Describe nephrogenic systemic fibrosis (NSF).**
Large areas of hardened skin in patients with chronic kidney disease that is likely associated with gadolinium-based MRI contrast agents. Histopathologic examination reveals disruption of normal collagen bundles with increased dermal mucin deposition.

230. **What is IgG4-related disease?**
An immune-mediated collection of disorders that typically occur more in men > 50 years that have commonly shared features of tumor-like swelling of certain organs, lymphoplasmacytic infiltrate enriched with IgG4-positive plasma cells, and varying degrees of fibrosis organized in a storiform pattern. Elevated IgG4 serum levels occur in 60–70% of patients. Common presentations include type 1 autoimmune pancreatitis, salivary gland disease, orbital disease, and chronic periaortitis.

RHEUMATOLOGIC MANIFESTATIONS IN SYSTEMIC DISEASES

231. **Describe amyloidosis.**
Extracellular tissue deposition of fibrils composed of subunits of various proteins. One or more organs may be involved, and the classification is based on the major component of fibril. The two most common categories are systemic AL amyloidosis (50–60%) and systemic AA amyloidosis (5–20%). Persons with AL amyloidosis typically have symptoms of fatigue, weight loss, overall pain, and proteinuria. AA amyloidosis may occur as a complication of chronic inflammatory conditions such as RA, seronegative spondyloarthropathies, IBD, and FMF.

232. **What is a Charcot joint?**
Joint changes found in the foot or ankle that occurs in type 1 or type 2 diabetics with longstanding, poorly controlled disease often complicated by diabetic neuropathy. Classic presentation is a sudden onset of unilateral warmth, redness, and edema with minor trauma history. Progression of disease may lead to midtarsal collapse. It is important to rule out infections such as cellulitis and osteomyelitis.

233. **What is the *prayer sign*, and what does it represent?**
The *prayer sign* is a physical examination sign that reflects the inability to fully extend the joints of the fingers when the palms are put together. This occurs in patients with diabetic cheiroarthropathy or diabetic stiff hand syndrome when there is development of insidious flexion contractures along the DIP and PIP joints. This may occur in both type 1 and type 2 diabetics.

234. **Describe the typical presentation of diabetic amyotrophy.**
Diabetic amyotrophy, a lumbosacral plexopathy, tends to occur in recently diagnosed type 2 diabetics or type 2 diabetics in good glycemic control. Patients present with acute, asymmetric pain along the proximal muscles of the pelvis and thigh. Associated weight loss, anorexia, and unsteady gait due to muscle weakness may occur. In contrast, diabetic muscle infarction occurs in type 1 diabetics and involves spontaneous infarction of muscle. Patients have an acute onset of pain and swelling in the thigh over the period of days or weeks.

235. **What are rheumatologic manifestations of hypothyroidism?**
Proximal muscle weakness, generalized myalgias, arthralgias, carpal tunnel syndrome, and Raynaud phenomenon.

236. **Describe thyroid acropathy.**
A rare complication of Graves disease with digital clubbing, diffuse soft tissue swelling of the hands, and periosteal new bone formation in the metacarpal bones or phalanges.

237. **Which rheumatologic conditions are associated with hyperparathyroidism?**
Chondrocalcinosis, pseudogout, hyperuricemia, osteoporosis, painless proximal muscle weakness, and osteitis fibrosa cystica. Osteitis fibrosa cystica is a consequence of longstanding hyperparathyroidism. Patients present with bone pain and may have diffuse osteopenia and bony erosions in the DIP, MCP, carpal, and acromioclavicular (AC) joints, with "salt and pepper" skull appearance. *Brown tumors* represent lytic lesions due to osteoclast collections intermixed with fibrous tissue and poorly mineralized woven bone.

238. **What is the relationship between acromegaly and rheumatologic disease?**
Acromegaly is a rare disease that is due to persistent hypersecretion of growth hormone. Patients typically present with macrognathia and enlargement of hands, feet, and skull. Early degenerative disease is very common in the areas of the knees, shoulders, ankles, and lumbar and cervical spine. Other conditions include carpal tunnel syndrome, proximal muscle weakness, and Raynaud phenomenon.

Acknowledgment

The editor gratefully acknowledges contributions by Dr. Richard A. Rubin that were retained from a prior edition of *Medical Secrets*.

WEBSITES

1. www.rheumatology.org
2. www.niams.nih.gov

BIBLIOGRAPHY

1. Firestein GS, Budd RC, Harris ED, eds. *Kelley's Textbook of Rheumatology*. 9th ed. Philadelphia: WB Saunders; 2013.
2. Hochberg MC, ed. *Rheumatology*. 6th ed. St. Louis: Mosby; 2015.
3. Klippel JH, ed. *Primer on the Rheumatic Diseases*. 13th ed. Atlanta: Arthritis Foundation; 2008.
4. Koopman WJ, ed. *Arthritis and Allied Conditions: A Textbook of Rheumatology*. 15th ed. Philadelphia: Lippincott Williams & Wilkins; 2005.
5. Resnick D, ed. *Diagnosis of Bone and Joint Disorders*. 4th ed. Philadelphia: WB Saunders; 2002.
6. Sheon RP, ed. *Soft Tissue Rheumatic Pain: Recognition, Management and Prevention*. 3rd ed. Philadelphia: Lippincott Williams & Wilkins; 1996.
7. Wallace DJ, ed. *Dubois' Lupus Erythematosus*. 8th ed. Philadelphia: Lea & Febiger; 2013.

CHAPTER 11

ALLERGY AND IMMUNOLOGY

Alexander S. Kim, MD

Some men also have strange antipathies in their natures against that sort of food which others love and live upon. I have read of one that could not endure to eat either bread or flesh; of another that fell in a swooning fit at the smell of a rose .... [T]here are some who, if a cat accidentally come into the room, though they neither see it, nor are told it, will presently be in a sweat, and ready to die away.

Increase Mather (1639–1723), *Remarkable Providence*

THE INNATE IMMUNE SYSTEM

1. **What are the main characteristics of the innate immune system?**
   The innate immune system is the first line of defense against active infections, and the initial early response occurs within minutes to hours of exposure. The innate immune system recognizes shared motifs on related microbes but is nonspecific and does not develop memory.

2. **What are the main components of the innate immune system?**
   Blood proteins (complement), cells (natural killer (NK) cells, innate lymphoid cells (ILCs), dendritic cells, macrophages, neutrophils), chemicals (antimicrobials), and physical barriers (epithelia, mucosa).

3. **How does the innate immune system recognize microbes and danger?**
   Germline-encoded pattern recognition receptor (PRR) engagement of pathogen-associated molecular patterns (PAMPs) and danger-associated molecular patterns (DAMPs).

4. **What are the major PRRs?**
   Leucine-rich repeats (Toll-like receptors [TLRs] and nucleotide oligomerization domain [NOD]-like receptors), retinoic acid inducible gene (RIG)-like receptors, cytosolic DNA sensors (DDX), C-type lectin-like receptors (CLRs), and pyrin/HIN domain-containing (PYHIN) protein. TLRs and CLRs are localized to the cell surface, whereas RIG-like receptors and NOD-like receptors are present in the cytoplasm.

5. **What are the main features of TLRs?**
   Contain leucine-rich repeats and Toll/IL-1 receptor (TIR) domains.

6. **What are the functions of NK cells?**
   Cytotoxicity (killing infected or injured cells), cytokine production (interferon gamma [IFN-γ]), and costimulation.

7. **How do you measure NK cell cytotoxicity?**
   By chromium release assay. Target cells in the assay are labeled with chromium 51 (^{51}Cr) and then incubated with effector cells. The level of cellular cytotoxicity is calculated using a gamma counter, for example, to quantitate the amount of radioactivity released in supernatant via cytolysis.

8. **What are innate lymphoid cells (ILCs)?**
   Innate immune cells (lymphocytes) that do not express any known surface markers for NK, NKT, T, or B cells and are therefore lineage-negative.

9. **What are the main types of mast cells in humans?**
   - **MC_T (tryptase only):** concentrated in mucosal surfaces, allergic conjunctivae, bronchi, and alveoli and have a scroll-rich granule structure. MC_Ts are T-cell dependent.
   - **MC_{TC} (tryptase, chymase):** also release carboxypeptidase A3 and cathepsin G and have granules that are lattice-like in structure. They are increased in asthma and primarily located in skin, submucosal connective tissue, perivascular spaces, and at serosal surfaces. MC_{TC}S express CD88 (receptor for C5a).

10. **What are the major differences between mast cells and basophils?**
    See Table 11.1.

258

Table 11.1. Comparison of Mast Cells and Basophils

PARAMETER	MAST CELLS	BASOPHILS
Life span	Weeks to years	Days
Origin	Probably bone marrow	Bone marrow
Location	Tissues, noncirculating	Normally circulating
Size	8–20 mm	5–7 mm
Nucleus	Round to oval, may be indented	Multilobulated
Cytoplasmic granules	Smaller, more numerous	Larger, fewer granules
High-affinity IgE receptor	Present	Present
Histamine release	Yes	Yes
Major arachidonic acid metabolites	PGD_2, LTC_4, $-D_4$, $-E_4$	LTC_4
Staining characteristics		
Toluidine blue	Yes	Yes
Tryptase	Yes	No
Chloroacetate esterase	Yes	No

IgE, immunoglobulin E; LT, leukotriene; PG, prostaglandin.

11. **Describe the major subsets of dendritic cells (DCs).**
Myeloid, plasmacytoid, Langerhans, CD14+/interstitial and monocyte-derived. The transcription factor for both conventional myeloid and plasmacytoid DCs is Flt3-ligand. Conventional myeloid DCs express TLR 4/5/8, and plasmacytoid DCs express TLR 7/9. Langerhans DCs contain Birbeck granules and express CD1a.

THE ADAPTIVE IMMUNE SYSTEM

12. **What are the main components of the adaptive immune system?**
Humoral immunity and cell-mediated immunity.

13. **How does humoral immunity work?**
B lymphocytes, the main effectors of humoral immunity, respond to extracellular pathogens by producing antibodies capable of neutralizing them and preventing infection. These neutralizing antibodies are produced by terminally differentiated B cells known as plasma cells and can facilitate opsonization, phagocytosis, and complement activation through the classical pathway.

14. **How does cell-mediated immunity work?**
T lymphocytes, the main effectors of cell-mediated immunity, orchestrate antigen-specific cell-mediated immune responses and can be classified into CD4+ helper T cells and CD8+ cytotoxic T cells. Helper T cells kill phagocytosed microbes via macrophage and lymphocyte activation, and cytotoxic T cells kill intracellular pathogens.

15. **What are the major advantages and disadvantages of the adaptive immune system?**
The advantages are that humoral and cell-mediated immunity mechanisms are specific and induce memory. The disadvantage is that the required expansion process may take more than 2 weeks after the first encounter with antigen. Many infectious agents can cause death or severe disability in less time than it takes the adaptive immune system to mobilize a specific response. This disadvantage leaves a gap in the host defense system.

16. **Explain the role of vaccines in the adaptive immune system.**
Vaccines provide active immunity by inducing a pathogen-specific immune response and memory.

17. **Explain immunologic memory.**
After the initial humoral and cell-mediated immune responses, antigen-specific memory cells are produced allowing for a more rapid and robust response on second encounter with the specific antigen. The innate immune system is inherently involved with the establishment of immunologic memory via pattern recognition induction of antigen-specific memory.

THE MAJOR HISTOCOMPATIBILITY COMPLEX

18. What is the major histocompatibility complex (MHC)?
A complex of genes on chromosome 6 in humans that functions in antigen processing and presentation to T cells.

19. Name the three main classes of MHC molecules and their subtypes.
- Class I MHC molecules are found on almost all nucleated cells and include HLA-A (human leukocyte antigen A), HLA-B, and HLA-C molecules.
- Class II MHC molecules are found only on antigen-presenting cells (APCs), including dendritic cells, monocytes, macrophages, and B cells. The class II MHC molecules include HLA-DR, HLA-DQ, and HLA-DP. MHC "nonclassical" class I molecules include HLA-E, HLA-F, HLA-G, and may play a role in immunosuppression and immunoregulation.
- Class III MHC molecules include complement components C2, C4, and factor B, as well as tumor necrosis factor (TNF)-α and lymphotoxin (TNF-β and LTβ).

20. What are the function and structure of class I and II MHC molecules?
To facilitate antigen presentation and processing. MHC class I molecules are responsible for presenting antigenic peptides to CD8$^+$ T cells, and class II MHC molecules are responsible for presenting antigenic peptides to CD4$^+$ T cells. CD8$^+$ T cells recognize the α_3 domain of the class I MHC molecule, and CD4$^+$ T cells recognize the β_2 subunit of the class II MHC molecule. The peptide binding site for class I MHC molecules is composed of the α_1 and α_2 domains, and the peptide binding site for class II MHC molecules is composed of the α_1 and β_1 domains.

21. What two signals are required to activate naïve T cells?
Signal 1 in the activation process is the interaction of the MHC-antigenic peptide complex with the TCR. Signal 2 involves costimulatory molecules expressed by the APC in response to microbes, adjuvants and cytokines (IFN-γ, e.g., from T cells), and costimulatory receptors on T cells. If costimulatory signaling molecules are not expressed and do not interact with their corresponding receptors, the T cell–MHC interaction may induce the T cell to undergo anergy.

22. Describe the concept of cross-presentation.
In cross-presentation, viruses and tumors infecting non-APCs are presented for recognition by cytotoxic T cells via a non–class I pathway mediated by dendritic cells. Dendritic cells ingest the virus/tumor-infected cells, process their antigenic peptides, and present them via class I MHC molecules to CD8$^+$ T cells. Normally as aforementioned, endocytosed proteins are processed and presented via class II molecules.

23. What are superantigens, and how do they bind to MHC molecules and TCR?
Microbial products able to induce large-scale immune activation and function by binding to the Vβ-region of the TCR and to class II MHC molecules. Examples of *Staphylococcus aureus* superantigens include TSST-1, and the staphylococcal enterotoxin (SE) families, and SE-like. Group A streptococci can produce superantigens as well, such as SSA and the families SPE and SMEZ.

24. What viruses can target the production of class I MHC molecules?
Epstein-Barr virus (EBV) and cytomegalovirus (CMV) can inhibit proteasome activity, herpes simplex virus (HSV) can block TAP transport, adenovirus and CMV can block the MHC synthesis, and CMV can remove class I molecules from the endoplasmic reticulum.

T-CELL BIOLOGY

25. How does the thymus develop?
From the third and fourth pharyngeal pouches, thymus development is completed by the first trimester. FoxN1 and TBX1 are two important transcription factors involved with thymic organogenesis.

26. What is the function of autoimmune regulatory (AIRE) protein in the thymus?
To establish central tolerance. The AIRE protein is encoded by the *AIRE* gene and is present in the thymic medulla. It plays a role in establishing central tolerance. Medullary thymic epithelial cells (mTECs) express tissue-restricted antigens (TRAs) normally expressed outside the thymus. Normally, TRAs can be recognized by immature T cells, leading to destruction of autoreactive T cells via negative selection. However, in those with a mutation in AIRE there is a failure of central tolerance

resulting in an autosomal recessive disease called *autoimmune polyendocrinopathy candidiasis–ectodermal dystrophy* (APECED). Individuals with this mutation suffer from autoimmune endocrine disorders such as hypoparathyroidism, Addison disease, and diabetes mellitus type 1 (DM1), as well as mucocutaneous candidiasis, ectodermal dystrophy, and recurrent infections.

27. **Summarize the role of T cells and their maturation process (central tolerance).**
    T cells function as both effectors and regulators of the immune response and are derived from embryonic hematopoietic stem cells in the bone marrow. Unlike B cells, which complete their maturation in the bone marrow, T cells undergo maturation in the thymus. T-cell tolerance mechanisms at two levels (central and peripheral) help maintain immunologic tolerance and prevent autoimmunity. Central tolerance involves positive selection in the thymic cortex and negative selection in the medulla. Negative selection involves removal of T cells whose TCR binds with high affinity to TRA-MHC complexes on mTECs. T cells with TCR binding with low affinity to TRA-MHC complexes undergo apoptosis.

28. **What are T-cell receptor excision circles (TRECs)?**
    DNA segments excised out during intrathymic T-cell receptor gene rearrangement. TRECs are a markers of proliferation and recombination (most recombination produces TRECs) and can be measured by quantitative polymerase chain reaction (PCR). This is clinically relevant as TREC levels are determined in many states during the newborn screening process and are low or undetectable in individuals with severe combined immunodeficiency (SCID) or complete DiGeorge syndrome.

29. **Describe the mechanisms of peripheral T-cell tolerance.**
    Anergy, suppression, and apoptosis. Anergy occurs if the TCR is able to recognize a self-antigen but there is no costimulation (either because of a signaling block or inhibitory receptor such as PD-1 or CTLA-4 binding to their respective ligand). Suppression is mediated by regulatory T cells via cytokine production of interleukin 10 (IL-10) or TGF-β, for example. Apoptosis is described later.

30. **What are the major subtypes of T cells?**
    CD4$^+$ T cells and CD8$^+$ T cells.

31. **Describe the principal function of CD4$^+$ T cells.**
    As helper/inducer T cells that provide soluble and cognate signals to (1) B cells to stimulate antibody production, (2) CD8$^+$ cytolytic T cells, and (3) monocytes and macrophages to facilitate their ability to carry out cell-mediated immune responses.

32. **Describe the principal function of CD8 T cells.**
    To recognize class I MHC molecules, kill infected cells, and activate macrophages.

33. **Describe the main subsets of T helper cells (T$_H$, CD4$^+$) and their properties.**
    T$_H$1, T$_H$2, T$_H$17, T$_{FH}$ (also described are T$_H$9, T$_H$22). T$_H$1 cells have the master transcription factor T-bet; are induced by IL-12, STAT4, and STAT1; and produce IFN-γ. T$_H$2 cells have the master transcription factor GATA3; are induced by IL-4 and STAT6; and produce IL-4, IL-5, IL-9, and IL-13. T$_H$17 cells have the master transcription factor RORC2; are induced by IL-1β, IL-6, IL-23, and STAT3; and produce IL-17, IL-21, IL-22, and IL-26. T$_{FH}$ cells have the master transcription factor Bcl6 and IRF4; are induced by IL-6 and IL-21 and STAT3, STAT4, and STAT1; and produce IL-21, IL-10, and IL-4.

34. **Summarize the development of regulatory T cells (Tregs).**
    During negative selection, DP (DP = CD4$^+$ CD8$^+$ double positive) T cells expressing TCRs with high-affinity to self-peptide-MHC complexes normally undergo negative selection, but a select population of Foxp3$^+$ T cells matures into regulatory T cells capable of suppressing autoreactive T cells in the periphery. This is crucial as negative selection does not completely prevent the generation of autoreactive mature T cells, and peripheral immunologic tolerance mechanisms in the periphery are required.

35. **What are NKT cells?**
    Thymus-derived cells that are CD1d-restricted and capable of recognizing glycolipid antigens. The strongest stimulus for NKT cells is α-GalCer (α-galactosylceramide). NKT cells classically possess invariant chains Vα24, Jα18, and Vβ11. CD4$^+$ NKT cells can produce IL-4, TNF, and IFN-γ, whereas CD4$^-$ NKT cells produce TNF and IFN-γ.

36. **Describe the effect of aging on T-cell populations.**
    With aging, there is an increase in mature T cells (CD45RO) and T effector memory (TEM) cells and a decrease in T central memory (TCM) cells. Additionally, susceptibility to viral infections increases, vaccine responses decrease, and reactivation of latent viruses occurs.

B-CELL BIOLOGY

37. **What are B lymphocytes (B cells)?**

Circulating lymphocytes derived from hematopoietic stem cells that are the precursors of plasma cells, the antibody- or immunoglobulin (Ig)-producing cells in the body. They differentiate from stem cells and complete their development in the bone marrow (unlike T cells, which complete maturation in the thymus), and migrate through the blood, lymph, and secondary lymphoid tissues (spleen, lymph nodes, and respiratory and gastrointestinal [GI] submucosal tissues).

38. **Briefly describe the main stages of B-cell development.**

Human B-cell development is a continuum of checkpoints starting with pluripotent hematopoietic stem cells in the fetal liver during embryonic development and ending with mature B cells in the bone marrow after birth. Developing B cells undergo a series of antigen receptor constructs and modifications using hierarchical gene rearrangement and positive/negative selection. The main stages of B-cell development include the stem cell, pro–B cell, pre–B cell, immature B cell, mature B cell, and plasma cell. In the pro–B-cell stage, recombination proteins RAG-1 and RAG-2 are expressed, as are CD19 and CD10. Heavy-chain D and J gene segments undergo the first recombination, and then the V heavy-chain gene segment is combined with the DJ unit. The pre–B-cell stage is defined by the presence of a successful Ig μ heavy chain rearrangement and surrogate light chains (λ5 and V pre-B). Allelic exclusion can occur during this stage. In the immature B-cell stage, light chain rearrangement occurs (κ before λ), and the resultant κ light chain will combine with the already produced μ chain to generate an IgM protein. Mature B cells express both IgM and IgD, with IgD generated via alternative splicing of the VDJ-C RNA.

39. **What is the 12/23 rule?**

V(D)J recombination only involves gene segments with dissimilar recombination signal sequences (RSS-12 and RSS-23). The recombination sequences contain heptamer and nonamer motifs separated by spacers of 12 base pairs and 23 base pairs (RSS-12 and RSS-23, respectively). The RSS-23 signal flanks both V_H and J_H gene segments and the RSS-23 signal flanks either side of the D_H gene segments, and as such, the V_H and J_H gene segments cannot recombine together and must include a D_H gene segment.

40. **What is the importance of RAG-1 and RAG-2 in B-cell development?**

RAG-1 and RAG-2 are recombination proteins that regulate V(D)J recombination of immunoglobulins and T-cell receptors (TCRs) and are present in B and T lymphocytes only. Deficiencies in RAG-1 and RAG-2 lead to SCID (phenotype T-B-NK+) as signaling is precluded due to the lack of antigen receptors.

41. **What is allelic exclusion?**

A regulatory process by which only one heavy chain allele is rearranged successfully even though an individual can inherit two heavy chain alleles. Apoptosis can result if two nonproductive heavy chains are generated.

42. **What are the three main types of mature B cells?**

B-1 cells, marginal zone B cells, and B-2 cells. B-1 cells are produced in the fetus and produce natural antibodies. They are T-independent and produce short-lived plasma cells. Marginal zone B cells are localized to the marginal zone of the spleen, are also T-independent, and can respond rapidly to polysaccharides. They are able to generate IgM and IgG specificity toward polysaccharides and generate short-lived plasma cells. B-2 cells are conventional B cells produced in the bone marrow that are T-cell dependent and respond to protein antigens. They are capable of producing isotype-switched, high-affinity antibodies and long-lived plasma cells.

43. **What are the defects underlying B-cell deficiencies?**

An inability to produce immunoglobulins due to deficiencies in RAG, failure to produce the B-cell receptor (BCR) due to deficiencies in the components (surrogate light chains V pre-β or λ5, Igα or Igβ), failure to signal through the BCR (Bruton tyrosine kinase [BTK] deficiency leading to X-linked agammaglobulinemia, or B-cell linker protein [BLNK] deficiency), or failure to regulate RAG rearrangements (seen in Burkitt lymphoma and follicular lymphoma).

44. **What are regulatory B cells (Bregs)?**

A new subset of B cells that can induce tolerance via IL-10 production and have been shown to inhibit T_H2 responses in allergic individuals. These regulatory B cells also exhibit antigen specificity and have been found in higher numbers in the circulation of those undergoing venom immunotherapy.

IMMUNOGLOBULINS

45. Define and explain the basic structure of an immunoglobulin.

Ig molecules are composed of two identical heavy chains and two identical light chains. Each light and heavy chain combines to form an antigen-binding cleft at their amino terminus, and the two heavy chains associate with each other at their carboxy end. The combined variable regions of the amino terminus (antigen-binding fragment known as Fab) are functionally distinct from the heavy chain constant region at the carboxy terminus (crystallizable fragment known as Fc). V_L and V_H have three regions (complementarity determining regions) where the amino acid sequences are highly variable and confer specificity. Notably, CDR3 is the most variable. The Fc protion can bind to Fc receptors, structures largely found on effector cells of the immune systems. The Fab regions are linked to the Fc regions via hinge segments. See Fig. 11.1.

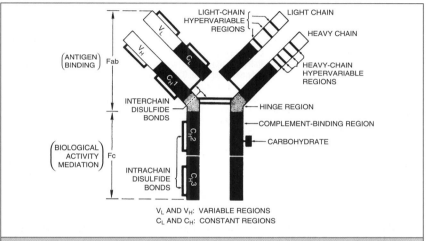

Fig. 11.1. Chain and domain structure of an immunoglobulin (Ig) molecule with hypervariable regions within variable regions of both H and L chains. Fab and Fc refer to fragments of the IgG molecule formed by protein cleavage. The former contains the VH and CH1 H chain regions and intact L chain; the latter consists of the CH2 and CH3 regions of two H chains linked to one another by disulfide bonds. *(From Wasserman RL, Capra JD. Immunoglobulin. In Horowitz MI, Pigman W, editors.* The Glycoconjugates. *New York: Academic Press; 1977, pp 323–348, used with permission.)*

46. Describe the process and function of immunoglobulin V(D)J rearrangement.

RAG-1 and RAG-2 first bind to the V and J genes and then cleave next to the RSS segments described earlier. Ku 70/80 protects the cleaved DNA and recruits DNA PK. DNA PK phosphorylates Artemis, which then opens the hairpins created by RAG-1 and RAG-2. Ligase IV, XRCC4, and Cernunnos/XLF complex catalyzes the ligation/repair of the ends. Terminal deoxynucleotidyl transferase (TdT) performs random modifications to the 3′ terminus of the DNA and provides junctional diversity. V(D)J is critical in generating antigen-independent diversity in the variable domains of immunoglobulin (and TCR genes).

47. How do papain and pepsin cleave immunoglobulins?

- **Papain:** into 2 Fab fragments and 1 Fc fragment
- **Pepsin:** into a bivalent F(ab′)$_2$ fragment and small Fc fragments

48. What are the members of the immunoglobulin superfamily?

MHC molecules, TCR, CD4/CD8, CD19, B7-1/B7-2, Fc receptors, KIR, VCAM-1.

49. Summarize the classes of the heavy chains and light chains of Ig.

There are five classes of heavy chains (mu, gamma, alpha, epsilon, and delta) that form the five isotypes or Ig classes: IgM, IgG, IgA, IgE, and IgD, respectively. There are two types of light chains, kappa and lambda, that are used by all Ig classes. IgG, IgA, and IgD each have three C_H domains, whereas IgM and E both have four C_H domains. IgA can polymerize into dimers and higher multimers. Secreted IgM is a pentamer of five basic subunits joined by a protein called "J," the joining piece. IgD, IgE, and IgG exist as monomers.

50. **Describe the process of class switch recombination.**
    Immunoglobulin class switch recombination is also known as *isotype switching* and allows for the generation of immunoglobulins with different isotypes. Different isotypes are stimulated by cytokines such as IFN-γ for IgG, IL-4 for IgE/IgG4, and TFG-β/IL-5/BAFF/APRIL for IgA, for example, and costimulation via signal 2 of the antigen-antibody complex (e.g., CD40-CD40L interaction). Germline transcription is initiated at switch regions upstream from the gene segments encoding the targeted constant region gene, leading to recombination of the VDJ exon with the desired gene segment exon. Unlike antigen receptor rearrangement in immunoglobulin and TCR genes, isotype switching utilizes activation-induced cytidine deaminase (AID) and uracil *N*-glycosylase (UNG) at switch regions rather than RAG-1 and RAG-2 (at RSS regions) to initiate DNA strand breaks. AID serves to deaminate cytosine residues to uracil residues and UNG excises uracil residues so that Ape I endonuclease can generate nicks that lead to double-stranded breaks. The notable exception is the isotype IgD, which is produced by alternative splicing due to the δ gene transcript's proximity to that of the μ gene.

51. **What are the features of primary and secondary antibody responses?**
    A primary antibody response occurs after the first exposure to an antigen, whereas a secondary antibody response occurs with the second and subsequent exposures. A secondary response is faster and bigger and contains antibodies that bind with higher affinity to antigen and a greater diversity of T cells that react with the target antigens. In a secondary response, the antibody levels increase, and new effector T cells enter the circulation within 1–2 days. In contrast, during a primary response, the emergence of these elements of an adaptive response can take a week or more. During a secondary response, the quantity of antibodies and the number of effector T cells are increased 10-fold or higher. The average affinity of the antigen-binding sites is also higher in a secondary response. Finally, during a secondary response, more of the antibodies belong to the IgG class, whereas in a primary response most of the antibodies are IgM. Major features of these two responses are illustrated in Figs. 11.2 and 11.3.

52. **What are the physical and biologic properties of the different classes of Ig?**
    See Table 11.2.

53. **What is the function of neonatal Fc receptor (FcRn) in humans?**
    To enable maternal IgG to be transported to the fetus. The FcRn resembles a class I MHC molecule and is localized in the placenta during pregnancy. In adults, endosomal FcRn functions to regulate serum IgG levels by sequestering IgG molecules intracellularly to protect against lysosomal degradation. The IgG half-life is high due to IgG binding to FcRn.

54. **Name and define the three main antigenic determinants.**
    The three main antigenic determinants are conformational, linear, and neoantigenic.
    - **Conformational:** Determinants are epitopes whose amino acids may be located far from one another and require protein folding for juxtaposition.

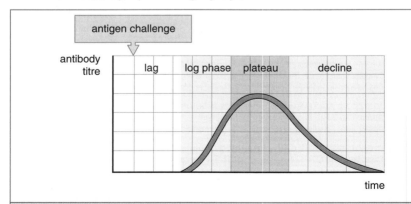

Fig. 11.2. After antigen challenge, the primary antibody response proceeds in four phases: (1) a lag phase when no antibody is detected; (2) a log phase in which the antibody titer rises logarithmically; (3) a plateau phase during which the antibody titer stabilizes; and (4) a decline phase during which the antibody is cleared or catabolized. *(From Roitt IM, Brostoff J, Male DK.* Immunology. *New York: Gower Medical; 1989, p 8.1, used with permission.)*

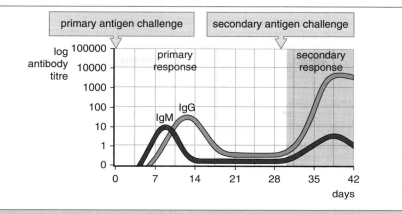

Fig. 11.3. Primary and secondary antibody responses. In comparison with the antibody response to primary antigenic challenge, the antibody level after secondary antigenic challenge in a typical immune response (1) appears more quickly and persists for longer, (2) attains a high titer, and (3) consists predominantly of IgG. In the primary response the appearance of IgG is preceded by IgM. *(From Roitt IM, Brostoff J, Male DK. Immunology. New York: Gower Medical; 1989, p 8.1, with permission.)*

Table 11.2. Physical and Biologic Properties of Human Immunoglobulins*

PROPERTY	IgG	IgA	IgM	IgD	IgE
Molecular form	Monomer	Monomer, polymer	Pentamer	Monomer	Monomer
Subclasses	IgG1, 2, 3, 4	IgA1, 2	None	None	None
Molecular weight	150,000 for IgG-1, 2, 4 180,000 for IgG3	160,000 + polymers	950,000	175,000	190,000
Serum level (mg/mL)	9, 3, 1, 0.5	2.1	1.5	4	0.03
Serum half-life (days)	23D for IgG1, 2, 4 7D for IgG3	6	5	3	3
Complement fixation	IgG1, 2, 3	(−)	+	(−)	(−)
Alternative pathway activation	IgG4	+	(−)	+	?
Placental transfer	+	(−)	(−)	(−)	(−)
Other properties	Secondary response	Abundant in mucous secretions	Primary response, rheumatoid factor	−	Binds to mast cells

*The plus and minus signs indicate whether the molecules have or do not have the indicated property.
Ig, immunoglobulin.
Modified from Paul WE. *Fundamental Immunology.* 2nd ed. New York: Raven Press; 1989; and Samter M, Talmage MM, Frank DF, et al, editors. *Immunological Diseases.* 4th ed. Boston: Little, Brown; 1988, p 44.

- **Linear:** Determinants are epitopes composed of linear stretches of consecutive amino acids in denatured or native proteins.
- **Neoantigenic:** Determinants are epitopes generated by proteolysis, phosphorylation or glycosylation.

55. Recognition of antigen by antibody requires which type of binding?
Noncovalent and reversible binding.

CHEMOKINES AND CYTOKINES

56. What is the cluster designation (CD) nomenclature for phenotyping cells?
The CD nomenclature is a system for the identification of cell surface antigens that have been defined by monoclonal antibodies. The development of a monoclonal antibody to a cell surface protein is one important step in its characterization. These antibodies allow identification of target proteins on cell surfaces. They can be used to help purify the proteins and illuminate their function. Over 200 CD antigens have been recognized thus far by international committees that assign these numbers. CD markers identify targets that can be used to remove whole classes of cells from the circulation by means of cytolytic monoclonal antibodies or by machines, called "cell sorters," that recognize and segregate cells expressing specific molecules identified by monoclonal antibodies.

57. How is the CD nomenclature used in clinical medicine?
Antibodies to CD3 and CD4 have been used to help control transplant rejection reactions by removing and inactivating the effector T cells. A few important CD markers are listed in Table 11.3.

58. What are cytokines, where are they made, and what do they do?
Proteins produced by many cells, not necessarily only cells of the immune system, that function as intracellular signaling molecules, usually within the radius of a few cell diameters. There are at present more than 38 cytokines (Table 11.4).

59. What are main interferons (IFNs)?
There are several main classes of interferons: IFN-α, IFN-β, IFN-γ, and IFN-λ. IFN-α and IFN-β were previously classified as type I, IFN-γ as type II, and IFN- λ as type III. IFN-β is divided into two major subtypes: IFN-β_1 and IFN-β_2.

60. How are IFN-α, IFN-β_1, and IFN-β_2 produced?
- **IFN-α:** by leukocytes, fibroblasts (to a lesser degree), and other cells and is composed of 20 or more subtypes.
- **IFN-β_1:** by fibroblasts, leukocytes (to a lesser degree), and many other cells.
- **IFN-β_2 (IL-6):** by fibroblasts, T cells, monocytes, and endothelial cells.

61. Summarize the major functions of IFN-α, IFN-β_1, and IFN-β_2.
Both IFN-α and IFN-β_1 modulate antibody production, graft rejection, and delayed-type hypersensitivity (DTH) reactions. They can induce autoimmune and inflammatory reactions, and they have important antiviral, antibacterial, antifungal, and antitumor activities. IFN-β_2 has important immunomodulatory activity and poor antiviral activity. It has also been called "B-cell differentiation factor" because it stimulates mature B cells to differentiate into Ig-secreting plasma cells. It also plays a role in early hematopoiesis and may be an important autocrine growth factor for B-cell malignancies. IRF3 and IRF7 (involved in the TLR signaling pathway) can promote type 1 interferon production.

62. What produces IFN-γ? Summarize its functions.
Activated T lymphocytes, NK cells, and lymphokine-activated killer (LAK) cells. IFN-γ is unrelated to the other IFNs in either structure or function. Its biologic effects include enhancing cytotoxic T-cell and NK-cell activity, induction of class II antigen expression on B cells and other APCs, and induction of IL-2 receptor expression on T cells. It downregulates collagen synthesis and inhibits IL-4–induced IgE synthesis.

63. Deficiency in IFN-γ leads to what clinical phenotype?
Mendelian susceptibility to bacillus Calmette-Guérin vaccine and nontuberculous mycobacterial infections.

Table 11.3. CD Markers, Isoforms, Sites of Expression, and Function

SURFACE MARKER	ISOFORMS	SITES OF EXPRESSION	COMMENTS
CD2	50-kD protein	Thymocytes, T cells, NK cells (large granular lymphocytes)	Adhesion molecule that binds to LFA-3, a ligand on APC. Ligation with LFA-3 activates T cells
CD3	γ: 25-kD glycoprotein δ: 20-kD glycoprotein ε: 20-kD protein	Thymocytes, T cells	Associated with TCR. Required for cell surface expression of TCR
CD4	57-kD glycoprotein	Thymocytes, T_H1 and T_H2 T cells, monocytes, and some macrophages	Coreceptor for MHC class II, and for HIV-1 + HIV-2 gp120
CD8	α: 32-kD glycoprotein β: 32–34 kD	Thymocytes, CD8 T cells	Coreceptor for MHC class I; anti-CD8 blocks cytotoxic T-cell responses
CD16	50–80 kD	NK cells, granulocytes, macrophages	Low-affinity Fc receptor (FcγRIII) that plays a role in antibody-dependent cell-mediated cytotoxicity and activation of NK cells
CD19	95 kD	B cells	Coreceptor for B cells involved in B-cell activation
CD28	44-kD homodimer	T-cell subsets Activated B cells	Binding to CD80 (on B cells) or CD86 (on macrophages or dendritic cells) sends costimulatory, differentiation-inducing signal
CD45RO	180-kD glycoprotein	Memory T cells, B-cell subsets, monocytes	See CD45RA
CD45RA	205–220-kD glycoprotein	Naïve T cells, B cells, monocytes	Role in signal transduction, tyrosine phosphatase
CD56	135–220-kD heterodimer	NK cells	Promotes adhesion of NK cells
CD80	60-kD protein	B-cell subset Ligand for CD28 on T cells	Costimulator involved in antigen presentation
CD86	80-kD protein	Activated B cells Monocytes, dendritic cells	Costimulatory ligand for CD28 on T cells, during antigen presentation

APC, antigen-presenting cell; HIV, human immunodeficiency virus; LFA, leukocyte function-associated antigen; MHC, major histocompatibility complex; NK, natural killer; TCR, T-cell receptor; T_H2, T helper 2 cell. From David J. Immunology. In Dale DC, Federman DD, editors. *Scientific American Medicine*. New York: Scientific American; 1996, p 6; and Janeway CA, Travers P, Walport M, Capra JD, editors. *Immunobiology*. 4th ed. London: Current Biology Publications; and New York: Garland Publishing; 1999.

COMPLEMENT SYSTEM

64. Describe the major functions of the complement system in host defense.

The complement system is an integral part of humoral immunity involved with complement-mediated cytolysis, inflammatory responses through anaphylatoxins and leukocyte recruitment, and opsonization/phagocytosis. C3b, generated by the cleavage of C3, binds to the surface of antigens and facilitates phagocytosis via recognition by neutrophils and monocytes expressing the C3b receptor. The binding of C3b to microbes and proteolysis of C5 leads to the release of anaphylatoxins C3a and C5a, respectively. C3a and C5a are termed *anaphylatoxins* as they are capable of inducing mast cell degranulation. C5a and, to some extent, C3a are chemotactic for neutrophils and

Table 11.4. Actions of Cytokines Relevant to Allergic and Immune Responses

CYTOKINE	EFFECTS
GM-CSF	Secreted by activated macrophages, T cells, mast cells, eosinophils, and other cells. Promotes differentiation of neutrophils and macrophages. Activates mature eosinophils. Prolongs eosinophil survival.
IFN-γ	Derived mainly from T_H1 lymphocytes, cytotoxic T cells, NK cells, but also macrophages. Represents the most important cytokine activator of macrophages. Increases expression of class I and II MHC antigens. Stimulates B-cell proliferation and differentiation. Inhibits IL-4–induced IgE synthesis. Inhibits T_H2 lymphocytes. Induces ICAM-1 expression.
IL-1	IL-1 family contains IL-1α, IL-1β, the IL-1 receptor antagonist (IL-1ra), and IL-18. Produced mainly by monocytes and macrophages but also by lymphocytes and other cells. Induced by endotoxin, microorganisms, antigens, and cytokines. Increases proliferation of B cells and antibody synthesis. Promotes growth of T_H cells in response to APCs. Stimulates production of T-cell cytokines and IL-2 receptors. Without IL-1, tolerance develops or immune response is impaired. Promotes formation of arachidonic acid metabolites, including PGE_2 and LTB_4. Induces proliferation of fibroblasts and synthesis of fibronectin and collagen. Increases ICAM-1, VCAM-1, E-selectin, and P-selectin expression. IL-1ra antagonizes proinflammatory effects of IL-1.
IL-2	Induces clonal T-cell proliferation. Enhances proliferation of cytotoxic T cells, B cells, NK cells, macrophages.
IL-3	Derived primarily from T_H cells but also from mast cells and eosinophils. Stimulates development of mast cells, lymphocytes, macrophages. Activates eosinophils. Prolongs eosinophil survival.
IL-4	Preformed peptide in mast cells and eosinophils. Also secreted by T_H2 cells, cytotoxic T cells, and basophils. Promotes growth of T_H2 cells, cytotoxic T cells, mast cells, eosinophils, basophils.
IL-4	Initiates IgE isotype switching. Upregulates expression of high- and low-affinity IgE receptors. Increases expression of class I and II MHC antigens on macrophages. Stimulates VCAM-1 expression.
IL-5	Produced by T_H2 cells and mast cells. Attracts eosinophils. Activates eosinophils. Prolongs eosinophil survival.
IL-6	Synthesized primarily by monocytes and macrophages but also by T, B, and other cells. Mediates T-cell activation, growth, differentiation. Induces B-cell differentiation into plasma cells. Inhibits TNF and IL-1 synthesis and stimulates IL-1ra synthesis.
IL-7	Necessary for development of B and T cells. Enhances growth of cytotoxic T and NK cells. Increases tumor killing by monocytes and macrophages.
IL-8	Produced mainly by monocytes, phagocytes, and endothelial cells. Exerts potent chemoattraction for neutrophils. Attracts activated eosinophils. Induces neutrophil degranulation and activation. Inhibits IL-4–mediated IgE synthesis.

Table 11.4. Actions of Cytokines Relevant to Allergic and Immune Responses *(Continued)*

CYTOKINE	EFFECTS
IL-9	Produced by T$_H$2 cells. Promotes mast cell and T-cell proliferation. Stimulates IgE synthesis. Produces eosinophilia. Induces bronchial hyperreactivity.
IL-10	Secreted primarily by monocytes and B cells. Inhibits monocyte/macrophage function. Stimulates growth of mast cells, B cells, and cytotoxic T cells. Induces permanent tolerance in T$_H$ lymphocytes. Decreases synthesis of IFN-γ and IL-2 by T$_H$1 cells. Inhibits IL-4–induced IgE synthesis and promotes IgG4 production. Decreases eosinophil survival.
IL-11	Produced in response to respiratory viral infections. Promotes generation of mast cells and B cells. Induces bronchial hyperreactivity.
IL-12	Synthesized by monocytes/macrophages, dendritic cells, B cells, neutrophils, mast cells. Induced by IFN-γ and microorganisms.
IL-12	Promotes T$_H$1 and inhibits T$_H$2 cell development. Inhibits IL-4–induced IgE synthesis. Enhances activity of cytotoxic T cells and NK cells.
IL-13	Produced by T$_H$1 and T$_H$2 cells, mast cells, and dendritic cells. Exerts effects similar to IL-4 on B cells and macrophages but does not affect T cells. Induces IgE isotype switching. Increases VCAM-1 expression. Promotes airway hyperreactivity and mucus hypersecretion. Suppresses production of proinflammatory cytokines and chemokines. Decreases synthesis of nitric oxide.
IL-16	Secreted by CD8$^+$ T cells, eosinophils, mast cells, and epithelial cells. Promotes growth of CD4$^+$ T cells. Provides major source of CD4$^+$ T-cell chemotactic activity after antigen challenge. Induces IL-2 receptors and class II MHC expression on CD4$^+$ T cells.
IL-18	Produced by lung, liver, and other tissues but not by lymphocytes. Stimulates secretion of IFN-γ and GM-CSF. Enhances IgE synthesis. Promotes T$_H$1 responses and activates NK cells (similar to IL-12). Induces synthesis of TNF, IL-1, Fas ligand. Decreases IL-10 synthesis.
IL-23	Induces secretion of IFN-γ.
TGF-α	Synthesized by macrophages and keratinocytes. Stimulates proliferation of fibroblasts. Promotes angiogenesis.
TGF-β	Secreted by platelets, monocytes, some T cells (T$_H$3), and fibroblasts. Stimulates monocytes and fibroblasts, inducing fibrosis and extracellular matrix formation. Attracts mast cells, macrophages, fibroblasts. Inhibits B cells, T$_H$ cells, cytotoxic T cells, NK cells, mast cells. Induces IgA isotype switching and secretory IgA synthesis in gut lymphoid tissue. Inhibits airway smooth muscle cell proliferation.

Continued

Table 11.4. Actions of Cytokines Relevant to Allergic and Immune Responses *(Continued)*

CYTOKINE	EFFECTS
TNF-α	Produced primarily by mononuclear phagocytes; stored preformed in mast cells. Induced by endotoxin, GM-CSF, IFN-γ, IL-1, and IL-3. Binds to cell surface receptors TNFR I and TNFR II. Enhances class I and II MHC expression. Activates neutrophils, modulating adherence, chemotaxis, degranulation, respiratory burst. Increases cytokine production by monocytes and airway epithelial cells.
TNF-α	Promotes ICAM-1, VCAM-1, and E-selectin expression. Stimulates COX-2 expression in airway smooth muscle. Induces bronchial hyperreactivity. Mediates toxic shock and sepsis. Produces cachexia associated with chronic infection and cancer.
TNF-β	Synthesized primarily by lymphocytes. Binds to cell surface receptors TNFR I and TNFR II. Mediates functions similar to TNF-α.

APC, antigen-presenting cell; COX-2, cyclooxygenase-2; GM-CSF, granulocyte macrophage–stimulating factor; ICAM-1, intercellular adhesion molecule-1; IFN, interferon; Ig, immunoglobulin; IL, interleukin; IL-1ra, interleukin-1 receptor antagonist; LT, leukotriene; MHC, major histocompatibility complex; NK, natural killer; PG, prostaglandin; TGF, tumor growth factor; T_H, T helper cell; TNF, tumor necrosis factor; VCAM, vascular cell adhesion protein.

From Hamilton ME. Immunology and pathophysiology of allergic disease. In Naguwa SM, Gershwin ME, editors. *Allergy and Immunology Secrets.* Philadelphia: Hanley & Belfus; 2001.

monocytes and serve to recruit leukocytes into sites of inflammation. The terminal complement components, C6, C7, C8, and C9, form the membrane attack complex (MAC), a tubular structure that generates pores in the plasma membrane leading to cytolysis. Fig. 11.4 summarizes specific functions of the complement system.

65. **Summarize the activation sequences of the classical complement pathways.**
Initiation of classical complement pathway activation occurs with the binding of the C1 complex to antigen-bound IgG or IgM and proceeds through the activation cascade shown in Fig. 11.5. C1 is a protein complex composed of C1q, C1r, and C1s, and activation requires binding of two of the five heads of C1q to Fc regions of IgG and IgM molecules. C1r is then activated and able to cleave C1s, which in turn cleaves C4 to generate C4b and releasing C4a (another anaphylatoxin like C3a and C5a described earlier). C4b remains cell surface bound and complexes with C2, which is cleaved by a neighboring C1s molecule to generate C2a, which remains bound to C4b (to generate C3 convertase) and C2b (function unknown). C4bC2a becomes the classical pathway C3 convertase and can proteolytically cleave C3.

66. **What factors cause activation of the classical complement pathway?**
Antibody-antigen (immune) complexes. C1q cannot readily bind free circulating antibodies as it requires two IgG molecules for activation. Similarly, the binding site for C1q in the IgM molecule undergoes a conformational change only when the antibody binds antigen. Therefore, free circulating IgM antibodies cannot activate complement. Certain viruses, urate crystals, DNA, and mitochondria that are released by damaged cells also activate the classical pathway by binding C1q.

67. **Which immunoglobulin isotypes are the most efficient activators of the classical complement pathway?**
IgM > IgG1/3 > IgG2. IgG4 cannot activate complement.

68. **Summarize the activation sequences of the alternative complement pathways.**
Activation of the alternative pathway is initiated by binding of C3b to the surface of antigens. C3 normally undergoes C3 "tickover" in plasma, a process whereby C3 undergoes low-level spontaneous cleavage leading to C3b formation. C3b can then bind covalently to microbial surfaces and binds factor B. Factor B is cleaved by factor D generating a Bb fragment and a Ba fragment. The

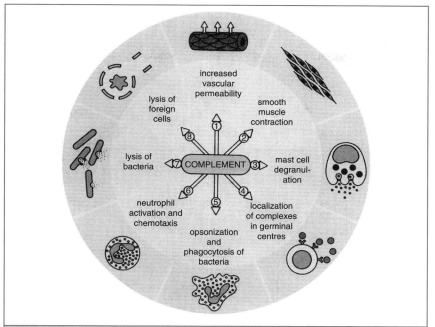

Fig. 11.4. Summary of the actions of complement and its role in the acute inflammatory response. Note how the elements of the reaction are induced. Increased vascular permeability (1) due to the action of C3a and C5a on smooth muscle (2) and mast cells (3) allows exudation of plasma protein. C3 facilitates both the localization of complexes in germinal centers (4) and the opsonization and phagocytosis of bacteria (5). Neutrophils, which are attracted to the area of inflammation by chemotaxis (6), phagocytose the opsonized microorganisms. The membrane attack complex, C5–9, is responsible for lysis of bacteria (7) and other cells recognized as foreign (8). *(From Roitt IM, Brostoff J, Male DK.* Immunology. *New York: Gower Medical; 1989, p 13.11, used with permission.)*

Bb fragment remains attached to C4b, forming the alternative pathway C3 convertase. The activation of C3 and the downstream participation of C5, C6, C7, C8, and C9 is the same for both classical and alternative complement pathways, and the biologic activities of opsonization, recruitment of inflammatory cells, mast cell degranulation, and cell lysis are identical for both pathways. The alternative pathways are depicted in Fig. 11.5.

69. **What factors cause activation of the alternative complement pathway?**
Charge differences, as seen in implantable objects such as Dacron grafts, as well as substances found on bacterial and yeast cell walls. C3 has a highly reactive thioester bond that allows activated C3 to bind covalently to a wide variety of substrates.

70. **Describe the lectin pathway complement activation.**
Circulating lectins, such as mannose-binding lectin (MBL), which structurally resemble C1q of the classical pathway, are a collection of collagen-like proteins that can bind to microbial polysaccharides. MBL binds to MBL-associated serine proteases (MASPs) MASP1 and MASP2, which are structurally homologous to C1r and C1s. MASP2 can cleave C4 and C2 in an activation pathway that is closely homologous to that utilized by the classical complement activation pathway.

71. **What is the common purpose of all of these activation cascades?**
To generate a C5 convertase that cleaves and activates C5 and the remaining elements of complement (C6–9) leading to the formation of the MAC capable of inducing cytolysis.

72. **How does liver disease affect complement levels?**
Because complement proteins are synthesized in the liver, severe liver disease leads to persistently low complement protein levels.

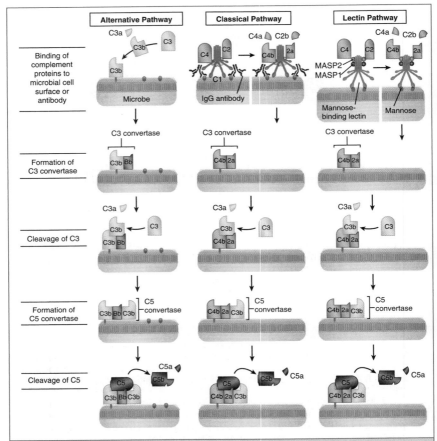

Fig. 11.5. An overview of the complement cascade shows the classical and alternative pathways. The central position of C3 in both pathways is indicated. *(From Samter M, editor.* Immunological Diseases. *4th ed. Boston: Little, Brown; 1998, p 205, used with permission.)*

73. What patterns of serum C3 and C4 levels are seen with activation of the classical and alternative complement pathways? Name at least one disease associated with each pattern.
    See Table 11.5.

Table 11.5. Serum Complement Levels in Disease

PATHWAY	C4	C3	DISEASE
Classical	↓	↓	Systemic lupus erythematosus, serum sickness
Classical (fluid phase)	↓	N	Hereditary angioedema
Alternative	N	↓	Endotoxemia (gram-negative sepsis)
Alternative (fluid phase)	N	↓	Type II membranoproliferative glomerulonephritis (C3 nephritic factor)

↓, decreased; N, normal.

74. Which complement proteins have the strongest association with systemic lupus erythematosus (SLE)?
C1q/r/s.

75. Atypical hemolytic uremic syndrome (aHUS) is associated with which complement proteins/factors?
C3, factor H, factor I, factor B, and MCP. aHUS is secondary to hyperactivation of the alternative complement pathway and has been treated with plasma exchange/infusion as well as kidney transplantation. Posttransplant recurrence in individuals has been treated with the terminal complement inhibitor monoclonal antibody eculizumab.
Noris M, Remuzzi G. Atypical hemolytic-uremic syndrome. *N Engl J Med*. 2009;361:1676–1687.

76. What are the four main complement receptors?
CR1 (CD35), CR2 (CD21), CR3 (Mac-1, CD11bCD18), and CR4 (p150,95, CD11cCD18). CR1 functions to promote phagocytosis of complement-coated particles and to clear circulating immune complexes. CR2 is a receptor involved with B-cell activation and is also a receptor for EBV. CR3 and CR4 are integrins involved with phagocytosis and adhesion.

T-CELL IMMUNODEFICIENCIES

77. Describe the common clinical phenotype of SCID.
Early-onset recurrent infections with low-grade or opportunistic infectious agents, such as fungi, viruses, or protozoa (e.g., *Pneumocystis jirovecii*), failure to thrive, diarrhea, growth retardation, graft-versus-host disease (GVHD) if given nonirradiated blood products or unmatched allogeneic bone marrow, high incidence of malignancy, and fatal infections after live virus vaccines and after vaccination with other attenuated microorganisms including bacille Calmette-Guérin (BCG).

78. Describe the common immunologic phenotypes of SCID.
SCID can be classified into immunologic phenotypes based on the presence or absence of T, B, or NK lymphocytes.
T⁻B⁺NK⁻ SCID is categorized into two main defects: (1) an X-linked SCID with defects in the IL-2 receptor γ gene *(IL2RG)* encoding the common gamma chain (γc—common to the receptors of IL-2, 4, 7, 9, 15, and 21) and (2) an autosomal recessive SCID with defects in *JAK3. JAK3* presents similarly to X-linked SCID due to its physical and functional relationship with γc in the T-cell signaling pathway.
T⁻B⁺NK⁺ SCID involves several defects involved with T-cell development and signaling, including IL-7Rα deficiency, CD3 subunit deficiency (δ, ε, ζ chains), CD45 tyrosine phosphatase deficiency, and more recently discovered coronin-1A deficiency involving defects in thymic egress of mature thymocytes (coronin-1A is an actin cytoskeleton regulator).
T⁻B⁻NK⁻ SCID results from two main defects with autosomal recessive inheritance: (1) adenosine deaminase (ADA) deficiency (ADA mediates conversion of the toxic metabolites adenosine and deoxyadenosine into inosine and deoxyinosine) leading to accumulation of the toxic metabolites, which lead to premature lymphoid progenitor apoptosis in the thymus and bone marrow and subsequent profound lymphopenia, and (2) reticular dysgenesis caused by defects in the mitochondrial enzyme adenylate kinase 2 *(AK2)*, which also leads to marked lymphopenia but also neutropenia and sensorineural deafness.
T⁻B⁻NK⁺ SCID results from defective antigen receptor rearrangement in B and T cells secondary to mutations in the proteins involved with recombination, leading to (1) recombinase-activating gene proteins RAG-1 and RAG-2 deficiency due to mutations in *RAG1* and *RAG2* genes; (2) Artemis deficiency (seen in Athebascan-speaking Native Americans and leads to increased radiation sensitivity); and (3) Cernunnos and DNA ligase IV deficiency resulting also in increased radiation sensitivity, microcephaly, and facial dysmorphisms. NK cells are not affected in this SCID phenotype.

79. Describe Omenn syndrome.
Hypomorphic mutations in *RAG1/RAG2*, IL-7Rα, ADA, Artemis, DNA ligase IV, γc, DiGeorge syndrome, cartilage hypoplasia leading to activated and oligoclonal T lymphocytes that can infiltrate tissue. The clinical presentation involves erythroderma, inflammatory GI disease, failure to thrive, opportunistic infections, hepatosplenomegaly, and lymphadenopathy. There is significant eosinophilia and elevations in IgE.

80. **Summarize the immunodeficiencies caused by thymic defects.**
FoxN1 SCID, DiGeorge syndrome, CHARGE syndrome (Coloboma [eye], Heart defects, Atresia, Retardation, Genital anomaly, Ear anomaly). FoxN1 SCID is associated with nail dystrophy and alopecia. DiGeorge syndrome is characterized by cardiac defects (tetralogy of Fallot, ventricular septal defect, interrupted aortic arch), facial dysmorphisms (short philtrum, low-set ears, hypoplastic mandible, high-arched/cleft palate), impaired development of the thymus and parathyroid glands (hypocalcemia), and psychiatric disorders. Most patients with DiGeorge syndrome possess hemizygous deletions (22q11.2 > 10p13-14). Those with complete DiGeorge syndrome have an SCID-like presentation and athymia, and partial DiGeorge syndrome is marked by oligoclonal T cells that can infiltrate tissue as seen in Omenn syndrome.

81. **Summarize the immunodeficiencies associated with elevated IgE levels.**
Autosomal dominant hyper-IgE syndrome (AD-HIES or Job syndrome): due to a mutation in *STAT3* resulting in a clinical presentation involving early-onset rash, recurrent skin abscesses (typically *Staphylococcus* aureus), recurrent pyogenic pneumonias with pneumatocele development (predisposing to secondary gram-negative and fungal infections), mucocutaneous candidiasis, eosinophilia and markedly elevated IgE levels, musculoskeletal abnormalities (hyperextensibility, scoliosis), vascular abnormalities (arterial involvement), facial dysmorphism (broad nose, prominent forehead), retained primary dentition, and increased risk of malignancy.
DOCK8 deficiency: involves autosomal recessive inheritance, recurrent viral infections (human papillomavirus [HPV], HSV, molluscum contagiosum, varicella), candidiasis, malignancy (lymphoma and squamous cell carcinoma), elevated IgE, low IgM, eosinophilia, and lymphopenia.
Omenn deficiency, atypical complete DiGeorge syndrome: described earlier
Wiskott-Aldrich syndrome: due to an X-linked defect in the *WASp* gene encoding WASp, a cytoskeleton regulator and characterized by early-onset eczema, thrombocytopenia, and recurrent infections (including opportunistic), high incidence of malignancy, and autoimmunity.
IPEX (immune dysregulation polyendocrinopathy enteropathy X-linked syndrome): characterized by early-onset enteropathy (diarrhea, villous atrophy), eczema, cytopenias, and polyendocrinopathy (early-onset DM1 and thyroiditis) due to a defect in the gene encoding FOXP3. Diagnosis includes flow cytometry looking for *FOXP3* expression in Tregs and mutational analysis. Treatment requires immunosuppression and hematopoietic stem cell transplantation (HSCT).
Netherton syndrome (ichthyosis linearis circumflexa): an autosomal recessive disorder characterized by erythroderma, fragile hair shafts, ichthyosis linearis circumflexa, and predisposition to atopy. The syndrome is caused by a mutation in the gene *SPINK5* encoding serine protease-inhibitor Kazal-type 5 (SPINK5/LEKTI) found in epithelial tissue and responsible for the regulation of epithelial desquamation and defense. Tacrolimus administration is a relative contraindication in these patients.

82. **What are the main features of ataxia telangiectasia?**
Ataxia developing in early childhood with onset of telangiectasia in late childhood. Patients are radiation sensitive as the AT protein is involved in DNA repair and blood analysis often reveals increased alpha fetoprotein (AFP) levels and decreased IgA levels.

83. **Summarize the immunodeficiencies associated with lymphoproliferation.**
Autoimmune lymphoproliferative syndrome (ALPS): due to defects in the apoptosis pathway and diagnosed by prominent nonmalignant lymphadenopathy, increased α/β DN T cells, in vitro evidence of defective lymphocyte apoptosis, and positive genetic testing. Clinical presentation includes the aforementioned lymphadenopathy, autoimmune cytopenias, and increased malignancy risk. The majority of ALPS patients have a mutation in the *FAS* gene (associated with increased IL-10, soluble Fas ligand, and vitamin B_{12}). Other mutations in *FASLG* (encoding Fas ligand) and *CASP10* (encoding caspase 10) have been described. RAS-associated leukoproliferative disorder (RALD) is a related disorder with overlap with ALPS, but these patients do not have any abnormal elevation in α/β DN T cells.
X-linked lymphoproliferative syndromes (XLP): associated with EBV-induced lymphoproliferation and categorized into two types:
- XLP1 due to an X-linked defect in the *SH2D1A/SAP* gene
- XLP2 due to an X-linked defect in the *XIAP* gene
XMEN syndrome: described later

Autosomal recessive lymphoproliferative syndrome with hepatosplenomegaly: due to a mutation in the *ITK* gene characterized by recurrent EBV infections and EBV-induced lymphoproliferation and hypogammaglobulinemia.

CD27 deficiency: a combined immunodeficiency associated with EBV-induced lymphoproliferation and hypogammaglobulinemia.

84. **How is hematophagocytic lymphohistiocytosis (HLH) diagnosed?**
    Either by molecular diagnosis that is consistent with HLH or the presence of five of the eight criteria:
    - Fever
    - Splenomegaly
    - Cytopenias affecting at least two of three lineages in peripheral blood
    - Triglycerides $\geq$ 265 mg/dL or fibrinogen $\leq$ 150 mg/dL
    - Ferritin $\geq$ 500 μ/L
    - Low or absent NK-cell activity
    - Soluble CD25 $\geq$ 2400 U/mL
    - Hemophagocytosis in bone marrow, lymph nodes, or spleen

    In addition, there should not be any evidence of malignancy.

85. **When are live vaccines contraindicated?**
    See Table 11.6.

Table 11.6. Patients in Whom Use of Live Vaccines Should Be Avoided

- Patients with primary immunodeficiency disorders (especially those with defective cell-mediated immunity such as SCID)
- Patients given immunosuppressive therapy (e.g., corticosteroids, cytotoxic drugs, radiation therapy)
- Patients with malignancies that cause immunosuppression (e.g., leukemia, lymphoma, Hodgkin disease)
- Patients with systemic immunoregulatory, inflammatory, or infectious diseases associated with defective cell-mediated immunity (e.g., SLE, diabetes mellitus, sarcoidosis, HIV-1 infections, atopic dermatitis)
- Children <1 year of age
- Patients with severe malnutrition or burns
- Pregnant women (because of potential harm to fetus)*

*The exception is yellow fever vaccine when the mother must travel to an endemic area. The risks of infection and detrimental effects without the vaccine are greater than the risks of receiving immunization.
HIV, human immunodeficiency virus; SCID, severe combined immunodeficiency disease; SLE, systemic lupus erythematosus.

B-CELL IMMUNODEFICIENCIES

86. **Name some of the characteristics of antibody-deficiency disorders.**
    See Table 11.7.

87. **What is the most common Ig deficiency disorder?**
    Selective IgA deficiency, which has a frequency of approximately 1 in 500–700 persons.

88. **How is selective IgA deficiency treated?**
    With supportive treatment. Even if patients have an increased incidence of infections, intravenous immunoglobulin (IVIG) therapy is unlikely to be effective because infused IgG will not be transported into secretions. Ig infusions also pose a risk because 50% of these patients may have the ability to develop antibodies to the small quantities of IgA present in most IVIG preparations. Life-threatening anaphylaxis can occur with the second and subsequent infusions of IVIG. A similar risk is associated with blood transfusions. IgA-deficient patients can develop antibodies to IgA in the plasma that accompanies packed red blood cells (RBCs). Subsequent transfusions, if needed, should be performed with well-washed RBCs to remove all traces of IgA.

Table 11.7. Characteristics of Antibody-Deficiency Disorders

1. Recurrent infections with extracellular encapsulated pathogens.
2. Relatively few problems with fungal or viral (except enteroviral) infections.
3. Chronic sinusitis and pulmonary disease; some patients may develop bronchiectasis.
4. Growth retardation is not a striking feature.
5. Low antibody levels measured in serum and secretions. Low Ig levels by themselves are not sufficient evidence of an antibody deficiency syndrome, and titers of specific antibodies should be measured.
6. The hallmark of these deficiency syndromes is the inability to make antibodies to new antigens when challenged with vaccines or following infection with one or another microbe.
7. Patients may or may not lack B lymphocytes. If they have B lymphocytes, these may lack surface Igs or complement receptors, indicating that they are arrested relatively early in ontogeny.
8. Absence of cortical follicles in lymph nodes and spleen are seen in X-linked agammaglobu-linemia.
9. Scanty cervical lymph nodes and small or absent tonsils and adenoids are characteristic of X-linked agammaglobulinemia.
10. Replacement therapy with IV Ig has greatly increased lifespan and reduced morbidity.

Ig, immunoglobulin; IV, intravenous.
From Wyngaarden JB, Smith LH, editors. *Cecil Textbook of Medicine.* 18th ed. Philadelphia: WB Saunders; 1988, p 1943.

89. **Which diagnostic tests should be interpreted with caution in those with IgA deficiency?**
    IgA deficiency can lead to false-positive pregnancy tests due to increased heterophile antibodies and lead to false-negative IgA-antihuman tissue transglutaminase tests (for celiac disease) due to absent IgA.

90. **What are secondary causes of isolated low IgG?**
    Protein-losing enteropathy (PLE), medications (corticosteroids, rituximab), malignancies (B-cell lymphoma, myeloma), and bone marrow failure.

91. **What is Good syndrome?**
    Combined immunodeficiency (hypogammaglobulinemia) with thymoma (most commonly spindle cell). Clinical presentation includes autoimmunity (pure RBC aplasia, myasthenia gravis, pernicious anemia), recurrent infections (sinopulmonary and opportunistic), and diarrhea. Patients have low B and CD4$^+$ T cells, neutropenia, no eosinophilia, and hypogammaglobulinemia. Thymectomy can improve autoimmunity but does not affect the immunodeficiency.

92. **Describe the different forms of agammaglobulinemia.**
    Agammaglobulinemia is a primary antibody deficiency characterized by low or absent levels of immunoglobulins and mature B cells. Mutation in BTK is seen in X-linked agammaglobulinemia (Bruton) which presents with recurrent sinopulmonary infections, CNS infections due to ECHO virus, and ecthyma or pyoderma gangrenosum. Autosomal recessive agammaglobulinemia can be secondary to mutations in μ heavy chain (most common), B-cell linker protein (BLNK), Igα/Igβ, λ5 (surrogate light chain), and leucine-rich repeat containing 8(LRRC8).

93. **What is common variable immunodeficiency (CVID) disease, and how is it diagnosed?**
    A common and heterogeneous primary immunodeficiency that presents generally in adulthood (20–40 years of age), involves both B- and T-cell abnormalities, and is often underdiagnosed, leading to delays in diagnosis (up to 8–9 years). The diagnosis of CVID requires significantly decreased levels of IgG, IgA, or IgM with specific antibody deficiency to two or more protein vaccines (tetanus, diphtheria, *Haemophilus* conjugate, MMR [measles-mumps-rubella]) and to pneumococcal polysaccharide vaccine. Antibody testing requires repeat testing 4 weeks after vaccination to document lack of significant increase in specific antibody titers. Primary and secondary causes of hypogammaglobulinemia must also be excluded, and specific antibody deficiency or low IgG alone are not sufficient for a diagnosis of CVID. Given difficulties in discerning transient hypogammaglobulinemia of infancy (THI) with early-onset CVID, diagnosis of CVID is not made until the age of 4.

94. **How does CVID present?**

Infectious complications include recurrent bacterial infections of the upper and lower respiratory tract with encapsulated bacteria (e.g., *Streptococcus pneumoniae, Haemophilus influenzae*) as well as mycobacterial, fungal, and protozoal (i.e., *Giardia lamblia*) infections due to defective cell-mediated immunity. Pulmonary complications include obstructive lung disease (bronchiectasis from recurrent pneumonias, asthma, bronchiolitis obliterans), restrictive lung disease (malignancy, granulomatous and lymphocytic interstitial lung disease [GLILD]). Autoimmune complications include autoimmune hemolytic anemia and immune thrombocytopenia purpura most commonly, as well as autoimmune hepatitis, thyroiditis, pernicious anemia, and others. GI complications include diarrhea, malabsorption, atrophic gastritis, and nodular lymphoid hyperplasia of the small intestine (can lead to portal hypertension and cholestasis). Granulomatous complications include noncaseating granulomas most commonly of the lungs, lymph nodes, and spleen (including GLILD), and patients with granulomatous disease have a higher incidence of autoimmune disease. Finally, there is an increased incidence of malignancy, particularly of the lymphoreticular system and the GI tract.

Cunningham-Rundles C. How I treat common variable immune deficiency. *Blood.* 2000;116:7–15.

95. **Discuss treatment and monitoring of CVID.**

IVIG replacement is the main treatment modality for CVID and can be given either intravenously or subcutaneously every 3–4 weeks or in shorter intervals via the subcutaneous route. Initial starting doses range from 400 to 600 mg/kg, with higher doses (600 mg/kg) and trough levels recommended for those with pulmonary complications including structural changes. The goal of IVIG infusions is to prevent infections, and target trough levels can vary because of baseline IgG levels as well as the presence of pulmonary complications. Severe adverse effects of IVIG include aseptic meningitis, thromboembolic disorders, acute renal failure, and anaphylaxis. Mild to moderate reactions include pruritus, headache, and nausea and usually resolve with slowing or stopping of the infusion.

Recommended monitoring of CVID patients includes complete blood counts (CBCs), comprehensive chemistry panel, albumin, serum IgG (and IgA/IgM as needed), spirometry and follow-up on an annual basis. High-resolution chest computed tomography (CT) is now recommended at diagnosis owing to the high mortality rate from interstitial lung disease and complete pulmonary function test recommended in those with lung disease. Those with malabsorption should be considered for bone density evaluation and nutrient intake, and those with GI complaints should be considered for upper and lower endoscopy (*Helicobacter pylori*, mucosal changes, etc.). Last, diagnostic testing of suspected infectious diseases should not be antibody-based but rather via culture or PCR.

Bonilla FA, Barlan I, Chapel H, et al. International Consensus Document (ICON): common variable immunodeficiency disorders. *J Allergy Clin Immunol Pract.* 2016;4:38–59.

96. **How is an abnormal specific antibody response to the pneumococcal polysaccharide vaccine defined?**

There are no set criteria for an abnormal response to pneumococcal polysaccharide vaccine although the presence of a twofold increase in > 70% of serotypes tested is commonly utilized for adults.

97. **What is transient hypogammaglobulinemia of infancy (THI)?**

An extended period of hypogammaglobulinemia in infancy beyond 6 months of age defined by IgG levels less than 2 SD (standard deviation) below age-matched control subjects. Patients can have impaired antibody production and increased infection susceptibility requiring antibiotic prophylaxis or IVIG. In terms of serum IgG levels, at birth serum IgG levels are similar to maternal IgG levels. At 3–6 months, serum IgG levels reach their nadir and slowly return to normal levels by 5 years of age.

98. **List the common secondary causes of hypogammaglobulinemia and the mechanism by which they cause disease.**

See Table 11.8.

99. **What immunologic defects are heralded by recurrent bacterial infections?**

Before the emergence of human immunodeficiency virus (HIV), the development of serial severe bacterial infections, defined as three or more episodes of bacterial sinusitis, pneumonia, or sepsis within the span of 1 year, was an indication to evaluate patients for a congenital or acquired

Table 11.8. Secondary Causes of Hypogammaglobulinemia

CAUSE	MECHANISM
Drugs a. Anticonvulsants (especially with phenytoin) b. Cytotoxic agents as used in cancer chemotherapy	Drugs a. Decreased B- and T-cell responses, often hypogammaglobulinemia b. Decreased Ig production and T-cell activity
Multiple myeloma	Decreased Ig production
Chronic lymphocytic leukemia	Decreased Ig production and T-cell activity
Myotonic dystrophy	Selective hypercatabolism of IgG
Nephrotic syndrome	Ig loss in urine (particularly IgG)
Intestinal lymphangiectasia	Ig loss through GI tract, increased Ig catabolism
Radiation therapy	Decreased Ig production

GI, gastrointestinal; Ig, immunoglobulin.

antibody-deficiency syndrome. Less commonly, recurrent bacterial infections may suggest complement deficiency or defective neutrophil function. Patients with antibody-deficiency syndromes commonly experience repeated infections with encapsulated organisms (e.g., *H. influenzae, S. pneumoniae*) that are common upper respiratory tract commensals.

COMPLEMENT DEFICIENCIES

100. **How do complement deficiencies present?**
   Isolated C3 deficiency typically presents at a very early age, most often shortly after birth. Because C3 deficiency has such a profound negative effect on leukocyte phagocytic function, patients experience recurrent life-threatening pyogenic infections. Deficiencies of the terminal complement components, with the possible exception of C9 deficiency, increase susceptibility to bacteremia with neisserial species, typically *Neisseria gonorrhoeae*. Deficiency of properdin, an alternative complement pathway component, may also be accompanied by recurrent pyogenic and neisserial infections. Complement deficiency can be evaluated by obtaining a CH50 (or CH100) and by measuring levels of specific complement components thereafter as indicated.

101. **Which is the only complement factor deficiency that is X-linked?**
   Properdin is the only known positive complement regulator. Deficiencies in properdin are associated with meningococcal infections, and treatment involves hypervaccination and antibiotics.

102. **Chronic or recurrent meningococcemia or gonococcemia are commonly associated with which host immune defects?**
   Deficiencies of the late components of complement (C6, C7, and C8) are the predominant defects associated with these disorders. Low C3, absent C5, or properdin deficiency has also been associated with such infections.

103. **What complication of gonococcal infection is of special concern in sexually active adults?**
   Acute monoarticular arthritis may be a consequence of bacteremia with *N. gonorrhoeae*. Such patients must be evaluated for complement deficiency after treatment of the septic joint. The intense neutrophilic infiltrate triggered by these infections is considered an orthopedic emergency requiring immediate drainage of the pus and irrigation of the joint to reduce the residence time of the inflammatory leukocytes in the joint space. The aim of this emergency treatment is to reduce the damage to the articular cartilage caused by leukocyte proteases and reactive oxygen products.
   Ross S, Densen P. Complement deficiency and infection: epidemiology, pathogenesis and consequences of neisserial and other infections in an immune deficiency. *Medicine.* 1984;63:243–273.

Table 11.9. Diseases Associated With Inherited Complement Deficiencies

DEFICIENT COMPONENT	REPORTED CASES	ASSOCIATED DISEASES
C1	31	Autoimmune diseases, SLE-like syndromes
C4	20	Autoimmune diseases, SLE-like syndromes
C2	109	Autoimmune diseases, SLE-like syndromes
C3	20	Bacterial infections, mild glomerulonephritis
C5	28	Gram-negative coccal infections
C6	76	Gram-negative coccal infections
C7	67	Gram-negative coccal infections
C8	68	Gram-negative coccal infections
C9	18	Gram-negative coccal infections
Properdin	70	Gram-negative coccal infections
Factor I	17	Bacterial infections
Factor H	13	Bacterial infections
Factor D	3	Bacterial infections
C4-binding protein	3	—
C1 inhibitor	100	Hereditary angioedema

SLE, systemic lupus erythematosus.
From David J. Immunology. In Dale DC, Federman DD, editors. *Scientific American Medicine*. New York: Scientific American; 1996. Section 6, Subsection VII, Table 6–9, p 26.

104. **What clinical conditions are associated with deficiencies of the various components of the complement system?**
See Table 11.9.

PHAGOCYTE BIOLOGY AND DISORDERS

105. **What are the main severe congenital neutropenias (SCNs)?**
- **Cyclic and severe congenital neutropenia:** Autosomal dominant mutations in *ELANE*
- **Kostmann syndrome:** Autosomal recessive mutations in *HAX1*

106. **What is chronic granulomatous disease (CGD)?**
A primary immunodeficiency disorder of phagocytes due to mutations in the structural genes of the nicotinamide adenine dinucleotide phosphate (NADPH) oxidase. Clinical presentation involves recurrent catalase-positive bacterial and fungal infections as well as granuloma formation. Both X-linked and autosomal recessive inheritances have been described. The organisms responsible for the majority of infections in CGD are *S. aureus*, *Serratia marcescens*, *Nocardia*, *Aspergillus*, and *Burkholderia cepacia*. Pathognomonic organisms include *Chromobacterium violaceum*. *Francisella philomiragia*, and *Granulibacter bethesdensis* (consider when no organism is identified).

107. **Describe the role of the NADPH oxidase in phagocyte function.**
The NADPH oxidase consists of structural (gp91^{phox}, p67^{phox}, p47^{phox}, p22^{phox}) and regulatory components (p40^{phox}, rac) that initiate the formation of superoxide via electron donation to molecular oxygen. Superoxide is converted to hydrogen peroxide via superoxide dismutase. Hydrogen peroxide in turn is converted into hypochlorous acid via myeloperoxidase and chlorine.
Holland SM. Chronic granulomatous disease. *Clin Rev Allergy Immunol.* 2010;38:3–10.

108. Summarize the three main types of leukocyte adhesion deficiencies (LADs).
   - **LAD type I:** autosomal recessive disorder due to mutations in CD18. Clinical presentation involves recurrent necrotizing infections, delayed umbilical separation, and baseline leukocytosis.
   - **LAD type II:** due to mutation *FUCT1* leading to defects in protein fucosylation. Clinical presentation involves mental retardation, short stature, and Bombay (Hh) blood type.
   - **LAD type III:** defect is in the gene *FERMT3* leading to defects in the inside-out signaling pathway involved with chemokine-mediated integrin activation. Bleeding diathesis can be seen in a subset of patients with the *KINDLIN3* mutation.

109. How is neutrophil function evaluated?
   The dihydrorhodamine (DHR) test is the preferred test for CGD and relies on flow cytometry to detect oxidation of dihydrorhodamine (DHR-123 test). Patients with CGD are unable to oxidize DHR because of impaired hydrogen peroxide generation. DHR testing can distinguish between X-linked, autosomal recessive CGD and identify mosaic and hypomorphic variants. If DHR testing is not available, a nitroblue tetrazolium test can be performed to assess neutrophil respiratory burst. LAD syndrome can be assessed functionally and by flow cytometric analysis for defects in cell surface expression of CD18-dependent beta integrins.

EOSINOPHILS

110. Describe the structure of the eosinophil.
   Eosinophils are bilobed granulocytes with granules that stain pink in the presence of eosin and nuclei that stain purple in the presence of hematoxylin. Eosinophils have primary granules which contain Charcot-Leyden–crystal proteins as well as distinct structures called *lipid bodies,* which are the sites of eicosanoid synthesis and release during eosinophil activation. Resting eosinophils have limited or no lipid bodies. Eosinophils are also characterized by their secondary granules, which contain eosinophilic cationic protein, eosinophilic-derived neurotoxin, eosinophil peroxidase, and major basic protein. They contain also chemokines such as RANTES (regulated on activation normal T cell expressed and secreted) and eotaxin.

111. Describe the functions of the eosinophil.
   Eosinophils contribute to the proinflammatory response via production and release of toxic mediators and are involved in allergic inflammation, tissue fibrosis, and thrombosis. They can also contribute to neuronal disease in hypereosinophilic syndrome and eosinophilic vasculitis. Eosinophils also play a role in protection and homeostasis, as they are involved with tissue repair and remodeling (i.e., during late pregnancy in uterine tissue), tumor surveillance, the innate immune response and plasma cell maintenance (via APRIL [a proliferation-inducing ligand]).

112. Where do eosinophils normally reside in healthy individuals?
   In tissues such as the lower GI tract, lymph organs, mammary glands, and the uterus. Eosinophils, however, if found in other locations, can signify the presence of a disease state because eosinophils can migrate along chemokine gradients on epithelial and endothelial surfaces to localized sites of inflammation.

113. How is eosinophilia defined?
   As an absolute eosinophil count greater than 450 cells/μL.

114. What factors can increase or decrease eosinophil counts?
   Increase
   - Allergic disorders (allergic rhinitis, atopic dermatitis, eosinophilic esophagitis, and related disorders and allergic asthma)
   - Drug hypersensitivity (DRESS [drug reaction with eosinophilia and systemic symptoms], quinine, quinolones, tetracycline, L-tryptophan)
   - Vasculitis (eosinophilic granulomatosis with polyangiitis [EGPA], Kawasaki disease)
   - Hypereosinophilic disorders (HES)
   - Idiopathic causes

   Decrease
   - Bacterial and viral infections
   - Fever states
   - During corticosteroid administration

   Additionally, there is a small degree of diurnal variation in eosinophil counts.

115. **What is the hypereosinophilic syndrome?**
     An idiopathic syndrome characterized by absolute peripheral eosinophilia of $1500/mm^3$ or greater, a lack of secondary causes for eosinophilia (parasitic infections, neoplasms, allergic disorders, drug hypersensitivity), and evidence of organ involvement. Although corticosteroids traditionally have been first-line therapy, there have been new variants described with severe phenotypes unresponsive to standard therapy. The myeloproliferative variant (M-HES) involves a mutation in the fusion tyrosine kinase *FIP1L1/PDGFRA* and is a form of chronic eosinophilic leukemia responsive to the tyrosine kinase inhibitor imatinib. A second variant, a lymphocytic variant (L-HES), is caused by aberrant T cells.

116. **Prior to initiating systemic corticosteroids in a patient with eosinophilia and recent travel history (to tropical and subtropical regions), what testing should be considered?**
     A *strongyloides* serologic test should be performed in patients with eosinophilia and potential exposure owing to the risk of inducing fatal strongyloidiasis (hyperinfection syndrome) with systemic corticosteroids.

117. **Describe Gleich syndrome and Well syndrome.**
     Both are forms of idiopathic eosinophilia. Gleich syndrome is episodic angioedema with eosinophilia. Patients can have elevated immunoglobulins, but there is no end organ involvement. Well syndrome is characterized by recurrent eosinophilic inflammatory dermatitis defined by histopathologic findings of eosinophilic dermal infiltration and free eosinophilic granules.

118. **What is the eosinophilic myalgia syndrome (EMS)?**
     EMS has been associated with contaminated L-tryptophan from a Japanese manufacturer, with peak incidence in the 1980s. Another drug association with eosinophilia includes tetracycline and eosinophilic hepatitis.

119. **Summarize the diagnostic work-up and treatment options for eosinophilic esophagitis (EoE).**
     EoE is a chronic inflammatory esophageal disease characterized by aeroallergen and food IgE sensitization and eosinophilic infiltration in the esophageal mucosa. EoE is part of a spectrum of eosinophilic disorders with similiar clinical, endoscopic and pathologic characteristics that includes gastroesophageal reflux disease (GERD) and proton pump inhibitor-responsive EoE (PPI-REE). EoE is a clinicopathologic diagnosis that depends on the presence of greater than 15 eosinophils per high-power field and nonresponsiveness to PPI trial. Treatment includes dietary modifications (elemental, six-food, or four-food elimination diet) and pharmacologic interventions (swallowed topical corticosteroid).
     Simon D, Cianferoni A, Spergel JM, et al. Eosinophilic esophagitis is characterized by a non-IgE-mediated food hypersensitivity. *Allergy.* 2016;71:611–620.

AUTOINFLAMMATORY DISORDERS

120. **What is the inflammasome?**
     An intracellular complex composed of proteins capable of sensing danger signals (and pathogens) and activating an inflammatory cascade culminating in the production of proinflammatory cytokines IL-1β and IL-18. Although the inflammasome is highly regulated, mutations in the genes encoding inflammasome proteins can lead to dysregulation and autoinflammatory disease.
     Hoffman HM, Broderick L. The role of the inflammasome in patients with autoinflammatory diseases. *J Allergy Clin Immunol.* 2016;138:3–14.

121. **What is the differential diagnosis for recurrent fever?**
     - **Autoinflammatory diseases:** cryopryin-associated periodic syndromes (Muckle-Wells, familial cold autoinflammatory syndrome, familial Mediterranean fever, and neonatal-onset multisystem inflammatory disease)
     - **Infection:** bacterial, viral, parasitic
     - **Autommunity/rheumatic diseases:** Still disease, Behçet disease, inflammatory bowel disease
     - **Malignancy:** lymphoma
     Autoinflammatory diseases are due to dysregulation in the inflammasome, and the main clinical signs suggesting autoinflammation are recurrent noninfectious febrile episodes (>3 episodes, >101° F)

with predictable patterns, family history of autoinflammation or amyloidosis, cold or vaccines as triggers, and significant systemic symptoms such as nonpruritic rash, joint pain, abdominal pain, and/or conjunctivitis.

Hoffman HM, Broderick L. The role of the inflammasome in patients with autoinflammatory diseases. *J Allergy Clin Immunol.* 2016;138:3–14.

122. **What is PLAID (PLCG2-associated antibody deficiency and immune dysregulation) syndrome?**
Syndrome of cold urticaria and hypogammaglobulinemia caused by mutations in PLCγ2. PLAID can be diagnosed in the clinical setting using the evaporative cooling test, which is positive (negative ice cube test). There is significant clinical overlap between PLAID and CVID as both can manifest with antibody deficiency, autoimmunity, granulomatous disease, decreased switched memory B cells.

Ombrello MJ, Remmers EF, Sun G, et al. Cold urticaria, immunodeficiency, and autoimmunity related to PLCG2 deletions. *N Engl J Med.* 2012;366:330–338.

TESTS OF IMMUNOLOGIC FUNCTION AND ALLERGY DIAGNOSIS

123. **Name common diseases associated with elevation of the total serum IgE level.**
    - **Atopic (allergic) diseases:** allergic rhinitis, allergic asthma, allergic bronchopulmonary aspergillosis (ABPA)
    - **Primary immunodeficiency disorders:** Wiskott-Aldrich syndrome, Nezelhof syndrome (cellular immunodeficiency with IgE), selective IgA deficiency with concomitant atopic disease, Job syndrome
    - **Infections:** parasitic; viral, including infectious mononucleosis; and fungal, including candidiasis
    - **Malignancies:** Hodgkin disease, bronchial carcinoma, IgE myeloma
    - **Dermatologic disorders:** atopic dermatitis and bullous pemphigoid, eczema
    - **Acute GVHD**

124. **How can antibody measurements be used to indicate an active infection?**
IgM antibodies are produced as new B cells are stimulated by the infection; their development indicates an active ongoing infection. IgG antibodies, though, can persist for years after an infection has resolved and cannot be used to prove active infection. The presence of a rising titer of antibodies also indicates an active response, regardless of antibody class. The first serum sample, typically called the *acute sample,* and a second sample, drawn 1 or more weeks later, typically called the *convalescent sample,* should be sent to the laboratory together for simultaneous testing. Many titrations—that is, antibody measurements—are done using serial twofold dilutions of serum. Results are not considered significant until there is a fourfold or greater rise in titer.

125. **How do H_1/H_2 antihistamines and corticosteroids affect the results of allergy skin-prick testing?**
H_1/H_2 antihistamines markedly inhibit skin-prick test reactivity. The wheal-and-flare reaction of a positive skin-prick test is primarily due to histamine stimulation of H_1 receptors in small blood vessels. H_2 antihistamines may occasionally depress skin-prick test reactivity as well and should also be avoided before skin testing. Antihistamines must be discontinued before skin-prick testing (length of discontinuation depends on antihistamine). Corticosteroids on the contrary do not affect mast cell degranulation, nor do they affect the biologic effects of histamine. Thus, corticosteroids do not alter allergy skin-prick test results.

126. **How does in vitro specific IgE testing compare with skin-prick testing in the diagnosis of allergy? When are they preferable to skin-prick testing?**
The in vitro immunoassay is less sensitive compared to skin-prick testing but is preferable in patients with diffuse skin disease, patients on immunosuppressive therapy, uncooperative patients, or a prior history or risk of anaphylaxis from skin-prick testing. In vitro IgE immunoassays do not have sufficient sensitivity for definitive penicillin/drug or venom allergy testing.

Bernstein IL, Li JT, Bernstein DI, et al. Allergy diagnostic testing: an updated practice parameter. *Ann Allergy Asthma Immunol.* 2008;100:S1–148.

127. **Is a positive aeroallergen-specific IgE in vitro test result diagnostic of allergy?**
No. The in vitro immunoassay test only identifies aeroallergen sensitization. Clinical relevance must be determined by the clinician based on clinical history.

128. **How is the enzyme-linked immunosorbent assay (ELISA) performed?**
Typically performed in plastic, flat-bottomed, 96-well, microtiter plates. The concentration of the substance to be measured is determined by comparing the optical density of the test samples against negative controls and a standard curve. The basic ELISA procedure used to test for antibody against specific antigen is:
1. Coat wells with antigen (by incubating appropriate concentration of antigen in the wells) and then wash.
2. Add test sample and incubate.
3. Wash.
4. Add enzyme-linked antispecies Ig and incubate.
5. Wash.
6. Add developing substrate and measure optical density.

129. **What is anergy?**
The lack of an immunologic response to an antigen under circumstances in which one would normally expect to see one. T-cell anergy, for example, is demonstrated by the lack of reaction to common DTH recall antigens. Clinically, this is seen frequently in patients with miliary tuberculosis, Hodgkin disease, or HIV infection. B-cell anergy is failure to develop a specific antibody response in a person who has been immunized with antigens that are known to routinely stimulate antibody responses in other individuals of the same species. Anergy may be temporary, as occurs during measles infection, or of indeterminate duration, as in sarcoidosis, acquired immunodeficiency syndrome (AIDS), and certain disseminated malignancies and overwhelming infectious diseases, including lepromatous leprosy.

With DTH skin testing, one typically employs four or five recall antigens to ensure a > 90% chance of using at least one antigen against which normal age-matched individuals would mount a DTH response. Recall antigens (tetanus toxoid, mumps, candida, purified protein derivative [PPD]) are antigens that a person has already encountered before; thus, during the test, the immune responses are asked to mount a secondary response.

ALLERGIC RHINITIS AND SINUSITIS

130. **What is the impact of house dust mite (HDM) allergy on asthma?**
Asthmatics who are not sensitized to HDM allergens (most commonly *Dermatophagoides pteronyssinus* and *Dermatophagoides farina*) have increased morbidity upon exposure. Asthmatics who have already been sensitized have more severe asthma, and HDM sensitization is a risk factor for recurrent asthma exacerbations.

131. **Describe the approach to treatment of allergic rhinitis, with specific attention to HDM allergy.**
There are three main treatment options for allergic rhinitis, and they are available for HDM allergy including allergen avoidance, pharmacologic intervention, and allergen immunotherapy (AIT). Intuitively, HDM avoidance measures would be expected to decrease HDM-related allergic rhinitis and asthma. However, a Cochrane review in 2015 was unable to conclusively determine the benefit of HDM reduction or avoidance measures. Treatment for HDM-related allergic rhinitis follows the ARIA (Allergic Rhinitis and its Impact on Asthma) and GINA (Global Initiative for Asthma) guidelines, and first-line treatment includes oral or intranasal antihistamines and corticosteroids. AIT is available in the United States subcutaneously (SCIT) and in sublingual form (SLIT). Meta-analyses have demonstrated the effectiveness of SCIT (and SLIT) in HDM-related allergic rhinitis and asthma (but considerable heterogeneity of the included studies).

Calderón MA, Kleine-Tebbe J, Linneberg A, et al. House dust mite respiratory allergy: an overview of current therapeutic strategies. *J Allergy Clin Immunol Pract.* 2015;3:843–855.

132. **Which biologic functions are mediated via H_1, H_2, or a combination of H_1 and H_2 histamine receptors?**
See Table 11.10.

Table 11.10. Biologic Functions Mediated by H_1, H_2, or a Combination of H_1 and H_2 Receptors

H_1 RECEPTORS	H_2 RECEPTORS	H_1 AND H_2 RECEPTORS
Smooth muscle contraction	Gastric acid secretion	Hypotension
↑ Vascular permeability	↑ Cyclic AMP	Tachycardia
Pruritus	Mucous secretion	Flushing
Stimulation of prostaglandin synthesis	Inhibits basophil but not mast cell histamine release	Headache
Tachycardia	Stimulates IL-5 production by T_H2 cells	
↑ Cyclic GMP production		

↑, increased; AMP, adenosine monophosphate; GMP, guanosine monophosphate; IL, interleukin; T_H, T helper cells.

Note that although the majority of histamine receptors in the skin are H_1, some H_2 receptors and recalcitrant cases of urticaria may require treatment with both H_1- and H_2-specific antihistamines.

133. **What are the available pharmacologic interventions available for allergic rhinitis and their relative effectiveness?**

- **Intranasal corticosteroid sprays:** First-line therapy that may take several weeks for full effectiveness. Effective also for ocular symptoms.
- **Intranasal H_1 antihistamine sprays:** Less effective as monotherapy compared to intranasal corticosteroids. Effective also for ocular symptoms. Dual intranasal corticosteroid and antihistamine administration is more effective compared to monotherapy of either for allergic rhinitis and is utilized as a step-up approach for patients on monotherapy with continued symptoms. There is no difference between intranasal H_1 antihistamines and intranasal corticosteroids with respect to ocular symptom reduction.
- **Oral H_1 antihistamines:** Less effective as monotherapy compared to intranasal corticosteroids. Combination therapy of an oral H_1 antihistamine and intranasal corticosteroid is not more effective compared to monotherapy with intranasal corticosteroid.
- **Leukotriene antagonist:** Less effective compared to oral H_1 antihistamines. Combination of leukotriene antagonist and intranasal corticosteroid is not more effective compared to monotherapy with intranasal corticosteroid.
- **Cromolyn sodium:** In patients who have ocular pruritus as part of their symptom complex, cromolyn sodium eye drops or some other mast cell stabilizer are necessary to control the problem fully.
- **Muscarinic antagonist nasal spray:** Effective for nonallergic rhinitis and significant rhinorrhea.
- **Sympathomimetics:** Effective in reducing congestion but limited applications (acute decongestion in treatment of reactions during aspirin-exacerbated respiratory disease [AERD] aspirin desensitization or prior to nasal endoscopy) due to rhinitis medicamentosa.

134. **Does systemic corticosteroid therapy have a role in the treatment of allergic rhinitis?**

Not used as first-line treatment for allergic rhinitis but can be used to control rhinitis complicated by nasal polyposis or in the treatment of allergic fungal sinusitis.

135. **Describe the immunoregulatory mechanisms of AIT.**

The exact mechanism of AIT has not been fully elucidated. There are, however, several proposed mechanisms of immune tolerance induced by AIT including the production of allergen-specific IL-10 producing Tregs and Bregs, increased IgG4, IgA, IL-10, and TGF-β. There is an early increase in IgE, but IgE levels decrease overall over the course of AIT. Additionally, there is a decrease in specific IgE, skin-prick test reactivity, and decreased mast cells, basophils, and eosinophils. IL-10 inhibits IgE production but can upregulate IgG4, which is a blocking antibody preventing the binding of allergen to IgE among other related roles including allergen presentation to T cells.

136. **What is vasomotor rhinitis, and how is it treated?**

    A form of nonallergic rhinitis that presents clinically with excessive rhinorrhea, congestion, and headache secondary to activation of transient receptor potential (TRP), A1, or V1 channels by nonspecific irritants. The TRP channels subsequently initiate neuronal reflexes leading to neuropeptide release including substance P. Treatment involves irritant avoidance and agents associated with TRP channels including muscarinic antagonists and intranasal antihistamines.

    Bernstein JA, Singh U. Neural abnormalities in nonallergic rhinitis. *Curr Allergy Asthma Rep.* 2015;15(4):18.

137. **What is rhinitis medicamentosa, and how is it treated?**

    Intense nasal congestion, often with complete obstruction of the nasal airway due to rebound vasodilatation secondary to chronic inhaled topical vasoconstrictor use. The causative agent is most commonly oxymetazoline. Alpha-adrenergic topical vasoconstrictors should not be prescribed for allergic rhinitis given the risk of rhinitis medicamentosa. However, in certain situations, oxymetazoline can be used including acute treatment of nasal congestion during AERD aspirin desensitization and prior to nasal endoscopy.

    Rhinitis medicamentosa is treated by maintaining avoidance of topical vasoconstrictors (oxymetazoline). Oral steroids are sometimes used to facilitate weaning off the vasoconstrictor.

138. **What are the clinical features of acute rhinosinusitis (ARS), and how is presumptive acute bacterial rhinosinusitis (ABRS) treated?**

    ARS is classified as having a duration < 12 weeks and involving some or all of the following symptoms: persistent upper respiratory infection (> 10 days or worsening following initial improvement), purulent rhinorrhea, postnasal drip, nasal congestion, facial pain, anosmia, headache, fever, cough. In some cases ABRS can present with acute upper dental pain and typically is unilateral. Recurrent ARS is defined as three or more episodes of ARS in a year. Of note, the term *ARS* is now preferred instead of acute sinusitis given that rhinitis generally accompanies and is prominent in sinusitis.

    Although most causes of ARS are viral in origin, treatment for presumptive ABRS should commence if symptoms have persisted for more than 10 days or if there is progression of symptoms after initial improvement. The Infectious Diseases Society of America (IDSA) recommends amoxicillin-clavulanate as the first-line therapy and no longer recommends macrolides. For penicillin-allergic patients, doxycycline, levofloxacin, and moxifloxacin can be considered. Recommendations are also to perform penicillin skin testing and graded oral challenge in presumptive penicillin-allergic patients due to resistance and complications.

139. **What are the indications for high-resolution CT imaging in chronic rhinosinusitis (CRS)?**

    Uncomplicated ARS and CRS.

140. **What are the indications for surgical intervention in ABRS and CRS? What measures should be performed if CRS is resistant to medical or surgical intervention?**

    Surgery should be considered in ABRS if symptoms are unresponsive to medical treatment or there is a threatened complication. Threatened complications include frontal bone osteomyelitis, cavernous sinus thrombosis, brain abscess, and meningitis. Surgical intervention in CRS is indicated if fungal rhinosinusitis is present, if unilateral disease (dental disease, suspected polyposis) is present, threatened complications, culture is needed, biopsy is needed (rule out neoplasm, ciliary dysfunction, granulomatous disease, fungal infection) and also if medical intervention has failed (allergic disease, nasal polyposis, anatomic defects). Considerations would include immunodeficiency, uncontrolled allergic or fungal rhinitis, cystic fibrosis, ciliary dysfunction, age, and malignancy.

    Peters AT, Spector S, Hsu J, et al. Diagnosis and management of rhinosinusitis: a practice parameter update. *Ann Allergy Asthma Immunol.* 2014;113:347–385.

141. **What are the features of fungal rhinosinusitis, and how is it evaluated and managed?**

    Three types of fungal rhinosinusitis have been described: acute fungal rhinosinusitis (AFRS), fungus ball, and invasive fungal sinusitis. Acute fungal rhinosinusitis presents in immunocompetent asthmatics who typically also have nasal polyposis. Diagnostic criteria vary (research or patient care focused) and can include:

- ≥12-week symptom course
- Characteristic symptoms (one or more of anterior/posterior nasal rhinorrhea, nasal obstruction, decreased sense of smell, facial pain/pressure)
- Positive fungal stain
- Characteristic CT sinus findings (heterogeneous opacification with high attenuation regions or bony erosion)
- Type 1 hypersensitivity to fungi (skin-prick positive or serum IgE positive), nasal polyposis, and eosinophilic mucin

    Treatment includes a combination of surgical intervention (débridement, polypectomy, mucin removal, enlargement of sinus ostia) and medical intervention (systemic and/or topical corticosteroids).

    Hoyt AEW, Borish L, Gurrola J, et al. Allergic fungal rhinosinusitis. *J Allergy Clin Immunol Pract.* 2016;4:599–604.

ASTHMA

See also Chapter 6, Pulmonary Medicine.

142. **What are the characteristic histopathologic findings in the sputum of asthmatics?**
     - **Charcot-Leyden crystals:** Composed of lysophospholipase, and their presence in tissue or secretions has been considered as specific for eosinophil activity; however, lysophospholipase is also found in basophils.
     - **Creola bodies:** Clumps of epithelial cells that suggest a desquamating disease process.
     - **Curschmann spirals:** Mucous plugs composed of mucus, proteinaceous material, and inflammatory cells in a swirling, spiraling pattern. They usually conform to the configuration of the involved airways.

     These three entities may be found alone or together as part of the clinical presentation of asthma. They are characteristically seen in patients who have died from status asthmaticus.

143. **Which aeroallergen has been associated with fatal asthma exacerbations?**
     Alternaria alternata.

144. **What factors determine the severity of the exacerbation?**
     Multiple factors, including age, severity of the underlying asthma, concurrent medical problems, site and severity of the infection, and specific infectious agent.

145. **How does GERD affect nocturnal exacerbations of asthma?**
     By microaspiration or reflex bronchoconstriction caused by stimulation of nerve endings by acid in the lower esophagus. GERD may be exacerbated by theophylline, which decreases lower esophageal sphincter tone. (See also Chapter 7, Gastroenterology.)

146. **What is the role of oral corticosteroids in asthma?**
     For use in acute asthma exacerbations but oral corticosteroids are not optimal for long-term treatment due to the significant side effects (immunosuppression, adrenal suppression, hypertension, glaucoma, decreased bone mineral density/aseptic necrosis, myopathy).

147. **Give the serum half-lives and relative potencies of the common glucocorticoids.**
     See Table 11.11.

148. **What is omalizumab?**
     An anti-IgE monoclonal antibody containing a mouse antibody against human IgE that has been "humanized." Omalizumab carries a black-box warning for anaphylaxis, which has been reported in at least 0.2% of patients treated.

149. **What are the approved indications for omalizumab?**
     Both moderate to severe persistent asthma (IgE level of 30–700 IU/mL and evidence for aeroallergen sensitization and inadequate control on inhaled corticosteroids) and chronic idiopathic urticaria (refractory to H_1 antihistamine treatment).

150. **What other biologic agents are approved for severe asthma?**
     The anti–IL-5 antibody mepolizumab, approved by the Food and Drug Administration (FDA) in 2015, and the anti-IL-5 receptor antibody benralizumab, approved by the FDA in 2017. Both mepolizumab and benralizumab target patients with severe persistent asthma with an eosinophilic phenotype.

Table 11.11. Relative Potencies and Effects of Common Glucocorticoids

PREPARATION	POTENCY RELATIVE TO HYDROCOR-TISONE	RELATIVE SODIUM-RETAINING POTENCY	APPROXIMATELY EQUIVALENT DOSE OF ACTION (MG)	DURATION OF ACTION
Hydrocortisone	1	1	20	Short
Cortisone	0.8	0.8	25	Short
Prednisolone	4	0.8	5	Intermediate
Prednisone	4	0.8	5	Intermediate
6α-Methylprednisolone	5	0.5	4	Intermediate
Triamcinolone	5	0	4	Intermediate
Dexamethasone	25	0	0.75	Long
Betamethasone	25	0	0.75	Long

From Schleimer RP. Glucocorticosteroids. In Middleton E, et al, editors. *Allergy: Principles and Practice*. 3rd ed. St. Louis: Mosby; 1988, p 742.

151. **What are two chronic respiratory diseases that predispose to allergic bronchopulmonary aspergillosis (ABPA)?**
Asthma and cystic fibrosis. (See also Chapter 6, Pulmonary Medicine)

ASPIRIN/NSAID-EXACERBATED RESPIRATORY DISEASE

152. **What is aspirin-exacerbated respiratory disease?**
Aspirin-exacerbated respiratory disease or nonsteroidal anti-inflammatory drug (NSAID)-exacerbated respiratory disease (AERD/NERD) is a type 2 inflammatory response that manifests clinically as CRS with nasal polyposis (CRSwNP), adult-onset asthma, and pathognomonic aspirin sensitivity. The CRSwNP is often progressive, persistent, and refractory to medical management and recurrent polypectomies, and systemic corticosteroid administrations are common. Additional clinical findings include anosmia as well as alcohol sensitivity. Reported prevalence rates vary, but the Centers for Disease Control and Prevention (CDC) estimates that approximately 9% of all adult asthmatics and 15% of patients with CRSwNP develop AERD/NERD. A 2015 meta-analysis found that among those with AERD, prevalence was approximately 7% in typical asthma patients and 15% in severe asthmatics. The gold standard of diagnosis remains the oral aspirin challenge although attenuations of both FEV_1 (forced expiratory volume in 1 second) reductions and extrapulmonary reactions (GI and laryngospasm) have been demonstrated with nasal ketorolac.
    Lee RU, White AA, Ding D, et al. Use of intranasal ketorolac and modified oral aspirin challenge for desensitization of aspirin-exacerbated respiratory disease. *Ann Allergy Asthma Immunol.* 2010;105:130–135.
    Rajan JP, Wineinger NE, Stevenson DD, et al. Prevalence of aspirin-exacerbated respiratory disease among asthmatic patients: a meta-analysis of the literature. *J Allergy Clin Immunol.* 2015;135:676–681.

153. **What is the underlying mechanism of AERD?**
The precise mechanisms involved in the pathogenesis of AERD/NERD are not yet fully elucidated, but environmental (active smoking, passive tobacco smoke) or viral factors may be clinically relevant. Although polymorphisms to genes encoding components of the 5-lipoxygenase-leukotriene C_4 pathway have been identified, replicate data have not yet been obtained, suggesting that a genetic basis may not be underlying AERD/NERD.
    With respect to underlying pathophysiology, one proposed mechanism involves an ILC2-mediated dysregulated type 2 immune response. There is evidence of robust T_H2 responses involving eosinophilic infiltration into the upper and lower airways and elevations of the T_H2 cytokine IL-5 compared to ASA (aspirin)-tolerant asthmatics. Additional evidence suggests aberrant arachidonic acid metabolism in aspirin-sensitive patients, with increased inflammatory lipid mediators such as prostaglandin D_2 (PGD_2)

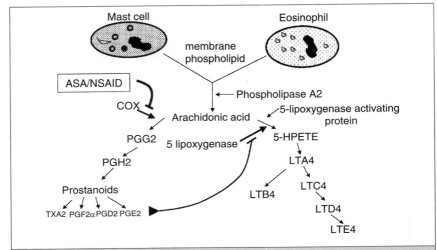

Fig. 11.6. Effects of aspirin and nonsteroidal anti-inflammatory drugs (NSAIDs) on the two major pathways of arachidonic acid metabolism. *(From Middleton E Jr, Reed CE, Ellis EF, et al, editors.* Allergy: Principles and Practice. *5th ed. Vol. II. St. Louis: Mosby; 1998, p 1229.)*

and cysteinyl leukotrienes (CysLTs) compared to non-AERD control subjects. Relatedly, aspirin-mediated reduction in the synthesis of PGE_2, a component of the cyclooxygenase (COX) pathway, inhibits 5-lipoxygenase, the enzyme responsible for the production of LTs from arachidonic acid, as well as mast cell activation. Disinhibition of the synthesis of downstream bronchoconstrictive metabolites in the 5-lipoxygenase pathway (Fig. 11.6) is thought to underlie the increased quantities of LTE_4 in the urine and LTC_4 in nasal and bronchial secretions during clinical reactions.

Laidlaw TM, Boyce JA. Aspirin-exacerbated respiratory disease: new prime suspects. *N Engl J Med.* 2016;374:484–488.

154. What are the two major pathways of arachidonic acid metabolism?
PGD_2 and thromboxanes A_2 and B_2 are the major products of the **COX pathway** of arachidonic acid metabolism. LTs, especially LTC_4, LTD_4, and LTE_4, are major products of the **lipoxygenase pathway.** These eicosanoids exhibit an array of potent inflammatory and immunoregulatory properties.

155. Which medications should be avoided in patients with AERD?
All nonslective NSAIDs must be avoided upon diagnosis of AERD/NERD. Additionally, acetaminophen in high doses (>1000 mg) can induce clinical reactions.

156. Which medications are tolerated in patients with AERD?
COX-2 inhibitors are usually tolerated by patients with AERD/NERD, as well as low doses of acetaminophen (<1000 mg).

157. How is AERD treated?
Outpatient aspirin desensitization is an effective treatment option and has become the standard of care for AERD/NERD patients. Current desensitization protocols involve graded administrations of nasal ketorolac (Toradol) and aspirin with target maintenance dose of 650 mg of aspirin twice daily to maintain the desensitized state. High-dose aspirin regimens have been shown to reduce the rate of polypectomies as well as oral corticosteroid dosing.

158. When is the optimal timing for aspirin desensitization in AERD/NERD patients?
Given that the recurrence rate of nasal polyposis in aspirin/NSAID-sensitive individuals can be rapid, and given that aspirin desensitization does not reduce existing polyposis, it is recommended that aspirin desensitization be performed 1 month after polypectomy for the best outcome. Additionally, prior studies have demonstrated marked reductions in lower airway reactions with leukotriene and

5-LO inhibitors (montelukast/zafirlukast and zileuton, respectively). Recommendations also include pretreatment with these agents prior to desensitization. Patients with uncontrolled asthma may need a course of an oral corticosteroid prior to desensitization.

159. **What is a silent desensitization?**
A negative aspirin challenge/desensitization in a patient with a strong clinical history of aspirin/NSAID sensitivity. The practicing allergist should consider a second confirmatory aspirin challenge in this situation.

White AA, Bosso JV, Stevenson DD. The clinical dilemma of "silent desensitization" in aspirin-exacerbated respiratory disease. *Allergy Asthma Proc.* 2013;34:378–382.

ANGIOEDEMA AND CHRONIC URTICARIA

160. **What clinical and laboratory findings are most important in illuminating the cause of angioedema?**
The majority of angioedema cases are idiopathic, and an extensive evaluation often fails to reveal a specific cause or associated underlying disease; however, a careful history is of the utmost importance. For example, allergic angioedema may be suggested by a temporal relationship to exposure to specific allergens (such as food). Cold urticaria/angioedema is indicated by onset after exposure to cold temperatures. A number of findings may indicate hereditary angioedema (HAE), including a positive family history, low C4 during and between attacks, and low antigenic or functional activity of C1 esterase inhibitor (C1INH). Because patients may have one gene producing functional C1INH and one gene producing a nonfunctional C1INH, it may be necessary to measure the quantity of functional or biologically active inhibitor as opposed to just the total quantity of C1INH protein.

161. **Describe angiotensin-converting enzyme inhibitor (ACEI)-mediated angioedema.**
ACEI may increase the risk of angioedema through bradykinin-mediated mechanisms and should be discontinued if angioedema has occurred while on the medication. Recurrent episodes of angioedema are possible months (common) to years (uncommon, but reported) after ACEI discontinuation.

162. **What are the pathophysiology and clinical presentation of HAE?**
HAE is an autosomal dominant disorder that clinically presents with unpredictable and potentially life-threatening episodes of angioedema and is often misdiagnosed (average delay in diagnosis is 8 years). There are three main types of HAE:
- **Type I (deficiency of C1 inhibitor: C1INH):** majority of HAE patients (~85%), mutation in *SERPING1* gene, low C4, low C1INH antigen and function
- **Type II (normal levels of C1INH but with functional deficiency):** affects ~15% of HAE patients, due to missense mutation, low C4, normal C1INH but low function
- **Type III (normal C1INH and function):** *F12* gene (factor XII) mutation in select cohort of patients
Clinically, type I and II HAE patients present similarly. There have been several triggers associated with angioedema attacks including trauma, stress, infections, and fatigue, but many episodes are without precipitating events. The angioedema in HAE is secondary to increased vascular permeability due to bradykinin generation and engagement of the bradykinin B2 receptor on endothelial cells. Decreased C1INH leads to unchecked activation of the classical complement pathway and decreased inhibition of Hageman factor–dependent activation of the kinin and plasmin pathways. This results in increased generation of bradykinin and other molecules that can increase vascular permeability.

163. **Summarize the treatment of type I and type II HAE.**
HAE treatment (type I and type II) involves both short-term and long-term prophylaxis, as well as access to on-demand treatment. Short-term prophylaxis is required for surgical procedures and significant dental procedures and involves plasma-derived C1INH given 1–12 hours prior to the procedure or anabolic steroid administration. Long-term prophylaxis involves both plasma-derived C1INH and anabolic steroids. HAE patients should have access to at least two doses of on-demand treatment. Approved on-demand treatments include IV administered plasma-derived and recombinant C1INH and subcutaneous administration of either a kallikrein inhibitor or bradykinin B2 receptor antagonist.

Zuraw BL, Christiansen SC. How we manage persons with hereditary angioedema. *Br J Haematol.* 2016;173:831–843.

164. **How is HAE distinguished from histaminergic urticaria/angioedema?**
Depressed serum C4 levels and absent urticaria are features of those with HAE. Although patients with HAE can have erythema marginatum prior to an exacerbation, these cutaneous lesions are markedly different from histaminergic urticaria.

165. **Describe acquired C1 inhibitor deficiency (ACID).**
Rare syndrome of:
- Recurrent angioedema without urticaria
- Acquired deficiency of C1 inhibitor (C1INH)
- Activation of the classical complement pathway and consumption of complement components (via neoplastic lymphatic tissue or inactivation/cleavage via its autoantibody)
- Approximately 1 ACID patient for every 10 HAE patients
  Castelli R, Zanichelli A, Cicardi M, et al. Acquired C1-inhibitor deficiency and lymphoproliferative disorders: a tight relationship. *Crit Rev Oncol Hematol.* 2013;87:323–332.
  Zuraw BL, Altman LC. Acute consumption of C1 inhibitor in a patient with acquired C1-inhibitor deficiency syndrome. *J Allergy Clin Immunol.* 1991;88:908–918.

166. **What elements in the history are important in the evaluation of a previously healthy 26-year-old patient who presents with a 2-week history of daily urticaria?**
Any potential exposures including underlying viral illness, medication, food ingestion, environmental exposure, or physical condition (e.g., heat, cold, water, sunlight, pressure, exercise). Acute urticaria is defined by urticaria of less than 6 weeks' duration. Urticaria for greater than 6 weeks is termed *chronic urticaria,* and the vast majority of chronic cases do not have an identifiable cause.

167. **What laboratory tests may be useful in patients with chronic urticaria?**
CBC with differential, urinalysis, erythrocyte sedimentation rate (ESR), and liver function tests. In patients older than 40 years, a serum protein electrophoresis should be obtained to rule out paraproteinemia.

168. **Which other tests may be helpful in specific cases?**
Cryoglobulins, screening for antinuclear antibodies (ANAs), thyroid function studies, complement C3 and C4, and rheumatoid factor (RF). In patients who have traveled abroad recently to developing countries, testing stool for ova and parasites may be helpful. Hepatitis B and C testing may be indicated. In patients from South or Central America, American trypanosomiasis (Chagas disease) should also be considered. Whether these and other tests for the evaluation for systemic diseases are obtained depends on the degree of clinical suspicion based on the history, physical examination, and initial laboratory results. Tests for specific types of the physical urticarias can be performed as indicated. Some investigations attribute a significant fraction of chronic urticaria cases to the development of autoantibodies either to the mast cell receptor for IgE or to IgE itself.

169. **Describe the first-line treatment for chronic urticaria.**
Nonsedating antihistamines (H_1 inverse agonists) are the first-line treatment for chronic urticaria. Those with severe persistent urticaria may need uptitration to higher doses in combination with sedating antihistamines such as diphenhydramine or hydroxyzine (of which cetirizine is a derivative).

170. **What other alternatives are available for the treatment of chronic idiopathic urticaria?**
H_2 antihistamines and if refractory to high-dose antihistamines, omalizumab can be considered. Omalizumab is an anti-IgE antibody that has been approved by the FDA for chronic idiopathic urticaria.

171. **When would a biopsy be indicated for urticaria?**
Urticarial lesions that are painful (as opposed to pruritic), persist longer than 24 hours, or produce hyperpigmentation and scarring should undergo skin biopsy due to the possibility of underlying urticarial vasculitis. Some of these cases are accompanied by hypocomplementemia and may require more aggressive medical therapy.

172. **What is Schnitzler syndrome?**
A rare syndrome involving chronic urticaria, periodic fever, bone or joint pain, and the presence of monoclonal IgM proteinemia.
Jain T, Offord CP, Kyle RA, et al. Schnitzler syndrome: an under-diagnosed clinical entity. *Haematologica.* 2013;98:1581–1585.

DRUG ALLERGY

173. What is the difference between type A and type B drug reactions?

Type A drug reactions (>80% of adverse drug reactions) tend to be dose-dependent reactions in healthy individuals and are predictable based on the pharmacologic action of the drug. Type A reaction examples include sedation from antihistamines and nephrotoxicity from aminoglycosides. Type B drug reactions (<20% of adverse drug reactions) are unpredictable dose-independent reactions in susceptible individuals. Type B drug reactions include drug allergy, drug intolerance, idiosyncratic drug reactions, and pseudoallergic reactions.

174. What are the risk factors for drug allergy?

Parenteral administration, large molecular weight, high frequency of administration, large dosage, female gender, pharmacogenetics (see next question), and age (decreased risk in infancy and in the geriatric population).

175. Distinguish between an immunologic anaphylactic reaction and a nonimmunologic anaphylactic reaction.

Immunologic anaphylaxis results from mast cell degranulation due to cross-linking of mast cell–bound high-affinity IgE. Degranulation caused by non-IgE mast cell activation (e.g., C3a or C5a) leads to nonimmunologic anaphylaxis (formerly called *anaphylactoid reactions*). Examples include reactions to radiocontrast, NSAIDs, vancomycin, and opioids.

176. What are the four types of hypersensitivity reactions?

See Table 11.12.

Table 11.12. Four Types of Hypersensitivity Reactions

TYPE	MECHANISM	TIMING TO ONSET	CLINICAL EXAMPLE
I	Mast cells and basophils, often involving IgE.	1–15 min	Atopy, hay fever, urticaria
II	Antibody reacts with host cells leading to phagocytosis or lysis. Stimulatory or blocking antibodies may also cause disease.	Hours	Autoimmune hemolytic anemia (lysis), diabetes (blocking antibodies), Graves disease (stimulatory antibodies)
III	Immune complexes of any specificity deposit in tissues (typically the walls of small vessels and the kidney), leading to frustrated phagocytosis and complement activation.	Hours	Arthus reaction, polyarteritis nodosa, serum sickness, small vessel vasculitis
IV	T-cell–mediated either by CD4 cells activating macrophages or by cytolytic CD8 cells.	36–48 hr	Granulomatous reactions in tuberculosis and sarcoidosis; PPD reaction

PPD, purified protein derivative.

177. Describe the Arthus reaction and serum sickness.

An acute, local inflammatory response involving complement and neutrophils mediated by antigen-antibody complexes (immune complexes with antigen excess) in previously immunized individuals with high serum levels of complement-fixing IgG antibodies. Arthus reactions occur at injection sites during reimmunization of some vaccines (e.g., tetanus and diphtheria). Serum sickness is a systemic response that occurs in nonimmunized individuals with a first reaction onset of days to weeks opposed to hours as seen in the Arthus reaction. The clinical presentation involves fever, arthralgias, rash, GI symptoms, and lymphadenopathy. Reactions in previously sensitized individuals occurs within hours. There are serum sickness–like reactions reported to penicillins, cephalosporins, phenytoin, sulfonamides, and monoclonal antibodies, for example.

178. **What are the four types of type IV hypersensitivity reactions?**
Type IVa (monocytes), type IVb (eosinophils), type IVc (CD4+/CD8+ T cells), and type IVd (neutrophils).

179. **How does pharmacogenetics play a role in delayed hypersensitivity drug reactions?**
Numerous HLA-associated delayed hypersensitivity drug reactions can cause severe hypersensitivity syndromes. Abacavir hypersensitivity syndrome is seen in those patients with HLA-B*57:01. Stevens-Johnson syndrome/toxic epidermal necrosis (SJS/TEN) can be seen in Han Chinese/European/Japanese patients with HLA-B*58:01 taking allopurinol, Han Chinese/Thai/Malaysian/Indian patients with B*15:02 taking carbamazepine (A*31:01 in northern Europeans), and dapsone hypersensitivity syndrome can be seen in Asian patients with HLA-B*13:01. See Table 11.13.

Table 11.13. Examples of Delayed Hypersensitivity Reactions

TIME TO TYPE	INDUCING ANTIGEN	PEAK	EXTERNAL SIGNS	HISTOLOGIC APPEARANCE
Tuberculin	Tuberculin	48 hr	Indurated, painful skin swelling	Intradermal lymphocyte and monocyte infiltration
Jones-Mote	Foreign proteins such as ovalbumin	24 hr	Slight skin thickening	Intradermal, lymphocyte and basophil infiltration
Contact	Urushiol, the antigen of poison ivy	48 hr	Eczema	Same as tuberculin
Granulomatous	Talcum powder silica, other substances that stimulate phagocytosis but cannot be metabolized	4 wk	Skin induration	Epithelioid cell and granuloma formation, giant cells, macrophages, fibrosis, necrosis

Modified from Klein J. *Immunology*. Oxford: Blackwell Scientific Publications; 1990.

180. **How do you test for penicillin hypersensitivity?**
Through skin-prick and intradermal testing to penicilloyl-polylysine (major determinant) and penicillin G (one of several minor determinants), followed by oral challenge to amoxicillin. Skin-prick testing is conducted first to penicilloyl-polylysine and penicillin G, and if negative, is followed by intradermal testing to both determinants. Negative predictive value using penicilloyl-polylysine and penicillin G alone is approximated at 96–99%, but 10–20% of penicillin-allergic patients only exhibit positive skin testing to penilloate and penicilloate—two minor determinants that are not commercially available.
Macy E. Penicillin and beta-lactam allergy: epidemiology and diagnosis. *Curr Allergy Asthma Rep.* 2014;14(11):476.

181. **What are the advantages of penicillin skin testing to the health care system in general?**
Performing skin testing and challenges to penicillin can prevent serious adverse complications resulting from unverified penicillin allergies including hospital-acquired infections and antibiotic resistance, as well as reduce health care utilization required for drug desensitizations. It is estimated that 8% of health care participants in the United States carry a penicillin allergy in their medical chart, but 90% of those with a history of reaction will test negative for penicillin allergy. Additionally, 80% of individuals will lose their penicillin-IgE after 10 years. With regard to infectious complications, 2014 data from the Kaiser Foundation hospitals in Southern California found that hospitalized patients with presumptive penicillin allergies were treated with significantly more antibiotics compared with control subjects, experienced 23.4% more *Clostridium difficile*, 30.1% more vancomycin-resistant enterococci (VRE), and 14.1% more methicillin-resistant *S. aureus* (MRSA) infections than expected compared to control subjects.
Macy E, Contreras R. Health care use and serious infection prevalence associated with penicillin "allergy" in hospitalized patients: a cohort study. *J Allergy Clin Immunol.* 2014;133:790–796.

182. **Can penicillin-allergic patients receive cephalosporins safely?**
Although the majority of penicillin-allergic patients with positive skin testing will not experience any reaction with cephalosporins, there have been fatal reactions. As such, penicillin-allergic patients with positive skin testing who require cephalosporins should undergo graded challenge to the desired cephalosporin. Patients with negative skin testing can safely receive cephalosporins.

183. **Summarize the usual prophylactic regimen for radiocontrast media (RCM) administration in patient with allergic history.**
   - Prednisone 50 mg orally at 13 hours, 7 hours, and 1 hour before the procedure.
   - H_1 antihistamines (diphenhydramine, 50 mg parenterally or orally 1 hour before RCM administration).

   Premedication does not prevent all RCM reactions, but reactions after prophylactic therapy are usually mild. However, it is important that the procedure be started at the scheduled time or the efficacy of the prophylaxis may be decreased. It has been suggested that in patients with a history of RCM reactions, nonionic RCM do not seem to offer a significant protective advantage over medical prophylaxis, but because the consequences of an adverse reaction are life threatening, it is wise to err on the side of caution and use both prophylaxis and the newer low-osmolar reagents.

   Patterson R, DeSwarte RD, Greenberger PA, et al. Drug allergy and protocols for the management of drug allergies. *N Engl Reg Allergy Proc.* 1986;7:325–342.

184. **Are there any validated indirect tests such as in vitro or skin testing for nonpenicillin antibiotics?**
No. There are published nonirritating concentrations for many antibiotics, but skin testing with these concentrations is not standardized. The negative predictive value of nonstandardized skin testing is poor, but a positive skin test to a nonirritating concentration may indicate that drug-specific IgE is present. For reference to nonirritating concentrations for antibiotics and nonantibiotic agents, see the ENDA/EAACI (European Network on Drug Allergy/European Academy of Allergy and Clinical Immunology) Drug Allergy Interest Group position paper.

   Brockow K, Garvey LH, Aberer W, et al. Skin test concentrations for systemically administered drugs—an ENDA/EAACI Drug Allergy Interest Group position paper. *Allergy.* 2013;68:702–712.

185. **Can patients with sulfonamide drug allergy receive other sulfonamide-containing medications?**
Yes, as the nonantibiotic sulfonamide-containing agents lack the aromatic amine group at the N4 position as well as a substituted ring at the N1 position. Patients can receive furosemide, thiazide diuretics, and celecoxib, for example.

186. **Describe the hybridoma process of monoclonal antibody production.**
Monoclonal antibodies can be produced by hybridoma or phage-display technology. Hybridoma technology starts with the immunization of a mouse with a target antigen in order to create an immune response. B cells are isolated from the immunized mouse's spleen and are fused with immortalized myeloma cells in hypoxanthine-aminopterin-thymidine (HAT) medium. Myeloma cells are preselected to be both nonantibody secreting and sensitive to HAT medium. The resultant fusion product (hybridomas) are thus antibody-secreting and immortal. Unfused myeloma cells die as they cannot survive in the HAT medium, and unfused B cells die as they are not immortal. These hybridomas are then diluted into single cell wells and undergo screening for specific antibodies. Those B cells are cloned and produce specific monoclonal antibodies.

187. **What are the different types of monoclonal antibodies and their nomenclature?**
Mouse monoclonal antibodies are denoted by the suffix "-omab" and are constructed of murine-variable and constant regions. Chimeric monoclonal antibodies are denoted with the suffix "-ximab" and are constructed of murine variable regions and human constant regions. Humanized monoclonal antibodies are denoted with the suffix "-zumab" and contain the murine hypervariable regions with the remaining portion of the human Ig molecule. Human monoclonal antibodies are denoted by the suffix "-umab" and involve phage-display libraries involving human heavy and light chain variable region genes. These antibodies possess affinities comparable to antibodies produced using hybridoma technology.

188. **Describe the reactions to chemotherapeutic agents.**

Chemotherapeutic agents can induce both immunologic and nonimmunologic anaphylaxis. Platinum compounds including cisplatin, carboplatin, and oxiplatin induce immediate IgE-mediated hypersensitivity reactions typically after seven treatment cycles. Skin testing is available to delineate those at elevated risk for reaction, and over half of patients who are skin test negative become skin test positive; 12-step (3-bag) and 16-step (4-bag) desensitization protocols have been widely published (selection of protocol dependent on severity of reaction) and are effective. Taxanes, which include docetaxel and paclitaxel, induce nonimmunologic anaphylaxis/reactions, which can be prevented by premedication with corticosteroids and antihistamines. Excipients such as the vehicle Cremophor EL can also induce nonimmunologic anaphylactic reactions.

Castells MC1, Tennant NM, Sloane DE, et al. Hypersensitivity reactions to chemotherapy: outcomes and safety of rapid desensitization in 413 cases. *J Allergy Clin Immunol.* 2008;122:574–580.

189. **What is drug desensitization?**

The process of inducing a state of unresponsiveness to a drug responsible for an immediate hypersensitivity reaction. Tolerance to the drug is short lived and is maintained only if the drug is continued. The mechanisms for drug desensitization are not fully elucidated, but it is thought that the frequent administration of escalating subtherapeutic doses can induce internalization of cross-linked $Fc\varepsilon RI$ receptors or lead to binding but not cross-linking of IgE. Desensitization protocols have been published for many drugs including antibiotics, chemotherapeutics, biologic agents, and insulin, for example.

190. **What are the indications and contraindications for drug desensitization?**

Indications include lack of alternative agent (pregnant women with syphilis requiring penicillin) or inferior alternative (AERD/NERD patient requiring aspirin). Relative contraindications to desensitization include unstable asthma ($FEV_1 < 70\%$ of the normal level), unstable cardiac disease, or hemodynamic instability. Contraindications include history of bullous skin disease such as DRESS, Stevens-Johnson syndrome (polymorphic eruptions, mucous membrane involvement, organ dysfunction, fever), and toxic epidermal necrosis (extensive painful eruptions, fever, mucous membrane involvement, organ dysfunction), as well as drug-induced organ dysfunction (hepatitis, nephritis, vasculitis).

FOOD ALLERGY

191. **What is the mechanism of food allergy?**

Ingested food antigens bind and cross-link IgE bound to surface IgE receptors on intestinal mast cells, inducing an immediate hypersensitivity reaction. Basophils may also participate if food antigens appear in the circulation. The most common food allergies are secondary to wheat, egg, milk, peanut, tree nuts, shellfish, fish, soy, and sesame. Cooking of certain foods can reduce allergenicity and expedite development of tolerance such as seen with milk and egg.

Bird JA, Lack G, Perry TT. Clinical management of food allergy. *J Allergy Clin Immunol Pract.* 2015;3:1–11.

192. **What can masquerade as food allergy?**

Examples include allergic as well as pharmacologic reactions to food additives, preservatives, dyes, and toxins. GI disorders such as eosinophilic gastroenteritis, malabsorption syndromes, enzyme deficiencies, gluten-sensitive enteropathy, gallbladder disease, peptic ulcer disease, and scombroid poisoning are among a long list of important nonimmunologic causes of adverse food reactions.

193. **Which test is the gold standard for diagnosis of food allergy?**

A double-blind, placebo-controlled oral food challenge (DBPCFC). In clinical practice, an open oral food challenge (open OFC) with graded doses is often utilized given the time and effort of performing a DBPCFC.

Bird JA, Lack G, Perry TT. Clinical management of food allergy. *J Allergy Clin Immunol Pract.* 2015;3:1–11.

194. **When and where should an oral food challenge be performed?**

Food challenge should only be performed in a controlled setting such as the allergist's office, because life-threatening anaphylaxis may occur and require advanced life support measures. Whether or not to perform an oral food challenge depends on the clinical judgment of the allergist and includes evaluation of the nature of the food reaction (anaphylaxis versus abdominal cramping) and available in vitro and skin-prick testing results. There are published cut-off levels for several major food allergens that indicate a 50% chance of a successful oral challenge as well as published cut-off levels determining the 90% probability of reaction.

195. What are the available treatments for food allergy?

For acute food-induced anaphylaxis, prompt epinephrine administration is required to avoid fatality (highest incidence with peanut and tree nuts and associated with delayed or absent epinephrine administration). Adjunctive treatment includes antihistamines, oxygen supplementation, volume replacement, vasopressors, and corticosteroids. Once a diagnosis of food allergy is made, a written food anaphylaxis/emergency action plan is required, and medical alert bracelets should be considered for severe allergies. Avoidance of the known food allergen is essential. Premedication is not an effective means of food allergy prevention.

196. Why is food allergy on the rise?

Considerations include delayed introduction of complementary foods and decreased microbial exposures. The LEAP (Learning Early About Peanut) study demonstrated that early introduction of peanut significantly reduced the development of peanut allergy in high-risk infants by 5 years of age, and the LEAP-ON study confirmed continued tolerance to peanut after discontinuation of continuous peanut ingestion.

Allen KJ, Koplin JJ. Prospects for prevention of food allergy. *J Allergy Clin Immunol Pract.* 2016;4:215–220.

197. What are the current recommendations on complementary food introduction in infants?

The current American Academy of Allergy, Asthma and Immunology (AAAAI) and American Academy of Pediatrics (AAP) both reversed an earlier 2000 AAP guideline that recommended the delayed introduction of complementary foods, and it is now recommended that introduction should commence at 4–6 months of age.

198. Should screening be performed for foods prior to introduction?

Current guidelines state that routine screening for foods prior to introduction is not recommended. Although food skin-prick and in vitro specific IgE testing is sensitive, there are poor specificity and high false-positive rates. High-risk infants (defined in the LEAP study described previously as having either egg allergy or severe eczema) can be considered for peanut skin-prick testing. In vitro IgE testing for peanut or its component proteins is not recommended.

199. What is scombroid poisoning?

An acute-onset histamine-mediated reaction to contaminated scombroid fish such as tuna and mackerel as well as nonscombroid fish such as amberjack, mahi-mahi, salmon, bluefish, sardines, and herring. Improperly refrigerated and stored fish undergo marked histamine production due to histidine decarboxylase production by bacteria. Histamine, through binding to various histamine receptors (H_1 through H_4), can induce symptoms including headache, dizziness, palpitations, flushing, nausea, vomiting, abdominal cramping, diarrhea, and urticaria. As histamine cannot be degraded by normal cooking temperatures, cooking poisoned fish properly cannot prevent symptoms. Symptoms can last 1 day or longer.

Greenberger PA, Lieberman P. Idiopathic anaphylaxis. *J Allergy Clin Immunol Pract.* 2014;2:243–250.

200. Describe pollen-food allergy syndrome (oral allergy syndrome).

An IgE-mediated syndrome due to cross-reactive proteins in certain foods and pollens. The class 2 allergen families profilins and Bet v1 can present as pollen-food allergy syndrome. The clinical presentation can involve paraesthesia, angioedema, and pruritus of the face, mouth, or throat upon contact with raw vegetables or fruits in pollen-allergic individuals. Severe symptoms including anaphylaxis are rare in this predominantly contact allergic reaction.

201. A patient presents with a history of delayed urticaria and anaphylaxis to ingestion of beef. What further information would be helpful, and what is the most likely diagnosis?

Pertinent information that would be helpful include prior history of tick bites (or chiggers) and recurrent allergic episodes 2–6 hours following red meat or organ ingestion (beef, pork, and lamb meats and various mammalian organs reported). Alpha-gal allergy is a novel food allergy characterized by delayed urticaria or anaphylaxis secondary to IgE directed against galactose-alpha-1,3-galactose (α-Gal) found in red meat. Sensitization to the oligosaccharide α-Gal is likely secondary to bites from ticks (or chiggers) that possess α-Gal in their alimentary tracts from prior feeding on mammals such as deer. Interestingly, patients with cat-pork syndrome can present with allergic reactions to pork ingestion due to cross-reactivity between cat and pork albumins. However, these reactions are not delayed and are limited to pork ingestion.

Commins SP, Satinover SM, Hosen J, et al. Delayed anaphylaxis, angioedema, or urticaria after consumption of red meat in patients with IgE antibodies specific for galactose-alpha-1,3-galactose. *J Allergy Clin Immunol.* 2009;123:426–433.

Tripathi A, Commins SP, Heymann PW, et al. Delayed anaphylaxis to red meat masquerading as idiopathic anaphylaxis. *J Allergy Clin Immunol Pract.* 2014;2:259–265.

202. **Describe food protein-induced enterocolitis syndrome (FPIES).**
A non–IgE-mediated food hypersensitivity presenting typically during infancy and characterized by profuse vomiting and lethargy 2–4 hours after allergen ingestion. Common inciting allergens include cow milk, soy, rice, and oat, although many other foods have been implicated. Adult-onset reactions to shellfish have been reported as well. Notably, skin-prick and in vitro allergen-specific IgE testing are generally negative. The gold standard diagnostic test is a physician-supervised oral food challenge (OFC), and an OFC can also be utilized to determine if tolerance has developed. OFCs should be performed in the hospital setting where full resuscitation equipment is available. The natural history of the common offending foods in FPIES is variable and not fully determined, but generally, solid food FPIES resolves by 5 years of age, and milk and soy typically take longer.

Caubet JC, Ford LS, Sickles L, et al. Clinical features and resolution of food protein-induced enterocolitis syndrome: 10-year experience. *J Allergy Clin Immunol.* 2014;134(2):382–389.

203. **What is Heiner syndrome?**
A non–IgE-mediated food hypersensitivity to cow milk characterized by variable clinical manifestations including pulmonary disease (infiltrates, hemoptysis, hemosiderosis), recurrent infections, and systemic symptoms (fever, failure to thrive, vomiting, diarrhea). Clinical improvement occurs with milk elimination.

Moissidis I, Chaidaroon D, Vichyanond P, et al. Milk-induced pulmonary disease in infants (Heiner syndrome). *Pediatr Allergy Immunol.* 2005;16(6):545–552.

204. **Describe food-dependent exercise-induced anaphylaxis (FDEIA).**
Anaphylaxis secondary to exercise preceded by food ingestion commonly to wheat and shellfish. Notably, food ingestion and exercise are independently tolerated, and clinical manifestations can include pruritus, urticaria, angioedema, respiratory and GI upset, and possible shock. The pathophysiology of FDEIA is not fully known but may include increased GI permeability—during exercise, for example.

Du Toit G. Food-dependent exercise-induced anaphylaxis in childhood. *Pediatr Allergy Immunol.* 2007;18:455–463.

VENOM ALLERGY

205. **How is venom allergy diagnosed?**
Clinical history remains the most important component in the evaluation of insect sting reactions, and diagnosis involves skin-prick and intradermal testing as well as in vitro IgE testing. Skin testing is generally the first step in evaluating a systemic reaction and performed using honeybee, wasp, and vespid (yellow and white-faced hornets, yellow jacket) venom. If skin-prick testing is negative, intradermal testing is performed. If both skin-prick and intradermal testing is negative, in vitro testing is recommended as 20% of skin testing can be falsely negative. If in vitro testing is also negative, repeat skin testing is recommended after 4–8 weeks.

Tankersley MS, Ledford DK. Stinging insect allergy: state of the art 2015. *J Allergy Clin Immunol Pract.* 2015;3:315–322.

206. **Which patients should undergo venom immunotherapy (VIT)? What are the considerations for VIT discontinuation?**
All patients with systemic reactions not limited to the skin and patients 17 years and older who have experienced systemic reactions limited to the skin should undergo skin testing and receive

epinephrine autoinjectors and VIT. There is a low risk of future systemic reactions in patients 16 years and younger who have had either a local reaction or systemic reaction limited to the skin. Currently immunotherapy exists for honeybee, wasp, mixed vespids, and fire ant, and patients usually will undergo immunotherapy to all venoms that were positive on testing. VIT is generally administered for 3–5 years and can reduce the risk of a systemic reaction to that of the general population (<5%). Patients who have had life-threatening initial reactions or recurrent systemic reactions while on VIT or have been diagnosed with mastocytosis or mast cell activation syndrome should be considered for lifelong therapy.

Tankersley MS, Ledford DK. Stinging insect allergy: state of the art 2015. *J Allergy Clin Immunol Pract.* 2015;3:315–322.

207. **In addition to skin testing to venom, what other test is recommended for patients presenting with venom anaphylaxis?**
Serum tryptase level is recommended to screen for indolent systemic mastocytosis, as anaphylaxis in those patients is most commonly due to insect stings.

Tankersley MS, Ledford DK. Stinging insect allergy: state of the art 2015. *J Allergy Clin Immunol Pract.* 2015;3:315–322.

ANAPHYLAXIS

208. **What are the main diagnostic criteria for anaphylaxis?**
There are three main clinical criteria for anaphylaxis (adapted from World Allergy Organization [WAO] criteria):
1. Acute onset (within minutes to several hours) of cutaneous and/or mucosal involvement AND at least one of the following:
    a. Respiratory distress (wheezing, shortness of breath, coughing, stridor, hypoxemia)
    b. Hypotension or end-organ dysfunction
2. Exposure to a likely allergen/trigger for the patient AND two or more of the following (within minutes to several hours):
    c. Cutaneous or mucosal involvement (diffuse urticaria, flushing, lip/tongue/uvula angioedema)
    d. Respiratory distress (wheezing, shortness of breath, coughing, stridor, hypoxemia)
    e. Hypotension or end-organ dysfunction
    f. GI distress (abdominal pain, vomiting, diarrhea)
3. Hypotension after exposure to known allergen to the patient

209. **A 20-year-old man presents with hypotension, wheezing, and urticaria 30 minutes after a bee sting. What is the first priority of treatment?**
Maintenance of cardiovascular and pulmonary function (advanced cardiovascular life support [ACLS]) and immediate treatment with epinephrine by either subcutaneous or intramuscular (IM) routes (0.01 mg/kg of a 1:1000 dilution IM) are crucial. With cardiovascular collapse, IV epinephrine may be indicated (0.01 mg/kg of a 1:10000 dilution IV).

210. **What other immediate steps should be taken?**
    - Maintain supine position unless actively vomiting to prevent cardiac hypoperfusion ("empty-heart syndrome").
    - Provide oxygen, airway support, and IV fluids for blood pressure.
    - If patient is beta-blocked, the first drug to administer is epinephrine. Glucagon can be considered after epinephrine administration.

211. **What is the best laboratory test to order during anaphylaxis?**
Serum tryptase level within 1–2 hours of the event. Notably, serum tryptase is not generally elevated during anaphylaxis due to food allergen but can be elevated in FDEIA.

212. **Which class of medications should be used with particular caution in patients prone to develop anaphylaxis?**
Beta blockers can accentuate the severity of anaphylaxis, prolong its cardiovascular and pulmonary manifestations, and dampen the effectiveness of epinephrine in reversing the life-threatening manifestations of anaphylaxis.

213. **What are the leading causes of perioperative anaphylaxis?**

The leading causes include neuromuscular blocking agents (NMBA), antibiotics, and latex. The most commonly identified causes are NMBAs and antibiotics.

MAST CELL DISORDERS

214. **What is the differential diagnosis for idiopathic anaphylaxis?**

Occult antigen (untested food antigen, excipient, preservative, latex), α-Gal, mast cell activation, mastocytosis, pheochromocytoma, vasointestinal polypeptide secreting tumors, carcinoid syndrome, vocal cord dysfunction/paradoxical vocal fold motion, panic attack, hyperventilation, Munchausen anaphylaxis (hidden self-induction of anaphylaxis due to known allergen), and somatoform reactions.

Greenberger PA, Lieberman P. Idiopathic anaphylaxis. *J Allergy Clin Immunol Pract.* 2014;2:243–250.

215. **What is systemic mastocytosis, and how is it diagnosed?**

One of two major primary mast cell disorders (mastocytosis and monoclonal mast cell activation syndrome) due to pathologic accumulation of mast cells in tissues and organs and in most cases is secondary to mutations in c-kit (most common is D816V in exon 17 found in almost all adults and 40% of children). The mutations in c-kit lead to derangement in the mast cell or multipotential hematopoetic progenitor. The most common clinical finding in mastocytosis is urticaria pigmentosa, although it is not sufficient for diagnosis. Diagnosis for systemic mastocytosis (based on World Health Organization [WHO] criteria) is 1 major criterion or 3 minor criteria. The major criterion is the presence of mast cell aggregates (>15 cells) in bone marrow or organ. The minor criteria include spindle shape or other atypical morphologic appearance in >25% of the mast cells in bone marrow or tissue, presence of the D816V c-kit mutation, CD2/CD25-positive mast cells, or baseline serum tryptase levels > 20 ng/mL.

Akin C. Mast cell activation disorders. *J Allergy Clin Immunol Pract.* 2014;2:252–257.

Yu JE, Akin C. Mast cell disorders. *J Allergy Clin Immunol Pract.* 2016;4:557–558.

216. **What is idiopathic mast cell activation syndrome (MCAS)?**

A syndrome consisting of symptoms of mast cell degranulation, increase in mast cell mediators (serum tryptase elevation of 20% plus 2 ng/mL from baseline, 24-hour urinary elevations at baseline or flare of PGD_2 or 11β-prostaglandin F2-alpha, N-methylhistamine, or leukotriene E4) and response to antihistamines, leukotriene antagonists or cromolyn. Patients do not have the D816V c-kit mutation.

Akin C. Mast cell activation disorders. *J Allergy Clin Immunol Pract.* 2014;2:252–257.

DERMATITIS AND OTHER CUTANEOUS DISORDERS

217. **What is the underlying immunopathology of atopic dermatitis (AD)?**

An impaired skin barrier (due to either a mutation in the gene encoding filaggrin, an epidermal structural protein, or to abnormalities in other epidermal proteins such as loricrin, involucrin, and hornerin) can lead to a proinflammatory type 2 response. Additionally, patients with atopic dermatitis have been found to have reductions in antimicrobial peptides such as defensins and cathelicidins.

Lio PA, Lee M, LeBovidge J, et al. Clinical management of atopic dermatitis: practical highlights and updates from the atopic dermatitis practice parameter 2012. *J Allergy Clin Immunol Pract.* 2014;2:361–369.

218. **What are the main treatment options for AD?**

Skin hydration (moisturizers), topical corticosteroids (1–2 weeks maximum due to adverse effects; evidence supports proactive treatment twice weekly to commonly affected areas with low potency corticosteroid), topical calcineurin inhibitors (effective and safe for patients 2 years and older; can use for proactive therapy; black-box warning for malignancy but large case-control study of 300,000 patients found no increased lymphoma risk), oral vitamin D (topical applications are not recommended owing to potential allergic and irritant properties), antibiotics (for skin infections, not colonization), bleach baths (can decrease AD severity with twice-weekly use), wet dressings (topical corticosteroid placed on soaked skin and under damp gauze and then a dry layer; can use up to 14 days; can lead to maceration of skin, secondary infections, topical corticosteroid adverse effects).

Lio PA, Lee M, LeBovidge J, et al. Clinical management of atopic dermatitis: practical highlights and updates from the atopic dermatitis practice parameter 2012. *J Allergy Clin Immunol Pract.* 2014;2:361–369.

219. **Summarize the clinical features, diagnosis, and treatment of contact dermatitis.**
Allergic and irritant contact dermatitis both can present with either an erythematous and pruritic skin rash or an eczematous rash with crusting. The distribution of the rash can provide clues leading to the potential allergen/irritant and the diagnosis. For example, eyelid dermatitis is typically secondary to either eye cosmetics or ectopic transfer from other sites including the nails, and women are at higher risk for facial contact dermatitis, which is most often allergic in nature. Systemic contact dermatitis ("baboon syndrome") can be seen in patients sensitized to Balsam of Peru, metal (nickel, mercury, gold), or neomycin who ingest or receive infusions to foods or medications containing those contactants. Patch testing should be considered in order to uncover contact sensitization. It is not clear whether atopic individuals are at higher risk of allergic contact dermatitis compared to nonatopic individuals.
Bernstein DI. Contact dermatitis for the practicing allergist. *J Allergy Clin Immunol Pract.* 2015;3:652–658.

220. **What are the clinical features of DRESS?**
DRESS, which is a potentially life-threatening syndrome of drug rash/reaction with eosinophilia and systemic symptoms, is most commonly secondary to anticonvulsants and antibiotics. Onset typically is between 2 and 8 weeks, although reactivation with EBV, human herpesvirus (HHV)-7, and HHV-6 has been associated with earlier onset disease. DRESS remains a clinical diagnosis with clinical manifestations including facial edema, lymphadenopathy, fever, rash (myriad manifestations including urticarial, vesicles, bullae, erythroderma), organ dysfunction (liver dysfunction, pneumonitis, myocarditis, pericarditis, nephritis, colitis), and hematologic abnormalities (eosinophilia, leukocytosis).

221. **What is erythema multiforme (EM)?**
An immunologic reaction of the skin and mucous membranes to a variety of antigenic stimuli including infection, collagen vascular disease, malignancy, hormonal changes, and medications. The lesions may be localized or widespread and consist of bullae, erythematous plaques, and epidermal cell necrosis. The lesions are usually bilaterally and symmetrically distributed on the extensor surfaces of the limbs, on the dorsal and volar aspects of the hands and feet, and on the trunk. The lesions, which resemble "targets" or "bull's eyes," are diagnostic. They appear as a central vesicle or dark purple papule, surrounded by a round, pale zone that is in turn surrounded by a round area of erythema.

222. **What is the Stevens-Johnson syndrome?**
A severe form of EM with fulminant, disseminated, multisystem involvement. Patients appear toxic, with fever, chills, malaise, tachycardia, tachypnea, and prostration. Diffuse vesicular, bullous, and ulcerative lesions of the skin and mucous membranes develop and desquamate, leading to secondary infections, which in turn may lead to sepsis and even death. It is associated with all causes of EM.

TRANSPLANTATION IMMUNOLOGY

223. **Explain the importance of HLA typing in solid organ and bone marrow transplantation (BMT).**
HLA compatibility of donor and recipient affects graft outcome in both solid organ transplantation (such as kidney, heart, lung, and liver) and BMT. For solid organs, HLA-DR mismatches are most important in the first 6 months after transplantation, whereas HLA-B mismatches are relevant in the first 2 years after transplantation. HLA-A mismatches negatively impact long-term graft survival. HLA incompatibility may lead to graft rejection of solid organ transplantation and to GVHD in BMT. In BMT HLA matching is performed to HLA-A, HLA-B, and HLA-DR.
Sheldon S, Poulton K. HLA typing and its influence on organ transplantation. *Methods Mol Biol.* 2006;333:157–174.

224. **Is HLA compatibility a major graft survival factor in corneal transplants?**
HLA compatibility is not a major graft survival factor for first-time nonvascularized corneal transplants.

225. **Explain how the mechanism of graft rejection differs from the mechanism of GVHD in BMT.**
In graft rejection, the graft is attacked by the recipient's immune system. In contrast, in BMT with GVHD, the immunocompetent cells from the donor attack the recipient, whose own immune system has been ablated prior to the transplant.

226. **Explain the importance of ABO typing in solid organ transplantation and BMT.**
ABO blood typing is critical in solid organ transplants because ABO antigens are expressed on all tissue cells of the transplanted organ and because type O, type A, or type B recipients almost always have preformed antibodies to these blood group antigens. Thus, transplantation of solid organ grafts at a minimum requires compatibility at ABO. However, ABO compatibility, oddly enough, is not a requirement for bone marrow grafting because the donor graft will thereafter supply all blood cells.

227. **List the four types of graft rejection and their immunologic mechanisms.**
See Table 11.14.

Table 11.14. Types of Solid Organ Graft Rejections

TYPE	ONSET	MAJOR EFFECTOR MECHANISMS
Hyperacute	Minutes to hours	Humoral: preformed cytotoxic antibody in the recipient against donor graft antigen(s) a. ABO system b. Anti-HLA class I
Accelerated	2–5 days	Cell-mediated: due to prior T-cell sensitization against donor antigen(s)
Acute	7–28 days	Principally cell-mediated immunity: allogeneic reactivity by recipient T cells against donor antigen(s) Humoral immunity to HLA antigens
Chronic	>3 mo	Principally cell-mediated immunity allogeneic reactivity by recipient T cells against donor antigen(s) Humoral immunity to HLA antigens

HLA, human leukocyte antigen.

228. **What is the mechanism of action of cyclosporine? What are its principal adverse effects?**
Cyclosporine inhibits calcineurin-dependent signal transduction and binds to cytoplasmic immunophilins. This interaction inhibits the phosphatase activity of calcineurin, resulting in a reduction of IL-2 production and T-cell activation. The main side effects include nephrotoxicity (25–75% of patients), hypertension, hirsutism, hepatotoxicity, gingival hyperplasia, seizures (5% of patients), and tremor (>50% of patients).

KEY POINTS: ALLERGY AND IMMUNOLOGY

1. Epinephrine/advanced life support should be the first interventions in suspected anaphylaxis.
2. Intranasal corticosteroids are the first-line treatment option for allergic rhinitis.
3. Aspirin desensitization is recommended in patients with AERD/NERD.
4. Drug desensitization or challenge should not be performed if there is a history of severe non-IgE–mediated reaction including SJS, TEN, hemolytic anemia, interstitial nephritis, or hepatitis.
5. Omalizumab is FDA approved for both moderate to severe persistent asthma and chronic idiopathic urticaria.
6. Amoxicillin-clavulanate is the first-line treatment for acute bacterial rhinosinusitis.
7. Smoking cessation is critical for successful management of asthma, COPD, and allergic rhinitis.
8. Mast cell activation disorders should be considered in patients presenting with idiopathic anaphylaxis.
9. The double-blind placebo-controlled food challenge is the gold standard for food allergy diagnosis.
10. CVID requires evidence of both decreased immunoglobulins (IgG, IgA, and/or IgM) as well as specific antibody deficiency.

AERD/NERD, aspirin-exacerbated respiratory disease/nonsteroidal anti-inflammatory drug–exacerbated respiratory disease; COPD, chronic obstructive pulmonary disease; CVID, common variable immunodeficiency; FDA, Food and Drug Administration; SJS, Stevens-Johnson syndrome; TEN, toxic epidermal necrosis.

BIBLIOGRAPHY

1. Abbas AK, Lichtman AH, Pillai S. *Cellular and Molecular Immunology*. 8th ed. Philadelphia: WB Saunders; 2014.
2. Adkinson NF, Middleton E, Busse W, eds. *Middleton's Allergy: Principles and Practice*. 8th ed. St. Louis: Mosby; 2013.
3. Murphy KP, Murphy KM, Travers P, eds. *Janeway's Immunobiology*. 7th ed. New York: Garland; 2008.
4. Klein J. *Immunology*. 2nd ed. Oxford: Blackwell Scientific Publications; 1997.
5. Paul WE, ed. *Fundamental Immunology*. 6th ed. Philadelphia: Lippincott Williams & Wilkins; 2008.
6. Rich RR, Fleisher TA, Shearer WT, eds. *Clinical Immunology, Principles and Practice*. 3rd ed. St. Louis: Mosby; 2008.

CHAPTER 12

INFECTIOUS DISEASES

Harrinarine Madhosingh, MD, FACP, FIDSA

ANTIBIOTICS AND RESISTANCE

1. **What is antimicrobial stewardship?**
   Coordinated interventions designed to improve and measure the appropriate use of antimicrobial agents by promoting the selection of the optimal drug, including dosing, duration of therapy, and route of administration.
   Society for Healthcare Epidemiology of America, Infectious Diseases Society of America, Pediatric Infectious Diseases Society. Policy Statement on Antimicrobial Stewardship by the Society for Healthcare Epidemiology of America (SHEA), the Infectious Diseases Society of America (IDSA), and the Pediatric Infectious Diseases Society (PIDS). *Infect Control Hosp Epidemiol.* 2012;33:322–327.

2. **Why is antimicrobial stewardship important?**
   Because effective stewardship:
   - Reduces emergence of resistant bacteria
   - Decreases rates of *Clostridium difficile* infections
   - Improves use of antibiotics in surgical prophylaxis
   - Ensures the proper and safest treatment of patients
   File TM Jr, Srinivasan A, Bartlett JG. Antimicrobial stewardship: importance for patient and public health. *Clin Infect Dis.* 2014;59:S93–S96.

3. **What are two core strategies of antimicrobial stewardship?**
   Prospective audit and feedback and formulary restriction with preauthorization for selected antimicrobials.
   Dellit TH, Owens RC, McGowan JE, et al. Infectious Diseases Society of America and the Society for Healthcare Epidemiology of America guidelines for developing an institutional program to enhance antimicrobial stewardship. *Clin Infect Dis.* 2007;44:159–177.

4. **What are commonly used antimicrobial stewardship metrics?**
   - DDD (defined daily dosing): a measure of the average daily dose of an antibiotic in a standard patient
   - DOT (days of therapy): the number of days a patient is on an antibiotic
   Both measures can be problematic and are usually standardized (hospitalized patient-days or 1000 patient-days).

5. **Is antimicrobial stewardship mandatory?**
   To date, the U.S. Centers for Medicare and Medicaid Services (CMS) does not require antimicrobial stewardship programs in hospitals, but a regulatory requirement for stewardship programs may be necessary by the end of 2017. Since 2008, the state of California has required acute care hospitals to review and monitor antibiotic utilization. In 2014, California Senate Bill 1311 was signed into law requiring antimicrobial stewardship programs in hospitals.
   Centers for Medicare & Medicaid Services, Hospital Infection Control Worksheet, Nov. 26, 2014. Available at: www.go.cms.gov/1B6NCSV [accessed 05.11.2016].
   President's Council of Advisors on Science and Technology: Report to the President on Combating Antibiotic Resistance, September, 2014. Available at: www.whitehouse.gov/sites/default/files/microsites/ostp/PCAST/pcast_carb_report_sept2014.pdf [accessed 05.11.2016].

6. **What antibiotics work by binding penicillin-binding proteins (PBPs)?**
   Beta-lactam antibiotics, which include penicillins, cephalosporins, carbapenems, and monobactams. These antibiotics inhibit cell wall synthesis and are generally considered bactericidal owing to their mechanism of action.

7. **What beta-lactam antibiotic could be safely used in patients allergic to penicillins?**
Aztreonam, which covers only aerobic gram-negative organisms. There is no cross-reactivity between aztreonam and pencillin; however, there are reports of cross-reactivity between aztreonam and ceftazidime due to an identical side chain.

   Adkinson NF Jr. Immunogenicity and cross-allergenicity of aztreonanm. *Am J Med.* 1990;88:S12–S15.

   Patriarca G, Shiavino D, Altomonto G, et al. Tolerability of aztreonam in patients with IgE-mediated hypersensitivity to beta-lactams. *Int J Immunopathol Pharmacol.* 2008;21:357–359.

8. **What is the antimicrobial spectrum of penicillins?**
Narrow spectrum for penicillin G including:
   * *Streptococcus pyogenes*
   * *Streptococcus pneumoniae* (except for those strains with beta-lactam resistance)
   * Oropharyngeal anaerobes
   * *Treponema pallidum*

   Broad spectrum for ticarcillin-clavulanate and piperacillin-clavulanate including:
   * Gram-positive organisms
   * Gram-negative organisms
   * Anaerobes

9. **Which penicillins are considered drugs of choice for methicillin-sensitive *Staphylococcus aureus* (MSSA)?**
Methicillin, nafcillin, oxacillin, and dicloxacillin with a very narrow spectrum of activity. Recently cefazolin has been compared to oxacillin for complicated bacteremia with MSSA and has been found to be similar for treatment with improved safety.

   Li J, Echevarria KL, Hughes DW, et al. Comparison of cefazolin versus oxacillin for treatment of complicated bacteremia caused by methicillin-susceptible *Staphylococcus aureus. Antimicrob Agents Chemother.* 2014;58:5117–5124.

10. **First- and second-generation cephalosporins are more effective than third-generation cephalosporins against which organisms?**
Gram-positive organisms.

11. **List cephalosporins and the generation to which they belong.**
   * **First:** cefazolin, cephalexin, cephradine, cefadroxil
   * **Second:** cefoxitin, cefotetan, cefuroxime, cefaclor
   * **Third:** ceftriaxone, cefotaxime, ceftizoxime, ceftazidime, cefixime, cefpodoxime, cefdinir
   * **Fourth:** cefepime

12. **Which cephalosporins have activity against methicillin-resistant *S. aureus* (MRSA)?**
   * Ceftaroline
   * Ceftobiprole (approved in some European countries)

   Laudano J. Ceftaroline fosamil: a new broad spectrum cephalosporin. *J Antimicrob Chemother.* 2011;66:iii11–iii18.

13. **What organism do cephalosporins *not* cover?**
Enterococcus.

14. **What is the spectrum of carbapenems?**
Broad-spectrum, including gram-positive, gram-negative, and anaerobic organisms.

15. **List specific deficiencies in carbapanem coverage.**
Ertapenem will not cover *Pseudomonas, Acinetobacter,* and *Enterococcus faecalis.* In general, carbapenems will not cover MRSA, *Stenotrophomonas, Legionella* or other atypicals, *Corynebacterium jeikeium, Burkholderia,* and *Enterococcus faecium.* Enterococcal coverage varies among the carbapenems and is typically bacteriostatic.

16. **How do fluoroquinolone antibiotics work?**
By directly inhibiting DNA synthesis through the inhibition of DNA gyrase and topoisomerase IV. These antibiotics are generally considered bactericidal.

   Hooper D. Mechanisms of action of antimicrobials: focus on fluoroquinolones. *Clin Infect Dis.* 2001;32:S9–S15.

17. **Which fluoroquinolones should not be used to treat pneumonia or urinary tract infections (UTIs)?**
Ciprofloxacin because of its poor activity against *Streptococcus pneumoniae*. Moxifloxacin should not be used to treat UTI owing to poor urinary concentrations of this drug. Moxifloxacin, unlike levofloxacin and ciprofloxacin, has no *Pseudomonas* activity. Other available fluoroquinolones include gemifloxacin, norfloxacin, and ofloxacin. Note that these drugs carry a black box warning about increased risk of tendonitis and tendon rupture.

18. **Which antibiotics inhibit protein synthesis at the 50S ribosomal subunit?**
Chloramphenicol, macrolides and letolides, lincosamides (clindamycin), oxazolidinones (linezolid, tedizolid), and streptogramins (quinupristin/dalfopristin).

19. **Which antibiotics inhibit protein synthesis by binding to the 30S ribosomal subunit?**
Tetracyclines and aminoglycosides.

20. **What is the mechanism of action of tigecycline?**
To block entry of tRNA by binding to the 30S ribosome. This glycylcycline antibiotic is an analog of minocycline and has a broad spectrum of activity including MRSA and vancomycin-resistant enterococci (VRE). Tigecycline does not cover *Pseudomonas* and certain *Proteus* species (including *P. mirabilis*).
    Doan, TL, Fung, HB, Mehta D, et al. Tigecycline: a glycylcycline antimicrobial agent. *Clin Ther*. 2006;28:1079–1106.

21. **What are the glycopeptide antibiotics?**
Vancomycin, telavancin, and teicoplanin (not available in the United States). Telavancin is a lipoglycopeptide and is approved for skin/skin structure infections and hospital-acquired/ventilator-acquired bacterial pneumonia due to *S. aureus*. The mechanism is similar to vancomycin in that it binds to terminal acyl-D-alanyl-D-alanine chains of the cell wall and inhibits cell wall synthesis.

22. **What antibiotic causes linear IgA bullous dermatosis?**
Vancomycin. Bullous dermatosis is an autoimmune disease caused by IgA deposition at the basement membrane zone, which eventually leads to loss of adhesion at the dermal-epidermal junction and blister formation. Vancomycin has also been reported to cause "red-man" syndrome (flushing/red rash affecting the face, neck, and torso), neutropenia, thrombocytopenia, nephrotoxicity and ototoxicity, toxic epidermal necrolysis, and fever.
    Bernstein E, Schuster M. Linear IgA bullous dermatosis associated with vancomycin. *Ann Intern Med*. 1998;129:508–509.

23. **What are the long-acting agents available for MRSA treatment?**
Dalbavancin and oritavancin. Both are lipoglycopeptides that can be dosed once weekly for treatment of gram-positive skin infections.

24. **What is the mechanism of action of daptomycin?**
Insertion of its lipophilic tail into the bacterial cell membrane causing rapid membrane depolarization and potassium ion efflux, a novel mechanism of action. Daptomycin is a cyclic lipopeptide that is active against many gram-positive organisms including MRSA, VRE, and some anaerobic gram-positive organisms.
    Steenbergen JN, Alder J, Thorne GM. Daptomycin: a lipopeptide antibiotic for the treatment of serious gram-positive infections. *Antimicrob Chemother*. 2005;55:283–288.

25. **What are the mechanisms of antibiotic resistance?**
    - Enzymatic degradaton of antibacterial drugs
    - Alteration of antimicrobial targets
    - Changes in membrane permeability to antibiotics
    Dever LA, Dermody TS. Mechanisms of bacterial resistance to antibiotics. *Arch Intern Med* 1991;151:886–895.

26. **What is TEM, SHV, CTX, and OXA?**
Beta-lactamases found in various organisms and responsible for hydrolysis of different antibiotics. Four molecular classes of beta-lactamases have been described (A, B, C, D). TEM, SHV, and CTX are class A beta-lactamases. OXA is a class D beta-lactamase.

27. **What is NDM-1?**

New Delhi metallo-beta-lactamase. Considered a class B beta-lactamase, this enzyme hydrolyzes a broad range of antibiotics including carbapenems and was first detected in a Swedish patient of Indian origin in 2008.

Walsh TR, Weeks J, Livermore DM, et al. Dissemination of NDM-1 positive bacteria in the New Delhi environment and its implications for human health: an environmental point prevalence study. *Lancet Infect Dis.* 2011;11:355–362.

28. **What is ESBL and KPC?**

ESBL or extended spectrum beta-lactamases hydrolyze extended spectrum cephalosporins. KPC or *Klebsiella pneumoniae* carbapenemase hydrolyzes carbapenem antibiotics.

29. **What is the mechanism of action of colistin (polymyxin E) and polymyxin B?**

To bind to lipopolysaccharides (LPS) and phospholipids in the outer cell membrane of gram-negative bacteria. They displace cations, calcium and magnesium, from the phosphate groups of the outer cell membrane, which disrupts the cell membrane and causes leakage of cellular contents with ensuing bacterial death.

Polymyxin B also binds to and inactivates endotoxin. Both these antibiotics are used as a last resort in gram-negative infections given their toxicities.

30. **What is *mcr-1*?**

A gene that can make bacteria resistant to polymyxins (including colistin) that exists on a plasmid, first described in China in late 2015. A patient in Pennsylvania was identified with this gene in 2016.

31. **What are the major antifungal classes and their mechanisms of action?**
    - **Azoles:** Inhibit 14-α-demethylase, which blocks demethylation of lanosterol thereby inhibiting ergosterol synthesis, which is essential for cell wall synthesis. Newest azoles include posaconazole and isavuconazole.
    - **Echinocandins:** Inhibit production of (1→3)-β-D-glucan by inhibiting the enzyme 1,3-β glucan synthase. This enzyme inhibits fungal cell wall synthesis.
    - **Polyenes:** Bind ergosterol in the fungal cell wall and disrupt cell wall permeability. Rapidly fungicidal. Amphotericin B is one of the broadest antifungals available. Nystatin is also a polyene but is used mostly topically because of its adverse effect profile.
    - **Flucytosine:** A pyrimidine analog that inhibits DNA synthesis and protein synthesis in the fungal cell. Unfavorable toxicity profile and rapid development of resistance when used as monotherapy limit its use.

32. **What electrolytes should be closely monitored with amphotericin B administration?**

Potassium, magnesium, and, to a lesser extent, calcium. Other severe reactions that occur during infusion include fever, chills, hypotension, headache, nausea, and tachypnea.

FEVER AND FEVER OF UNKNOWN ORIGIN (FUO)

33. **What is the definition of a fever?**
    - Oral temperature > 38° C (100.4° F)
    - Rectal or ear temperature > 38.3° C (101° F)

34. **What is FUO?**

A temperature of at least 38.3° C on several occasions lasting more than 3 weeks in duration with failure to reach a diagnosis despite 1 week of inpatient investigation or after two or more outpatient visits.

Hayakawa K, Ramasamy B, Chandrasekar PH. Fever of unknown origin: an evidence based review. *Am J Med Sci.* 2012;344:307–316.

Petersdorf RG, Beeson PB. Fever of unexplained origin: report on 100 cases. *Medicine (Baltimore).* 1961;40:1–30.

35. **What are the three major causes of FUO?**
    - Infection
    - Malignancy
    - Autoimmune syndromes

36. **What are some infectious causes of FUO?**
    - Cholangitis
    - Intra-abdominal or pelvic abscess
    - Acalculous cholecystitis
    - Tuberculosis
    - Typhoid fever
    - Epstein-Barr virus (EBV)
    - Cytomegalovirus (CMV)
    - Cat-scratch disease (due to *Bartonella henselae*)
    - Visceral leishmaniasis
    - Endocarditis (especially subacute bacterial endocarditis)
    - Toxoplasmosis
    - Q fever (*Coxiella burnetii*)
    - Brucellosis
    - Trichinosis
    - Histoplasmosis
    - Lymphogranuloma venereum (LGV)
    - Whipple disease

37. **List the noninfectious causes of FUO.**
    See Table 12.1.

Table 12.1. Noninfectious Causes of Fever of Unknown Origin

AUTOIMMUNE	MALIGNANCIES	MISCELLANEOUS
Temporal arteritis (giant cell arteritis)	Leukemia Lymphoma (especially Hodgkin)	Medications (drug fever) Venous thromboembolism and pulmonary embolism
Systemic lupus erythematosus	Myeloid metaplasis Renal cell carcinoma	Sarcoidosis Crohn disease
Adult Still disease	Hepatoma	Granulomatous disease
Polymyalgia rheumatica		Familial Mediterranean fever (FMF) Adrenal insufficiency
Polyarteritis nodosa		Thyrotoxicosis
Mixed connective tissue disease		Factious sources
Wegener granulomatosis		
Relapsing polychondritis		
Subacute thyroiditis		

38. **Is the cause of FUO always found?**
    No. Up to 10–30% of these patients do not have an identified cause, but the fever usually resolves with full recovery. Reevaluation of these patients will sometimes reveal a cause after an initial negative work-up.

GRAM-POSITIVE BACTERIA

39. **What test distinguishes *Staphylococcus* from *Streptococcus*?**
    Catalase. *Staphylococcus* is catalase positive whereas *Streptococcus* is catalase negative.

40. **What are some of the virulence factors of *Staphylococcus*?**
    - Leukocidin (including Panton-Valentine leukocidin): A toxin that lyses cells and promotes spread of the bacteria in tissues and also damages cell membranes.
    - Catalase: Helps the bacteria survive in phagocytes
    - Coagulase
    - Protein A
    - Other exotoxins and enterotoxins

41. **What mechanisms allow *S. aureus* to develop antibiotic resistance?**
    - Enzyme production (beta-lactamases)
    - Altered penicillin-binding proteins (PBPs), which lower binding affinity of beta-lactam antibiotics
    - Altered cell wall thickness
    - Acquisition of *VanA* gene from *Enterococcus*

    Hiramatsu K, Okuma K, Ma XX, et al. New trends in *Staphylococcus aureus* infections: glycopeptide resistance in hospital and methicillin resistance in the community. *Curr Opin Infect Dis*. 2002;15:407–413.

    Sieradzki K, Tomasz A. Alterations of cell wall structure and metabolism accompany reduced susceptibility to vancomycin in an isogenic series of clinical isolates of *Staphylococcus aureus*. *J Bacteriol* 2003;185:7103–7110.

42. **Which of the coagulase-negative staphylococci has been reported to behave as virulently as *S. aureus*?**
    Staphylococcus lugdunensis, which has been reported in cases of native valve endocarditis, wound infection and abscess, and infection of intravascular catheters and other medical devices. A clue to this species is the antibiotic susceptibility pattern that shows sensitivity to beta-lactam antibiotics including oxacillin. Many of the other coagulase-negative staphylococci are resistant to beta-lactams.

    Frank KL, Del Pozo JL, Patel R. From clinical microbiology to infection pathogenesis: how daring to be different works for *Staphylococcus lugdunensis*. *Clin Microbiol Rev*. 2008;21:111–133.

43. **Which form of *Staphylococcus* causes UTIs in young women?**
    Staphylococcus saprophyticus, a coagulase-negative organism that accounts for up to 15% of cases of cystitis in young, sexually active women. Clinical findings are identical to those found in UTIs caused by other typical pathogens such as *Escherichia coli*, *Proteus*, and *Klebsiella*.

44. **Which coagulase-negative *Staphylococcus* may have higher minimal inhibitory concentrations (MICs) to vancomycin and resistance to multiple other antibiotics?**
    Staphylococcus haemolyticus, occurring in approximately 10% of clinical coagulase-negative staphylococcus isolates. Studies have shown relative resistance to vancomycin, teicoplanin, and other antibiotics. Newer agents such as linezolid and daptomycin may be useful in treating infections caused by this organism.

    Frogatt JW, Johnston JL, Galetto DW, et al. Antimicrobial resistance in nosocomial isolates of *Staphylococcus haemolyticus*. *Antimicrob Agents Chemother*. 1989;33:460–466.

45. **What toxin-mediated syndromes are caused by *S. aureus*?**
    - **Toxic shock syndrome:** Fever, rash with desquamation, hypotension, and abnormalities in the gastrointestinal, central nervous, musculoskeletal, renal, hepatic, or hematologic systems associated with toxin 1 (TSST-1)
    - **Scalded skin syndrome:** Separation of the epidermis from the dermis—the basis for the Nikolsky sign—caused by exfoliative toxins (A and B)
    - **Food poisoning:** Severe gastroenteritis that is usually self-resolving caused by enterotoxins

46. **What are two toxin-mediated syndromes caused by *Streptococcus*?**
    - Toxic shock syndrome
    - Scarlet fever

47. **What gram-positive coccus is catalase negative and considered intrinsically resistant to vancomycin?**
    Leuconostoc. Many *Lactobacillus* species also demonstrate resistance to vancomycin, but lactobacilli are gram-positive rods.

    Carr FJ, Chill D, Maida N. The lactic acid bacteria: a literature survey. *Cit Rev Microbiol*. 2002;28:281–370

48. **What are the clinically relevant gram-positive rods?**
    - *Clostridium* species (including *C. perfringens, C. difficile, C. tetani, C. botulinum, C. novyi, and C. sordellii*)
    - *Listeria monocytogenes*
    - *Actinomyces* (multiple species, most commonly *A. israelii*)
    - *Bacillus* (*B. anthracis, B. cereus*)
    - *Corynebacteria* (*C. diphtheriae, C. jeikeium*)
    - *Erysipelothrix rhusiopathiae*
    - *Nocardia*
    - Mycobacteria (also acid-fast)

49. What is the causative organism of erythrasma?

    Corynebacterium minutissimum. Erythrasma is a skin condition that affects the superficial layers of the skin and typically manifests with scaly patches of brown skin in the intertriginous areas (groin, armpits, and intergluteal fold as well as submammary areas).

GRAM-NEGATIVE BACTERIA

50. What are the SPACE/SPICE organisms?
    - **SPACE:** *Serratia, Pseudomonas, Acinetobacter, Citrobacter, Enterobacter*
    - **SPICE:** *Serratia, Pseudomonas,* indole-positive *Proteus, Citrobacter, Enterobacter*

      These organisms can produce beta-lactamases of the AmpC type and can express resistance to antibiotics such as penicillins, cephalosporins, and monobactams.

      MacDougall C. Beyond susceptible and resistant, Part I: treatment of infections due to gram-negative organisms with inducible β-lactamases. *J Pediatr Pharmacol Ther.* 2011;16:23–30.

51. What gram-negative bacteria is associated with cat-scratch fever?

    Bartonella henselae.

52. What are other diseases caused by *Bartonella* species?
    - **B. bacilliformis:** Verruga peruana, Oroya fever (Carrion disease)
    - **B. quintana:** Trench fever, bacillary angiomatosis/visceral peliosis, fever/bacteremia, endocarditis
    - **B. henselae:** Lymphadenopathy, fever/bacteremia, bacillary angiomatosis/visceral peliosis, cat-scratch disease, endocarditis
    - **B. elizabethae:** Endocarditis
    - **B. clarridgeiae:** Cat-scratch disease
    - **B. vinsonii subsp. berkhoffi:** Endocarditis
    - **B. vinsonii subsp. arupensis:** Fever
    - **B. grahamii:** Neuroretinitis

53. What gram-negative bacteria are oxidase positive?

    Pseudomonas, Aeromonas, Burkholderia cepacia, Neisseria, Moraxella, Helicobacter, Vibrio, Campylobacter, Legionella, Brucella, Pasteurella, Alcaligenes, Kingella, Eiknella, Plesiomonas, Achromobacter, and *Chryseobacterium.*

54. Which gram-negative organism has been associated with MALT (mucosa-associated lymphoid tissue) lymphoma?

    Helicobacter pylori. Patients with MALT lymphoma and early stage gastric disease could be treated by eradication of *H. pylori* infection alone; therefore, early diagnosis of *H. pylori* is imperiative.

    Fischbach W, Goebeler ME, Ruskone-Fourmestraux A, et al. Most patients with minimal histological residuals of gastric MALT lymphoma after successful eradication of *Helicobacter pylori* can be managed safely by a watch and wait strategy: experience from a large international series. *Gut.* 2007;56:1685–1687.

55. What infections are classically attributed to *Pseudomonas*?
    - Malignant (necrotizing) otitis externa: Occurs in diabetics with symptoms of pain and discharge from the ear
    - Otitis externa (swimmer's ear): Frequent in children
    - Endocarditis: Commonly seen in intravenous (IV) drug abusers due to contamination of drug paraphernalia
    - Osteomyelitis: Associated with puncture wounds of the foot through sneakers, usually seen in young, healthy patients with calcaneal bone osteomyelitis
    - Cystic fibrosis exacerbations: Due to chronic airway colonization
    - Nosomocomial infection: Including ventilator-associated pneumonia
    - Noma neonaturum: Necrotizing mucosal and perianal infection of newborns
    - "Green nail syndrome": Paronychia caused by frequent immersion of hands into water

56. What diseases are caused by *Vibrio* species?
    - **V. cholerae:** Cholera (severe diarrheal disease)
    - **V. vulnificus:** Necrotizing wound infections, sepsis/shock (typically in patients with chronic liver disease), gastroenteritis
    - **V. parahaemolyticus:** Self-limited gastroenteritis
    - **V. alginolyticus:** Otitis, wound infections

57. **What is ecthyma gangrenosum?**
Skin lesions associated with gram-negative bacteremia, most commonly in neutropenic patients. *Pseudomonas aeruginosa* is the most commonly implicated bacteria, but other species have produced this lesion, including *Aeromonas hydrophila and E. coli.* The lesions typically begin as painless erythematous macules that rapidly progress to papules and develop central vesicles or bullae. Eventually, they ulcerate to form gangrenous ulcers. The characteristic histologic appearance demonstrates large numbers of bacteria in and around blood vessels, but with an absence of an inflammatory response.

58. **List three clinically relevant species of *Burkholderia*?**
- *B. cepacia:* Associated with disease exacerbation in cystic fibrosis patients
- *B. pseudomallei:* Agent of melioidosis, a disease of both humans and animals with a wide variety of clinical symptoms such as skin ulcer, abscess, chronic pneumonia, fulminant septic shock with abscesses in internal organs
- *B. mallei:* Cause of glanders, a disease of animals, but a potential zoonosis

59. **What gram-negative bacillus has been implicated in skin and soft tissue infections and bacteremia in soldiers serving in Iraq?**
Acinetobacter baumannii, reported to cause bacteremia and skin/soft tissue infections in service members following Operation Iraqi Freedom and typically resistant to multiple drug classes.
Centers for Disease Control (CDC). *Acinetobacter baumannii* infections among patients at military medical facilities treating injured U.S. service members, 2002-2004. 2004;53:1063–1066.

60. **Which species of *Achromobacter* are most often associated with infections?**
A. xylosoxidans and *A. dentrificans,* most frequently isolated in patients with pneumonia and bronchitis. These bacteria are typically multidrug resistant and seen in patients with cystic fibrosis, cancer, chronic kidney disease, and other immunocompromised conditions.
Swenson C, Sadikot R. Achromobacter respiratory infections. *Ann Am Thorac Soc.* 2015;12:252–258.

61. **What bacteria species has been associated with cat bites?**
Pasteurella multocida. These gram-negative coccobacilli and facultative anaerobes are one of the most commonly isolated pathogens in the mouths of cats (and dogs).
Freshwater A. Why your housecat's trite little bite could cause you quite a fright: a study of domestic felines on the occurrence and antibiotic susceptibility of *Pasteurella multocida. Zoonoses Public Health.* 2008;55:507–513.

VIRUSES

62. **What is Zika virus (ZKV)?**
A flavivirus first discovered in Uganda. Symptoms of Zika infection include fever, rash, conjunctivits, muscle and joint pain, malaise, and headache that usually last 2–7 days then resolve. Over 80% of patients infected with Zika virus will have no symptoms. There is no current treatment.

63. **What syndromes are associated with Zika virus?**
Microcephaly in infants and Gullain-Barré syndrome. Because of its association with microcephaly, the virus is particularly worrisome for pregnant women or those who intend to become pregnant.

64. **How is Zika virus transmitted?**
Through the bite of the *Aedes aegypti* (or *A. albopictus*) mosquito, which typically bites during the day. Other modes of transmission include sexual intercourse. Blood transfusion is also a potential source of transmission but is a low risk in the United States. During an outbreak in French Polynesia, 2.8% of blood donors tested positive for Zika virus.
Oster AM, Brooks JT, Stryker JE, et al. Interim guidelines for prevention of sexual transmission of Zika virus—United States. *MMWR Morb Mortal Wkly Rep.* 2016;65:120–121.

65. **What diseases other than Zika virus are spread by the bite of the *Aedes* mosquito?**
Dengue, Chikungunya, and yellow fever.

66. **How can dengue fever be differentiated from Chikungunya?**
Polyarthralgia and severe arthritis appears more likely with Chikungunya. Both diseases cause an acute febrile illness with myalgia, headache, and rash.

67. What is MERS?

Middle East respiratory syndrome (MERS), caused by a coronavirus (MERS-CoV) and first encountered in Jordan in 2012. Symptoms include fever, cough, and shortness of breath and possibly gastrointestinal symptoms (nausea, vomiting, diarrhea). Incubation time is about 5–6 days. Severe cases of MERS are typically seen in patients with comorbid conditions. No vaccine or treatment exists to date. The case fatality rate is around 36%.

68. What is SARS?

Severe acute respiratory syndrome (SARS), also caused by coronavirus, SARS-CoV, reported initially in 2003 in Asia.

69. What is reassortment?

The process by which influenza viruses swap gene segments, resulting in different strains of the influenza A virus, including the 2009 H1N1 virus. Two glycoproteins of the influenza virus membrane, hemagglutinin and neuraminidase, are involved in infection of the host.

Steel J, Lowen AC. Influenza A virus reassortment. *Curr Top Microbiol Immunol.* 2014;385: 377–401.

70. What is H1N1 influenza?

A reassortment of the influenza virus detected in 2009 when it caused a worldwide pandemic. This virus is known as the *swine flu* due to its similarity to influenza found in pigs in Europe and Asia.

71. What treatments are available for influenza?

Currently, five antiviral agents are available in the United States. Neuraminidase inhibitors include oseltamivir, zanamivir, and peramivir. These are active against both influenza A and B. The adamantanes (amantadine and rimantadine) are active only against influenza A. The adamantanes are not recommended for treatment or prophylaxis of influenza owing to a high level of resistance.

72. What are the clinically significant flaviviruses and what diseases do they cause?

- Mosquito-borne flaviviruses: Yellow fever, dengue fever, Japanese encephalitis, West Nile virus infection, Zika virus infection, and St. Louis encephalitis
- Tick-borne flaviviruses: Tick-borne encephalitis (TBE), Kyasanur forest disease (KFD), Alkhurma disease, Powassan virus, and Omsk hemorrhagic fever

  Goro K, Gwong-Jen J, Tsuchiya RK, et al. Phylogeny of the genus Flavivirus. *J Virol.* 1998;72:73–83.

73. What are the clinical manifestations of parvovirus B19 infection?

- Erythema infectiousum: "Fifth disease"
- Arthropathy: Particularly in adults
- Transient aplastic crisis: In patients with sickle cell anemia
- Pure red blood cell aplasia: Associated acquired immunodeficiency virus (AIDS)
- Virus-associated hemophagocytic syndrome
- Hydrops fetalis

74. With what syndromes are the various herpesviruses associated?

- **Herpes simplex virus (HSV):** Mucocutaneous lesions and encephalitis.
- **Varicella-zoster virus:** Chickenpox and shingles.
- **CMV:** Mononucleosis syndrome, meningoencephalitis, transverse myelitis, hepatitis, myocarditis, pneumonitis, esophagitis, colitis, and retinitis, usually in immunocompromised patients.
- **EBV:** Infectious mononucleosis, Burkitt lymphoma, nasopharyngeal carcinoma, and EBV-related lymphoproliferative syndromes.
- **Human herpesvirus 6 (HHV-6):** Roseola (exanthem subitum) and nonspecific febrile illnesses in young children; mononucleosis-like syndrome in adults; febrile seizures, meningoencephalitis, and encephalitis; hepatitis; and opportunistic infections (interstitial pneumonitis) in immunocompromised patients. There may be an association with chronic fatigue syndrome, lymphoproliferative disorders, and histiocytic necrotizing lymphadenitis (Kikuchi syndrome).
- **HHV-7:** Possibly exanthum subitum–like illness, hepatitis, and encephalitis.
- **HHV-8:** Kaposi sarcoma, primary effusion (body cavity based), lymphoma, and multicentric Castleman disease. There may be an association with primary pulmonary hypertension.
- **Herpes B virus:** Myelitis and hemorrhagic encephalitis following primate bites and scratches.

75. **What causes hand, foot, and mouth disease (HFMD)?**
Usually a virus of the picornavirus family, most often coxsackievirus A16. Outbreaks have occurred with coxsackieviruses A4, A5, A9, A10, B2, and B5 and enterovirus 71.

76. **What are the clinical findings of HFMD?**
An ulcerative exanthem, usually occurring on the buccal mucosa, followed by a vesicular exanthem on the hands and feet.

77. **What animal is the reservoir for the agent causing the hantavirus pulmonary syndrome (HPS)?**
The deer mouse, *Peromyscus maniculatus*, which harbors the Sin Nombre hantavirus.
Childs JE, Ksiazek TJ, Spiropoulou CF, et al. Serologic and genetic identification of *Peromyscus maniculatus* as the primary rodent reservoir for a new hantavirus in the southwestern United States. *J Infect Dis*. 1994;169:1271–1280.

78. **List the more common viral hemorrhagic fevers.**
- Rift Valley fever
- Crimean-Congo hemorrhagic fever
- Lassa fever
- Ebola hemorrhagic fever
- Marburg hemorrhagic fever
- Dengue hemorrhagic fever

79. **Describe the Ebola virus, including incubation and clinical presentation.**
Ebola virus is a member of the filoviridae family, consisting of five species: *Zaire, Bundibuyo, Sudan, Reston,* and *Tai Forest* that spreads from human to human via contact with blood and body fluids. The incubation period is 2 to 21 days. Symptoms include fever, fatigue, muscle pain, headache, and sore throat, followed by vomiting, diarrhea, rash, and kidney and liver dysfunction. Bleeding can be seen in some patients. Case fatality rate for Ebola approaches 50%. The virus has caused multiple outbreaks in Africa and was described for the first time in the United States in 2014 in a patient who had traveled from Liberia to Dallas, Texas.

80. **What is fifth disease or erythema infectiosum?**
A viral illness more frequent in children caused by parvovirus B19 with symptoms of fever, runny nose, headache, and rash that is usually seen on the cheeks. The rash is called the *slapped cheek* rash.

81. **What is sixth disease?**
A viral illness caused by HHV-6. Also known as *roseola infantum* and *exanthema subitum*, sixth disease is characterized by high fever, usually lasting 3–5 days then resolving. Rash appears usually at the resolution of fever.

FUNGI

82. **What is the beta-D-glucan assay?**
A component of fungal cell walls with the exception of *Cryptococcus* and *Zygomycetes*. The beta-D-glucan assay is helpful for the diagnosis of invasive fungal infections.
Karageorgopoulos DE, Vouloumanou EK, et al. β-D-glucan assay for the diagnosis of invasive fungal infections: a meta-analysis. *Clin Infect Dis*. 2011;52:750–770.

83. **What are the dematiaceous fungi?**
Brown-pigmented fungi that are widespread in the environment and found in soil, wood, and decomposing wood. They cause a wide range of infections including phaeohyphomycosis, chromoblastomycosis, and eumycotic mycetoma. Clinically relevant species include *Alternaria, Cladophialophora, Curvularia, Exophiala, Madurella, Fonsecaea, Wangiella,* and *Scedosporium*.
Brandt ME, Warnock DW. Epidemiology, clinical manifestations and therapy of infections caused by dematiaceous fungi. *J Chemother* 2003;15:36–47.

84. **How can *Aspergillus* be differentiated from *Mucor*?**
Aspergillus is a mold that demonstrates hyphae with 45-degree branching with distinct septae by direct examination. *Mucor* typically has broad, ribbon-like hyphae that are nonseptate. *Mucor* typically branches at an angle close to 90 degrees.

85. **What disease should be considered in a diabetic with ketoacidosis and black eschar in the nasal mucosa?**
Rhinocerebral mucormycosis. The zygomycete fungi (*Rhizopus, Mucor, Rhizomucor,* and *Absidia*) can cause this clinical entity, which is rapidly progressive with a mortality rate up to 50%. Therapy includes aggressive surgical débridement and amphotericin B.

86. **List the clinical settings and risk factors associated with *Candida* infections.**
   - Chronic mucocutaneous infections
   - Defects in T-lymphocyte immunity: either congenital or acquired (e.g., AIDS)
   - Deeply invasive, disseminated infections
   - Peripheral neutrophil count < 500/mm^3
   - Mucosal barrier breakdown: burn, cytotoxic agents, gastrointestinal surgery, or IV catheter sites
   - Broad-spectrum antibiotic use with *Candida* overgrowth
   - Indwelling catheter
   Pappas PG, Rex JH, Sobel JD, et al. Guidelines for the treatment of candidiasis. *Clin Infect Dis.* 2004;38:161–189.

87. **Which species of *Candida* are considered resistant to the -azole class of antifungals?**
C. krusei, which is inherently resistant, and *C. glabrata,* which demonstrates dose-dependent resistance.

88. **Which species of *Candida* is considered resistant to amphotericin B?**
C. lusitaniae.

89. **What is a dimorphic fungus?**
One that grows both mycelia and yeast forms depending on conditions.

90. **List the clinically important dimorphic fungi and the diseases they cause.**
See Table 12.2.

Table 12.2. Diseases Caused by Dimorphic Fungi

FUNGUS	DISEASE
Histoplasma	Pneumonia Disseminated disease with bone marrow and adrenal involvement Ulcers and polyploidy masses in mouth, esophagus, stomach, small and large intestines, and colon; cutaneous lesions Meningitis, encephalitis
Blastomyces	Pneumonia Skin lesions (typically a verrucous lesion), osteomyelitis Prostatitis Disseminated disease
Coccidioides	Valley fever Pneumonia (with symptoms similar to community-acquired pneumonia) Cutaneous disease Meningitis Osteomyelitis Arthritis
Sporothrix	Cutaneous (lymphocutaneous) disease Pneumonia (with symptoms similar to tuberculosis) Joint infection
Paracoccidioides	Pneumonia with or without cavitary lesions Cutaneous disease (ulcerative lesions that may infiltrate the skin) Ulcerative lesions of the mucosa of the mouth, nose, or larynx
Penicillium	Pneumonia Cutaneous lesions Keratitis, endophthalmitis

KEY POINTS: INFECTIONS CAUSED BY DIMORPHIC FUNGI

1. *Penicillium marneffei* can cause disease in patients with AIDS and other forms of immunosuppression.
2. Consider histoplasmosis in patients with adrenal insufficiency.
3. Sporotrichosis is also called "alcoholic rose gardener's disease."

AIDS, acquired immunodeficiency syndrome.

91. **What are the major pulmonary syndromes associated with *Aspergillus* spp.?**
    - **Allergic bronchopulmonary aspergillosis (ABPA):** Occurs in patients with asthma who have eosinophilia, transient pulmonary infiltrates thought to be due to bronchial plugging, with elevated serum IgE and IgG antibody to aspergillus.
    - **Aspergilloma (fungus ball):** Results from colonization and growth of aspergillus, usually within a preexisting pulmonary cavity.
    - **Invasive aspergillosis:** Usually occurs in individuals with profound granulocytopenia, and it is being described more frequently in patients with AIDS.
    - **Chronic necrotizing aspergillosis:** Slowly progressive form of invasive aspergillosis that occurs in patients with an underlying lung disease (chronic obstructive pulmonary disease, sarcoid, pneumoconiosis, or inactive tuberculosis) or mild systemic immunocompromising illness (low-dose corticosteroids, diabetes mellitus, alcoholism). These patients usually have a chronic infiltrate that may slowly progress to cavitation of aspergilloma formation.

    Latge JP. Aspergillus fumigatus and aspergillosis. *Clin Microbiol Rev.* 1999;12:310–350.

92. **How are pulmonary syndromes associated with *Aspergillus* spp. treated?**
    - **ABPA:** Corticosteroids traditionally, although anecdotal reports suggest itraconazole may have a role.
    - **Aspergilloma:** No specific treatment unless significant hemoptysis occurs, in which case surgical excision is performed.
    - **Invasive aspergillosis:** Amphotericin B or one of the newer liposomal preparations (caspofungin or voriconazole), with or without surgical excision. Many experts recommend voriconazole as preferred therapy for *Aspergillus* infections.

93. **Which fungi has yeast forms with "broad-based" budding?**
    Blastomyces dermatitidis, which causes lung infections due to inhalation of spores and is endemic to the Ohio and Mississippi river valleys. Other sites of infection include the skin (papules, nodules, verrucous lesions or draining lesions). Bones, joints, and prostate may also be infected.

94. **Which mold was described to cause infection of the sacroiliac and peripheral joints as well as meningitis?**
    Exserohilum rostratum, the main pathogen involved in an outbreak of meningits and epidural, paraspinal, and joint infections. An outbreak in 2012 was traced back to contaminated lots of methylprednisolone.

    Pettit AC, Kropski JA, Castilho JL, et al. The index case for the fungal meningitis outbreak in the United States. *N Engl J Med.* 2012;367:2119–2125.

95. **What is a prion?**
    An infectious misfolded protein. Prions do not have nucleic acids (DNA, RNA).

96. **What are the human prion diseases and their clinical manifestations?**
    See Table 12.3.

97. **How can one differentiate the dementia of Creutzfeldt-Jakob disease (CJD) from that of Alzheimer disease (AD)?**
    By careful assessment of associated movement disturbances. Ataxia is most often associated with CJD and hypokinesis with AD.

    Edlar J, Mollenhauer B, Heinemann U, et al. Movement disturbance in the differential diagnosis of Creutzfeldt-Jakob disease. *Mov Disord.* 2009;24:350–356.

98. **What microbial agents are considered potential biologic warfare agents?**
    See Table 12.4.

Table 12.3. Clinical Manifestations of Human Prion Disease

DISEASE	CLINICAL MANIFESTATIONS
Sporadic Creutzfeldt-Jakob disease	Rapid mental decline toward dementia Myoclonus
Variant Creutzfeldt-Jakob disease	Sensory disturbances (paresthesia) Psychiatric symptoms (depression, anxiety, psychosis) Neurologic symptoms (ataxia, mental decline)
Gerstmann-Sträussler-Scheinker syndrome	Cerebellar degeneration (ataxia, lack of coordination) Dementia Myoclonus Dysarthria Nystagmus Visual disturbances
Fatal familial insomnia	Progressive insomnia Disturbances in autonomic nervous system (hyperthermia and tachycardia) Endocrine disorders (decreased ACTH secretion and increased cortisol)
Kuru	Tremors Ataxia Myoclonus Choreoathetosis Dementia Indifference

ACTH, adrenocorticotropic hormone.

Table 12.4. Infectious Agents With Potential Use in Biologic Warfare and Their Symptoms and Diseases

INFECTIOUS AGENT	SYMPTOMS AND DISEASES
Bacteria	
Bacillus anthracis	Inhalational and cutaneous anthrax
Brucella spp.	Debilitating flulike illness
Burkholderia mallei	Usually causes glanders in horses but can cause skin and pulmonary infections and sepsis
Coxiella burnetii	Flulike illness, pneumonia, hepatitis
Francisella tularensis	Various forms including pneumonic
Clostridium botulinum	Visual symptoms and muscle weakness leading to respiratory muscle paralysis
C. perfringens	Watery diarrhea, gangrene
Salmonella spp.	Inflammatory diarrhea, typhoid fever
Shigella dysenteriae	Inflammatory diarrhea
Yersinia pestis	Plague (bubonic, pneumonic, septicemic)
Escherichia coli O157:H7	Bloody diarrhea, hemolytic uremic syndrome
Vibrio cholerae	Cholera with severe diarrhea and dehydration
Cryptosporidium parvum	Diarrhea, cholecystitis
Multidrug-resistant tuberculosis	Tuberculosis symptoms
Viruses	
Alphaviruses (Venezuelan and eastern and western equine)	Encephalitis
Hantaviruses	Hemorrhagic fever with renal syndrome, Hantavirus cardiopulmonary syndrome

Table 12.4. Infectious Agents With Potential Use in Biologic Warfare and Their Symptoms and Diseases *(Continued)*

INFECTIOUS AGENT	SYMPTOMS AND DISEASES
Tick-borne encephalitis	Fever, myalgia, meningitis, encephalitis
Nipah virus	Encephalitis
Arenaviruses (Lassa, Junin)	Lassa fever, hemorrhagic fever
Filoviruses (Ebola and Marburg)	Hemorrhagic fever
Smallpox	Rash, following prodrome of fever and headache/myalgia
Yellow fever	Fever, jaundice, renal failure, and hemorrhage

From Centers for Disease Control and Prevention. Biological and chemical terrorism: Strategic plan for preparedness and response. Recommendations of the CDC Strategic Planning Workgroup. *MMWR Morb Mortal Wkly Rep* 2000;49(RR-4):1–14.

PARASITIC INFECTIONS

99. **Which species of *Plasmodium* have a dormant phase in the liver (hypnozoites)?**
    P. vivax and *P. ovale*. These species also need to be treated differently from other malarial infections to avoid relapse because of the hypnozoite phase.

100. **Why is malaria caused by *Plasmodium falciparum* more severe than that caused by other species?**
    Because *P. falciparum* can infect red blood cells of any age and size, leading to red blood cell clumping and blockage of small vessel blood flow. The diminished blood flow can lead to severe hypoxic damage, especially in the brain and kidneys.

101. **What are the malaria-causing *Plasmodium* species?**
    P. falciparum, P. vivax, P. ovale, P. malariae, and *P. knowlesi*.

102. **What is "blackwater fever"?**
    Intravascular hemolysis, hemoglobulinuria, and renal failure due to tubular necrosis seen in patients with falciparum malaria exposed to quinine. The urine appears dark owing to hemoglobin deposition.

103. **What parasite causes a chronic infection that appears as linear calcifications seen in the wall of the urinary bladder on a roentgenogram?**
    Schistosoma haematobium. The eggs are deposited in the submucosa and mucosa of the bladder. The subsequent inflammatory response leads to scarring and calcium deposition.

104. **What is the "hyperinfection" syndrome associated with *Strongyloides stercoralis*?**
    Symptoms of abdominal pain, diarrhea, vomiting, shock, fever, cough, and decreased mental status due to dissemination of the filariform larval stage. Hyperinfection syndrome due to *S. stercoralis* is the result of systemic dissemination by the filariform larva in individuals who are immunocompromised, primarily with defects in cell-mediated immunity. Bacteremia occurs frequently, usually with enteric organisms that are thought to accompany the larvae as they migrate through the bowel wall.

105. **What is kala-azar?**
    Visceral leishmaniasis, caused by various species of *Leishmania* (*L. donovani, L. infantum,* and *L. chagasi*). The *Leishmania* are transmitted by the bite of a sandfly, which transfers promastigotes of the organism to the host. Clinical findings include fever and splenomegaly with or without hepatomegaly. The diagnosis is made by a splenic or bone marrow aspirate showing amastigotes.

106. **Infection with which species of *Trypanosoma* can lead to dilated cardiomyopathy, conduction abnormalities, and megacolon?**
    Trypanosoma cruzi, the causative agent of Chagas disease, which can lead to the complications described if untreated. In addition, megaesophagus and achalasia have been described. *T. brucei* causes African sleeping sickness.

107. **Which nematodes (roundworms) are able to infect the host by penetration of the skin?**
S. stercoralis, Ancylostoma duodenale, and *Necator americanus.*

108. **What is the clinical manifestation of pinworm infection?**
Rectal or perirectal area itching that is worse at night. Infection by *Enterobius vermicularis* is usually acquired by ingestion of eggs. The eggs hatch and mature in the host, and the adult female worm migrates to the rectal area to lay eggs.

109. **What is Katayama fever?**
A manifestation of acute schistosomiasis that includes fever, urticarial rash, and hepatosplenomegaly. *Schistosoma japonicum* is most commonly associated with this clinical syndrome.

110. **List the tissue flukes and their typical associations.**
- ***Fasciolopsis buski:*** Infectious stage (metacercariae) found in aquatic plants such as water chestnuts, lotus roots, and water bamboo.
- ***F. hepatica:*** Large liver fluke of sheep that infects humans through ingestion of a meal that contains infected watercress, chestnuts, or bamboo shoots.
- ***Clonorchis sinensis:*** Liver fluke that blocks bile ducts and leads to jaundice and cholangitis, just as caused by *Fasciola. Clonorchis* is acquired by ingestion of metacercaria in undercooked or raw freshwater fish.
- ***Paragonimus westermani:*** Lung fluke, acquired by ingestion of the organism in raw or pickled crawfish or freshwater crabs.

111. **What is tungiasis?**
A disease of the skin, caused by infestation by the flea, *Tunga penetrans.* The disease is endemic in areas of Africa and South and Central America. Treatment consists of surgical removal of the flea; antiparasitic medications are not effective.

112. **What is the causative agent of "river blindness"?**
Onchocerca volvulus, transmitted by the bite of a black fly that deposits the larvae onto the skin. Onchocerciasis initially presents with an itchy, erythematous rash with formation of fibrous skin nodules later in the disease. Eye lesions also occur that lead to blindness. The incidence of onchocerciasis has been markedly reduced in central African countries through vector control and oral medication use.

113. **Which infectious agents have been reported to be transmitted by blood transfusion?**
See Table 12.5.

Table 12.5. Infectious Agents That Can Transmit Disease Through Blood Transfusion

VIRAL	NONVIRAL
Hepatitis (A, B, C, and D) Hepatitis G	*Treponema pallidum* (syphilis)
HIV-1 and HIV-2	*Babesia microti*
HTLV I and II	*Plasmodium* spp. (malaria)
CMV	*Trypanosoma cruzi* (Chagas disease)
Human herpes virus 8	*Leishmania* spp.
West Nile virus	*Toxoplasma gondii*
Anelloviridae (TT virus or *Thetatorquevirus* and its variant, SEN virus)	*Yersini enterocolitica* *Serratia* spp. *Pseudomonas* spp.
EBV	*Bacillus cereus*

CMV, cytomegalovirus; EBV, Epstein-Barr virus; HIV, human immunodeficiency virus; HTLV, human T-lymphotrophic virus.
Adapted from Chamberland ME. Emerging infectious agents: do they pose a risk to the safety of transfused blood and blood products? *Clin Infect Dis.* 2002;34:e797–e805.

114. What occupations are associated with an increased risk of *Chlamydia psittaci* infection?
    - Pet shop employees
    - Pigeon fanciers
    - Zoo workers
    - Veterinarians
    - Poultry processors
    These workers usually present with fever, headache, myalgias, and dry cough that can progress to severe disease involving multiple organ systems.

115. Extrusion of "sulfur granules" from a draining wound is characteristic of which infection?
    Actinomyces spp. that characteristically form external sinuses, which discharge "sulfur granules" consisting of conglomerate masses of branching filaments cemented together and mineralized by host calcium phosphate stimulated by tissue inflammation. The name is a misnomer because the granules do not contain sulfur.

116. List the infectious causes of adrenal insufficiency.
    - *Mycobacterium tuberculosis*
    - Fungi: *Histoplasma capsulatum, Cryptococcus neoformans, Coccidioides immitis, Sporothrix schenckii, Blastomyces dermatitidis, Paracoccidioides brasiliensis*
    - *Neisseria meningitidis*: in Waterhouse-Friderichsen syndrome
    - Other organisms causing shock
    - Human immunodeficiency virus (HIV) infection
    - *Mycobacterium avium* complex (MAI)
    - CMV
    Painter BF. Infectious causes of adrenal insufficiency. *Infect Med.* 1994;11:515–520.

117. Which organisms most commonly cause infectious complications after bites?
    Human bites:
    - Streptococci (alpha and group A beta-hemolytic)
    - *S. aureus*
    - *Eikenella corrodens*
    - *Peptostreptococcus* spp.
    - *Bacteroides* spp.
    - *Fusobacterium* spp.
    Cat or dog bites:
    - *Pasteurella multocida*
    - *Capnocytophaga canimorsus* (DF-2)
    - Rabies
    Cat bites:
    - Tularemia
    Dog bites:
    - Brucellosis
    - EF-4
    - Blastomycosis
    Goldstein EJC. Bite wounds and infection. *Clin Infect Dis.* 1992;14:633–640.

118. What are the infectious causes of parotitis?

Viral	*Bacterial*
Mumps	*S. aureus*
Influenza	*S. peumoniae*
Parainfluenza types 1 and 3	Enteric gram-negative bacilli
Coxsackievirus A and B	*Haemophilus influenzae*
Echovirus	*Actinomyces* spp.
Lymphocytic choriomeningitis virus	*M. tuberculosis*
HIV	*Salmonella typhi*
Anaerobic organisms	*B. pseudomallei*

119. What is the differential diagnosis of exudative pharyngitis?
    - Streptococci groups A, C, and G
    - *Arcanobacterium hemolyticum*
    - *Neisseria gonorrhoeae*
    - *Corynebacterium diphtheriae*
    - Anaerobic bacteria
    - HIV-1
    - *Yersinia enterocolitica*
    - *Mycoplasma pneumoniae*
    - Adenovirus
    - HSV
    - EBV

120. What are the most common pathogens seen in months 2–6 after solid organ transplantation?
    - CMV
    - *Aspergillus*
    - EBV
    - *Nocardia*
    - VZV
    - *Toxoplasma*
    - Papovavirus (BK and JC)
    - *Cryptococcus*
    - Adenovirus
    - *Pneumocystis jiroveci*
    - HSV
    - *Legionella* spp.
    - Non-A, non-B hepatitis
    - *L. monocytogenes*

121. What is the differential diagnosis of monocytosis?

Infectious	*Noninfectious*
Tuberculosis	Myeloproliferative disorders
EBV mononucleosis	Lymphomas
Rocky Mountain spotted fever (RMSF)	Solid tumors
Diphtheria	Gaucher disease
Subacute bacterial endocarditis	Regional enteritis
Histoplasmosis	Ulcerative colitis
Typhus	Sprue
Brucellosis	Rheumatoid arthritis
Kala-azar	Systemic lupus erythematosus
Malaria	Polyarteritis nodosa
Syphilis	Following splenectomy
Recovery from neutropenia	Sarcoidosis
Recovery from chronic infection	

122. What is the differential diagnosis of atypical lymphocytosis in patients with > 20% atypical lymphocytes?
Mononucleosis caused by EBV or CMV.

123. What is the differential diagnosis of atypical lymphocytosis in patients with < 20% atypical lymphocytes?

Infectious	*Noninfectious*
Rubella	Drug fever
HSV	Dermatitis herpetiformis
VZV	Radiation therapy
Tuberculosis	Stress

Infectious	*Noninfectious*
Brucellosis	Lead intoxication
Smallpox	Drug hypersensitivity reaction
Babesiosis	
Ehrlichiosis	
Rubeola	
Roseola infantum (HHV-6)	
Influenza	
Syphilis	
Toxoplasmosis	
Malaria	
RMSF	

124. **If a patient with no prior history of tetanus vaccination recovers from an episode of tetanus, is she or he at risk for a second episode?**
Yes. The occurrence of tetanus does not prevent second episodes of clinical disease from occurring because the amount of toxin needed to produce the clinical syndrome is so small that it is usually not immunogenic. Persons recovering from tetanus should be vaccinated with tetanus toxoid against future episodes of the disease.

MYCOBACTERIAL INFECTIONS

125. **What is an interferon gamma release assay?**
A blood test that measures release of interferon gamma by CD4 cells (as a response to infection with *M. tuberculosis*) and which can be used as an alternative to tuberculin skin testing (TST) for detection of latent or active tuberculosis.

126. **What is scrofula?**
Cervical lymphadenitis, which is the most common presentation of extrapulmonary tuberculosis. Scrofula refers to painless swelling of the cervical and supraclavicular lymph nodes that is most often caused by *M. tuberculosis* in adults and nontuberculous mycobacteria in children. *M. avium-intracellulare* (MAI), *M. scrofulaceum*, and *M. bovis* have been reported in cases on scrofula.

127. **What is a Ghon complex?**
The lung lesion of primary tuberculosis that consists of the area of initial infection with the bacilli and associated lymphadenopathy. The lesion will decrease in size over time and may become calcified, allowing it to be visible on chest radiograph.

128. **Which mycobacterial species should be considered when a patient who works in an aquarium presents with nodular skin lesions?**
M. marinum, found in both salt and fresh water environments causing localized granulomas, often associated with lymphangitic spread. Treatment is usually prolonged (several weeks) and includes surgical débridement when necessary. The organism is notably resistant to isoniazid, which is a mainstay of therapy for infection with other mycobacteria, particularly *M. tuberculosis*.

129. **What is Lady Windermere syndrome?**
A specific pulmonary syndrome caused by MAI, named after the title character of Oscar Wilde's play, "Lady Windermere's Fan," who was extremely genteel and unlikely to cough in public. The syndrome results from cough suppression and is more commonly seen in women. Pulmonary involvement is typically limited to lingula or middle lobe. These patients usually have no underlying lung disease and present with symptoms of bronchitis.
Tryfon S, Angelis N, Klein L, et al. Lady Windermere syndrome after cardiac surgery procedure: a case of *Mycobacterium avium* complex pneumonia. *Ann Thorac Surg.* 2010;89:1296–1299.

130. **List the mycobacteria that most commonly cause pulmonary disease in patients with HIV.**
- *M. tuberculosis*
- MAI
- *M. kansasii*

131. **What is Pott disease?**
An extrapulmonary manifestation of *M. tuberculosis* infection that affects the spine. Complications of this disease include collapse of vertebral bodies (gibbus) as well as chest wall and psoas abscesses.

132. **What is XDR tuberculosis?**
Extensively drug-resistant tuberculosis, which includes resistance to the first-line agents (isoniazid, rifampin, pyrazinamide, and ethambutol) as well as resistance to second-line agents (fluoroquinolones) and at least one of three other agents (amikacin, kanamycin, or capreomycin).

KEY POINTS: TUBERCULOSIS

1. Consider genitourinary tuberculosis in the patient with sterile pyuria.
2. Most tuberculosis cases are due to reactivation of primary infection.
3. John Keats, Frederick Chopin, and Robert Louis Stevenson all had tuberculosis.

---

133. **What is Hansen disease?**
Leprosy, caused by *M. leprae*. Patients have visible skin lesions as well as lesions of the peripheral nervous system.

134. **Which nontuberculous mycobacteria (NTM) are considered photochromogens (develop pigments in or after exposure to light)?**
M. kansasii, M. simiae, M. marinum, and *M. asiaticum.*

135. **Which NTM are considered scotochromogens (become pigmented in darkness)?**
M. szulgai, M. scrofulaceum, and *M. gordonae.*

136. **Which NTM are considered nonchromogens?**
MAI, *M. ulcerans, M. xenopi, M. malmoense, M. terrae, M. haemophilum,* and *M. genavense.*

137. **Which NTM are considered "rapid growers"?**
M. chelonae, M. abscessus, M. fortuitum, and *M. peregrinum.*

HEAD AND NECK INFECTIONS

138. **What is Ludwig angina?**
Cellulitis involving the sublingual and submaxillary spaces, usually arising from a dental infection. Patients often appear quite ill with swelling below the angle of the jaw. Airway obstruction is frequently a concern and is due to edema in the sublingual space that forces the tongue into a superior and posterior position. Cervical lymphadenopathy does not usually occur.

139. **What is Vincent angina?**
A severe form of gingivitis (also called *acute ulcerative gingivitis* or *trench mouth*) that leads to ulceration and necrosis of the gingiva with pain and bleeding of the gums. Unlike Ludwig angina, lymphadenopathy is common. The causative organisms are usually oral anaerobes that are treated with penicillin plus metronidazole.

140. **What is Lemierre syndrome?**
Jugular vein septic thrombophlebitis. Also called *postanginal sepsis*, this syndrome typically starts with tonsillitis or a peritonsillar abscess that affects the deep pharyngeal space and drains into the lateral pharyngeal space. Septic emboli to the lung and other sites may occur. The initial infection is classically associated with *Fusobacterium necrophorum*, although other organisms, including *S. aureus, Bacteroides fragilis, Peptostreptococcus,* and anaerobic streptococci, have been reported.
      Puymirat E, Biais M, Camou F, et al. A Lemierre syndrome variant caused by *Staphylococcus aureus. Am J Emerg Med.* 2008;26:380.e5–e7.
      Riordan T. Human infection with *Fusobacterium necrophorum* (necrobacillosis), with a focus on Lemierre's syndrome. *Clin Microbiol.* 2007;20:622–659.

141. **What infection, associated with airway compromise, has decreased since the advent of *H. influenzae* type B (HiB) vaccine?**
Acute epiglottitis, a rapidly progressive cellulitis of the epiglottis classically caused by *H. influenzae.*

142. **What is Pott puffy tumor?**
Subperiosteal abscess that results from edema of the frontal bone as a complication of frontal sinusitis.

143. **List the complications of frontal, ethmoid, and sphenoid sinusitis.**
See Table 12.6.

Table 12.6. Complications of Sinusitis

SINUS INVOLVED	COMPLICATION
Frontal	Pott puffy tumor; epidural, subdural, or brain abscess
Ethmoid	Periorbital and orbital cellulitis, orbital abscess, cavernous sinus thrombosis, meningitis
Sphenoid	Septic cavernous sinus thrombosis, meningitis

144. **What are the clinical manifestations of sinusitis?**
- Nasal congestion
- Rhinorrhea (which may be purulent)
- Facial pain or pressure
- Maxillary tooth pain

145. **What is the most common cause of acute sinusitis?**
Viruses including adenoviruses, influenza virus, and parainfluenza virus, making antibiotics generally ineffective.
Gwaltney JM Jr. Acute community-acquired sinusitis. *Clin Infect Dis*. 1996;23:1209–1223.

146. **List the frequency of the most common bacterial causes of acute sinusitis in adults.**
See Table 12.7.

Table 12.7. Frequency of Isolation of Bacteria in Sinusitis

ORGANISM	FREQUENCY (%)
Streptococcus pneumoniae	31–35
Haemophilus influenzae (unencapsulated)	12–40
Moraxella catarrhalis	8–20
Mixed	5
Staphylococcus aureus	4
Anaerobic bacteria (*Bacteroides, Peptococcus, Fusobacterium*)	2–6
Streptococcus pyogenes	2

From Brook I. Acute and chronic bacterial sinusitis. *Infect Dis Clin North Am.* 2007;21:427–428.

147. **What are causes of eosinophilic meningitis?**
See Table 12.8.

148. **What drugs cause aseptic meningitis?**
- Antibiotics: trimethoprim-sulfamethoxazole, trimethoprim, sulfamethoxazole, penicillin, cephalosporins, metronidazole
- Cetuxamib
- Carbamazepine
- IV immunoglobulin (IVIG)
- Nonsteroidal anti-inflammatory drugs (NSAIDs)
- OKT3 antibodies
- Ranitidine
- Rofecoxib

Table 12.8. Causes of Eosinophilic Meningitis

Infectious	
Bacterial	*Mycobacterium tuberculosis, Rickettsia rickettsii, Treponema pallidum*
Viral	LCM, coxsackievirus B4
Fungal	*Coccidioides immitis*
Parasitic	*Angiostrongylus catonensis, Gnathstoma, Baylisascaris, Paragonimus westermanii, Trichinella spiralis, Toxocara canis, Taenia soleum, Fasciola hepatica, Trypanosoma, Toxoplasma gondii, Schistosoma japonicum*
Noninfectious	
Drugs	Ciprofloxacin, intraventricular vancomycin, gentamicin, ibuprofen
Malignancy	Non-Hodgkin lymphoma, Hodgkin disease, leukemia
Other	Sarcoidosis, ventriculoperitoneal shunts

LCM, lymphocytic choriomeningitis virus.
From Re V, Lo II, Gluckman SJ. Eosinophilic meningitis. *Am J Med.* 2003;144:217–223.

149. **Which bacteria most commonly cause community-acquired meningitis?**
   - *S. pneumoniae*
   - *N. meningitidis*
   - *L. monocytogenes*
   - Streptococci other than *S. pneumoniae*
   - *S. aureus*
   - *H. influenzae*

150. **Who should receive adjunctive steroids when being treated for meningitis?**
   Patients with meningitis due to *S. pneumoniae* and admitted with a Glasgow Coma Scale (GCS) score of 8–11. Note that steroids may be harmful in some subsets of patients, and many experts would not use steroids in meningitis caused by other bacteria.
   Van De Beek D, de Gans J, Tunkel AR, et al. Community-acquired bacterial meningitis in adults. *N Engl J Med.* 2006;354:44–53.

151. **What antibiotic could be used to treat *Listeria* meningitis in a patient allergic to penicillin?**
   Trimethoprim-sulfamethoxazole.

152. **Who should receive postexposure prophylaxis for *Neisseria* meningitis?**
   - Health care workers with close contact to the infected patient or exposure to oral secretions (i.e., performing intubation)
   - Household contacts
   - Contacts residing in close quarters such as military barracks, nursery schools, and college dormitories

153. **What are some characteristics of human cestode infections?**
   See Table 12.9.

ENDOCARDITIS

154. **What are the major and minor Duke criteria for diagnosing infective endocarditis?**
   Major criteria
   - Positive blood cultures with an organism typical for endocarditis (viridans streptococci, *S. aureus*, enterococci, or HACEK (see Question 157) in at least two separate cultures drawn 12 hours apart
   - Evidence of endocardial involvement (positive echocardiogram or new/worsening regurgitant murmur)

Table 12.9. Common Human Cestode Infections

SPECIES	STAGE FOUND IN HUMANS	COMMON NAME	PATHOLOGY	THERAPY
Diphyllobothrium latum	Adult	Fish tapeworm	Pernicious anemia	Niclosamide, praziquantel
Hymenolepis nana	Adult	Dwarf tapeworm	Rarely symptomatic	Niclosamide, praziquantel
Taenia saginata	Adult	Beef tapeworm	Rarely symptomatic	Niclosamide, praziquantel
T. solium	Adult	Pork tapeworm	Rarely symptomatic	Niclosamide, praziquantel
	Larva	Cysticercosis	Brain and tissue cysts	Albendazole, praziquantel, surgery
Echinococcus granulosus	Larva	Hydatid cyst disease	Solitary tissue cysts	Surgery, albendazole
E. multilocularis	Larva	Alveolar cyst disease	Multilocular cysts	Surgery, albendazole
Taenia multiceps	Larva	Bladderworm, coenurosis	Brain and eye cysts	Surgery
Spirometra mansonoides	Larva	Sparganosis	Subcutaneous larvae	Surgery

From King CK. Cestode Infections. In Goldman L, Ausiello D, editors. *Cecil Textbook of Medicine*. 23rd ed. Philadelphia: WB Saunders; 2008.

Minor criteria
- Predisposition (predisposing heart condition or IV drug abuse)
- Fever (>38° C)
- Vascular phenomena: Janeway lesions, septic pulmonary emboli, major arterial emboli, mycotic aneurysm, conjunctival hemorrhages
- Immunologic phenomena: Osler nodes, glomerulonephritis, positive rheumatoid factor, Roth spots
- Microbiologic evidence: positive blood culture not meeting major criteria

Endocarditis is *definitely* diagnosed by the presence of:
1. Histologic evidence of endocarditis from abscess or valve vegetations *or*
2. Gram stain or culture evidence of endocarditis from surgical or autopsy specimen *or*
3. Presence of two major clinical criteria *or*
4. Presence of one major and three minor clinical criteria *or*
5. Five minor criteria

Endocarditis is *possibly* diagnosed by the presence of:
1. One major and one or two minor criteria *or*
2. Three minor criteria

155. **Endocarditis with which organisms should prompt a work-up for a gastrointestinal malignancy?**
Streptococcus bovis (now called *Streptococcus gallolyticus*) and *Clostridium septicum*.
Ridgway EJ, Grech ED. Clostridial endocarditis: report of a case caused by *Clostridium septicum* and review of the literature. *J Infect.* 1993;26:309–313.

156. **What organisms are most commonly associated with prosthetic valve endocarditis?**
- Late (>12 months after surgery)
- *Staphylococcus epidermidis*
- *Streptococcus*
- HACEK

- Early (<12 months after surgery)
- *S. aureus*
- Gram-negative bacilli

157. What are the HACEK organisms?
- *Haemophilus aphrophilus*
- *Actinobacillus actinomycetemcomitans*
- *Cardiobacterium hominis*
- *Eikenella corrodens*
- *Kingella kingae*

Recently, *A. actinomycetemcomitans* and *H. aphrophilus* have been placed into the new genus *Aggregatibacter*. These organisms can be isolated from blood cultures that are held for at least 5 days.

158. Which organism is associated with endocarditis in IV drug users?
P. aeruginosa. The organism is thought to contaminate water used to mix drugs or store drug paraphernalia. Right-sided endocarditis with *S. aureus* is also well described in IV drug abusers.

159. What organisms have been implicated in culture-negative endocarditis?
- *Coxiella burnetti* (also the agent of Q fever)
- *Tropheryma whipplei*
- *Abotrophia elegans*
- *Granulicatella*
- *Mycoplasma hominis*
- Nutritionally deficient streptococci
- *Brucella* spp.
- Intracellular organisms (*Rickettsia* and *Chlamydia* spp.)
- Fungi
- Anaerobic organisms

Houpikian P, Raoult D. Blood culture-negative endocarditis in a reference center: etiologic diagnosis of 348 cases. *Medicine (Baltimore).* 2005;84:162–173.

160. What are the nutritionally variant streptococci?
Gram-positive cocci that include *Abiotrophia defectiva, Granulicatella adiacens,* and *Granulicatella elegans.* These bacteria are important causes of bacteremia and infective endocarditis (IE).

Alberti MO, Hindler JA, Humphries RM. Antimicrobial susceptibility of *Abiotrophia defectiva, Granulicatella adiacens,* and *Granulicatella elegans. Antimicrob Agents Chemother.* 2016;60:1411–1420.

161. What organisms cause myocarditis?
Typically viruses. Patients usually have fevers, joint pain, and malaise. Chest pain, chills, and sweats may also occur. A variety of viruses including coxsackieviruses A9 and B3 have been found as causes. Other viruses implicated include enterovirus, adenovirus, CMV, influenza, EBV, HIV-1, and hepatitis viruses. RSV along with mumps, rubeola, varicella, parvovirus, yellow fever, HSV-1, rabies, and arboviruses may also be to blame. Other organisms include parasites, spirochetes, and *Rickettsia* spp. along with many bacteria. Pericarditis appears to have similar infectious causes as myocarditis.

PULMONARY INFECTIONS

162. Which organisms cause severe disease in asplenic patients?
Encapsulated organisms such as *S. pneumoniae, H. influenzae,* and *N. meningitidis.* Asplenic patients have decreased ability to clear opsonized antigens, decreased IgM levels, and poor antibody production. Gram-negative organisms such as *Klebsiella* spp. and *E. coli, Capnocytophaga canimorsus, Babesia microti,* and *Plasmodium falciparum* may all pose a higher risk in this patient population.

Cadili A, de Gara C. Complications of splenectomy. *Am J Med.* 2008;121:371–375.

163. What organisms most frequently cause community-acquired pneumonia?
- *S. pneumoniae*
- *M. pneumoniae*

- *Chlamydophila pneumoniae*
- Anaerobic bacteria
- *H. influenzae*
- *Legionella pneumophila*
- Respiratory viruses
- *S. aureus*

164. What organisms cause postinfluenza bacterial pneumonia?
- *S. pneumoniae*
- *S. aureus* (including CA-MRSA)
- *H. influenzae*
  Rothberg MB, Haessler SD, Brown RB. Complications of viral influenza. *Am J Med.* 2008;121:258–264.

165. What constitutes an adequate sputum sample in the diagnosis of pneumonia?
One with <10 epithelial cells and >25 polymorphonuclear leukocytes (PMNs) on Gram stain per low-power field.

166. What are the clinical findings and treatment of diphtheria?
Fever, pharyngitis, and cervical adenopathy associated with adherent pharyngeal membranes are the findings. Patients may present with stridor, hoarseness, and paralysis of the palate as well. Cultures on special media (Tindale media reveals black colonies with halos) and detection of toxin are used to confirm the diagnosis. Erythromycin and penicillin G are recommended antibiotics.

KEY POINTS: CLNICAL CLUES FOR DIPHTHERIA

1. Mildly painful tonsillitis or pharyngitis associated with gray palatal membrane
2. Cervical lymphadenopathy and neck swelling
3. Hoarseness and stridor
4. Unilateral palatal paralysis
5. Moderate temperature elevation
6. Serosanguineous nasal discharge with associated mucosal membrane

167. What organisms are responsible for most infections in patients with cystic fibrosis?
S. aureus and *P. aeruginosa. B. cepacia* is also commonly seen, particularly in adult patients with cystic fibrosis. Various other bacteria, including nontypeable *H. influenzae, S. pneumoniae,* and some of the Enterobacteriaceae, are occasionally isolated. The most important fungal pathogen is *Aspergillus fumigatus*, which causes ABPA in this patient population.
  Gilligan PH. Microbiology of airway disease in patients with cystic fibrosis. *Clin Microbiol Rev.* 1991;4:35–51.

GASTROINTESTINAL INFECTIONS

168. Which organisms most frequently cause traveler's diarrhea?
See Table 12.10.

169. Which patients should be treated with antibiotics for diarrhea caused by *Salmonella*?
Those with:
- Severe diarrhea (>10 stools/day)
- Need for hospitalization
- Immunosuppression due to HIV infection, organ transplantation, chemotherapy, corticosteroids, or other immunosuppressive agents
- Age > 50 years
- Sickle cell disease and other hemoglobinopathies

Table 12.10. Frequency of Organisms Isolated in Cases of Traveler's Diarrhea

ORGANISM	FREQUENCY ISOLATED (%)
Bacteria	
Enterotoxigenic *Escherichia coli*	20–50
Enteroinvasive *E. coli*	5–15
Enteroaggregative *E. coli*	5–15
Campylobacter jejuni	5–30
Salmonella spp.	5–25
Shigella spp.	5–15
Aeromonas spp.	0–10
Plesiomonas shigelloides	0–5 (very rare)
Vibrio spp.	≤5
Viruses	
Norovirus	0–10
Rotavirus	0–10
Protozoa	
Giardia spp.	0–10
Entamoeba histolytica	0–10
Cryptosporidium parvum	1–5
Cyclospora cayetanensis	0–5
No Pathogen	10–50

Adapted from Diemert DJ. Prevention and self-treatment of traveler's diarrhea. *Clin Microbiol Rev.* 2006;19:583–594.

170. **List the strains of *E. coli* and associated toxins and the diarrheal disease each causes.**
See Table 12.11.

Table 12.11. Strains of *Escherichia coli* and the Associated Toxins and Illnesses

STRAIN	TOXIN	ILLNESS	OTHER FEATURES
Enterotoxigenic (ETEC)	Cholera-like	Traveler's diarrhea	
Enteroaggregative (EAggEC)	Enterotoxin	Watery diarrhea	Adheres to colonic mucosa
Enteropathogenic (EPEC)	Secretes proteins, not toxins	Diarrhea	Adheres and binds to colonic mucosa
Enterohemorrhagic (EHEC)	Shiga-like cytotoxins and verotoxins	Hemorrhagic colitis; hemolytic uremic syndrome	Most pathogenic strain (OI57:H7)
Enteroinvasive (EIEC)	None	Inflammatory colitis	Requires large inoculum to cause illness

171. **What is the infectious agent causing cholera?**
Vibrio cholerae, a small, curved, gram-negative rod, which produces an enterotoxin. Patients typically develop a profuse watery diarrhea (often described as "rice-water" stool) that can lead to life-threatening dehydration.

172. **What are the clinically relevant microsporidia?**
Enterocytozoon bienusi and *Encephalitozoon intestinalis*. Both can cause chronic diarrhea in patients with AIDS.

173. **List the more common parasitic causes of diarrhea.**
- *Cryptosporidium*
- *Isospora*
- *Cyclospora*
- *Microsporidium*
- *Giardia*
- *Entamoeba histolytica*

174. **What organism causes diarrhea, mesenteric adenitis, and reactive arthritis and has been the cause of needless appendectomy in the past?**
Y. enterolitica. This organism can cause mesenteric adenitis, which clinically mimics appendicitis—fever, leukocytosis, and right lower quadrant abdominal pain.

175. **What organism causes diarrhea, malabsorption, and endocarditis?**
T. whipplei, a gram-positive organism that is the causative agent of Whipple disease. Whipple disease is a multisystem disorder characterized by migratory polyarthritis, diarrhea, malabsorption, weight loss, generalized lymphadenopathy, hyperpigmentation, and occasional neurologic abnormalities. Cases of endocarditis alone have been reported.
   Dutly F, Altwegg M. Whipple's disease and *Tropheryma whippelii. Clin Microbiol Rev.* 2001;14:561–583.
   Marin M, Sanchez M, del Rosal M, et al. *Tropheryma whipplei* infective endocarditis as the only manifestation of Whipple's disease. *J Clin Microbiol.* 2007;45:2078–2081.

176. **What pathogens are associated with consumption of contaminated fish and shellfish?**
- Hepatitis A virus
- *V. cholerae* O-1 and non-O-1
- *V. parahaemolyticus*
- *V. vulnificus*
- *C. botulinum*
- Norwalk virus
- *Giardia lamblia*
- *Diphyllobothrium*
- *Anisakis*

177. **What toxin-induced syndromes are caused by ingestion of seafood?**
- Ciguatera poisoning
- Paralytic shellfish poisoning due to *Gonyaulax* spp. of dinoflagellates
- Scombroid poisoning
- Tetrodotoxication due to eating puffer fish (also called *Fugu* or *blowfish*)
- Neurotoxic shellfish poisoning due to the toxic dinoflagellate *Ptychodiscus brevis*
- Diarrheic shellfish poisoning
   Eastaugh J, Shepherd S. Infectious and toxic syndromes from fish and shellfish consumption: a review. *Arch Intern Med.* 1989;149:1735–1740.

178. **What is possible estuary-associated syndrome (PEAS)?**
A toxin-mediated illness due to dinoflagellates such as *Pfiesteria* that are found in the estuaries of the Tar-Pamlico and Neuse Rivers in North Carolina and the Maryland Eastern Shore.
   Morris JG Jr. Pfiesteria, "the cell from hell," and other toxic algal nightmares. *Clin Infect Dis.* 1999;28:1191–1196.

179. **What laboratory test predicts spontaneous bacterial peritonitis (SBP)?**
A PMN count of 250 cells/mm^3 in an ascetic fluid sample which has > 90% specificity and sensitivity in diagnosing SBP.

SEXUALLY TRANSMITTED DISEASES

180. What is the causative agent of condyloma acuminatum?
Human papillomavirus (HPV), a double-stranded DNA virus with multiple serotypes. Types 6 and 11 are more commonly associated with anogenital warts. Types 16 and 18 are strongly linked to cervical cancer.

181. What is the causative agent of condyloma latum?
T. pallidum. Condyloma latum is a manifestation of secondary syphilis in which the generalized maculopapular rash becomes flat and broad with whitish lesions.

182. What is the difference between nontreponemal and treponemal tests?
Nontreponemal tests (reactive plasma reagin [RPR] and Venereal Disease Research Laboratory [VDRL]) are not specific for syphilis and can be falsely positive under many conditions. These tests are used to screen for syphilis and to assess therapeutic response because the titers return to normal over time after therapy is initiated. Treponemal tests are specific for syphilis and include the microhemagglutination assay for *T. pallidum* (MHA-TP) and the fluorescent treponemal antibody absorption (FTA-Abs) test. These tests are used to confirm the diagnosis of syphilis and, once positive, will remain positive for life and never return to normal.

183. What are the causes of false-positive serologic tests for syphilis?
See Table 12.12.

Table 12.12. Causes of False-Positive Nontreponemal and Treponemal Tests for Syphilis	
<6 MO AFTER EXPOSURE	**>6 MO AFTER EXPOSURE**
Nontreponemal Tests (RPR, VDRL)	
Pneumonia (viral, mycoplasma, pneumococcal)	Liver disease
Hepatitis	Malignancy
Tuberculosis	Intravenous drug abuse
Mononucleosis	Aging
Chancroid	Connective tissue disorders
Chickenpox	Multiple blood transfusions
HIV	
Measles	
Malaria	
Immunizations	
Pregnancy	
Laboratory error	
Treponemal tests (FTA, MHA-TP)	
Mononucleosis	SLE
Lyme disease	
Malaria	
Leprosy	

FTA, fluorescent treponemal antibody; HIV, human immunodeficiency virus; MHA-TP, microhemagglutination assay—*Treponema pallidum*; RPR, reactive plasma reagin; SLE, systemic lupus erythematosus; VDRL, Venereal Disease Research Laboratory.

184. What are the indications for lumbar puncture in a patient with latent syphilis?
- Neurologic signs or symptoms
- Ophthalmic signs or symptoms

- Tertiary syphilis without neurologic symptoms
- Treatment failure of secondary syphilis
- HIV infection and late latent syphilis or syphilis of unknown duration
- Patient preference (in immunocompetent patients)

185. **What is the earliest manifestation of syphilis?**
Painless ulceration at the site of inoculation (penis, vagina, anus, and throat) often associated with regional lymphadenopathy.

186. **What other sexually transmitted diseases (STDs) present as ulcers with lymphadenopathy?**
- **Chancroid:** *Haemophilus ducreyi* causes these ulcers and is usually associated with suppurative inguinal lymphadenopathy.
- **Genital herpes:** HSV type 1 or type 2 causes multiple vesicular or ulcerative painful genital ulcers, often associated with inguinal lymphadenopathy. HSV-2 is classically associated with this presentation, but HSV-1 may be causative in up to 50% of cases.
- **Granuloma inguinale:** *Klebsiella granulomatis* (formerly *Calymmatobacterium granulomatis*) causes painless, genital ulcerative disease. The lesions are highly vascular, bleed easily on contact, and rarely occur in the United States.
- **LGV:** *Chlamydia trachomatis* serovars L1, L2, and L3 cause tender inguinal or femoral lymphadenopathy that is typically unilateral.
  Workowski KA, Bolan GA. Centers for Disease Control and Prevention: sexually transmitted diseases treatment guidelines, 2015. *MMWR Recomm Rep.* 2015;64:1–138.

187. **What is a Bartholin cyst?**
An obstruction of the Bartholin glands leading to cystic dilatation. Bartholin glands are located on each side of the vaginal opening. Bartholin cyst abscess can occur and usually develops rapidly over 2–4 days. Symptoms include acute vulvar pain, dyspareunia, and pain during walking. Local symptoms of acute pain and tenderness are secondary to rapid enlargement, hemorrhage, or secondary infection. The signs are those of a classic abscess: erythema, acute tenderness, edema, and, occasionally, cellulitis of the surrounding subcutaneous tissue.

188. **How is a Bartholin cyst treated?**
By observation or antibiotics, depending on the severity of symptoms. Without therapy, most abscesses tend to rupture spontaneously by the third or fourth day. Asymptomatic cysts in women older than 40 years do not need treatment. The therapy for acute adenitis without abscess formation is broad-spectrum antibiotics and frequent hot sitz baths. In one series, 80% of cultures from the abscess was sterile; however, organisms such as *C. trachomatis* and *E. coli* have been reported. STDs do not play a major role in causing Bartholin abscess.

189. **What is the Fitz-Hugh–Curtis syndrome? What organisms cause it?**
Perihepatitis usually caused by either *N. gonorrhoeae* or *C. trachomatis*, thought to occur by spread of organisms from the fallopian tubes to the surface of the liver. Fitz-Hugh–Curtis syndrome is part of the differential diagnosis of right upper quadrant pain in young, sexually active women and has been occasionally reported in males, probably as a result of bacteremic spread.

ZOONOSES

190. **What tick-borne diseases are found in the United States?**
- Lyme disease (*Borrelia burgdorferi*)
- Q fever (*Coxiella burnetii*)
- Human ehrlichiosis (*Ehrlichia chaffeensis, E. ewingii, Anaplasma phagocytophilum*)
- RMSF (*Rickettsia rickettsii*)
- Tularemia (*Francisella tularensis*)
- Babesiosis (*Babesia microti*)
- Relapsing fever (*Borrelia hermsii*)
- Tick-borne encephalitis (flavivirus)
- Colorado tick fever (orbivirus)

191. What organism shares a common epidemiologic niche and the same tick vector as *B. burgdorferi*?

    B. microti, a protozoan that parasitizes human erythrocytes. *Ixodes scapularis* is the most important tick vector, with *Dermacentor variabilis* being a less frequent vector. Some of this same geographic distribution is also shared by one of the agents causing human granulocyte ehrlichiosis, *Anaplasma phagocytophilum*, for which *I. scapularis* (the black-legged tick) is also the vector. Consequently, it is theoretically possible to see simultaneous infection with all three agents.

192. What is the newest *Borrelia* species discovered?

    B. mayonii, which is closely related to *B. burgdorferi* and was described by scientists at the Mayo Clinic in Rochester, Minnesota. Six patients were treated for an illness similar to that caused by *B. burgdorferi*; however, *B. mayonii* infections were associated with diffuse rash as well as nausea and vomiting.

    Pritt B, Mead PS, Johnson DK, et al . Identification of a novel pathogenic *Borrelia* species causing Lyme borreliosis with unusually high spirochaetaemia: a descriptive study. *Lancet Infect Dis*. 2016;16:556–564.

193. What organism causes louse-borne relapsing fever?

    Borrelia recurrentis, frequently found in areas of overcrowding and poverty. Relapsing fever transmitted by the body louse is not seen in the United States and is more frequent in Africa or South America.

194. What organism causes tick-borne relapsing fever?

    B. hermsii, found in the United States in Western mountain states typically during late spring and summer. *Borrelia turicatae* has also been reported in the Southwest.

    Davis H, Vincent JM, Lynch J. Tick-borne relapsing fever caused by *Borrelia turicatae*. *Pediatr Infect Dis J*. 2002;21:703–705.

195. List the *Rickettsia* species, the diseases they cause, and the common geographic distribution.

    See Table 12.13.

Table 12.13. Diseases Caused by Rickettsial Species and Their Geographic Distribution

DISEASE	RICKETTSIAL SPECIES	GEOGRAPHIC DISTRIBUTION
African tick-bite fever	*Rickettsia africae*	Sub-Saharan Africa, Caribbean
Boutonneusse fever (Mediterranean spotted fever)	*R. conorii*	Southern Europe, Africa, southern and western Asia
Murine typhus	*R. typhi*	Coastal tropical and subtropical regions
Scrub typhus	*Orientia tsutsugamushi*	Southern and eastern Asia, western Pacific islands, northern Australia
Louse-borne typhus	*R. prowazekii*	Potentially worldwide
Queensland tick typhus	*R. australis*	Eastern Australia
North Asian tick typhus	*R. sibirica*	North Asia
Rocky Mountain spotted fever	*R. rickettsii*	North, Central, and South America

196. What questions are helpful in determining the risk of acquiring Lyme disease from a tick bite?
    - ***What is the size of the tick?*** Disease is typically spread by the nymph stage of *I. scapularis*, which is quite small.
    - ***Was the tick attached and for how long?*** Ticks that do not attach to the skin cannot transmit disease; therefore, the risk of transmission is low with ticks that have been attached for <24 hours.
    - ***Was the tick engorged when removed?*** Engorgement suggests a prolonged attachment and thus higher risk of transmission.

197. **What organism causes tick paralysis?**
None. Tick paralysis is not caused by an infectious agent but rather by a toxin secreted in tick saliva. Patients present with ascending flaccid paralysis that may be mistaken for other neurologic disorders. Treatment for this condition is quite simple—remove the tick.
Edlow JA, McGillicuddy DC. Tick paralysis. *Infect Dis Clin North Am*. 2008;22:397–413.

198. **What species of *Ehrlichia* have been associated with human disease?**
   - *E. chaffeensis*: Human monocytic ehrlichiosis (HME)
   - *E. ewingii*: Human granulocytic ehrlichiosis (HGE)
   - *A. phagocytophilum*: Human granulocytic anaplasmosis (HGA)
   - *E. sennetsu*: Mononucleosis-like illness in Japan and Malaysia
   - *E. canis*: One case report in Venezuela

199. **How does human disease due to *Dirofilaria immitis* usually present?**
As a solitary, noncalcified pulmonary nodule. Because humans are unsuitable hosts for *D. immitis*, the dog heartworm, larvae that mature in subcutaneous tissues after inoculation by infected mosquitoes enter veins and travel to the heart. From the heart, they embolize to the pulmonary arteries, resulting in infarcts.
Nicholson CP, Allen MS, Trastek VF, et al. Dirofilaria immitis: a rare, increasing cause of pulmonary nodules. *Mayo Clin Proc*. 1992;67:646–650.

200. **Most cases of RMSF occur in what regions of the United States?**
The south Atlantic states (most frequently in North Carolina) and south-central region (Oklahoma, Missouri, and Arkansas). Despite its name, few cases of RMSF occur in the Rocky Mountain states.

201. **What is the Jarisch-Herxheimer reaction?**
A self-limited systemic reaction occurring within 1–2 hours after the initial treatment of syphilis with antimicrobial agents. The reaction occurs most frequently in patients treated for secondary syphilis but can occur during treatment of any syphilitic stage and with other spirochete infections. The reaction consists of the abrupt onset of chills, fever, myalgias, tachycardia, hyperventilation, vasodilatation with associated flushing, and mild hypotension. The symptoms are probably due to the release of pyrogens from the spirochetes and one study found elevated levels of tumor necrosis factor (TNF), interleukin 6 (IL-6), and IL-8.
Negussie Y, Remick DG, DeForg LE, et al. Detection of plasma tumor necrosis factor, interleukins 6, and 8 during the Jarisch-Herxheimer reaction of relapsing fever. *J Exp Med*. 1992;175:1207–1212.

MISCELLANEOUS INFECTIONS

202. **What organisms can cause infections associated with medicinal use of leeches?**
Aeromonas hydrophila, which has the same freshwater habitat as the medicinal leech, *Hirudo medicinalis*. Leeches are used in microvascular surgical procedures because of their anticoagulant properties and *Aeromonas* infections may occur as postoperative infections.
Abrutyn E. Hospital-associated infection from leeches. *Ann Intern Med*. 1988;109:356–358.

203. **What is typhlitis?**
Necrotizing enterocolitis or neutropenic enterocolitis, a fulminate, necrotizing process that occurs in the gastrointestinal tract of individuals with profound neutropenia. Symptoms of the disease include fever, abdominal pain and distention, rebound tenderness in the right lower quadrant, and diarrhea. The cecum and terminal ileum are characteristically involved.

204. **What is CAUTI? CLABSI?**
   CAUTI: Catheter-associated urinary tract infection referring to infection involving any organ or structure of the urinary tract in the presence of a urinary catheter that has been in place for >2 days on the date of the event
   CLABSI: A bloodstream infection that is confirmed and in which a central line or umbilical catheter has been in place for >2 days on the date of the event

205. **What is differential time to positivity (DTP)?**
The time difference to a positive result of blood cultures drawn from a catheter suspected to be infected and peripheral culture by venipuncture. DTP ≥ 120 minutes is a sensitive and specific marker in the diagnosis of catheter-related infection.
Park KH, Lee MS, Lee SO, et al. Diagnostic usefulness of differential time to positivity for catheter-related candidemia. *J Clin Microbiol*. 2014;52:2566–2572.

WEBSITES

1. Centers for Disease Control: www.cdc.gov
2. Infectious Diseases Society of America: www.idsociety.org
3. National Institute of Allergy and Infectious Diseases: www.niaid.nih.gov

BIBLIOGRAPHY

1. Kaspar DL, Fauci AS, Hauser S, eds. *Harrison's Principles of Internal Medicine*. 19th ed. New York: McGraw-Hill Medical; 2015.
2. Gorbach SL, Bartlett JG, Blacklow NR, eds. *Infectious Diseases*. 3rd ed. Philadelphia: Lippincott Williams & Wilkins; 2004.
3. Bennett JE, Dolin R, Blaser MJ, eds. *Mandell, Douglas, and Bennett's Principles and Practice of Infectious Diseases*. 9th ed. Philadelphia: Saunders; 2014.
4. Southwick F. *Infectious Diseases: A Clinical Short Course*. 3rd ed. New York: McGraw-Hill Education/Medical; 2013.

ACQUIRED IMMUNODEFICIENCY SYNDROME AND HUMAN IMMUNODEFICIENCY VIRUS INFECTION

Daniel Lee, MD, Ankita Kadakia, MD, and Amy M. Sitapati, MD

Drawing largely on the work that Donna Mildvan and Dan Williams started in New York City in early 1981, the Morbidity and Mortality Weekly Report [May 12, 1982] on "Generalized Lymphadenopathy Among Homosexual Males" was released from Atlanta, the first MMWR publication on any aspect of the epidemic in nine months.... Doctors should be alert for the symptoms, the article concluded, most notably fatigue, fever, unexplained weight loss, and, of course, night sweats.

Randy Shilts
And the Band Played On (1987)

BASIC PRINCIPLES AND EPIDEMIOLOGY

1. **What is human immunodeficiency virus (HIV), and how many virions are typically made per day?**
   HIV is a single-stranded RNA lentivirus that integrates into the host cell DNA and attacks the immune system, in particular, CD4 cells, also known as *T cells*. If not treated, approximately 10^{12} virions are produced each day.

2. **Describe the difference between HIV infection and acquired immunodeficiency syndrome (AIDS).**
   HIV infection refers to the detection of HIV antibodies or HIV RNA in a person's serum. In order to make the diagnosis of AIDS in a person with HIV infection, at least 1 of 21 indicator diseases must be diagnosed. AIDS is also diagnosed in the presence of HIV infection if the CD4 count is <200 cells/mL or CD4 is < 14% even if symptoms of the indicator diseases are absent.

3. **What are the AIDS indicator diseases?**
   See Table 13.1.

4. **What is a T-cell count? What is its use?**
   A T-cell count is synonymous with a CD4 lymphocyte count, a laboratory measurement of the CD4 lymphocyte or the helper-inducer cells in the peripheral blood that is used to assess the degree of immunosuppression. HIV targets these T cells and their progressive death accounts for the immunosuppression caused by HIV infection. By measuring the T-cell count, a clinician can stage a patient's HIV infection according to the CDC classification system for HIV infection. A normal T-cell count (CD4) is 500–1600 cells/mL. Various opportunistic infections occur at or below certain CD4 counts. A T-cell count can be used to identify patients at high risk for opportunistic infections who require prophylactic treatment against specific infections. The CD4 count thus has prognostic and therapeutic value.

5. **How much time elapses between HIV infection and the diagnosis of AIDS?**
   This period is not easily defined. Studies of large patient cohorts indicate that in the absence of treatment, 50% of HIV-positive patients progress to AIDS in approximately 10 years. The rate of disease progression is not stable over this period because few develop disease early after exposure

Table 13.1. Acquired Immunodeficiency Syndrome Indicator Diseases

Candidiasis
Cervical cancer (invasive)
Coccidioidomycosis, cryptococcosis, cryptosporidiosis
Cytomegalovirus disease
Encephalopathy (HIV-related)
Herpes simplex (severe infection)
Histoplasmosis
Isosporiasis
Kaposi sarcoma
Lymphoma (certain types)
Mycobacterium avium complex
Pneumocystis jiroveci pneumonia
Pneumonia (recurrent)
Progressive multifocal leukoencephalopathy
Salmonella septicemia (recurrent)
Toxoplasmosis of the brain
Tuberculosis
Wasting syndrome

HIV, human immunodeficiency virus.
Data from Centers for Disease Control and Prevention: 1993 Revised classification system for HIV infection and expanded surveillance case definition for AIDS among adolescents and adults. *MMWR Morb Mortal Wkly Rep.* 41(RR-17), 1992. Available at: http://wonder.cdc.gov/wonder/help/AIDS/ MMWR-12-18-1992.html.

and proportionally more develop AIDS with each passing year. Several studies indicate that the average loss of CD4 lymphocytes is 80 cells/year. With the development and use of antiretroviral treatments, the natural progression of HIV infection to AIDS can be decreased or even halted if patients begin treatment sooner than later in their disease course.

Lifson AR, Rutherford GW, Jaffe HW. The natural history of human immunodeficiency virus infection. *J Infect Dis.* 1988;158:1360–1367.

6. **Have the number of new HIV infections increased in the past few years?**
No. According to the Joint United Nations Program on HIV/AIDS (UNAIDS) the number of new HIV infections continues to fall worldwide with a 35% decrease since 2000. However, 2 million people are infected globally every year. The incidence of HIV infections in the United States has remained stable with an estimated 50,000 new HIV infections per year, according to The Centers for Disease Control and Prevention (CDC). A disproportionate number of these new HIV cases represent minorities including blacks/African Americans and Hispanics/Latinos. Young black men who have sex with men represent the greatest number of new infections.

7. **How many people are living with HIV and AIDS worldwide and in the United States?**
36.9 million people worldwide and 1.2 million people in the United States. In the United States, almost 1 in 8 people are unaware of their HIV infection.

HIV in the United States. At A Glance. 2017. Available at: http://www.cdc.gov/hiv/statistics/overview/ataglance.html.

UNAIDS/AIDS by the Numbers 2015. Available at: http://www.unaids.org/en/resources/documents/2015/AIDS_by_the_numbers_2015.

TRANSMISSION, PREVENTION, AND DIAGNOSIS

8. **What is the most common form of HIV transmission in the United States?**
Unprotected anal sex. The second highest transmission form is unprotected vaginal sex. In the United States, 63% of new HIV infections are reported in men who have sex with men (MSM). In addition, infection can be spread via sexual intercourse (vaginal, anal, and oral), percutaneous blood exposure

(injection use and needlesticks), blood transfusion, perinatal maternal-fetal transmission, and breast feeding. Globally, blood transfusions are the highest risk of HIV transmission followed by maternal-fetal transmission.

Centers for Disease Control and Prevention. Prevalence of Diagnosed and Undiagnosed HIV Infection—United States 2008-2012. *MMWR Morb Mortal Wkly Rep.* 2015;64:657–664.

Patel P, Borkowf CB, Brooks JT, et al. Estimating per-act HIV transmission risk: a systematic review. *AIDS.* 2014;28:1509–1519.

9. **What increases the risk of HIV transmission between heterosexual partners?**
HIV viral load. Other risk factors found to increase the risk for HIV transmission include exposure volume; presence of other sexually transmitted diseases (STDs) such as syphilis, herpes simplex, gonorrhea, and chlamydia infection; and lack of circumcision. Although circumcision appears to be protective in heterosexuals in Africa, circumcision has not been found to be protective in MSM.

Galvin SR, Cohen MS. The role of sexually transmitted diseases in HIV transmission. *Nat Rev Microbiol.* 2004;2:33–42.

Quinn TC, Wawer MJ, Sewankambo N, et al. Viral load and heterosexual transmission of human immunodeficiency virus type 1. Rakai Project Study Group. *N Engl J Med.* 2000;342:921–929.

10. **Have studies definitively shown that treatment of other STDs reduces the risk of HIV transmission?**
No. Treatment of STDs has not been found to effectively reduce the risk for HIV transmission. Multiple studies have shown that despite aggressive measures to control STDs the rates of HIV infection remained the same; however, screening for STDs can help to assess someone's risk for getting HIV.

Gregson S, Adamson S, Papaya S, et al. Impact and process evaluation of integrated community and clinic-based HIV-1 control: a cluster-randomised trial in eastern Zimbabwe. *PLoS Medicine.* 2007;4:e10. https://doi.org/10.1371/journal.pmed.0040102.

Vellozzi C, Brooks JT, Bush TJ, et al. The Study to Understand the Natural History of HIV and AIDS in the Era of Effective Therapy (SUN study). *Am J Epidemiol.* 2009;169:642–652.

Wawer MJ, Sewankambo NK, Serwadda D, et al. Control of sexually transmitted diseases for AIDS prevention in Uganda: a randomized community trial. *Lancet.* 1999;353:525–535.

11. **Should HIV treatment reduce the risk for HIV transmission?**
Yes. Risk of HIV transmission is greatly reduced when an HIV-positive person on antiretrovirals has an undetectable HIV viral load in his or her bloodstream. One study used mathematical modeling to predict infections and found that increasing the number of individuals on highly active antiretroviral therapy (HAART) from 50% to 75%, 90%, and 100% would reduce the number of annual new HIV infections by 30%, 50%, and 60%, respectively.

Lima VD, Johnson TK, Hogg RS, et al. Expanded access to highly active antiretroviral therapy: a potentially powerful strategy to curb the growth of the HIV epidemic. *J Infect Dis.* 2008;198:56–67.

12. **Is HIV treatment effective in preventing perinatal HIV transmission from mother to child (vertical transmission)?**
Yes. All pregnant women should be tested for HIV infection so that early treatment can be initiated. Without treatment, perinatal transmission rates are 20–33%. With combination therapy treatment of the pregnant mother, transmission rates were lowered to less than 2%. In general, therapy recommendations are the same during pregnancy as in the nonpregnant patient, but efavirenz should be avoided in the first trimester owing to significant teratogenicity manifested as neural tube defects. Zalcitabine and delavirdine are also potential teratogens. The combination of didanosine and stavudine can lead to fatal lactic acidosis and should be avoided in pregnancy unless there are no alternative regimens. When used as part of combination therapy in pregnant women with CD4 counts > 250 cell/mm^3, nevirapine has been associated with fatal hepatotoxicity.

13. **What is the risk of HIV transmission via needlestick?**
~0.3% among health care workers. However, each exposure needs to be evaluated individually. There is tremendous variation in the degree of exposure, which affects the likelihood of infection. Exposure to a large volume of infectious material (or material with a high viral load), a deep injury, visible blood on the device causing the injury, prolonged contact with the infectious material, and the portal of entry are important factors. Intramuscular injection, exposures via hollow needles (as opposed to suture needles and pins), and exposure to material from a viremic HIV-infected patient also increase the transmission risk.

Tokars JI, Marcus R, Culver DH, et al. Surveillance of HIV infection and zidovudine use among health-care workers after occupational exposure to HIV-infected blood. *Ann Intern Med.* 118:913–919.

14. **What is postexposure prophylaxis (PEP), when do you give it, what do you give, and for how long?**
PEP is given for HIV transmission risks associated with occupational and nonoccupational exposure to HIV. Animal studies have shown optimal benefit when antiretroviral therapy (ART) is administered within the initial 3 hours, but the benefit of PEP continues for the initial 72 hours after exposure. No randomized, controlled trial has been performed, and, most likely, none will be done in the future. However, a retrospective case-control study involving 31 exposed and infected health care workers and 679 exposed, uninfected workers found that postexposure zidovudine reduced the risk of HIV infection by 79%. Therapy recommendations include combination ART given for 28 days based on the treatment status of the source patient including consideration for possible drug resistance.

Centers for Disease Control and Prevention. Case-control study of HIV seroconversion in health-care workers after percutaneous exposure to HIV-infected blood—France, United Kingdom, and United States, January 1988–August 1994. *MMWR Morb Mortal Wkly Rep.* 1995;44:929–933.

Centers for Disease Control and Prevention. Updated U.S. Public Health Service Guidelines for the management of occupational exposures to HBV, HCV, and HIV and recommendations for postexposure prophylaxis. *MMWR Morb Mortal Wkly Rep.* 2001;50:1–67.

Centers for Disease Control and Prevention, U.S. Department of Health and Human Services. Updated guidelines for antiretroviral postexposure prophylaxis after sexual, injection drug use, or other nonoccupational exposure to HIV—United States. 2016. Available at: https://stacks.cdc.gov/view/cdc/38856.

15. **A discordant couple (i.e., one partner is HIV-positive and the other partner is HIV-negative) experiences a condom break during sexual intercourse. What window of time has been shown to be effective for initiating ART and reducing the risk of HIV transmission?**
72 hours. ART given to reduce the risk for sexual transmission of HIV is called "n-PEP" or nonoccupational PEP, and includes individuals exposed during intercourse, sexual abuse, and rape and follows a similar guideline as outlined for occupational PEP.

Centers for Disease Control and Prevention, U.S. Department of Health and Human Services. Updated guidelines for antiretroviral postexposure prophylaxis after sexual, injection drug use, or other nonoccupational exposure to HIV—United States. 2016. Available at: https://stacks.cdc.gov/view/cdc/38856.

16. **Is there a vaccine available that might reduce the risk for HIV transmission?**
No. Despite much global research and effort, an effective HIV vaccine has not yet been developed. A placebo-controlled trial involving over 3000 subjects was halted in 2007 because of lack of vaccine efficacy at the interim analysis (the Step Study). Subsequent data analysis suggests that certain populations may actually have an increased risk of HIV acquisition after vaccination. The data from the STEP trial did have a few confounding factors in their analysis. A more recent study shows some possible efficacy of a vaccine and plans for future trials continue.

Buchbinder SP, Mehrota DV, Duerr A, et al. Efficacy assessment of a cell-mediated immunity HIV-1 vaccine (the Step Study): a double-blind, randomised, placebo-controlled, test-of-concept trial. *Lancet.* 2008;372:1881–1893.

McElrath MJ, De Rosa SC, Moodie Z, et al. HIV-1 vaccine-induced immunity in the test-of-concept Step Study: a case-cohort analysis. *Lancet.* 2008;372:1894–1905.

Rerks-Ngarm S, Pitisuttithum P, Nitayaphan S, et al. Vaccination with ALVAC and AIDSVAC to prevent HIV-1 infection in Thailand. *N Engl J Med.* 2009;361:2209–2226.

17. **Who should have HIV testing? How might testing reduce HIV transmission?**
The CDC recommends screening all patients aged 13–64 years in all health care settings once as part of routine health care and more frequently in individuals with certain risk factors. Risk factors include MSM, more than one sex partner, sex with an HIV positive person, injecting drugs or sharing needles, exchanging sex for money, or being tested or treated for STDs, hepatitis, or tuberculosis (TB). The U.S. Preventive Services Task Force recommends screening from ages 15–64. Currently, 1 in 8 people (12.8%) with HIV are unaware of his or her status. Once patients are aware of their HIV status, 53% will modify their high-risk behavior. A recent study estimated that 91.5% of new infections were transmitted

by persons unaware of their HIV diagnosis or persons not retained in follow-up care for their HIV infection. Early identification of HIV infection can lead to early treatment and transmission prevention.

Centers for Disease Control and Prevention. Revised recommendations for HIV testing of adults, adolescents, and pregnant women in health-care settings. *MMWR Morb Mortal Wkly Rep.* 2006;55:1–17.

Moyer V, LeFevre M, Siu A, et al. U.S. Preventive Services Task Force (USPSTF): screening for HIV. *Ann Intern Med.* 2013;159:51–60.

Skarbinski J, Rosenberg E, Paz-Bailey G. Human immunodeficiency virus transmission at each step of the care continuum in the United States. *JAMA Intern Med.* 2015;175:588–596.

18. **What are the problems with rapid tests for HIV?**
Inaccurate results. Rapid tests are immunoassays that give quick results, usually in less than 30 minutes. Rapid HIV tests use saliva, serum, or whole blood samples to look for HIV antibodies. If a rapid HIV test is conducted during the window period (the period after exposure but before antibodies are present) a false-negative test can result. Also, an increased number of false-positive results have been reported with the oral rapid tests. Any positive rapid test result must be confirmed by traditional blood test.

ACUTE HIV INFECTION

19. **List the symptoms of acute HIV infection along with their frequency.**
    - Fatigue: 80%
    - Lymphadenopathy: 75%
    - Pharyngitis: 70%
    - Rash: 70%
    - Myalgias/arthralgias: 55%
    - Nausea, vomiting, diarrhea: 30%
    - Headache: 30%
    - Weight loss: 15%
    - Oral candidiasis (thrush): 15%
    - Central/peripheral neurologic symptoms: 10%
      Perlmutter B, Glaser J, Oyugi S. How to recognize and treat acute HIV syndrome. *Am Fam Physician.* 1999;60:535–542.

20. **How soon after acute HIV infection do symptoms develop? How long do the symptoms persist?**
1–8 weeks after the initial infection, believed to result from specific immune responses to HIV. Patients presenting with these symptoms should have a specific risk history taken for possible recent exposure to HIV. The symptoms that develop are transient and generally are present for 1–3 weeks; however, cases have been reported with symptoms lasting up to 8 weeks.

21. **How can acute primary HIV infection be diagnosed?**
By using a fourth-generation Ag/Ab combination enzyme immunoassay (EIA) test for the presence of HIV-1 or HIV-2 antibodies and HIV-1 p24 antigen. Early in HIV infection, the host has not yet made antibodies that can be detected reliably with older antibody-based screening. Fourth-generation EIA is a two-step test that initially looks for Ag/Ab, and, if positive, a second differentiation test to distinguish HIV-1 infection from HIV-2 infection is done. If the second test is indeterminate or nonreactive, then an HIV-1 nucleic acid test (NAT) is performed. A positive NAT indicates acute HIV infection. If fourth-generation EIA testing is not available, then testing for HIV RNA (also known as a viral load) can be done. A result of > 5000 copies of HIV can be presumptively positive for acute HIV infection, but Ag/Ab testing should be repeated 3 or more weeks later.

Centers for Disease Control and Prevention and Association of Public Health Laboratories. Laboratory Testing for the Diagnosis of HIV Infection: Updated Recommendations. Available at http://stacks.cdc.gov/view/cdc/23447. Published June 27, 2014 [accessed 05.09.16].

VIRAL LOAD AND HIV LIFE CYCLE

22. **What is a "viral load" test? How is it used in patients with HIV?**
A test that measures the amount of HIV RNA in the plasma and indicates the degree of viral replication. Viral load testing is the single best prognostic indicator in HIV infection, with a higher

level of mRNA indicative of a poorer prognosis. The test is routinely performed as part of the initial assessment of newly diagnosed HIV infection. Once therapy has been initiated, the viral load is used to assess the efficacy and durability of ART. There should be at least a 1.0-log decrease in the viral load within 8 weeks of the start of therapy. Within 24 weeks, the viral load should be below detectable limits.

23. **Does "undetectable" viral load mean "cured" or "not infectious"?**
   No. An undetectable viral load means only that the ART has effectively halted viral replication below the threshold that can be detected by the assay being used.

24. **Do patients with undetectable HIV still need to use condoms to prevent HIV transmission during sexual activity?**
   Yes. HIV infection is still present, and HIV infection is, most importantly, still transmissible even though the risk for transmission may be reduced. This appears to be true for sexual, needlestick, and perinatal transmissions. However, a recent study showed that early initiation of ART in the HIV-positive partner among discordant heterosexual couples led to a 96% reduction in HIV transmission to the HIV-negative partner.
   Cohen M, Chen Y, McCauley M, et al. Prevention of HIV-1 infection with early antiretroviral therapy. *N Engl J Med.* 2011;365:493–505.

KEY POINTS: HUMAN IMMUNODEFICIENCY VIRUS INFECTION

1. HIV infection is currently a lifelong condition without cure.
2. Persons living with HIV infection are infectious regardless of HIV viral load.
3. Lifestyle changes including condom use, using clean needles, and adherence to antiretroviral therapy can decrease HIV transmission risk.
4. Many persons living with HIV live long and healthy lives; but delayed diagnosis and poor adherence to therapy can increase the risk for AIDS-related illnesses and death.
5. HIV tests include fourth-generation HIV Ag/Ab immunoassay, HIV antibody tests, and HIV RNA tests. All rapid HIV test results should be confirmed by a blood test.
6. HIV resistance testing should be done early in the disease, usually prior to starting antiretroviral therapy.
7. Initiation of antiretroviral therapy is now recommended to be started as soon as possible in all HIV-infected individuals regardless of CD4 count except in certain opportunistic infections for which treatment may be shortly deferred.

AIDS, acquired immunodeficiency syndrome; HIV, human immunodeficiency virus.

---

25. **Describe the HIV life cycle.**
   See Fig. 13.1.

26. **What stages of the HIV life cycle are targets of currently available therapy?**
   - Cell entry
   - Reverse transcription
   - Integrase and maturation
   - Protease

   Current therapy can attack these steps in the HIV life cycle. The first point of contact preceding entry of a virion into a new cell is the CD4 receptor and CXCR4 or CCR5 coreceptor. Cell entry can be blocked by an injectable fusion inhibitor, which binds gp41, thereby preventing fusion of viral and cellular membranes or an oral CCR5 receptor antagonist. Reverse transcription enzyme inhibition can be achieved through either nucleoside analogs (NRTIs, or "nucs") or non-nucleoside analog reverse transcriptase inhibitors (NNRTIs, or "non-nucs"). Next, the insertion of HIV proviral DNA into the host can by inhibited by integrase strand transfer inhibitors (INSTI). Finally, protease inhibitors (PIs) can interrupt mature cleavage of virions.

HIV TREATMENT AND RESISTANCE TESTING

27. **Describe the mechanism of action of the reverse transcriptase inhibitors (RTIs).**
   The RTIs block the function of viral reverse transcriptase during the transcription of viral RNA to host complementary DNA. There are two kinds of RTIs: NRTIs and NNRTIs. NRTIs mimic nucleoside bases and are incorporated into the DNA chain stopping further chain extension. The NNRTIs bind to the enzyme reverse transcriptase near the active site, sterically obstructing function of the enzyme.

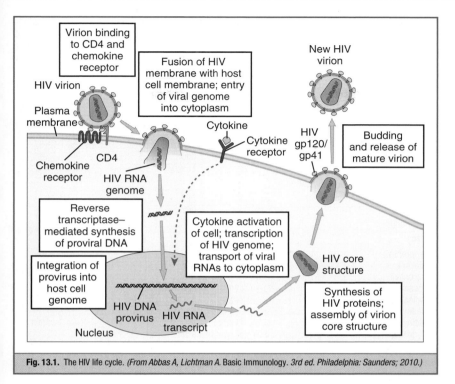

Fig. 13.1. The HIV life cycle. *(From Abbas A, Lichtman A.* Basic Immunology. *3rd ed. Philadelphia: Saunders; 2010.)*

28. **How do PIs work?**
    By preventing the cleavage of HIV polyproteins by HIV-1 protease that is required to make a mature viral core during the final stages of virion synthesis. Virions that subsequently bud from the surface of the cell in the presence of PIs lack a mature developed core. These immature virions are unable to infect new host cells.

29. **How do INSTIs work?**
    By preventing the integration of viral DNA with host DNA by blocking the HIV enzyme, integrase.

30. **What is HAART?**
    Highly active antiretroviral therapy. The term originated from the development of combination of at least three medications that could suppress HIV viral replication below the level of detection by a viral load test. Optimally, targeted ART should include three active drugs from at least two different classes. Commonly, HAART includes two NRTIs combined with either an NNRTI, a PI, or an INSTI.
        Panel on Antiretroviral Guidelines for Adults and Adolescents. Guidelines for the use of antiretroviral agents in HIV-1–infected adults and adolescents. Department of Health and Human Services. Available at: www.aidsinfo.nih.gov/ContentFiles/AdultandAdolescentGL.pdf [accessed 28.01.16].

31. **What antiretroviral drugs are currently available?**
    See Table 13.2.

32. **At what threshold of CD4 cell count in an HIV-infected individual should one consider initiating ART?**
    ART is recommended for all HIV-positive individuals regardless of CD4 count in order to reduce morbidity and mortality rates.

Table 13.2. Antiretroviral Drugs for Treatment of Human Immunodeficiency Virus Infection

DRUG	ABBREVIATION
NRTIs	
Abacavir	ABC
Didanosine	ddI
Emtricitabine	FTC
Lamivudine	3TC
Stavudine	d4T
Tenofovir	TDF, TAF
Zalcitabine	ddC
Zidovudine	ZDV, AZT
NNRTIs	
Delavirdine	DLV
Efavirenz	EFV
Nevirapine	NVP
PIs	
Amprenavir	APV
Atazanavir	ATV
Darunavir	DRV
Fosamprenavir	FPV
Indinavir	IDV
Nelfinavir	NFV
Ritonavir	RTV
Saquinavir	SQV
Tipranavir	TPV
Fusion Inhibitor	
Enfuvirtide	T-20
INSTI	
Elvitegravir	EVG
Dolutegravir	DTG
Bictegravir	BTG
Raltegravir	RAL
CCR5 Antagonist	
Maraviroc	MVC

CCR5, chemokine coreceptor type 5; INSTI, integrase strand transfer inhibitor; NNRTIs, non-nucleoside reverse transcriptase inhibitors; NRTIs, nucleoside reverse transcriptase inhibitors; PIs, protease inhibitors.

33. Why consider early treatment of HIV infection?

To reduce the risk for HIV transmission and theoretically reduce the risk for AIDS-defining illnesses, malignancy, and cardiovascular disease. Newer data, including two large clinical trials, have shown that earlier treatment is better before further decline in CD4 cell counts. Earlier suppression of viral replication may also preserve immune function.

International Network for Strategic Initiatives in Global HIV Trials (INSIGHT) START Study Group. Strategic Timing of AntiRetroviral Treatment (START) study, Available at https://clinicaltrials.gov/ct2/show/NCT00867048ClinicalTrials.gov [accessed 05.09.16].

The TEMPRANO ANRS 12136 Study Group. A trial of early antiretrovirals and isoniazid preventive therapy in Africa. *N Engl J Med*. 2015;373:808–822.

34. What are the preferred initial treatments for HIV infection?

Two NRTIs with an INSTI is considered a first-line regimen. A PI-based regimen with darunavir and two NRTIs, preferably tenofovir and emtricitabine, is also considered a first-line regimen. Alternative regimens include two NRTIs plus an NNRTI, or an alternative PI, or a CCR5 antagonist.

Panel on Antiretroviral Guidelines for Adults and Adolescents: Guidelines for the use of antiretroviral agents in HIV-1–infected adults and adolescents. Department of Health and Human Services. Available at: www.aidsinfo.nih.gov/ContentFiles/AdultandAdolescentGL.pdf. Accessed January 28, 2016.

35. What are the goals of HIV treatment?

To suppress the HIV viral load also knowns as HIV RNA. Suppressing the viral load helps to preserve the immune system and decrease HIV transmission. Acceptable viral load suppression is HIV RNA to <50 copies, but this number is dependent on the assay used. Currently ultrasensitive assay can detect virus to 20 copies; however, most viral load tests will range from <40 to <20 copies/mL. If a specimen has an amount of HIV RNA below the limit of detection on a viral load assay, it is said to be "undetectable" or, more accurately, "below the limits of detection." A repeat viral load should be performed within 2–4 weeks, and not more than 8 weeks, of initiation of therapy and should be at least 1.0-log less (down by 90%) than the baseline level. At 48 weeks after beginning treatment, the viral load should be <50 copies.

36. List the predictors of long-term virologic success (or reduction of viral load to <50 copies) in HIV therapy.

- Low baseline viral load
- High baseline CD4 count
- Rapid reduction of viral load to undetectable levels
- Patient adherence to prescribed therapy

37. How does patient adherence to prescribed ART affect treatment efficacy?

See Table 13.3.

Table 13.3. Level of Adherence in Relation to Efficacy of Therapy

LEVEL OF ADHERENCE (%)	PATIENTS WITH UNDETECTABLE VIRAL LOAD AT 48 WK (%)
95–100	84
90–95	64
80–90	47
70–80	24
<70	12

38. List the reasons for virologic or treatment failure of ART.

- Insufficient drug potency
- Poor adherence to ART
- Pharmacokinetics including lack of adequate penetration into compartments such as central nervous system (CNS)
- Decline of immunologic function
- Emergence of resistance to one or more drugs in ART regimen

39. Is there evidence that interrupted therapy (taking a break from ART) is poor for health?

Yes. The Strategies for Management of Antiretroviral Therapy (SMART) study clearly showed that the risk of disease progression and death was increased by 2.6 times in the group that interrupted therapy.

The Strategies for Management of Antiretroviral Therapy (SMART) Study Group. CD4+ count–guided interruption of antiretroviral treatment. *N Engl J Med.* 2006;55:2283–2296.

40. What is tropism?

The identification of the specific coreceptor used by the infecting virus in an individual patient and use of that knowledge to select antiviral therapy for that patient. HIV primarily binds to the CD4 receptor on the cell surface but also requires a chemokine (CCR5 or CXCR4) coreceptor for cell entry that resides beside the CD4 receptor on the cell surface. When HIV envelope glycoprotein gp120 attaches to the CD4 receptor, the virus uses the CCR5 or CXCR4 coreceptors to facilitate cell entry. Some HIV viruses use the CCR5 coreceptor (particularly in early HIV infection), some use the CXCR4 coreceptor, and some use both. Currently, a drug called maraviroc is effective only against HIV viruses that use the CCR5 coreceptor.

KEY POINTS: HUMAN IMMUNODEFICIENCY VIRUS THERAPY

1. HIV therapy is complicated but generally well tolerated despite toxicities.
2. Good adherence (≥95%) is required to secure durable viral control.
3. Suboptimal adherence promotes viral replication and resistance to anti-HIV medications.
4. Optimal time to initiate HIV therapy is early in the diagnosis or as soon as possible regardless of CD4 count.

AIDS, acquired immunodeficiency syndrome; HIV, human immunodeficiency virus.

41. **How can HIV resistance be measured?**
    Through genotypic or phenotypic resistance testing and tropism testing. A genotypic resistance test will report specific sequences of mutations in the form of letters and numbers such as an M184V or K103N, which can infer resistance to certain antiretrovirals or certain ART classes. A phenotypic resistance test will report an x-fold change for a medication to report whether a specific medication may have activity. Phenotypes tend to provide more useful information when complex genetic evolution of the virus has occurred. Tropism assays are similar to resistance tests but look at the coreceptors used by the virus to enter CD4$^+$ cells.

42. **When should an HIV resistance test be ordered?**
    At the time of initial HIV diagnosis. Approximately 10–17% of untreated HIV-infected patients already have resistant HIV at the time of diagnosis in higher income countries and an even greater amount of transmitted resistance is predicted in lower income countries according to the WHO based on multiple studies. A traditional genotype resistance test cannot be accurately done when a viral load is suppressed on therapy to < 500 copies/mL. Newer genotype resistance testing can detect mutations below 500 copies/mL but is used in certain situations such as changing therapy for virally suppressed patients owing to adverse reactions. After treatment begins, failure of a patient to suppress viral load to undetectable by 48 weeks on a new regimen or failure to maintain a viral load < 400 copies/mL on two consecutive tests would also indicate the need for resistance testing.
    WHO HIV Drug Resistance Report 2012. Available at: www.who.int/hiv/pub/drugresistance/report2012/en/ [accessed 05.09.16].

43. **If the HIV develops resistance to one medication, will other medications have increased activity or effectiveness?**
    Yes. In the push-and-pull antagonistic development of mutations by the HIV, some mutations can increase the effectiveness of specific medications. For example, zidovudine becomes more effective in the presence of lamuvidine resistance with an M184V mutation.

PULMONARY INFECTIONS

44. **What is PJP (also known as PCP)?**
    Pneumocystis jiroveci pneumonia (previously called *Pneumocystis carinii* pneumonia). Before routine prophylactic treatments for PCP in HIV-infected patients, PCP was the presenting diagnosis in > 60% of patients with AIDS and was eventually seen in 80% of patients with AIDS at some time during their illness. Without secondary prophylaxis after initial PCP diagnosis and effective HIV therapy, the recurrence rate of PCP is 40% within 6 months. With more proactive HIV testing before depletion of immune function and the initiation of effective primary PCP prophylaxis, the incidence of PCP should approach zero.

45. **What clinical features in an HIV-infected patient indicate increased risk for PCP?**
    - CD4 count < 200 or < 14% of total lymphocyte count
    - Diagnosis of thrush
    - Concomitant use of immunosuppressive medications for conditions such as organ transplantation

46. **Describe the typical signs and symptoms of PCP.**
    - Nonproductive cough or cough productive of clear sputum
    - Dyspnea on exertion (may have insidious onset)
    - Fever

- Malaise
- Sensation of chest tightness or inability to deeply inspire
- Normal physical examination or signs of tachypnea or dry rales
  Krajicek BJ, Thomas CF, Limper AH. *Pneumocystis* pneumonia: Current concepts in pathogenesis, diagnosis, and treatment. *Clin Chest Med.* 2009;30:265–278.

47. What laboratory findings are associated with PCP?
Hypoxemia with an elevated alveolar-arterial (A-a) oxygen partial pressure gradient (Pao_2–Pao_2) and elevated serum lactate dehydrogenase (LDH) levels, although these findings lack sensitivity and specificity. High or rising LDH in PCP suggests increased mortality risk but should not solely be used for diagnosis.

Zaman MK, White DA. Serum lactate dehydrogenase levels and *Pneumocystis carinii* pneumonia: diagnostic and prognostic significance. *Am Rev Respir Dis.* 1988;137:796–800.

48. How is PCP diagnosed?
By sputum analysis for *P. jiroveci*, with Giemsa stain, cytologic silver stain, or direct fluorescence antibody (DFA). Sputum is sometimes induced, but most centers rely on bronchoscopy with bronchoalveolar lavage (BAL) for diagnosis. Lavage alone has a sensitivity of > 95% and is considered the gold standard. An experienced HIV clinician may make an empirical diagnosis of PCP in HIV-infected patients with appropriate signs and symptoms.

KEY POINTS: *PNEUMOCYSTIS JIROVECI* PNEUMONIA

1. PCP is preventable.
2. Diagnosis of PCP represents a failed opportunity to diagnose HIV infection or use appropriate prophylaxis.
3. Onset of PCP is insidious and progressive.
4. Typical community-acquired "broad-spectrum" antibiotic coverage will not cover PCP.

HIV, human immunodeficiency virus; PCP, *Pneumocystis carinii* (former name of *P. jiroveci*) pneumonia.

---

49. Describe the chest radiograph findings in PCP.
Diffuse, bilateral, and interstitial infiltrates, often more pronounced in the hilar region (called a *butterfly distribution*). Areas of focal consolidation are less common, as are cystic and cavitary changes. Normal chest radiographs are common, especially in patients presenting early in the illness. Pleural effusion and hilar adenopathy are rare and, if present, should raise the suspicion of another diagnosis.

50. How is PCP treated?
See Table 13.4. For primary treatment, oral trimethoprim-sulfamethoxazole (TMP-SMX) for 21 days is considered the best first-line therapy. In severe infection with hypoxia as determined by a Pao_2 < 70 mm Hg or an A-a gradient > 35 mm Hg, corticosteroids may be needed in addition to antibiotics.

51. When is atovaquone used?
When patients have mild to moderate PCP and are allergic or intolerant of TMP-SMX. Compared with TMP-SMX, atovaquone has less bone marrow suppression and rash; however, it is also less effective than TMP-SMX and must be taken with food to ensure absorption. The dosing regimen with the oral suspension is 750 mg twice daily, taken with a fatty meal, for 21 days.

52. What are the side effects of medications used to treat moderate to severe PCP?
TMP-SMX
- Rash
- Stevens-Johnson syndrome
- Fever
- Leukopenia
- Nausea
- Hyperkalemia
- Elevated liver function tests

Table 13.4. Standard and Alternative Therapies for *Pneumocystis jiroveci* Pneumonia

DRUG	DOSAGE	ADDITIONAL INFORMATION
Standard Therapy		
TMP-SMX	TMP: 15–20 mg/kg plus SMX: 75–100 mg/kg divided into three or four doses daily IV or orally for 21 days	Preferred treatment: Desensitization available for patients with sulfa allergy Adjust dose in renal insufficiency
Alternative Therapies		
Pentamidine	4 mg/kg IV daily for 21 days	Similar efficacy to TMP-SMX but greater toxicity (nephrotoxicity, pancreatitis, glucose dysregulation, cardiac arrhythmias) Reserved for patients with severe disease who require IV therapy
Dapsone + trimethoprim	Dapsone* 100 mg orally daily plus trimethoprim 15 mg/kg orally (3 divided doses) daily for 21 days	Appropriate for mild to moderate disease
Clindamycin + primaquine	Clindamycin 600–900 mg IV every 6–8 hr (or 300–450 mg orally every 6–8 hr) plus primaquine* base 15–30 mg orally once daily for 21 days	Appropriate for mild to moderate disease
Atovaquone	750 mg orally twice daily for 21 days	For mild to moderate PCP only; not as potent as TMP-SMX
Trimetrexate (+ leucovorin)	Trimetrexate 45 mg/m^2 (or 1.2 mg/kg) IV daily plus leucovorin 25 mg orally every 6 hr for 21 days	Not as potent as TMP-SMX. Leucovorin must be continued for 3 days beyond completion of trimetrexate

*Confirm G6PD status prior to use when appropriate.
G6PD, glucose-6-phosphate dehydrogenase; IV, intravenously; PCP, *Pneumocystis carinii* (former name of *P. jiroveci*) pneumonia; TMP-SMX, trimethoprim-sulfamethoxazole.
From Centers for Disease Control and Prevention: Guidelines for prevention and treatment of opportunistic infections in HIV-infected adults and adolescents. Recommended from CDC, the National Institutes of Health, and the HIV Medicine Association of the Infectious Diseases Society of America. *MMWR Morb Mortal Wkly Rep.* 58, 2009. Available at: www.cdc.gov/mmwr/pdf/rr/rr5804.pdf.

Rash, fever, or leukopenia may occur in as many as 30–40% of patients.
Intravenous (IV) pentamidine
- Progressive renal insufficiency
- Pancreatitis
- Hypoglycemia or hyperglycemia
- Nausea
- Taste disturbances
- Cardiac arrhythmias
- Hypocalcemia

Atovaquone
- Rash (rare)
- Nausea

53. List the indications for primary PCP prophylaxis.
- CD^{4+} count < 200/mm^3 or < 14% of total lymphocytes
- Oral candidiasis
- Immunosuppressive agents such as organ transplant agents
  The use of PCP prophylaxis after the initial episode of PCP is considered secondary prophylaxis.

54. What drugs are used for PCP prophylaxis?

TMP-SMX (one double-strength daily) remains the drug of choice for prophylaxis but may be given as a single strength dose or three times a week. Alternatives include dapsone, atovaquone, and aerosolized pentamidine, but all efforts should be made, including desensitization, to allow use of TMP-SMX (Table 13.5).

Table 13.5. Regimens for *Pneumocystis jiroveci* Pneumonia Prophylaxis

TMP-SMX

- TMP 160 mg, SMX 800 mg daily (one DS tablet)
- Side effects similar to but less common than with primary PCP treatment
- Decreasing dose by 50% (1 DS tablet three times/wk or single-strength daily) may limit side effects while preserving efficacy
- Also provides prophylaxis against CNS toxoplasmosis

Dapsone (+ Pyrimethamine)

- 100 mg/day or 50 mg twice daily
- Provides prophylaxis against toxoplasmosis with addition of pyrimethamine

Aerosolized Pentamidine

- 300 mg once monthly via nebulizer
- Transient taste alterations and coughing or wheezing (can be minimized by pretreatment with inhaled bronchodilators)
- Evaluate patients for active TB before starting therapy—administer in negative pressure room or booth

Atovaquone

- 1500 mg/day
- Gastrointestinal discomfort is main adverse event
- Also covers toxoplasmosis

CNS, central nervous system; DS, double-strength; PCP, *Pneumocystis carinii* (former name of *P. jiroveci*) pneumonia; TB, tuberculosis; TMP-SMX, trimethoprim-sulfamethoxazole.

Centers for Disease Control and Prevention. Guidelines for prevention and treatment of opportunistic infections in HIV-infected adults and adolescents. Recommended from CDC, the National Institutes of Health, and the HIV Medicine Association of the Infectious Diseases Society of America. *MMWR Morb Mortal Wkly Rep.* 2009;58:1–198. Available at: www.cdc.gov/mmwr/preview/mmwrhtml/rr5804a1.htm [accessed 05.09.16].

55. Describe the relationship between HIV and TB.

In 1986, the number of new TB cases increased for the first time since nationwide reporting was initiated in 1953, concurrent with the beginning of widespread HIV infection. Until the mid-1980s, there had been a steady and rapid decline in the morbidity and mortality rates attributed to TB. HIV patients are highly susceptible to primary TB, and there is a high rate of progression from latent to active TB in HIV patients with preexisting latent TB. In fact, approximately 30% of TB patients have HIV.

56. How is this relationship explained?

Control of TB depends on cell-mediated immunity which is profoundly affected in HIV infection. The incidence of TB in an HIV-infected population can be expected to mirror that population's previous exposure to *Mycobacterium tuberculosis* (MTb). Immigrants, inner-city minorities, and IV drug users, groups with a high prevalence of both HIV and previous TB infection, will develop a high number of active TB cases unless prophylaxis is used. HIV strongly promotes the development of active TB from latent infection. With HIV infection, a person with latent TB is at a 5–9% risk per year of developing active disease compared with an HIV-negative person who carries a lifetime risk of 5%.

Shafer RW, Edlin BR. Tuberculosis in patients infected with human immunodeficiency virus: perspective on the past decade. *Clin Infect Dis.* 1996;22:683–704.

57. Does TB differ in presentation in HIV-infected patients?

Yes. Although the common pulmonary symptoms of TB (cough, hemoptysis, fever, and weight loss) may be present in HIV patients, the incidence of extrapulmonary disease is much higher with frequent miliary and disseminated disease. Progressive fevers and wasting are common presenting symptoms. Cough for > 3 weeks or fever after antibiotic therapy for bronchitis in an HIV-infected patient should be considered TB until proved otherwise. Atypical or less common TB presentations are much more frequent in HIV patients, especially those with poor immunity (CD4 count < 200 cells/mL). Radiographically, TB may atypically present with lower lobe disease (as opposed to upper lobe disease) in individuals with CD4 < 200/mL.

58. **How is the diagnosis of pulmonary TB made in an HIV-infected patient?**
Four symptoms describe pulmonary TB:
- Cough with or without hemoptysis
- Fever
- Night sweats
- Weight loss
Radiograph appearance is variable, but mediastinal adenopathy is highly suggestive of pulmonary TB. Clinical suspicion alone may warrant therapy whereas the sputum cultures are held in the microbiology laboratory for 8–12 weeks before final reporting. Induced sputum collection for acid-fast bacilli (AFB) smear and culture × 3 are suggested. Mycobacterial DNA probing (*M. tuberculosis* direct [MTD] test) can be useful to detect organisms at a lower load.

59. **Describe the treatment of TB in an HIV-infected patient.**
Multiple drugs given for 2 months, including:
- Isoniazid (INH) 300 mg/day with vitamin B_6 (to prevent neuropathy)
- A rifamycin (such as rifabutin with less potential interaction with ARTs than rifampin)
- Pyrazinamide (PZA) 15–30 mg/kg/day
- Ethambutol 15–25 mg/kg/day.
This regimen is then followed by 4 months of INH and a rifamycin. Directly observed therapy (DOT, or observation of the patient actually swallowing pills) with a health care provider or responsible person is preferred. Sometimes, medications can be given two or three times a week for DOT or DOT is provided only Monday through Friday. Treatment is extended beyond 6 months if cultures are still positive after the initial 2 months of therapy. TB is a curable infection in HIV patients. The recommended treatment is currently similar for both HIV-infected and non–HIV-infected patients.

KEY POINTS: TUBERCULOSIS AND HUMAN IMMUNODEFICIENCY VIRUS

1. All TB patients need to be tested for HIV infection.
2. All HIV patients without prior history of TB need to have the tuberculin skin test (PPD) or a blood test measuring IFN-γ.
3. PPD induration of 5 mm in HIV is positive, and treatment for LTBI should be strongly considered.
4. Risk of TB reactivation from LTBI is higher than the risk of significant toxicity from treatment.
5. Rifamycins such as rifampin have drug interactions with many ARTs. Therefore, use of rifabutin, a less potent CYP450 inducer, is preferable.
6. IRIS is common in TB and can paradoxically present as a clinical worsening despite appropriate therapy.

ARTs, antiretroviral therapies; CYP450, cytochrome P-450; HIV, human immunodeficiency virus; IFN-γ, interferon-γ; IRIS, immune reconstitution inflammatory syndrome; LTBI, latent tuberculosis infection; PPD, purified protein derivative; TB, tuberculosis.

60. **Is tuberculin skin testing (TST) with purified protein derivative (PPD) of any use in HIV-infected patients?**
Yes. TST may be helpful, but a negative PPD TST result does not rule out TB exposure or infection. The accuracy of TST depends on the prevalence of underlying TB infection in the screened population and the degree of immunosuppression present in the screened patient. About half of active TB cases are secondary to reactivation, and, therefore, treatment of latent TB infection (LTBI) would significantly reduce new outbreaks of active tubercular disease. TST is recommended in all patients diagnosed with HIV infection. Patients with a reaction > 5 mm should receive INH prophylaxis

for 9 months, regardless of age at the time of diagnosis. Anergy is common, so patients with a documented exposure to TB should be given INH prophylaxis even when the TST is negative. An interferon-releasing assay (known as *QuantiFERON test*), which detects the release of interferon-γ (IFN-γ) in response to MTb peptides is a newer technology available to screen for LTBI. Although commercially available, the clinical use of these assays is still under review, and they likely will be used in combination with TST to improve specificity and sensitivity. These assays also have high false-negative rates in immunodeficient patients.

61. Define *immune reconstitution inflammatory syndrome* (IRIS).
    Inflammation related to a "rebooted" immune system that may occur with initiation of HAART treatment and commonly reported in patients with a poor immune status before initiating ART. Patients with TB may develop similar symptoms when antituberculosis therapy is started. The IRIS results in symptomatic inflammatory responses to subclinical opportunistic infections present in the patient. The most common findings are lymphadenitis due to *Mycobacterium avium* complex (MAC), paradoxical reactions of TB (fever, malaise, weight loss, worsening of chest x-ray finding), and exacerbations of cryptococcal meningitis or cytomegalovirus (CMV) retinitis. In severe cases, steroid therapy is temporarily given to diminish the inflammation but is administered cautiously.
    Shelburne SA, Hamill RJ. The immune reconstitution inflammatory syndrome. *AIDS Rev.* 2003;5:67–79.

62. What other mycobacterial infections in addition to MTb are seen in HIV-infected patients?
    MAC and *Mycobacterium kansasii*. MAC may have a prevalence of 50% in autopsy findings of death from AIDS, and clinical studies have shown an annual risk of ~20% in patients with AIDS.
    Nightingale SD, Bird TL, Southern PM, et al. Incidence of *M. avium*–intracellulare complex bacteremia in human immunodeficiency virus-positive patients. *J Infect Dis.* 1992;165:1082–1085.

63. What are the symptoms and laboratory findings of MAC infection?
    - Fever
    - Night sweats
    - Weight loss
    - Fatigue
    - Malaise
    - Diarrhea (may be chronic with resulting malabsorption)
    - Abdominal pain
    - Anemia
    - Elevated liver function tests
    - CD4 cell count < 50/mL

64. Describe the standard therapy for MAC in patients with AIDS.
    At least two oral medications with good activity against MAC. One of these agents should be either azithromycin (500 mg/day) or clarithromycin (500 mg twice daily). The second drug is usually ethambutol (15 mg/kg/day). Other active agents include rifabutin (300 mg/day) and ciprofloxacin (750 mg twice daily). When AFB are initially seen in a specimen and not yet identified, therapy for both MTb and MAC is given with a regimen of RIPE (rifampin or rifabutin, INH, pyrazanimide, ethambutol) + azithromycin.
    Centers for Disease Control and Prevention. Guidelines for prevention and treatment of opportunistic infections in HIV-infected adults and adolescents. Recommended from CDC, the National Institutes of Health, and the HIV Medicine Association of the Infectious Diseases Society of America. *MMWR Morb Mortal Wkly Rep.* 2009;58:1–198. Available at: www.cdc.gov/mmwr/preview/mmwrhtml/rr5804a1.htm.

65. Which drugs are used as prophylaxis against MAC?
    Rifabutin, clarithromycin, and azithromycin. Primary prophylaxis is initiated when the CD4 cell count reaches < 50/mL. Because of ease of dosing and lack of drug interactions, most practitioners use azithromycin (1200 mg once/week). Rifabutin may cause cross-resistance to rifampin in a patient with MTb who is inadequately evaluated and then treated with this single drug inadvertently.

SYPHILIS

66. **Which HIV-infected patients should have a serologic test for syphilis (STS)?**
Every HIV-infected patient. In addition, a detailed history for all STDs and past treatments should be obtained. Most literature in the pre-HAART era suggested an accelerated course and unusual progression of syphilis in patients also infected with HIV. Transmission routes for HIV and syphilis are similar and both infections are likely to be transmitted simultaneously. Patients with a positive serologic test for one infection should be tested for the other. If the initial HIV test is negative in a patient with primary syphilis, a second test should be done in 3 months to evaluate for the possibility of early HIV infection with the absence of antibodies at the initial visit.

67. **Which HIV-infected patients with syphilis need a lumbar puncture (LP)?**
Those with syphilis of > 1 year's duration or with any clinical signs or symptoms of CNS involvement. Although a few authorities recommend an LP in all HIV-infected patients with syphilis, most agree that those with a clear episode of adequately treated primary or secondary syphilis do not need an LP. Patients with early syphilis whose serologic titers increase or fail to decrease fourfold in 6 months also should undergo an LP to evaluate for CNS involvement with syphilis before re-treatment. A prospective study of 231 HIV-infected individuals with newly diagnosed syphilis found that risk factors for developing neurosyphilis included a CD4 count of < 350 cells/mL, an RPR titer > 1:128, and male gender.
Ghanem KG, Moore RD, Rompalo AM, et al. Neurosyphilis in a clinical cohort of HIV-1-infected patients. *AIDS*. 2008;22(10):1145–1451.

68. **What is the treatment for neurosyphilis in HIV-infected patients?**
Aqueous crystalline penicillin G, 3–4 million units (mU) IV every 4 hours (18–24 mU/day) for 10–14 days. Patients with penicillin allergy should undergo desensitization in order to allow appropriate treatment with penicillin.

69. **If a chancre is present, is initial therapy for syphilis changed?**
No. The recommended regimen remains one dose of benzathine penicillin G, 2.4 mU intramuscularly (IM), but many authorities treat primary syphilis more aggressively in patients coinfected with HIV and administer a total of 7.2 mU (2.4 mU benzathine penicillin G IM weekly for 3 consecutive weeks).

70. **How should patients with HIV infection and primary syphilis be followed?**
With repeat STS at 1, 3, 6, and 12 months. If at any time there is a fourfold increase in titer, an LP should be done. If by 6 months, the titer has not decreased fourfold, an LP should be done to evaluate the cerebrospinal fluid (CSF) for CNS syphilis.

CNS DISORDERS AND INFECTIONS

71. **What is the most common cause of meningitis in AIDS patients?**
Cryptococcus neoformans. Although only 5–10% of AIDS patients present with cryptococcal infection, up to 15% are subsequently found to have infection.

72. **How does cryptococcal infection present?**
See Table 13.6.

73. **What findings in a patient with suspected cryptococcal infection suggests the need for an urgent LP?**
- Undiagnosed fever and headache with CD4 count < 100 cells/mL
- Altered mental status, lethargy, psychosis, and vomiting (symptoms of increased intracranial pressure) with CD4 count < 100 cells/mL
- Positive serum cryptococcal antigen (CrAg) or blood culture positive for cryptococcus
Repeat LPs should be performed in patients in whom the initial opening pressure was elevated (>25 cm H_2O), sometimes as often as daily, to relieve increased intracranial pressure and prevent neurologic damage. LP should also be repeated after 2 weeks of therapy to help evaluate microbial response.

74. **What CSF findings are seen in cryptococcal meningitis?**
- Elevated total protein
- Mild white blood cell (WBC) elevation

Table 13.6. Frequency of Signs and Symptoms of Cryptococcal Meningitis

SIGNS AND SYMPTOMS	FREQUENCY (%)
Symptoms	
Malaise	76
Headache	73
Fever	65
Nausea or vomiting or both	42
Cough or dyspnea or both	31
Stiff neck	22
Diarrhea	21
Photophobia	18
Reported symptomatic focal neurological deficits	5
Seizures	4
Signs	
Fever	56
Meningeal signs	27
Altered mentation	17
Focal deficit on neurologic examination	15

Adapted from Chuck SL, Sande MA. Infections with *Cryptococcus neoformans* in acquired immunodeficiency syndrome. *N Engl J Med.* 1989;321:794–799.

- Low glucose
- Positive India ink preparation
- Positive CrAg
- Positive fungal culture
  CSF findings may also be relatively normal.

75. **What treatment is recommended for cryptococcosis in AIDS?**
    IV amphotericin B, or its liposomal preparations, and oral flucytosine for 14 days, followed by oral fluconazole at a dose of 400 mg/day for 8 weeks for consolidation therapy. Maintenance therapy at a dose of 200 mg/day is continued lifelong. In complicated disease or in the presence of high CrAg titers, treatment with IV amphotericin B may be extended beyond 14 days and oral doses of fluconazole increased.

76. **Are serum CrAg levels good indicators of response to therapy?**
    No. Although the serum antigen test can be very helpful in the diagnosis of cryptococcal infection, it cannot be used to judge therapeutic response. In most cases of meningitis, the CSF antigen titer should be determined by repeat LP. If the serum titer does revert to very low titer or is negative after therapy, an increasing titer in the future should raise concern about a relapse. High serum CrAg titers suggest a poorer prognosis. CSF fungal cultures should also be obtained after 2 weeks of induction antifungal therapy to confirm sterilization of the CSF, even in individuals who are improved clinically.

77. **What is progressive multifocal leukoencephalopathy (PML)?**
    A CNS demyelinating disease resulting from infection with a prion, Jakob-Creutzfeldt (JC) virus. Although spread throughout the population, JC virus requires profound immunosuppression to cause disease; in HIV, the CD4 count is typically < 50 cells/mL. Any part of the CNS can be involved, and, therefore, patients often present with cognitive decline, ataxia, aphasia, and other focal motor weaknesses. As the name implies, lesions are multifocal and result in focal neurologic defects. Diagnosis is based on clinical findings, classic findings on magnetic resonance imaging (MRI) of T2 flair, and positive CSF JC virus polymerase chain reaction (PCR). Although there is no specific treatment for PML, HAART is indicated.

78. **What are HIV-associated neurocognitive disorders (HAND)?**
    HAND is an umbrella term used to describe various cognitive, behavioral, and motor dysfunction associated with HIV infection. The range of these deficits is typically defined by abnormal performance on standardized neuropsychological testing. If there are no symptoms or

impairment, but poor performance on standardized testing, then an individual is described as having asymptomatic neurocognitive impairment (ANI). Individuals who progress with mild deficits along with minor symptoms or impairment are described as having mild neurocognitive disorder (MND). HIV-associated dementia refers to severe neurocognitive deficits that lead to substantial functional impairment. HAND is believed to be caused by direct CNS infection by HIV, and a diagnosis can be made after ruling out other opportunistic infections (e.g., cryptococcosis, toxoplasmosis, and TB). Patients may first complain of mild cognitive dysfunction including difficulties with memory, concentration, or focus. Family and friends may also note personality changes. Treatment should focus on using HAART therapy with good CSF penetration.

79. **What are the most common causes of CNS mass lesions in AIDS?**
Cerebral toxoplasmosis and primary CNS lymphoma. Other causes include PML, cryptococcomas, tuberculomas, bacterial and fungal abscesses, and metastatic disease such as lung and breast cancer.

80. **What computed tomography (CT) scan findings differentiate CNS toxoplasmosis from lymphoma?**
See Table 13.7. Centers with access to single-photon emission CT (SPECT) scanning can identify likely lymphoma when an increased signal ratio is demonstrated.

Table 13.7. Brain Computed Tomography (CT) Findings in Central Nervous System Toxoplasmosis and Lymphoma

CT FINDING	TOXOPLASMOSIS	LYMPHOMA
Area involved	Deep gray matter and basal ganglia	White matter, periventricular areas
Mass effect	Yes	Yes
Enhancement	Ring enhancement	Weakly, not ring-shaped
Number of lesions	Multiple	1–2

81. **How is CNS toxoplasmosis treated?**
Most clinicians recommend treatment for a presumptive diagnosis of toxoplasmosis with pyrimethamine, 200-mg loading dose, then 75 mg/day; sulfadiazine, 4–6 g/day in divided doses; and folinic acid, 10–25 mg/day. CNS toxoplasmosis usually readily responds to this treatment with rapid improvement on CT or MRI within 3–5 days. If no response is seen within 10–14 days, another cause should be investigated via stereotactic brain biopsy of a lesion.

82. **Should primary toxoplasmosis prophylaxis be given?**
Yes. Patients positive for *Toxoplasma* antibodies who also have a CD4+ count < 100 cells/mL but no symptoms of toxoplasmosis should receive primary prophylaxis. Oral TMP-SMX 160/800 mg is the preferred daily regimen, providing protection against both PCP and toxoplasmosis. If this regimen is not tolerated, oral dapsone-pyrimethamine or atovaquone can be given.
    Centers for Disease Control and Prevention. Guidelines for prevention and treatment of opportunistic infections in HIV-infected adults and adolescents. Recommended from CDC, the National Institutes of Health, and the HIV Medicine Association of the Infectious Diseases Society of America. *MMWR Morb Mortal Wkly Rep.* 2009;58:1–198. Available at: www.cdc.gov/mmwr/preview/mmwrhtml/rr5804a1.htm.

HEPATITIS B AND C VIRAL INFECTIONS

83. **What are the best treatment combinations for hepatitis B virus (HBV) and HIV infections?**
Tenofovir with emtricitabine or lamivudine. Much like treatment of HIV, monodrug therapy for the treatment of HBV has been associated with development of hepatitis B resistance including the YMDD mutation, occurring in ~13% of patients after 1 year. For this reason, HBV therapy should include more than one active agent. Another combination would be entecavir with one of the

following: lamivudine or emtricitabine or tenofovir. If lamivudine is withdrawn from an HIV treatment regimen, hepatitis may flare if there is a coinfection with HBV. Successful therapy is often marked by immunoconversion with development of a surface antibody (HBsAb). The HBV DNA level is a prognostic marker for the risk for hepatocellular carcinoma and cirrhosis.

Centers for Disease Control and Prevention. Guidelines for prevention and treatment of opportunistic infections in HIV-infected adults and adolescents. Recommended from CDC, the National Institutes of Health, and the HIV Medicine Association of the Infectious Diseases Society of America. *MMWR Morb Mortal Wkly Rep.* 2009;58:1–198. Available at: www.cdc.gov/mmwr/preview/mmwrhtml/rr5804a1.htm.

84. **Is there an interaction between HIV and hepatitis C virus (HCV) infections?**
Probably. Most studies have shown a more rapid course of HCV infection in the HIV-infected patient, but some studies have not. The positive studies have shown an increased percentage of patients developing cirrhosis and a shorter time from infection to cirrhosis. Patients coinfected with HIV and HCV have an increased risk for liver disease–related death.

85. **How common is HIV/HCV coinfection?**
Very common. Many HIV clinics have reported coinfection rates in the range of 15–30%.

86. **What are the best treatments currently available for HCV infection in the presence of HIV infection?**
The management of HCV in HIV-coinfected patients has been rapidly evolving. Recent data suggest that HIV/HCV-coinfected patients can now be treated with all-oral regimens. In the past, patients were treated with combination injectable peginterferon and oral ribavirin therapy. Now, there are many oral direct-acting antiviral (DAA) agents that target the HCV replication cycle and have been shown to achieve high sustained virologic response (SVR) rates compared to previous drugs. The first-generation DAA agents that were approved for HCV infection were the HCV PIs boceprevir and telaprevir. However, these DAAs still were often used in combination with peginterferon and ribavirin, thus leading to issues of high pill burden, increased dosing frequency, and side effects. The first-generation DAA agents have now been replaced by newer combination regimens that do not require peginterferon and ribavirin. The currently Food and Drug Administration (FDA)-approved second-generation DAA agents include daclatasvir, grazoprevir/elbasvir, ledipasvir, ledipasvir/sofosbuvir, paritaprevir/ritonavir/ombitasvir + dasabuvir, simeprevir, and sofosbuvir. In addition, the duration of HCV treatment has been significantly shortened. Most individuals can be treated for HCV infection with these newer DAAs for 12 weeks and achieve SVR. The selection of DAAs and length of therapy still depend on the HCV genotype. Some DAAs also have drug-drug interactions with HIV ART and may require alteration of HIV ART prior to initiation of HCV treatment.

AIDSInfo: Guidelines for the use of antiretroviral agents in HIV-1-infected adults and adolescents. Available at: https://aidsinfo.nih.gov/contentfiles/lvguidelines/adultandadolescentgl.pdf.

87. **What factors are associated with poorer response to HCV therapy in patients coinfected with HIV?**
- Low CD4 cell counts
- HCV genotype 1
- HCV viral load > 800,000 IU/mL
- Presence of cirrhosis
- Active alcohol use

88. **What is the major toxicity of ribavirin (RBV)?**
Hemolytic anemia that is dose-dependent. In the AIDS Pegasys Ribavirin International Coinfection Trial (APRICOT) of pegylated IFN-α plus RBV and a randomized controlled trial of Pegylated-Interferon-alfa-2b plus Ribavirin vs. Interferon-alfa-2b plus Ribavirin for the Initial Treatment of Chronic Hepatitis C in HIV Co-infected Patients (RIBAVIC) trial, 10–16% of patients required dose reductions in RBV because of anemia. Decreasing the dose of RBV has been associated with higher rates of virologic failure.

Chung RT, Andersen J, Volberding P, et al. Peginterferon alfa-2a plus ribavirin versus interferon alfa-2a plus ribavirin for chronic hepatitis C in HIV-coinfected persons. *N Engl J Med.* 2004;351:2340–2341.

Torriani FJ, Rodriguez-Torres M, Rockstroh JK, et al. Peginterferon alfa-2a plus ribavirin for chronic hepatitis C virus infection in HIV-infected patients. *N Engl J Med.* 2004;351:438–450.

89. **What are the potential interactions between RBV and antiretroviral medications?**
    RBV interacts with didanosine, zidovudine, and abacavir. Didanosine is absolutely contraindicated for patients taking ribavirin. Ribavirin increases didanosine phosphorylation and increases risk for mitochondrial toxicity leading to lactic acidosis, hepatic decompensation, and death. RBV decreases zidovudine phosphorylation, leading to impaired HIV control. RBV and abacavir share common phosphorylation pathways (guanosine analogs), which can lead to decreased response to HCV therapy.

DERMATOLOGIC DISORDERS

90. **How would you describe Kaposi sarcoma (KS)?**
    Thickened and edematous woody skin with erythematous purple nodules and plaques. Retention hyperkeratosis can look warty in appearance with surrounding purple color or erythema. Bacillary angiomatosis from *Bartonella henselae* can mimic KS. The human herpesvirus-8 (HHV-8) is the cause of KS, which occurs as a result of abnormal T-cell responses. ART is the backbone of treatment of limited infection. Biopsy-proven disease will usually be required in order to institute chemotherapy. Lymphedema is a sign of systemic involvement. In this instance, ART may not be adequate and liposomal doxorubicin will likely be required for treatment. Facial lesions may be treated with vincristine by injection or radiation therapy. Hemoptysis and hematochezia may indicate that patients will likely require chemotherapy.

91. **What skin conditions can be a marker of a low immune system?**
    - Prurigo nodularis (generally with CD4 count < 100 cells/mL)
    - Molluscum contagiosum
    - Cryptococcal infection
    - KS

92. **What is the appearance of toxic epidermal necrolysis?**
    Triangular blisters that represent shearing of the skin due to the separation of the epidermis from the dermis. The disorder is usually drug-induced (trimethoprim, sulfa, and vancomycin). Dermatologic consultation and treatment with IV immunoglobulin (IVIG) are indicated. Toxic epidermal necrolysis is a life-threatening condition.

93. **What common ART has been described to cause skin eruptions?**
    NNRTI therapy such as efavirenz and nevirapine. These medications can cause erythema multiforme and in some cases, Stevens-Johnson syndrome. Once skin eruptions have occurred, do not rechallenge the patient with the offending drug. Abacavir has also been described to have allergic reaction with rash in 5–8% of patients, and patients with human leukocyte antigen (HLA)-B*5701 are most likely to show hypersensitivity reactions. The FDA now recommends that patients be screened with HLA-B5701 typing before the initiation of therapy when abacavir is prescribed.

RENAL DISORDERS

94. **What is HIVAN?**
    HIV-associated nephropathy. Case reports of HIVAN were first described in 1984 as a rapidly progressive form of focal segmental glomerulosclerosis (FSGS). What differentiates HIVAN from other forms of FSGS is the hallmark finding of a collapsing glomerulonephropathy and the presence of microcystic tubular dilatation and interstitial inflammation. HIVAN primarily affects blacks of African descent, although other HIV-infected patients with low CD4 counts (<200 cells/mL) and high HIV viral load (>4000 copies/mL) are at risk for developing HIVAN.

95. **How does HIVAN present, and how is it diagnosed?**
    HIVAN presents as proteinuria with either normal or abnormal glomerular filtration rate (GFR). There are recent reports of HIVAN presenting with microalbuminuria, but all of these reports are in uncontrolled HIV infection with low CD4 cell counts and high HIV viral load. HIVAN is diagnosed by renal biopsy. The following clinical findings are suggestive of HIVAN: nephrotic range proteinuria, abnormal renal function for > 3 months (estimated GFR [eGFR] < 60 mL/min), echogenic normal size or large unobstructed kidneys, and absence of diabetes mellitus, hypertension, pregnancy, collagen vascular disease, cirrhosis, or organ transplant.

96. **How is HIVAN managed?**

With HAART. Since December 2007, the diagnosis of HIVAN by renal biopsy is an AIDS-defining illness; therefore, the initial treatment includes HAART. As in other proteinuric renal disease, angiotensin-converting enzyme (ACE) inhibitors and angiotensin receptor blockers may be beneficial. The adjunctive use of corticosteroids has not been proved, but small uncontrolled studies have suggested some benefit with regards to decreasing proteinuria and improving the clinical course of HIVAN. If chronic kidney disease stage 3 or worse has developed at the time of diagnosis, it is very likely that HIVAN will progress to end-stage renal disease (ESRD) rapidly. HIV-infected patients with ESRD will benefit from dialysis support. Renal transplant should be considered as long as the HIV infection is well controlled. Although most reports show that acute rejection in the first year after renal transplant is higher in patients with HIV infection, the overall survival after the first year is almost equal to that in non–HIV-infected patients.

97. **Which HAART medications need to be adjusted based on eGFR?**

All NRTIs except abacavir.

98. **How does tenofovir nephrotoxicity present?**

With proximal tubular acidosis (renal tubular acidosis type 2) and global proximal tubular dysfunction, also known as *Fanconi syndrome*. Fanconi syndrome can manifest as non–anion-gap metabolic acidosis, hypophosphatemia, hypokalemia, glucosuria, aminoaciduria, and proteinuria. Tenofovir has also been associated with acute tubular necrosis.

MISCELLANEOUS DISORDERS

99. **What is thrush?**

Oropharyngeal pseudomembranous candidiasis, which often presages AIDS. Thrush usually presents as white plaques called *pseudomembranes* on areas of less friction such as under the tongue and the posterior buccal wall. The lesions from *Candida albicans* easily rub off, leaving a red base. Fluconazole is the treatment of choice. Resistant forms of thrush (*Candida glabrata*) require non–azole-based therapy, such as echinocandins and amphotericin B. Thrush can be confused with oral hairy leukoplakia, a whitish corrugated growth along the margins of the tongue found in HIV-infected patients and caused by the Epstein-Barr virus (EBV).

100. **Explain the significance of thrush.**

Thrush often indicates significant immunosuppression and, if found during an initial examination, suggests the need for HIV-related medical interventions for prophylaxis of opportunistic infections regardless of CD4 cell count. If the patient is not known to be HIV-infected, the diagnosis of thrush warrants HIV testing.

101. **What is the most common cause of blindness in AIDS?**

CMV infection leading to chorioretinitis. Although formerly experienced by 5–10% of patients with AIDS during the course of their illness, the incidence of this AIDS-defining diagnosis has declined dramatically during the era of more effective ART.

102. **How is CMV retinitis diagnosed?**

By funduscopic examination. Retinal examination usually reveals large white granular areas with hemorrhage (described as "cottage cheese in ketchup") with CMV retinitis. Symptoms may include blurred vision, decreased visual acuity, increasing "floaters," or a clear visual field cut. All patients with advanced HIV infection (CD4 counts < 100 cells/mL) should undergo routine retinal screening on a quarterly basis.

103. **In addition to chorioretinitis, what are the other manifestations of CMV infection in HIV infection?**
   - Interstitial pneumonia
   - Colitis
   - Esophagitis
   - Adrenal insufficiency
   - Encephalitis

104. **Define HIV wasting syndrome.**

Weight loss of > 10% of body weight with either chronic diarrhea or weakness and fever for > 30 days. HIV wasting syndrome is an AIDS-defining diagnosis. One should always evaluate a patient with suspected HIV wasting syndrome for other HIV-related causes of chronic diarrhea, weakness, and fever, but in the absence of other secondary causes, a diagnosis of HIV wasting syndrome can be made.

105. **In addition to KS and non-Hodgkin lymphoma, what other malignancies are seen in HIV infection?**

See Table 13.8.

Table 13.8. Malignancies Associated With Human Immunodeficiency Virus and Changes in Incidence Since 1998

MALIGNANCY	INCIDENCE CHANGE
Kaposi sarcoma	↓
Central nervous system lymphoma	↓
Lymphoma (non-Hodgkin)	↑
Lymphoma (Hodgkin disease)	↑
Cervical cancer	↑
Anal cancer	↑
Lung cancer	↑
Prostate	↔
Breast	↔
Hepatoma	↔

From Patel P, Hanson DL, Sullivan PS, et al. Incidence of types of cancer among HIV-infected persons compared with the general population in the United States, 1992–2003. *Ann Intern Med.* 2008;148:728–736.

106. **How often does HIV infection result in anemia or thrombocytopenia?**

Frequently, in untreated patients. Anemia occurs in up to 80%, neutropenia in 85%, and thrombocytopenia in 65% of cases. HIV-infected but asymptomatic patients are much less frequently cytopenic. Clinically significant thrombocytopenia indistinguishable from that seen in idiopathic thrombocytopenic purpura (ITP) may be a presentation of HIV infection. Typically, bone marrow is normal with adequate numbers of megakaryocytes. The disorder behaves much like classic ITP in that patients respond to steroids and splenectomy. An HIV antibody test is recommended in patients presenting with ITP. Of interest is the recent recognition of thrombotic thrombocytopenic purpura in association with HIV infection.

107. **What metabolic complications are associated with HIV treatments?**
- **Alterations in glucose metabolism:** insulin resistance, glucose intolerance, diabetes mellitus
- **Hyperlipidemia:** hypercholesterolemia, hypertriglyceridemia
- **Hyperlactatemia** and **lactic acidosis**
- **Fat redistribution:** visceral fat accumulation, subcutaneous fat atrophy
- **Osteoporosis**

108. **Describe the sensory neuropathy seen in HIV.**

Many patients with HIV experience a distal sensory polyneuropathy that may be due to HIV infection or HIV treatment with certain neurotoxic nucleoside analogs such as zalcitabine, didanosine, and stavudine. Patients present with paresthesias, numbness, or pain in the distal extremities. Symptoms are symmetrical and move proximally with progression. The temporal relationship of symptoms to initiation of medication is the only way to implicate a drug side effect as the cause of the neuropathy. HIV-related neuropathy often responds to effective anti-HIV therapy, but this response is not uniform and can be delayed.

109. **How are rheumatologic studies affected by HIV infection?**

Patients with HIV make increased nonspecific antibodies, resulting in both an increased frequency of autoimmune disorders as well as an increased number of false-positive antibody based tests. Laboratory evaluations often reveal low titers of rheumatoid factor (RF), antinuclear antibodies (ANAs), and anticardiolipin antibodies. Generalized hypergammaglobulinemia is also seen, as are elevated creatine kinase (CK) levels of uncertain significance.

Mody GM, Parke FA, Reveille JD. Articular manifestations of human immunodeficiency virus infection. *Best Prac Res Clin Rheum.* 2003;17:580–591.

PRIMARY CARE OF HIV-INFECTED PATIENTS

110. **What vaccines are recommended in HIV-infected patients?**
     - Hepatitis A, one complete series of two doses
     - Hepatitis B, one complete series of three doses
     - Pneumococcal conjugate vaccine–13 (PCV13) first, followed 12 months later by a dose of pneumococcal polysaccharide vaccine–23 (PPSV23) in individuals who have not previously received PCV13. In those individuals who have already received one or more doses of PPSV23, the dose of PCV13 should be given at least 1 year after the most recent dose of PSV23.
     - Inactivated influenza vaccine (intramuscular) annually
     - Tetanus toxoid, reduced diphtheria toxoid, and acellular pertussis vaccine (Tdap) as a single dose followed by tetanus diphtheria toxoid (Td) every 10 years
     - For men or women aged 13–26, human papillomavirus (HPV) vaccine, as a complete series of three doses

111. **What vaccines should be avoided in persons with HIV infection?**
     - Combined measles-mumps-rubella vaccine (MMR) or any of its individual components
     - Shingles vaccine (herpes zoster)
     - Oral typhoid vaccine
     - Smallpox vaccine

     These are all live or partially live vaccines and should not be given because of the risk for disseminated disease.

112. **How well do HIV-infected patients respond to the influenza vaccine?**
     Not as well as non–HIV-infected subjects, but administration of the influenza vaccine is indicated for all persons infected with HIV. CD4+ counts < 100 cells/mL are associated with poor antibody responses. Studies showing increased HIV viral load and decreased CD4+ counts in study participants receiving influenza vaccine compared with placebo-injected control subjects have raised concerns, but no adverse clinical events have been demonstrated.

     Tasker SA, O'Brien WA, Treanor JJ, et al. Effects of influenza vaccination in HIV-infected adults: A double-blind placebo-controlled trial. *Vaccine.* 1998;16:1039–1042.

113. **Do HIV-infected patients respond to the pneumococcal polysaccharide vaccine?**
     Partially. The response is impaired compared with normal control subjects. HIV-infected patients mount an adequate antibody response to fewer of the serotypes contained in the 23-valent vaccine, and this response rate decreases with decreasing CD4+ counts. As with influenza vaccination, there appears to be increased HIV viral activity after pneumococcal vaccination, but because morbidity due to pneumococcal disease is clearly and substantially increased in HIV-infected patients, the risk-to-benefit ratio supports vaccination.

     Moore D, Nelson M, Henderson D. Pneumococcal vaccination and HIV infection. *Int J STD AIDS.* 1999;9:1–7.

114. **Are there any travel restrictions for persons living with HIV?**
     Yes. In 1992, the International AIDS Conference moved outside the United States because of visa restrictions for persons with HIV who enter the United States at that time. In January 2010, all restrictions for entering or migrating to the United States for people with HIV infection were lifted. Country-specific information can be obtained at www.hivtravel.org.

Acknowledgment

The editor gratefully acknowledges contributions by Dr. Christopher J. Lahart, Dr. Amy Sitapati, Dr. Alfredo Tiu, and Dr. Joseph Caperna that were retained from the previous edition of *Medical Secrets.*

WEBSITES

1. The AIDS Education and Training Center (AETC): http://www.aids-ed.org
2. AIDSInfo: http://www.aidsinfo.nih.gov/Guidelines
3. The American Academy of HIV Medicine (AAHIVM): http://aahivm.org
4. HIV Medicine Association (HIVMA): http://www.hivma.org
5. International AIDS Society (IAS-USA): http://www.iasusa.org
6. Stanford HIV RT and Protease Sequence Database: http://hivdb.stanford.edu/hiv

BIBLIOGRAPHY

1. Bennett JE, Dolin R, Blaser MJ, eds. *Mandell, Douglas, and Bennett's Principles and Practice of Infectious Diseases.* 8th ed. Philadelphia: Saunders; 2014.
2. Sande MA, Volberding PA. *The Medical Management of AIDS.* 6th ed. Philadelphia: WB Saunders; 1999.

CHAPTER 14

HEMATOLOGY

Damian Silbermins, MD, and Ara Metjian, MD

HYPOPROLIFERATIVE ANEMIAS AND IRON METABOLISM

1. **What is the definition of anemia?**

   In practice, anemia is defined as a reduction in the hemoglobin (Hb) or hematocrit (Hct). The World Health Organization (WHO) definition is Hb < 13 g/dL (men) and < 12 g/dL (nonpregnant women). The appropriate threshold may depend on gender, race, and other medical conditions (such as chemotherapy).

   Beutler E, Waalen J. The definition of anemia: what is the lower limit of normal of the blood hemoglobin concentration? *Blood.* 2006;107:1747–1750.

2. **How are anemias classified?**

   According to cause: underproduction, destruction (hemolysis), or blood loss. In addition, anemia can be acute or chronic. Most anemias are chronic and allow the body time to compensate. A low reticulocyte count (young red blood cells [RBCs] that still have ribonucleic acid [RNA] in their cytoplasm) is pathognomonic of anemia of underproduction.

3. **How are mean cell volume (MCV) and red blood cell distribution width (RDW) used in the evaluation of anemias?**

   The RDW is an index of the heterogeneity of cell size. In iron deficiency anemia (IDA), RBCs have been produced during periods of iron sufficiency and varying degrees of deficiency; thus, cell size in IDA is more heterogeneous than in spherocytosis, in which all of the cells are small (Table 14.1).

Table 14.1. Classification of Anemias Based on Mean Cell Volume and Red Blood Cell Distribution Width*

RDW VALUES	MCV LOW	MCV NORMAL	MCV HIGH
RDW normal	Chronic disease Nonanemic heterozygous thalassemia	Normal Chronic disease Nonanemic or enzyme abnormality	Aplastic anemia
	Children	Splenectomy CLL (except extreme high-lymphocyte number) Acute blood loss	
RDW high	Iron deficiency	Early or mixed nutritional deficiency	Folate or vitamin B_{12} deficiency
	HbS–α- or β-thalassemia	Anemic abnormal hemoglobin	Sickle cell anemia (one third of cases)
		Myelofibrosis	Immune hemolytic anemia
		Sideroblastic anemia	Cold agglutinins
		Myelodysplasia	Preleukemia

*Chronic liver disease, chronic myelogenous leukemia, and cytotoxic chemotherapy may be associated with high or normal MCV and high or normal RDW.

CLL, chronic lymphocytic leukemia; HbS, hemoglobin S; MCV, mean cell volume; RDW, red blood cell distribution width.

From Bessman JD. *Automated Blood Counts and Differentials: A Practical Guide.* Baltimore: Johns Hopkins University Press; 1986, p 11.

4. Summarize the symptoms and signs of iron deficiency.

Symptoms include fatigue, dyspnea on exertion, and signs of congestive heart failure or angina if cardiac disease present. Patients may be fatigued even **before** the erythron synthesis is impaired, which can be ameliorated by prompt iron supplementation. **Pica,** or craving of nonfood items such as ice, starch, or even dirt, may occur in adults and is increased in iron deficiency. Other findings include **esophageal webs** (sometimes causing dysphagia), painless stomatitis, spooning of the fingernails (**koilonychia**), **beeturia** (red urine occurring from the ingestion of beets), and restless leg syndrome. The association of IDA, dysphagia, and esophageal webs is known as the *Plummer-Vinson syndrome.*

Allen RP, Auerbach S, Bahrain H. The prevalence and impact of restless legs syndrome on patients with iron deficiency anemia. *Am J Hematol.* 2013;88:261–264.

Anker SD, Colet JC, Filippatos G, et al. Ferric carboxymaltose in patients with heart failure and iron deficiency, *N Engl J Med.* 2009;361:2436–2448.

5. How is the diagnosis of IDA made? How does it differ from functional iron deficiency (FID)?

Multiple laboratory tests can suggest IDA. The gold standard is bone marrow biopsy, but this is rarely necessary, although biopsy can be useful if serum ferritin > 1200 µg/dL and IDA is suspected. Interobserver variability can be present for bone marrow biopsy interpretation and this method is not useful for diagnosis after replacement with parenteral iron therapy. A ferritin level < 30 µg/dL is diagnostic of iron deficiency, but relying only on this cut-off would miss milder forms of iron deficiency. Ferritin < 12 µg/dL indicates absent iron stores. Body iron stores < 8 mg/kg is diagnostic of iron deficiency and can be calculated as follows:

$$- [\log \; (\text{Soluble transferrin receptor/serum ferritin}) - 2.8229]/0.1207$$

FID is a state in which there is insufficient iron incorporation into erythroid precursors in the face of apparently normal iron stores. The percentage of hypochromic RBCs (% HRC) is the preferred method for identification of FID. HRC > 6% is consistent with FID. Reticulocyte Hb content (CHr) is the next option. CHr < 29 pg predicts FID in patients on erythropoiesis-stimulating agents (ESAs). A reticulocyte Hb equivalent (Ret-He) < 25 pg is suggestive of IDA. A Ret-He < 30.6 pg predicts response to intravenous (IV) iron in patients on hemodialysis.

Thomas DW, Hinchliffe RF, Briggs C, et al. Guideline for laboratory diagnosis of functional iron deficiency. *Br J Haematol.* 2013;61:639–648.

6. In the treatment of IDA, how much iron should be administered, in what form, and for how long?

Typically, patients take oral iron (each tablet about 60–70 mg elemental iron) three times/day on an empty stomach (180–200 mg/day). The benchmark for successful treatment is a 2 g/dL increase in Hb in 3 weeks. The major side effects are dyspepsia, constipation, and blackening of the stool. Only 10–15% of iron is absorbed this way and likely the nonabsorbed component is contributing to the side effects. The understanding of hepcidin metabolism has raised the question whether high oral iron doses upregulate hepcidin and prevent further absorption from subsequent doses. Hence an interesting alternative dose of **2 tablets (120–140 mg) on an empty stomach three times a week** might be as efficacious with fewer side effects. IV iron therapy can be used in patients undergoing renal dialysis to optimize the response to ESAs. Certain patients with ongoing blood loss (e.g., inflammatory bowel disease or Osler-Weber-Rendu syndrome) who cannot tolerate oral iron or cannot absorb enough iron from the gut (e.g., celiac disease) also benefit from IV iron replacement.

Moretti D, Goede JS, Zeder C, et al. Oral iron supplements increase hepcidin and decrease iron absorption from daily or twice-daily doses in iron-depleted young women. *Blood.* 2015;126:1981–1989.

7. Describe the major steps in iron absorption.

- Heme and elemental iron are absorbed in the diet. Heme iron requires gastric acidity to release it from its apoprotein.
- Ferric iron (Fe^{3+}) is transformed into ferrous iron (Fe^{2+}) by duodenal ferric reductase enzyme (duodenal cytochrome *b*, Dcytb), which allows DMT1 (divalent metal transporter) to transfer the Fe^{2+} into the enterocyte (mostly in duodenum).
- Iron is stored as ferritin inside the enterocyte.

- Fe^{2+} is converted back to Fe^{3+} by hephaestin and other enzymes to allow transportation out of the cell into circulation.
- Fe^{3+} is transported into the circulation by ferroportin. Only a limited amount of the iron goes into circulation. The remaining intracellular iron is lost with enterocyte shedding.

Fleming RE, Bacon BR. Orchestration of iron homeostasis. *N Engl J Med.* 2005;352:1741–1744.

8. **What is the role of hepcidin?**
To inhibit iron egress from the cells. Hepcidin is an acute phase reactant produced by the liver and filtered by the kidney that binds to ferroportin and causes internalization, ubiquitinization, and degradation of the transporter.

Hentze MW, Muckenthaler MU, Galy B, et al. Two to tango: regulation of mammalian iron metabolism. *Cell.* 2010;142:24–38.

9. **What causes iron overload?**
Chronic administration of iron to non–iron-deficient persons, chronic transfusion therapy, and disorders associated with increased absorption of dietary iron (hemochromatosis, thalassemia intermedia or major, and certain refractory anemias, such as sideroblastic anemia).

10. **List the consequences of iron overload.**
   - Cardiomyopathy and arrhythmias
   - Hepatic dysfunction and cirrhosis
   - Hepatoma
   - Endocrine dysfunction (hypothyroidism, hypogonadotrophic hypogonadism, hyperpigmentation, diabetes mellitus)
   - Arthropathy (chondrocalcinosis, synovial fluid containing calcium pyrophosphate or hydroxy-apatite crystals)
   - Osteopenia and subcortical cysts

   If the transferrin saturation is > 75%, the percentage of labile iron (non–transferrin-bound iron) increases significantly. This form of iron has a greater potential to cause end-organ damage.

11. **What test is frequently used to screen for hemochromatosis?**
Ferritin. A value > 300 ng/mL in males and > 200 ng/mL in females suggests hemochromatosis. Causes of increased ferritin not related to iron overload include alcoholism, metabolic syndrome, inflammatory conditions (usually with an elevated C-reactive protein [CRP]), and acute or chronic hepatitis. Other rare causes include macrophage activation syndrome (hemophagocytic syndrome), Gaucher disease, and the ferritin/cataract syndrome. Once iron overload is suspected, documentation of visceral iron deposition is needed (i.e., T2-weighted magnetic resonance imaging [MRI] of the liver or liver biopsy with Perls staining). The serum transferrin saturation (serum iron/total iron-binding capacity) is also used to screen for hemochromatosis. Because of the diurnal variation in serum iron, a fasting morning sample is best. A serum transferrin saturation > 50% for women and > 60% for men suggests the possibility of iron overload.

12. **Summarize the genetic link to hemochromatosis.**
Homozygosity for C282Y or the combination of C282Y and another mutation, H63D, in *HFE* gene, can be detected by the polymerase chain reaction (PCR) assay. Not all patients who have mutations develop clinical iron overload. In presence of iron overload, absent *HFE* mutation in a young (<30 years old), non-Caucasian patient suggests hemojuvelin or hepcidin mutation. In older patients ferroportin or transferrin receptor 2 mutation is possible. When iron overload is present in patients with normal or low transferrin saturation, a plasma ceruloplasmin should be drawn to exclude **hereditary aceruloplasminemia.** If normal, then genetic testing for ferroportin mutation (type 4A hemochromatosis) should be undertaken to detect V162del and A77D mutations.

Brissot P, Troadec MB, Bardou-Jacquet E, et al. Current approach to hemochromatosis. *Blood Rev.* 2008;22:195–210.

13. **How is hemochromatosis treated?**
Usually with phlebotomy in two phases:
   - **Induction phase:** Weekly as long as ferritin (checked monthly) is above normal (>300 ng/mL in males and > 200 ng/mL in females) then continued every other week until the ferritin level is < 50 ng/mL.
   - **Maintenance phase:** Every 2–4 months to keep ferritin < 50 ng/mL.

The transferrin saturation should be checked twice yearly. Phlebotomy is contraindicated in the presence of anemia (Hb < 11 g/dL) and in this scenario iron chelators can be considered. Patients should **avoid** vitamin C, excessive ethanol, and uncooked seafood. Patients are at risk for certain infections with bacteria that thrive on the increased plasma iron concentrations such as *Vibrio vulnificus* (found in uncooked seafood), *Listeria monocytogenes,* and *Yersinia enterocolitica.*

Bacon BR, Adams PC, Kowdley KV, et al. Diagnosis and management of hemochromatosis: 2011 practice guideline by the American Association for the Study of Liver Diseases. *Hepatology.* 2011;54:328–343.

14. When is it appropriate to order hemoglobin electrophoresis to evaluate hypochromic microcytic anemia?

When iron stores are normal to detect β-thalassemia minor and the so-called thalassemic hemoglobinopathies (including hemoglobin [Hb] E in Asians). β-Thalassemia minor is marked by an increased HbA_2 and sometimes increased fetal Hb. Iron deficiency results in a decreased pool of alpha chains, for which the beta chain of HbA and the delta chain of HbA_2 must compete. Beta chains are more successful, resulting in diminished HbA_2 during iron deficiency. For this reason, a search for β-thalassemia may be thwarted when patients are also iron deficient.

Beutler E. The common anemias. *JAMA.* 1988;259:2433–2437.

15. Which diseases are usually associated with the anemia of chronic disease (AOCD)?

Typically inflammatory states, including malignancy, rheumatologic disease, and infection. However, a study of hospitalized patients showed that the laboratory pattern of AOCD occurs in a significant number of anemic patients who do not have inflammatory conditions such as patients with complications of diabetes, renal failure, and hypertension. AOCD is a subtype of underproduction anemia compounded by decreased RBC life span, typified by a low serum iron, low total iron-binding capacity, and low percent saturation but increased iron stores, as evidenced by an increased ferritin.

Spivak J. The blood in systemic disorders. *Lancet.* 2000;355:1707–1712.

16. What causes macrocytosis?

See Table 14.2.

17. How is cobalamin (vitamin B_{12}) deficiency diagnosed?

By measuring vitamin B_{12}, methylmalonic acid (MMA), or homocysteine. In 97% of the cases vitamin B_{12} level is low (<200 ng/L or <148 pmol/L). Subclinical vitamin B_{12} deficiency can exist with levels of 250–350 ng/L (185–258 pmol/L). In clinical cobalamin deficiency, **MMA** is elevated in 98% of the cases and **homocysteine,** in 96%. The MMA is most accurate if the blood sample is centrifuged within an hour of venipuncture as levels can increase as much as 10% per 1 hour delay. MMA can be elevated in chronic kidney disease.

Carmel R, Green R, Rosenblatt DS, et al. Updated on cobalamine, folate, and homocysteine. *ASH Education Book.* 2003;2003:62–81.

Table 14.2. Causes of Macrocytosis

Megaloblastic anemia (macro-ovalocytosis)	Sideroblastic anemia*
Alcoholism	Chronic obstructive pulmonary disease
Malignancy	Artifacts and idiopathic
Hemolysis (usually poorly compensated)	Pregnancy
Aplastic anemia	Liver disease
Hypothyroidism	Drugs (zidovudine, hydroxyurea, azathioprine,
Refractory anemias (myelodysplasia)	anticonvulsants)
	Arsenic poisoning

*Often marked by dual populations of red blood cells—one hypochromic microcytic and the other macrocytic. From Colon-Otero G, Menke D, Hook CC. A practical approach to the differential diagnosis and evaluation of the adult patient with macrocytic anemia. *Med Clin North Am.* 1992;76:581–596; and Savage DG, Ogundipe A, Allen RH, et al. Etiology and diagnostic evaluation of macrocytosis. *Am J Med Sci.* 2000;319:343–352.

18. What processes may interrupt vitamin B_{12} absorption?
    - **Loss of intrinsic factor (IF):** *Pernicious anemia* associated with gastric atrophy due to an autoimmune-mediated attack on the gastric mucosa
    - **Gastrectomy:** Occurring 5–6 years after total gastrectomy
    - **Disorders of the small intestine:** Ileal resection, Crohn disease, sprue
    - **Competition with intestinal flora:** Blind-loop syndrome, fish tapeworm *(Diphyllobothrium latum)*
    - **Pancreatic disease:** Deficiency of R-binders with chronic pancreatitis
    - **Dietary:** Vegans (no meat, eggs, or milk) and breastfed infants of vegans
    - **Drug induced:** Aspirin, neomycin, colchicines, slow-release potassium chloride, cholesty-ramine, and others

19. Describe the pattern of neurologic disease associated with vitamin B_{12} deficiency.
    - **Posterior column:** Paresthesia, disturbed vibratory sense, loss of proprioception
    - **Pyramidal:** Spastic weakness, hyperactive reflexes
    - **Cerebral:** Dementia, psychosis (megaloblastic madness), optic atrophy

20. Is the severity of anemia a good predictor of neurologic involvement?
    No.
    Lindebaum J, Healton EB, Savage DG, et al. Neuropsychiatric disorders caused by cobalamin deficiency in the absence of anemia or macrocytosis. *N Engl J Med.* 1988;318:1720–1728.

21. What disorders are detected through bone marrow biopsy and aspiration?
    - **Pancytopenia:** Myelodysplasia, aplastic anemia (AA), myelophthisic states, hypersplenism, megaloblastic anemia
    - **RBC abnormalities:** Sideroblastic anemia, refractory anemia, pure RBC aplasia
    - **Staging of malignancy:** Hodgkin disease, leukemias, non-Hodgkin lymphoma, multiple myeloma
    - **Thrombocytopenia:** Idiopathic thrombocytopenic purpura
    - **Neutropenia**
    - **Infectious diseases:** Typhoid, tuberculosis, pancytopenia seen in acquired immunodeficiency syndrome (AIDS), brucellosis, and fever of unknown origin
    - **Lipid-storage diseases:** Gaucher disease

22. Why is bone marrow biopsy essential to the diagnosis of sideroblastic anemia?
    To detect the presence of ringed sideroblasts.

23. How is aplastic anemia (AA) defined?
    By findings on bone marrow examination:
    - **Moderate aplastic anemia (MAA):**
      - Bone marrow cellularity < 30%
      - Absence of severe pancytopenia
      - Depression of at least two of three blood elements below normal
    - **Severe aplastic anemia (SAA):**
      - A bone marrow biopsy showing < 25% of normal cellularity, or
      - A bone marrow biopsy showing < 50% normal cellularity in which fewer than 30% of the cells are hematopoietic **and**
      - At least two of the following are present: absolute reticulocyte count < 40,000/μL; absolute neutrophil count (ANC) < 500/μL; or platelet count < 20,000/μL.
    - **Very severe aplastic anemia (vSAA):**
      - Criteria for SAA are met **and**
      - ANC is < 200/μL
      Rozman C, Marín P, Nomdedeu B. Criteria for severe aplastic anaemia. *Lancet.* 1987;2:955–957.

24. What tests should be ordered in the work-up of AA?
    - CBC (complete blood count) with differential, reticulocyte count, blood film, and HbF (in children it can be a marker of myelodysplastic syndrome [MDS])
    - Bone marrow biopsy and aspirate
    - Blood chromosomal breakage analysis to exclude Fanconi anemia if < 50 years old

- Flow cytometry to rule out paroxysmal nocturnal hemoglobinuria (PNH)
- Vitamin B_{12} and folate
- Viral studies (hepatitis A, B, and C, Epstein-Barr virus [EBV], human immunodeficiency virus [HIV], and cytomegalovirus [CMV])
- Antinuclear antibody (ANA) and anti–double-stranded DNA (anti-dsDNA) antibodies
- Chest radiograph to evaluate for the presence of a thymoma
- Abdominal scan and echocardiogram
- Peripheral blood gene mutation analysis for dyskeratosis congenital *(DKC1, TERC, TERT)* if there are clinical features or lack of response to immunotherapy

  Marsh JC, Ball SE, Cavenagh J, et al. Guidelines for the diagnosis and management of aplastic anaemia. *Brit J Haematol.* 2009;147:43–70.

25. **What is the differential diagnosis for pancytopenia and a hypocellular marrow?**
    - Hypocellular: MDS/acute myelogenous leukemia (AML)
    - Hypocellular: Acute lymphocytic leukemia (ALL)
    - Hairy cell leukemia (HCL)
    - Lymphomas
    - Mycobacterial infections
    - Anorexia nervosa or prolonged starvation

26. **What supportive measures should be taken in the care of AAs?**
    - Prophylactic platelet transfusion (<10,000 or <20,000 if the patient is febrile)
    - **Irradiated** blood products
    - Prophylactic antibiotics and antifungals for patients with ANC < 200/μL
    - Human leukocyte antigen (HLA) typing should be done as soon as possible (both for bone marrow donor search as well as platelet transfusion if there is refractoriness)
    - Iron chelation if serum ferritin > 1000 ng/dL

27. **What is the best therapy for AA in a young person (under age 40)?**
    Bone marrow transplantation (BMT) from an HLA-identical sibling. If there is not an HLA-identical sibling, cyclosporine and antithymocyte globulin (ATG) should be started. High-resolution HLA-identical but nonrelated donors may be used for such patients. If a PNH clone is detected, immunosuppression is preferred. Responses to ATG/cyclosporine will take **months.**

28. **What types of donors are available for BMT?**
    - **HLA-matched sibling:** Probability of matching is 25% per sibling.
    - **Matched unrelated donor** (MUD): HLA-A, HLA-B, HLA-C, DRB1
    - **Unrelated cord blood:** Chances of HLA matching are much smaller than with MUD but because T-cell dose is much smaller, the probability of graft-versus-host disease (GVHD) is less for cord blood. Allele disparities worsen cord engraftment and increase transplant-related mortality risk.
    - **Related donors identical for one HLA haplotype (haploidentical):** Available to anyone with a first-degree relative. Donors with greater than one HLA locus disparity require modified protocols given greater chance of graft failure, GVHD, and death.

      Eapen M, Klein JP, Ruggieri A, et al. Impact of allele-level HLA matching on outcomes after myeloablative single unit umbilical cord blood transplantation for hematologic malignancies. *Blood.* 2014;123:133–140.

29. **What are the most important causes of death in patients undergoing BMT?**
    Infections, interstitial pneumonitis, and veno-occlusive disease. After conditioning, patients become pancytopenic during the 3 weeks or so required for engraftment. The objective of the myeloablative preparation is both to eradicate the cancer and induce immunosuppression to allow engraftment. During that time, these patients are prone to **infections** and require prophylactic treatment with antibiotics and transfusions. Blood products must be irradiated to prevent **GVHD** from donor lymphocytes. After engraftment, **interstitial pneumonitis** is a possible complication, with a high mortality rate. Some of these deaths are due to infectious agents such as CMV. Recently, a severe form of **veno-occlusive disease** of the liver has emerged as a cause of morbidity and death after BMT. Defibrotide has been recently approved by the Food and Drug Administratin (FDA) for this indication. Because of the high mortality rate of conditioning regimens, some patients may benefit

from reduced-intensity conditioning (RIC), although it can be offset by a higher rate of relapse. RIC has been most effective in slow-growing cancers (chronic lymphocytic leukemia [CLL] and low-grade non-Hodgkin lymphoma). If transplantation is urgent and a match cannot be found, cord blood can be safely used. The transplantation of cord blood requires less stringent HLA matching but is complicated by a longer time to engraftment.

Copelan EA. Hematopoietic stem cell transplantation. *N Engl J Med*. 2006;354:1813–1826.

30. **What are the characteristics of acute GVHD?**

Acute GVHD arises during the first 100 days after transplant, with donor T cells targeting the host's skin, liver, and gastrointestinal tract. Patients may have mild skin rashes or more severe disease resulting in toxic epidermal necrolysis. Diarrhea and transient elevation of liver enzymes may occur and, in some patients, are more severe, resulting in massive diarrhea and liver failure. Immunologic competence is also delayed by GVHD so that patients are susceptible to new infections, including those mediated by encapsulated organisms such as pneumococci. A regimen of total lymphoid irradiation and an antithymocyte regimen (i.e., T-cell depletion) has been shown to reduce acute GVHD but may be associated with higher relapse rates.

Lowsky R, Takahashi T, Lui YP, et al. Protective conditioning for acute graft versus host disease. *N Engl J Med*. 2005;353:1321–1331.

31. **Describe chronic GVHD.**

Almost 40–60% of survivors of allogenic BMT will develop chronic GVHD, affecting the same organs as acute GVHD, with the additional features of a scleroderma-like illness. Dry eyes, dry mouth, myasthenia, bronchiolitis, and infections are also observed. Three variables have been associated with shortened survival: extensive skin involvement (>50% of the body surface), platelet count < 100,000/μL, and progressive onset. The main treatment is immunosuppression, although patients are best treated under investigational protocols.

Filipovich AH, Weisdorf D, Pavletic S, et al. National Institutes of Health consensus development project on criteria for clinical trials in chronic graft-versus-host disease: I. Diagnosis and staging working group report. *Biol Blood Marrow Transplant*. 2005;11:945–956.

32. **What is the principal indication for ESAs therapy in the treatment of anemia?**

Chronic renal failure, AZT (azidothymidine)-treated HIV patients, cancer patients on chemotherapy (palliative only), and MDS.

33. **What concomitant studies should be checked prior to initiation of ESAs?**

Iron studies. ESAs should be started only after iron replacement has taken effect. In practice, a ferritin level > 100 ng/dL and an iron saturation > 20% is necessary. For patients with MDS, the pretreatment erythropoietin (EPO) level should be < 500 mIU/mL.

34. **What are the potential adverse events of ESAs?**

Hypertension, fever, and local reactions. Other rare events include vascular thrombotic events, increased mortality rate in certain cancers, splenic rupture, and pure RBC aplasia. The TREAT investigators found a higher risk of stroke in diabetic patients treated for anemia of chronic kidney disease. A rapid raise in the Hb (>1 g/dL per week) is an adverse prognostic factor.

Pfeffer MA, Burdmann EA, Chen CY, et al. A trial of darbopoetic alpha in type 2 diabetes and chronic kidney disease. *N Engl J Med*. 2009;361:2019–2032.

35. **What are the current indications for ESA use in chemotherapy-induced anemia?**

An Hb concentration that is approaching or falling below 10 g/dL. In patients with a higher risk of vascular events (elderly, uncontrolled hypertension, limited cardiopulmonary reserve, underlying coronary artery disease, or frail patients), watchful waiting is recommended until the Hb has dropped below 10 g/dL. We would also advocate caution in patients who are at a high risk for venous thromboembolism (pancreatic and stomach cancer, thrombocytosis, leukocytosis, and morbid obesity). ESAs should only be used in patients receiving **palliative chemotherapy** and not in those undergoing **adjuvant** chemotherapy.

Khorana AA, Kuderer NM, Culakova E, et al. Development and validation of a predictive model for chemotherapy associated thrombosis. *Blood*. 2008;111:4902–4907.

Rizzo JD, Brouwers M, Hurley P, et al. ASCO/ASH clinical practice guideline update on the use of epoetin and darbepoetin in adult patients with cancer. *J Clin Oncol*. 2010;28:4996–5010.

HEMOLYTIC ANEMIAS

36. **How can hemolytic anemia be conceptualized?**
    There are a number of ways to think of the causes of hemolytic anemia. One such schema is the following:
    - Immunologic causes
    - Disorders of the RBC membrane
    - Disorders of RBC enzymes
    - Disorders of globin synthesis
    - External causes (pathogens [e.g., malaria], mechanical [e.g., valves])

37. **List the complications of chronic hemolytic anemias.**
    - Aplastic crises (associated with parvovirus B19)
    - Hemolytic crises
    - Megaloblastic crises (due to increased demand for folate)
    - Pigment gallstones
    - Splenomegaly
    - Stasis ulcers
    - Pulmonary artery hypertension
    - Thrombosis, arterial or venous.

38. **What supplement is mandatory in all hemolytic anemias?**
    Folate 1 mg by mouth daily.

39. **What are the immunologic causes of hemolytic anemia?**
    Alloimmune and autoimmune processes. The **alloimmune** causes occur after the receipt of incompatible blood such as an immediate reaction mediated by preformed IgM antibodies due to inappropriately cross-matched blood (i.e., type A patient receiving type B blood). Delayed hemolytic transfusion reactions occur when the patient has been sensitized to a foreign RBC antigen, which can be from pregnancy or a prior transfusion. Eventually, the alloantibody decreases in titer and is no longer detected on a typical type and cross. However, if blood containing that same RBC epitope is transfused again, the patient develops a rapid immune response against the transfused RBCs. **Autoimmune** causes include warm antibody mediated, cold antibody mediated, and drug induced.
    Gehrs BC, Friedberg RC. Autoimmune hemolytic anemia. *Am J Hematol*. 2002;69:258–271.

40. **What is warm autoimmune hemolytic anemia, and what are the causes?**
    Warm autoimmune hemolytic anemia is characterized by an antibody, usually IgG, which is able to bind to the RBCs at 37° C, hence the "warm" designation. Cold antibodies, on the other hand, are typically IgM and bind to RBCs at much lower temperatures. Warm autoimmune hemolytic anemia can be seen in a variety of conditions, including autoimmune disease such as systemic lupus erythematous (SLE); lymphoproliferative disorders (CLL, Hodgkin disease, non-Hodgkin lymphomas); or following infections; or it may be idiopathic.
    Barros MM, Blajchman MA, Bordin JO. Warm autoimmune hemolytic anemia: recent progress in understanding the immunobiology and the treatment. *Transfus Med Rev*. 2010;24:195–210.

41. **With which disorders are cold antibody-mediated immune hemolytic anemias associated?**
    Mycoplasma infection (usually anti-I) or infectious mononucleosis (usually anti-i). Chronic cold agglutination disease may be an idiopathic syndrome or associated with a lymphoproliferative disorder.

42. **What is paroxysmal cold hemoglobinuria (PCH)?**
    The appearance of red or brown urine after exposure to cold association with the **Donath-Landsteiner** autoantibody. Although PCH is classically associated with syphilis, it is now more common in children following infections. PCH is diagnosed based upon the "biphasic hemolysin" properties, which means the autoantibody will bind to RBCs without lysing them at 0° C. However, when the sample is warmed to 37° C, hemolysis will occur.

43. **Explain the direct Coombs test used to evaluate autoimmune hemolytic anemia.**
    The Coombs test is used to detect antibodies on RBCs (direct Coombs or direct antiglobulin test positive [DAT]) or in plasma. In the direct test, the RBCs are washed and incubated with an antiglobulin serum (rabbit or other species) and then examined for agglutination.

44. Explain the indirect test.

Serum is mixed with a panel of RBCs bearing antigens of interest. Antibodies, if present in the sera, bind to the RBCs bearing the relevant antigen. The panel cells are washed to reduce nonspecific binding, and then incubated with an antiglobulin serum to detect agglutination. The antiglobulin reagent is necessary because antibodies attached to RBCs are usually IgG in low numbers and cannot ordinarily cross-link to agglutinate. The antiglobulin serum bridges these antibodies, favoring agglutination.

45. How is the Coombs test used to evaluate autoimmune hemolytic anemia?

In autoimmune hemolytic anemia, the direct test is usually positive, indicating the presence of an autoantibody on the RBCs. The indirect test, indicating the presence of the same antibody in serum, also may be positive. Persons who have been exposed to blood or have had pregnancy losses may develop antibodies to certain antigens on the transfused RBCs that do not exist on native RBCs. Later, they have a positive indirect Coombs test and negative direct Coombs test.

46. What are some of the disorders of RBC membranes that lead to anemia?

- Hereditary spherocytosis (HS)
- Hereditary elliptocytosis (HE)
- Hereditary pyropoikilocytosis
- Rh deficiency
- Dehydrated hereditary stomatocytosis (formerly known as xerocytosis)
- Overhydrated hereditary stomatocytosis.

47. Describe the underlying protein deficiency associated with HS.

Decreased amounts of spectrin, the principal membrane protein found in erythrocytes. Spectrin has self-associative properties and forms a lattice with other RBC membrane proteins and actin. This supportive lattice on the inner aspect of the lipid bilayer gives the RBC its unique properties of strength and suppleness. Deficiency of spectrin correlates with the degree of hemolysis, changes in osmotic fragility, and response to splenectomy.

An X, Mohandas N. Disorders of the red cell membrane. *Br J Haemotol.* 2008;141:367–375.

48. What is the differential diagnosis of spherocytosis in the peripheral blood film?

Hemoloytic anemias including:
- Glucose-6-phosphate dehydrogenase (G6PD) deficiency or HbH
- ABO incompatibility
- Phospholipases, venoms, or clostridial sepsis
- Microangiopathic hemolytic anemias
- Autoimmune hemolytic anemias

49. What are the indications for splenectomy in patients with HS?

Symptomatic anemia or growth restriction. The risks of splenectomy include infections, vascular events, and pulmonary hypertension.

Schilling RF. Risks and benefits of splenectomy versus no splenectomy for hereditary spherocytosis—a personal view. *Br J Haemotol.* 2009;145:728–732.

50. What is hereditary elliptocytosis (HE)?

A broad spectrum of disorders that result in an elliptical RBC shape and hemolysis. In general, HE results from genetic defects that arise in the horizontal interaction of the RBC membrane cytoskeleton that depends on alpha spectrin–beta spectrin association and interaction of spectrin with band 4.1 protein to form a high-molecular-weight oligomeric structure. Most patients with HE and its variants have a structural abnormality of the spectrin protein that results in failure of the protein to self-associate into higher-order tetramers and oligomers.

51. What are the most important subsets of HE?

- **Mild common HE:** Normal Hct and mild reticulocytosis.
- **Common HE with chronic hemolysis:** More striking degree of hemolysis, anemia, and more bizarre RBC morphologic appearance.
- **Infantile poikilocytosis:** Present at birth; later associated with striking hemolysis, bizarre RBCs, and jaundice.
- **Homozygous HE:** Rare subset accompanied by severe anemia.

- **Hereditary pyropoikilocytosis:** Rare subset in which the spectrin is abnormally sensitive to heat. The peripheral blood picture resembles that seen in hemolysis associated with severe burns.
- **Spherocytic elliptocytosis:** Unusual autosomal dominant disorder in which the elliptocytes are rounded. Spherocytes and increased osmotic fragility are also found.
- **Southeast Asian ovalocytosis**

52. **What RBC enzyme defects lead to anemia?**
    - **Hexokinase:** Rare, autosomal recessive
    - **Glucose-6-phosphate isomerase:** Second most common enzyme deficiency
    - **Phosphofructokinase:** Rare, autosomal recessive
    - **Aldolase:** Only six cases have been reported
    - **Triosephosphate isomerase:** Another very rare autosomal recessive disease
    - **Phosphoglycerate kinase**
    - **Pyruvate kinase:** The most common enzyme deficiency leading to hemolysis
    - **G6PD**
    Mutations have been described in almost all enzymes of the glycolytic and NADPH (nicotinamide adenine dinucleotide phosphate, reduced form) pathways.

53. **How is G6PD deficiency characterized?**
    As an X-linked disease, so the majority of symptomatic individuals are male. G6PD deficiency is considered to be the most common enzyme deficiency in the world, with an estimated 400 million affected individuals. The enzyme catalyzes the rate-limiting step in the generation of NADPH by converting glucose 6-phosphate to 6-phosphoglucono-δ-lactone. NADPH is necessary for the reduction of glutathione-containing disulfides (GSSG to GSH) in the reduction of oxidative species. Therefore, reduced or absent stores of NADPH in the RBC make it vulnerable to oxidative stress. In addition to hemolysis, oxidation results in precipitation of hemoglobin, which can be detected as Heinz bodies by supravital staining with crystal violet.
    G6PD deficiency is categorized into five groups:
    - **Class I:** Severe deficiency in enzyme activity associated with a chronic nonspherocytic hemolytic anemia
    - **Class II:** 1–10% enzyme activity
    - **Class III:** Moderate deficiency with 10–60% enzyme activity
    - **Class IV:** Normal activity (60–150%)
    - **Class V:** Elevated level of enzyme activity (>150%)

54. **How do patients with G6PD present?**
    Early in life, typically with jaundice and hemolytic anemia. However, many patients with G6PD deficiency may go through life without any symptoms. Patients typically present after some stress to their RBCs, whether by ingestion of medications, certain foods, or illness.

55. **How is G6PD deficiency diagnosed?**
    By measuring the enzymatic activity of G6PD by quantitative spectrophotometric analysis of the rate of NADPH production from NADP.
    Cappellini MD, Fiorelli G. Glucose-6-phosphate dehydrogenase deficiency. *Lancet.* 2008;371:64–74.

56. **What is favism?**
    An acute hemolytic crisis in patients with G6PD deficiency that occurs after eating fava beans. Compounds within the beans are thought to increase the activity of the erythrocytic hexose monophosphate shunt, leading to hemolysis.

57. **What else can cause hemolysis in G6PD deficiency?**
    Mainly medications or drugs including:
    - Antimalarials (primaquine and possibly chloroquine)
    - Sulfonamides
    - Nitrofurantoin
    - Acetanilide and possibly aspirin
    - Naphthalene

58. **What are the disorders of globin synthesis?**
    Thalassemias, sickle cell syndromes, and the unstable hemoglobins, commonly referred to as the hemoglobinopathies.

59. **What is thalassemia?**
Any disorder in which the synthesis of a globin chain required for the production of hemoglobin is disrupted. In adults, RBCs contain mostly hemoglobin A (HbA), typically > 96%, with a minimal amount of hemoglobin A2 (HbA2), and rare amounts of hemoglobin F (HbF). Whereas HbA is composed of two α and β chains apiece ($\alpha_2\beta_2$), HbA2 is $\alpha_2\delta_2$ and HbF is $\alpha_2\gamma_2$. Normally, the ratio of α and β chains in the RBC is tightly regulated to be 1:1.

60. **What is α-thalassemia?**
A series of defects that lead to a decrease in the synthesis of α-globin. Normal adults have two copies of the α-globin gene on each copy of chromosome 16, denoted $\alpha\alpha/\alpha\alpha$. α-Thalassemia results from the deletion of one ($-\alpha/\alpha\alpha$), two ($-\alpha/-\alpha$ or $--/\alpha\alpha$), three ($--/-\alpha$), or four ($--/--$) of the α-globin genes.

61. **What are the different α-thalassemias and how do they manifest?**
Unfortunately, there are a variety of names in the literature, which often leads to confusion. These are the basic names/forms of the α-thalassemias:
- Loss of one α-globin gene is termed α^+-*thalassemia* or α-thalassemia trait ($-\alpha/\alpha\alpha$) and occurs in approximately one third of African Americans. The majority of patients are "silent carriers," meaning they are clinically normal. RBC morphologic appearance and indices can be normal, along with a normal Hb electrophoresis.
- Loss of two α-globin genes on one chromosome alone, is α-thalassemia-1 or α^0-thalassemia ($--/\alpha\alpha$), also referred to as being in *cis-*. This form is common in patients of Asian descent and is characterized by a mild, hypochromic, microcytic anemia. The Hb EP can be normal and care must be taken not to mistake this for IDA. Of concern is that two parents can potentially have a child who may inherit no α-globin genes, leading to hydrops fetalis *(see later)*.
- One α-globin gene deleted from both chromosomes ($-\alpha/-\alpha$) is α-thalassemia-2, α^+-thalassemia, or α-thalassemia minima, also referred to as being in *trans-*. It is commonly seen in patients of African or Mediterranean descent. Like α-thalassemia-1, it is associated with a mild, hypochromic, microcytic anemia and a normal Hb EP.
- When a total of three α-globin genes are missing ($--/-\alpha$), this leads to the production of HbH. Because very little α-globin is made, β_4 tetramers form RBC inclusions, which can be visualized by staining with brilliant cresyl blue. The resulting hemolytic anemia is characterized by a marked anisopoikilocytosis, hypochromia, and reticulocytosis. Hb EP shows the presence of HbH.
- Deletion of all four α-globin genes ($--/--$) causes the total absence of α-chains; therefore, HbA, HbA2, or HbF cannot be made, resulting in Hb Bart (γ_4). The peripheral blood smear is remarkable for a marked anisopoikilocytosis, hypochromia, target cells, reticulocytosis, and NRBCs. The Hb EP shows ~80% Hb Bart and ~20% Hb Portland ($\zeta_2\gamma_2$). These hemoglobins have a left-shifting oxygen dissociation, leading to significant fetal hypoxia, often causing death in utero or shortly thereafter. The *cis-* mutations are needed for the deletions to occur and are common in Asian populations.

62. **What is β-thalassemia?**
A spectrum of diseases caused by the imbalance of available β-globin chains. Unlike α-thalassemia, β-thalassemia is characterized not by whole gene deletions but of mutations within the β-globin genes. Fortunately, the nomenclature for β-thalassemia is not as confusing, because there is only one β-globin gene on chromosome 11.

63. **What are the different types of β-thalassemia?**
- **β-Thalassemia minor:** β-Thalassemia trait that refers to patients with a single defect in the β-globin gene, causing reduced expression of the β chains. Patients are mildly anemic, hypochromic, and microcytic. The hallmark of β-thalassemia minor is an Hb EP with an elevated HbA2. As with the α-thalassemias, it is important to not inappropriately diagnose or treat these patients as iron deficient.
- **β-Thalassemia intermedia:** A broad spectrum of mutations and clinical symptoms caused by mutations in both β-globin genes. Those who are able to make some β-globin are sometimes referred to as β^+-thalassemia. Symptoms range between that of β-thalassemia minor and β-thalassemia major. Patients usually exhibit microcytic, hypochromic anemia. The Hb EP will also show an increase in the HbA2 levels.
- **β^0-Thalassemia, β-thalassemia major, or Cooley anemia:** These terms all refer to conditions in which no β-globin chains are made. This absence of β-globin causes the formation of α_4 tetramers that are highly toxic to the RBC membrane. Because no β-globin chains can be made, no HbA or HbA2 will be seen on the Hb EP. Developing RBCs perish in the marrow or limp

out to live a short, withered existence in the circulation. Erythropoiesis is highly ineffective, and patients have tremendous expansion of the bone marrow and extramedullary hematopoiesis, as evidenced by marked hepatosplenomegaly. Affected children are transfusion-dependent; if not transfused aggressively, they develop pathologic fractures and significant growth retardation.

Oliveri N. The beta-thalassemias. *N Engl J Med*. 1999;341:99–109.

64. What is sickle cell disease?

A disorder with hemoglobin S (HbS) resulting from a substitution of a valine for glutamic acid at the sixth amino acid of the β-globin chain. Sickle cell disease is caused by mutations in the β-globin chain, which produces polymers that are poorly soluble when deoxygenated.

65. What other abnormal hemoglobins are associated with sickle hemoglobin?

Sickle hemoglobin coexists with other β-chain variants to produce a spectrum of disorders from clinically insignificant conditions such as sickle cell trait (AS and S-hereditary persistence of fetal hemoglobin) to severe disease represented by homozygous sickle syndrome (SS). Other forms of sickle cell disease include S-β-thalassemia, SC, SD-Punjab, SO-Arab, S-Lepore-Boston, and S-Antilles.

66. What is the incidence of sickle hemoglobinopathies in births among African Americans?

1. AS 8.0% (1 of 12)
2. AC 3.00%
3. SS 0.16%
4. SC 0.12%
5. Sβ⁰ 0.03%

Note that the incidence of Sβ⁰ and SC is approximately that of SS. In adults, as many patients with sickle β-thalassemia or SC will be seen as homozygous S patients. Although Sβ⁰ is clinically similar to SS disease, Sβ⁺ and SC patients are more likely to have palpable spleens and may experience splenic sequestration/infarct crises as adults rather than in early childhood, as is the case with SS disease. SC patients also tend to have higher hematocrits. They may present with blindness due to retinopathy or aseptic necrosis of the hip.

67. Is any morbidity truly associated with sickle trait?

Yes. The following abnormalities have been associated with sickle trait:
- Splenic infarction at high altitude
- Sudden death following exertion
- Bacteremia in women
- Pulmonary embolism (PE)
- Hyposthenuria
- Medullary renal carcinoma
- Glaucoma, anterior chamber bleeds
- Bacteriuria and pyelonephritis in pregnancy

Tsaras G, Owusu-Ansah A, Boateng FO, et al. Complications associated with sickle cell trait: a brief narrative review. *Am J Med*. 2009;122:507–512.

68. What are sickle crises?

Sudden, unheralded vaso-occlusive events. The most common event is a simple pain crisis affecting the limbs, low back, chest, or abdomen. Sometimes specific organs are affected by definite infarcts, including the bone and spleen (if splenic tissue has been preserved).

69. What is acute chest syndrome?

Symptoms of dyspnea, fever, pain, and sudden appearance of an infiltrate on chest radiograph consistent with pneumonia. Although an overt pneumonia may not exist, a number of patients may have atypical infections, notably *Chlamydia pneumoniae*. Recent studies of chest syndrome have emphasized the role of fat embolism from bone marrow infarcts and infections. Splinting while the patient is suffering a rib infarct may lead to hypoventilation and pulmonary vaso-occlusion. Incentive spirometry has been advocated to reduce the risk of chest syndrome in patients hospitalized with sickle crises and chest pain. Among older patients and those with neurologic dysfunction, the symptoms can progress to respiratory failure. In a large multicenter trial neurologic events occurred in 11% of patients. Acute chest syndrome progressed to respiratory failure in 13% of the patients, and 3% of the cohort died.

Vichinsky EP, Neumayr LD, Earles AN, et al. Causes and outcomes of the acute chest syndrome in sickle cell disease. *N Engl J Med.* 2000;342:1855–1865.

70. **How are patients in a sickle crisis managed? How often do crises occur?**
Patients with acute chest syndrome often receive antibiotics and require oxygen. When hypoxemia continues despite oxygen therapy, exchange transfusions are helpful. The pathophysiology of the pain crisis is not well understood. Strict adherence to National Institutes of Health (NIH) guidelines in the treatment of vaso-occlusive episodes is recommended. Careful history review of prior hospitalizations is necessary for prompt pain relief and to recognize subtle changes that may require more aggressive therapy.

National Heart, Lung, and Blood Institute. The management of sickle cell disease, 2004. Available at: www.nhlbi.nih.gov/health-pro/guidelines/current/management-sickle-cell-disease [accessed 21.10.16].

71. **How often do crises occur?**
Relatively infrequently—once every year or two. About 20% of patients, however, are troubled by more frequent crises and may visit the emergency department or hospital monthly. Why some patients with sickle cell disease do poorly, while others do relatively well is one of the mysteries of sickle cell disease. Similarly, it is not known what initiates crises or what mechanisms of spontaneous recovery terminate crises while patients are receiving only supportive care. The severity and duration of crises are variable. Hospitalization stays vary from 3 to 10 days.

Platt OS, Thorington BD, Brambilla DJ, et al. Pain in sickle cell disease: rates and risk factors. *N Engl J Med.* 1991;325:11–16.

72. **Summarize routine health maintenance for adults with sickle cell anemia.**
Genetic counseling about the risk of sickle cell disease in relatives or children, supplementation with folic acid, and periodic ophthalmoscopic examinations. All adults should receive pneumococcal (both pneumococcal conjugate [PCV13] and pneumococcal polysaccharide [PPS23]), *Haemophilus influenzae* b (Hib), and meningococcal vaccines, if not already received during childhood, and annual influenza vaccine. As patients get older, periodic review of renal function is prudent but standard calculations of glomerular filtration **cannot** be used reliably in patients with sickle cell disease. In the acute setting, an increase of 0.3 mg/dL in creatinine should prompt avoidance of nephrotoxic agents. If there has been a history of blood transfusions, evaluating for iron overload is recommended.

National Heart, Lung, and Blood Institute. Evidence-based management of sickle cell disease. Expert Panel Report, 2014. Available at: www.nhlbi.nih.gov/health-pro/guidelines/sickle-cell-disease-guidelines [accessed 21.10.16].

73. **What are the main complications of sickle cell disease?**
Painful episodes, strokes (can be silent and lead to cognitive impairment), acute chest syndrome, priapism, liver disease (from iron overload, hepatitis B and C, etc.), splenic sequestration, miscarriages, leg ulcers, osteonecrosis, proliferative retinopathy, renal insufficiency, pulmonary hypertension, cholelithiasis, gout, venous thrombosis, acute aplastic episodes, osteomyelitis, alloimmunization, hyperhemolysis, and functional asplenia.

74. **Is RBC transfusion routinely recommended for the treatment of typical pain crises?**
No.

75. **Under what circumstances should RBC transfusion be considered in the treatment of sickle cell disease?**

Strong Indications	Relative Indications
Aplastic crises	Before general anesthesia
Hypoxemia and acute chest syndrome	During pregnancy
Heart failure	Baseline anemia
CNS events, stroke	Simple surgery
Sequestration crises	Priapism
Intractable pain	

CNS, central nervous system.

Wanko SO, Telen MJ. Transfusion management in sickle cell disease. *Hematol Oncol Clin North Am.* 2005;19:803–826.

76. **How is pulmonary arterial hypertension (PAH) defined in sickle cell disease?**
Either by a tricuspid regurgitation (TR) jet $\geq$ 2.5 m/s or pulmonary artery pressures by right-sided cardiac catheterization of 25 mm Hg or more. PAH occurs in about 30% of adult patients homozygous for HbSS and confers an increased risk of death (about 20% mortality rate at 2 years).
    Gladwin MT, Sachdev V, Jison ML, et al. Pulmonary hypertension as a risk factor for death in patients with sickle cell disease. *N Engl J Med.* 2004;350:886–995.

77. **What protocol is recommended for RBC transfusion in sickle cell disease before general anesthesia?**
Simple transfusions to an arbitrary level of hemoglobin. A national study found that this protocol enabled patients to undergo general anesthesia with no worse outcome than patients who had exchange transfusions according to a national study. Because less blood was used, the conservative transfusion protocol was complicated less often by alloimmunization.
    Claster S, Vichinsky EP. Managing sickle cell disease. *BMJ.* 2003;327:1151–1155.

78. **A patient with sickle cell disease presents with a history of a viral syndrome, followed by dramatic worsening of the anemia. What entity needs to be strongly considered?**
Aplastic crisis. Typically, patients have a flulike illness, with or without an evanescent rash, fever, and myalgias, followed 5–10 days later by weakness and dyspnea. The patient presents with a sharply reduced Hct and nearly absolute absence of reticulocytes. This disorder is in fact a transient pure RBC aplasia. The platelet and white blood cell (WBC) counts are usually unaffected. Bone marrow shows the absence of erythroid progenitors, except for a few "giant pronormoblasts."

79. **What is the most common cause of aplastic syndrome?**
Infection with parvovirus B19, which has a unique tropism for erythroid progenitors.

80. **Explain the physiologic and clinical significance of parvovirus-induced aplasia.**
In patients with a compensated chronic hemolytic disorder, parvovirus-induced aplasia is significant because the duration of aplasia (5–10 days) coincides with the half-life of RBCs. Thus, cessation of RBC production for 10 days in a patient with Hct of 22% and RBC life span of 9 days spells trouble. Transfusions of packed RBCs are lifesaving. The 10-day cessation of erythropoiesis caused by the parvovirus goes unnoticed in a normal person with Hct of 40% and an RBC life span of 120 days. The parvovirus may be the cause of fifth disease, arthritis, and spontaneous abortions.
    Saarinen UM, Chorba TL, Tattersall P, et al. Human parvovirus B19-induced epidemic acute red cell aplasia in patients with hereditary hemolytic anemia. *Blood.* 1986;67:1411–1417.

81. **What is the the the role of hydroxyurea in the treatment of patients with severe (more than three crises/year) sickle cell anemia?**
Perhaps the greatest therapeutic advance in sickle hemoglobinopathy was the recognition that certain chemotherapeutic agents can reverse the developmental "switch" from fetal to adult hemoglobin synthesis. The rise in HbF in each RBC suppresses sickling and offers the promise of reduced hemolysis and vaso-occlusive phenomena. A double-blinded trial of hydroxyurea was halted early when it was shown to reduce the rate of crises by about 40% and to reduce the incidence of acute chest syndrome and frequency of transfusions and, in a follow-up study, prolonged survival.
    Charache S, Terrin ML, Moore RD, et al. Effect of hydroxyurea on the frequency of painful crises in sickle cell anemia. *N Engl J Med.* 1995;332:317–322.

82. **Is hydroxyurea leukemogenic?**
In some cases. Reports of leukemia and other cancers have been described in patients who have received hydroxyurea. However, this has been observed in patients with other blood conditions (e.g., polycythemia vera [PCV] or essential thrombocytosis), which can progress to leukemia on their own. Although cases of leukemia and other cancers have been described in sickle cell patients treated with hydroxyurea, they are rare and are no more common than seen in the regular population. At this point there are no data to support the theory of leukemogenicity of hydroxyurea in practice.
    Steinberg MH, McCarthy WF, Castro O, et al. The risks and benefits of long-term use of hydroxyurea in sickle cell anemia: A 17.5 year follow-up. *Am J Hematol.* 2010;85:403–408.

83. **What are some features of intravascular hemolysis?**
During hemolysis, the bone marrow responds to the premature destruction of RBCs by increasing its production of RBCs, which can be ascertained by increased reticulocytosis. Other clues to accelerated RBC destruction are:
- Indirect hyperbilirubinemia-acholuric jaundice (because unconjugated bilirubin is not secreted in urine)
- Hemoglobinuria
- Fall of hemoglobin > 1 g over 7 days in the absence of bleeding or massive hematoma

84. **Give examples of intravascular hemolytic disorders.**
Hemolytic transfusion reactions, paroxysmal nocturnal hemoglobinuria, march hemoglobinuria, and RBC fragmentation syndromes.

85. **What are some other causes of major acquired hemolytic disorders?**
Malaria, hypersplenism, and physical agents such as heat, copper, and certain oxidants.

86. **What is the appearance of fragmentation hemolysis of a peripheral smear?**
Schistocytes, helmet cells, burr cells (echinocytes), and spherocytes. The hemolysis is intravascular and can be associated with a wide variety of conditions.

87. **What are some of the causes of microangiopathic hemolytic anemia?**
- Cavernous hemangiomas (Kasabach-Merritt syndrome)
- Thrombotic thrombocytopenic purpura (TTP)
- Hemolytic uremic syndrome (HUS)
- Atypical hemolytic uremic syndrome (AHUS)
- Shiga toxin producing *Escherichia coli* (STEC-HUS)
- Eclampsia/preeclampsia
- Malignant hypertension
- Scleroderma
- Valve hemolysis
- Disseminated carcinomatosis
- Disseminated intravascular coagulation (DIC)

88. **What is the classic pentad of TTP?**
- Microangiopathic hemolytic anemia with schistocytes on the peripheral smear.
- Thrombocytopenia
- Renal insufficiency
- Fever
- Neurologic changes

  Most patients will **not** present with the classic pentad in the modern era. Currently TTP is a diagnosis of exclusion. A platelet count of less than $100 \times 10^9/L$ and lactate dehydrogenase (LDH) levels greater than 1.5 times the upper limit of normal are necessary for diagnosis.

89. **How does HUS differ from TTP?**
In HUS, renal failure is the predominant organ syndrome associated with thrombocytopenia and fragmentation hemolysis. Metalloprotease activity, absent in TTP, is present in HUS, indicating a different pathogenesis; 90% of HUS is associated with shiga-like toxin producing bacteria (STEC-HUS). In some families a deficiency in plasma factor H, a complement control factor, is associated with recurrent HUS. Another small population with AHUS may carry a mutation in thrombomodulin.

90. **What is ADAMTS13, and how is it implicated in TTP?**
*A D*isintegrin *A*nd *M*etalloproteinase with *T*hrombo*S*pondin-1 like motif, member *13* that cleaves the ultra-large von Willebrand factor (vWF) multimers produced by endothelial cells. Some patients with TTP have a deficiency in ADAMTS13, and therefore have a high concentration of the ultra-large vWF multimers. This leads to extensive microvascular platelet deposition with thrombocytopenia and blockage of small vessels. Activity of ADAMTS13 but not antibodies against ADAMTS13 has been associated with relapse of TTP. Although the effectiveness of plasma exchange had been attributed to removal of antibodies against ADAMTS13 and replacement of this critical enzyme, it has also been demonstrated to be useful in patients without a severe deficiency.
  Sadler JE. VWF, ADAMTS13 and TTP. *Blood*. 2008;112:11–18.

91. How is TTP treated?

With plasma exchange, which has radically decreased the mortality rate of this disease. Patients are typically exposed to 11 to 22 units of plasma per day for 1 to 3 weeks with a high number of expected allergic reactions (~66%). Prednisone 1 mg/kg/day is often added as adjuvant and rituximab has been used in refractory cases. Further immunosuppression with cyclosporine or mycophenolate can also be considered.

Reutter JC, Sanders KF, Brecher ME, et al. Incidence of allergic reactions with fresh frozen plasma or cryo-supernatant plasma in the treatment of thrombotic thrombocytopenic purpura. *J Clin Apher.* 2001;16:134–138.

Rock GA, Shumak KH, Buskard NA, et al. Comparison of plasma exchange with plasma infusion in the treatment of thrombotic thrombocytopenic purpura. *N Engl J Med.* 1991;325:393–397.

92. When is it safe to discontinue plasmapheresis in TTP?

When the platelets are above 150×10^9/L for 2 days and the LDH is normal or near normal, **daily** plasma exchanges can be discontinued. Although most centers use some form of taper from pheresis, additional plasma exchanges has the potential theoretical concern of removing both platelets and thrombopoietin.

Scully M, Hunt BJ, Benjamin S, et al. Guidelines on the diagnosis and management of thrombotic thrombocytopenic purpura and other thrombotic microangiopathies. *Br J Haematol.* 2012;158:323–335.

LEUKOCYTES

93. What is the lower limit for the ANC?

1.8×10^9/L (1800/mm^3). African Americans may have a lower mean neutrophil count, which may be encountered during routine examinations; however, they do not have an increased incidence of infections, nor do they have increased severity of infectious diseases. When the neutrophil count is $< 0.5 \times 10^9$/L (500/mm^3), neutropenia is severe, and there is a greater propensity for compromised response to infection.

Grann VR, Ziv E, Joseph CK, et al. Duffy (Fy), DARC, and neutropenia among women from the United States, Europe and the Caribbean. *Br J Haemotol.* 2008;143:288–298.

94. What disorders cause decreased production of neutrophils?

- Drug-induced disorders
- Hematologic diseases: Idiopathic disease, cyclic neutropenia, Chediak-Higashi syndrome, AA, infantile genetic disorders
- Tumor invasion, myelofibrosis
- Nutritional deficiencies: Vitamin B_{12}, folate (especially in alcoholics)
- Infections: Tuberculosis, typhoid fever, brucellosis, tularemia, measles, dengue fever, mononucleosis, malaria, viral hepatitis, leishmaniasis, AIDS

95. Which drugs commonly cause neutropenia?

Cytotoxic chemotherapeutic agents (including alkylating agents and antimetabolites) as well as immunosuppressive drugs are obvious choices, but other drugs such as phenothiazines, antithyroid drugs, or chloramphenicol may cause neutropenia in a dose-dependent fashion by inhibiting cell replication. Immune-related neutropenia may be seen with penicillins, cephalosporins, and other agents. The following list names the drugs with the highest odds ratio for causing drug-induced neutropenia in a descending order: methimazole, pyrithyldione, ticlopidine, calcium dobesilate, sulfasalazine, dipyrone, trimethoprim-sulfamethoxazole.

Tesfa D, Keisu M, Palmblad J. Idiosyncratic drug induced agranulocytosis: possible mechanisms and management. *Am J Hematol.* 2009;84:428–434.

96. Describe the features of lymphocytosis caused by infections.

When infections (usually viral) cause lymphocytosis, the lymphocyte morphologic appearance is unusual or atypical. In EBV infection, B cells are penetrated by the virus, eliciting a polyclonal T-cell response manifested in the peripheral blood as atypical lymphocytosis. Cold agglutinin disease also may occur in EBV infection. The IgM antibodies are usually directed against the i antigen. An acute lymphocytosis may be associated with primary infection with HIV-1, adenovirus, rubella, or herpes simplex II. These disorders are usually self-limited.

97. **What do granulocyte colony-stimulation factor (G-CSF) and vitamin B$_3$ have in common?**

G-CSF binds to its receptor inducing NAMPT (nicotinamide phosphoribosyltransferase) leading to increased NAD (nicotinamide dinucleotide) levels. NAD-dependent sirtuin 1 (SIRT1) then increases transcription of C/EBP transcription factors (CCAAT/enhancer binding protein alpha) thereby inducing proliferation and differentiation. Recent work suggests that vitamin B$_3$ (nicotinamide) can enter the cell and through NAMPT be converted to nicotinamide mononucleotide (NMN). NMN can be converted to NAD with the use of ATP thereby increasing levels of NAD. In a recent pilot protocol, Skokowa and colleagues administered 10–20 mg/kg of vitamin B$_3$ to healthy individuals, showing an increase in the neutrophil counts by day 3 which returned to normal after the vitamin discontinuation.

Skokowa J, Lan D, Kumar Thakur B, et al. NAMPT is essential for the G-CSF induced myeloid differentiation via NAD$^+$-sirtuin-1 dependent pathway. *Nature.* 2009;2:151–158.

MYELOPROLIFERATIVE DISORDERS

98. **What criteria should be present before considering a diagnosis of polycythemia?**
    - Hct > 48% in females, 52% in males or Hb > 16 g/dL in females, 18.5 g/dL in males
    - No hypoxia (Pao$_2$ > 92%)
    - No elevation of erythropoietin

99. **List the major and minor criteria widely used to diagnose PCV.**

PCV diagnosis requires the presence of both major criteria plus one minor criterion or one major criterion and two minor criteria:

Category A (major criteria)
- Increased RBC mass (>25% above normal mean for sex) or Hb > 18.5 g/dL for men, > 16.5 g/dL for women or > 99th percentile of method-specific reference range for age, sex, and altitude of residence
- Presence of JAK2 (janus kinase 2) mutation or other functional similar mutations such as exon 12

Category B (minor criteria)
- Endogenous erythroid colony formation in vitro
- Bone marrow biopsy showing panmyelosis with prominent erythroid and megakaryocytic proliferation
- Low serum erythropoietin level

Tefferi A, Thiele J, Orazi A, et al. Proposals and rationale for revision of the World Health Organization diagnostic criteria for polycythemia vera, essential thrombocythemia, and primary myelofibrosis: recommendations from an ad hoc international expert panel. *Blood.* 2007;110:1092–1097.

100. **What secondary causes of polycythemia must be considered?**

Smoking and genetic disorders. Carboxyhemoglobin should be measured if the patient is a heavy smoker, and in certain families a high-affinity Hb may be identified by determining the P$_{50}$ (oxygen half-saturation pressure). Several kindreds have alterations in the gene for the erythropoietin receptor, resulting in familial erythrocytosis. Mutations in hypoxia-inducing factor alpha have also been identified in a hereditary condition known as *Chuvash polycythemia*. Finally, a neoplasm-producing ectopic erythropoietin also may result in erythrocytosis.

101. **What particular situation warrants the thorough search for an occult myeloproliferative disorder (MPD)?**

Abdominal vein thrombosis (Budd Chiari, portal, mesenteric, or splenic vein thrombosis).

102. **How are patients with PCV risk stratified?**

By age and history. Patients who are older (age > 60 years) or have had thromboembolic events should be considered high risk and may warrant cytoreductive therapy. Although leukocytosis has recently been found to be a potential adverse prognostic factor, similar findings have yet to be confirmed in other studies. Thrombocytosis is **not** a risk factor in PCV.

Bonicelli G, Abdulkarim K, Mounier M, et al. Leucocytosis and thrombosis at diagnosis are associated with poor survival in polycythaemia vera: a population-based study of 327 patients. *Br J Haematol.* 2013;160:251–254.

103. **Once the diagnosis of PCV is established, how are patients treated?**

Initially, with phlebotomy of 500 mL of blood every other day as tolerated until the Hct is reduced to a normal range. In the elderly or those with cardiovascular disease, phlebotomies of 200–300 mL twice a week might be preferred. Treatment of PCV is important because untreated patients are uncomfortable and at risk for life-threatening thrombotic events. Once the target has been reached, maintenance phlebotomies can be scheduled in order to keep the Hct in the desired range.

Di Nisio M, Barbui T, Di Gennaro L, et al. The haematocrit and platelet target in polycythemia vera. *Br J Haematol.* 2007;136:249–259.

Marchioli R, Finazzi G, Specchia G, et al. Cardiovascular events and intensity of treatment in polycythemia vera. *N Engl J Med.* 2013;368:22–33.

104. **What is the role of aspirin in PCV?**

To reduce mortality rate. Low-dose aspirin is recommended in all (both low- and high-risk) PCV patients without history of gastrointestinal bleeding or gastric intolerance.

Landolfi R, Roberto Marchioli, Jack Kutti, et al. Efficacy and safety of low-dose aspirin in polycythemia vera. *N Engl J Med.* 2004;351:114–124.

105. **How are high-risk PCV patients managed?**

By offering cytoreductive therapy. Although there are no hydroxyurea (HU) placebo-controlled randomized trials in PCV, extrapolations from studies in patients with high-risk essential thrombocytemia found HU effective in the prevention of thrombosis and should be considered the drug of choice in high-risk patients. The starting dose of HU is 15–20 mg/kg/day until response is obtained without reducing WBC count to less than 3×10^6/dL.

Cortelazzo S, Finazzi G, Ruggieri M, et al. Hydroxyurea in the treatment of patients with essential thrombocytemia at high risk of thrombosis: a prospective randomized trial. *N Eng J Med.* 1995;332:1132–1136.

106. **How is pruritus from PCV managed?**

With anhistamines. If unsuccessful paroxetine, 20 mg/day, and phototherapy with psoralen and ultraviolet A light (UVA) might be of use. Interferon may be successful as well.

Tefferi A, Fonseca R. Selective serotonin re-uptake inhibitors are effective in the treatment of polycythemia vera-associated pruritus. *Blood.* 2002;99:2627.

107. **How are pregnant patients with PCV managed?**

HU is currently class D (teratogenic and embryotoxic). If PCV patients desire to become pregnant, a wash-out period is mandatory for conception. In **low-risk** pregnancies, the target Hct should be kept below 45% and low-dose aspirin should be given throughout the pregnancy. Low-molecular-weight heparin (LMWH) prophylaxis should be offered in the postpartum period for at least 6 weeks. In **high-risk** pregnancies (either previous thrombotic complications or pregnancy complications), LMWH prophylaxis akin to the one given to antiphospholipid syndrome patients can be offered. Furthermore, if myelosuppression is desired and there are no contraindications, interferon should be considered.

108. **How is chronic phase chronic myeloid leukemia (CML) treated?**

With tyrosine kinase inhibitor (TKI), one of most successful treatments ever conducted in cancer. CML patients may need to continue TKI indefinitely. Nilotinib, dasatinib, and bosutinib can produce higher rates of deeper molecular responses but overall survival rate is generally the same (>90%).

Kalmanti L, Saussele S, Lauseker M, et al. Safety and efficacy of imatinib in CML over a period of 10 years: data from the randomized CLM-study IV. *J Clin Oncol.* 2014;32:415–442.

109. **What are the definitions of response in CML?**

- **Complete hematologic response** (CHR): WBC count $< 10 \times 10^6$/dL, with no immature granulocytes, less than 5% basophils, platelets $< 450 \times 10^6$/dL, and a nonpalpable spleen
- **Complete cytogenetic response** (CCgR): No Philadelphia positive (Ph+) metaphases
- **Partial cytogenetic response** (PCgR): 1–35% Ph+ metaphases
- **Minor cytogenetic response** (mCgR): 36–65% Ph+ metaphases
- **Minimal cytogenetic response** (minCgR): 66–94% Ph+ metaphases
- **No cytogenetic response** (NoCgR): >95% Ph+ metaphases
- **A major molecular response** (MMolR): BCR/ABL transcripts of $< 0.1\%$ on the international scale (IS, also known as 3-log reduction)
- **Complete molecular response** (CMolR): Undetectable BCR/ABL transcript by quantitative PCR

110. What are the warning signs of treatment failure in chronic-phase CML?
High risk at baseline according to the Sokal score or other chromosomal abnormalities in Ph+ cells at baseline or detected at any time through treatment, less than a MMolR at **12 months**, or rise in the transcript levels. Data from multiple trials show that a rapid decline of BCR/ABL transcripts in peripheral blood at 3 (<10% IS) or 6 months (<1% IS) correlates with subsequent MMolR and better overall survival.

Hanfstein B, Muller MC, Hochhaus A. Response-related predictors of survival in CML. *Ann Hematol.* 2015;94:227–239.

111. What are the criteria for treatment failure with frontline TKIs?
- No CHR and/or Ph+ > 95% at 3 months
- BCR/ABL > 10% IS and/or Ph > 35% at 6 months
- BCR/ABL > 1% and/or Ph+ detectable at 12 months
- Loss of hematologic response, cytogenetic response, or new mutations at any given point in time
- Loss of MMolR in consecutive samples

Baccarani M, Deininger MW, Rosti G, et al. European LeukemiaNet recommendations for the management of CML. *Blood.* 2013;122:872–884.

112. What are the warnings of a suboptimal response?
- BCR/ABL > 10% and/or Ph 35–95% at 3 months
- BCR/ABL 1–10% and/or Ph 1–35% at 6 months
- BCR/ABL 0.1–1% at 12 months
- Clonal chromosomal abnormalities (Ph−, −7, or del7q)

Alvarado Y, Kantarjian H, O'Brien S, et al. Significance of suboptimal response to imatinib, as defined by the European LeukemiaNet, in the long-term outcome of patients with early chronic myeloid leukemia in chronic phase. *Cancer.* 2009;115:3709–3718.

113. Is a bone marrow biopsy needed at diagnosis?
Yes, to identify other potential cytogenetic defects.

114. How are patients followed?
With real-time quantitative polymerase chain reaction (qPCR) for BCR/ABL every 3 months until an MMolR has been achieved and every 3 to 6 months thereafter. This test should be done in a laboratory that reports transcripts in IS.

O'Brien S, Radich JP, Abboud CN, et al. CML, version 1.2015. *J Natl Compr Canc Netw.* 2014;12:1590–1610.

115. When should a mutation analysis be ordered?
In the presence of consistent raise in BCR/ABL transcripts. Point mutations in the BCR/ABL gene have been shown to be associated with certain responses to TKIs. For example, T315I or E255V mutations are refractory to imatinib. A mutation analysis may also help in choosing the second line of therapy. Very sensitive tests may pick up clinically irrelevant signals. Compound mutations (two or more mutations in the same gene) can confer resistance to all currently approved TKIs.

O'Hare T, Zabriskie MS, Eiring AM, et al. Pushing the limits of targeted therapy in CML. *Nat Rev Cancer.* 2012;12:513–526.

116. Describe the clinical features of accelerated CML and CML blast phase.
Accelerated CML: 10–19% blasts in the peripheral blood or bone marrow, peripheral basophilia > 20%, persistent thrombocytopenia (<100 × 10^6/dL) unrelated to therapy or persistent thrombocytosis (>1000 × 10^6/dL) unresponsive to therapy, increasing spleen size or WBC count unresponsive to therapy or cytogenetic evidence of clonal evolution.
CML blast phase: 20% or more blasts in the peripheral blood or bone marrow or by the presence of extramedullary blast cell disease. In most chemotherapy studies, the criterion was 30% or more blasts.

Swerdlow SH, Campo E, Harris NL, et al. *World Health Organization Classification of Tumours of Haematopoietic and Lymphoid Tissues.* Lyon: IARC Press; 2008.

117. How is CML in blast crisis treated?
With imatinib at higher doses (600 mg/day) or dasatinib. AML induction chemotherapy with another TKI is also a possible option. After blast crisis has been diagnosed, the patient should be considered for bone marrow transplant.

Palandri F, Castagnetti F, Testoni N, et al. Chronic myeloid leukemia in blast crisis treated with imatinib 600mg: outcome of the patients alive after a 6 year follow-up. *Haematologica.* 2008;93:1792–1796.

118. **How is imatinib metabolized, and why is it important?**
Through cytochrome P450 (CYP450). Inhibitors such as clarithromycin and grape juice and fruit may increase imatinib levels, whereas inducers such as dexamethasone and St. John's wort may decrease them.

119. **How do nilotinib and dasatinib toxicities differ in general?**
Nilotinib can cause corrected QT interval (QTc) prolongation and an increase in amylase and lipase. Electrolytes monitoring is recommended. Dasatinib is known to cause fluid retention and pleural/pericardial effusions. Daily dosing (100 mg daily) is recommended. In the event of an effusion, a short course of steroids with further dose modification is recommended.

120. **Patients presenting with large spleens, fibrotic marrows, and teardrop-shaped erythrocytes on the peripheral blood film have what MPD?**
Idiopathic myelofibrosis (IMF), a myeloproliferative disease with a leukoerythroblastic blood picture. Extramedullary hematopoiesis is usually present in the liver and spleen. Patients may have neutrophilia, thrombocytosis, and anemia, but other patients, typically with massively enlarged spleens, may be cytopenic instead. Patients with enlarged spleens and neutrophilia resemble patients with CML. Determination of the presence of Ph chromosome may distinguish the two.

121. **How is IMF risk stratified?**
Several models have been proposed which include the severity of cytopenias, constitutional symptoms, and blast percentage. The most widely used model is the DIPSS-plus which stratifies patients into four risk groups with a median survival of 185, 78, 35, and 16 months. Most recently two genetic enhanced scores have been proposed (GPSS and MIPSS).
Ganga N, Caramazza D, Vaidya R, et al. DIPSS plus: a refined DIPSS for primary myelofibrosis that incorporates prognostic information from karyotype, platelet count and transfusion status. *J Clin Oncol.* 2011;29:392–339.

122. **How is myelofibrosis treated?**
With **allogeneic bone marrow transplant,** currently the only treatment that might offer the potential for cure. Other treatment modalities are palliative and include splenectomy, thalidomide, lenalidomide, pomalidomide, ruxolitinib, epigenetic modifiers (panobinostat, azacitidine), androgens, and hydroxyurea. **JAK2 inhibitors** (ruxolitinib, pacritinib, and momelotinib) have been very successful in reducing splenomegaly and ameliorating disease-related symptoms. **Telomerase inhibitors** (imetelstat) were found to be active in IMF but with the potential of significant myelosuppression.
Tefferi A, Lasho TL, Begna KH, et al. A pilot study for the telomerase inhibitor imetelstat for myelofibrosis. *N Engl J Med.* 2015;373:908–919.

123. **A patient without massive splenomegaly has a platelet count above 1,000,000/mL ("platelet millionaires"). What myeloproliferative disease may be present?**
Severe **iron deficiency** with concurrent hemorrhage or inflammatory disease have platelet counts > 1,000,000/mL. Once iron deficiency is corrected or the inflammatory disorder resolves, platelet counts return to normal levels. Another MPD, **essential thrombocythemia (ET),** should be considered when the platelet count rises above 600,000/mL.

124. **What are the signs and symptoms of ET?**
Modest splenic enlargement and purpura and, if platelets are high enough, hemorrhage due to acquired von Willebrand deficiency. Purpura, epistaxis, and gingival bleeding are typical manifestations that can be exacerbated by aspirin. Erythromelalgia is characterized by a localized burning pain and warmth of the distal extremities and is dramatically relieved with small doses of aspirin. Neurologic manifestations include dizziness, seizures, and transient ischemic attacks.
Chiusolo P, La Barbera EO, Laurenti L, et al. Clonal hematopoiesis and risk of thrombosis in young female patients with essential thrombocytemia. *Exp Hematol.* 2001;29:670–676.

Lambert JR, Everington T, Linch DC, et al. In essential thrombocytemia, multiple JAK2-V617F clones are present in most mutant-positive patients: a new disease paradigm. *Blood.* 2009;114:3018–3023.

125. What are the criteria for ET?
    - Sustained platelet count > 450×10^9/L
    - Bone marrow biopsy specimen showing proliferation mainly of the megakaryocytic lineage with increased numbers of enlarged, mature megakaryocytes; no significant increase or left-shift of neutrophil granulopoiesis or erythropoiesis
    - Not meeting WHO criteria for other MPD or myeloid neoplasm
    - Demonstration of JAK2 617V>F or other clonal marker, or in the absence of a clonal marker, no evidence for reactive thrombocytosis

    Rumi E, Pietra D, Ferretti V, et al. JAK2 or CALR mutation status defines subtypes of essential thrombocythemia with substantially different clinical course and outcomes. *Blood.* 2014;123:1544–1551.

126. List the causes of thrombocytosis.
    - Reactive disease
    - MPDs
    - Malignancy
    - ET
    - Iron deficiency
    - PCV
    - Splenectomy
    - CML (Ph[1]+)
    - Inflammatory bowel disease
    - Myelofibrosis
    - Infection
    - Collagen vascular diseases
    - MDS

127. What is the most likely complication in a patient with a myeloproliferative disease who presents with a swollen, hot ankle?
    Gout. Patients with myeloproliferative syndromes (PCV, CML, myelofibrosis, ET) may develop hyperuricemia. Thus, arthritis in such patients should be investigated thoroughly, including arthrocentesis and examination for intracellular, negatively birefringent crystals under polarized light.

128. What is the long-term outcome of patients with essential thrombocytemia?
    Although it is generally safe to observe low-risk patients, long-term follow-up suggests that even after an uneventful first decade the mortality rate is worse when compared to their normal counterparts. In high-risk patients, despite cytoreductive therapy and appropriate management, there is a small but very important potential of transformation into an acute leukemia, and an approximate 10% risk of venous thromboembolic events at 10 years.

    Montanaro M, Latagliata R, Cedrone M, et al. Thrombosis and survival in essential thrombocythemia: a regional study of 1,144 patients. *Am J Hematol.* 2014;89:542–546.

MYELODYSPLASTIC SYNDROMES

129. What is SF3B1, and why is it important?
    A distinct gene expression pattern associated with ringed sideroblasts. Patients with ringed sideroblasts but not meeting the 15% threshold to be classified as refractory anemia with ringed sideroblasts (RARS) will be diagnosed with RARS if an SF3B1 mutation is present and there are at least 5% ringed sideroblasts.

    Patnaik MM, Hanson CA, Sulai NH, et al. Prognostic irrelevance of ring sideroblast percentage in WHO defined MDS without excess blasts. *Blood.* 2012;119:5674–5677.

130. What are the MDSs?
    A group of malignant hematopoietic stem cell disorders characterized by dysplasia, ineffective blood cell synthesis, and an inherent risk of transformation to leukemia.

131. What is ICUS?
    Idiopathic cytopenia of undetermined significance designed to describe patients in whom MDS is possible but not proved. Clonality is not necessary for the diagnosis.

132. **What is CHIP?**
Clonal hematopoiesis of indetermined potential identifies a group of people at risk of developing hematologic malignancies. Hence, CHIP would be to hematologic cancers what MGUS is to myeloma.

133. **Why is a karyotype essential?**
Because an abnormal chromosome abnormality supports clonality. Specific abnormalities are diagnostic of MDS in cases with subtle morphologic changes (e.g., 5q−, monosomy 7).

ACUTE MYELOGENOUS LEUKEMIA (AML)

134. **What are the symptoms of leukostasis?**
Dyspnea, limitation in activity, tinnitus, headache, dizziness, visual disturbances, confusion, priapism, cardiac ischemia, ischemic necrosis, and strokes. Patients with AML and WBC count > 100,000/dL or > 50,000/dL and symptoms of leukostasis should undergo leukapheresis.
Novotny JR, Müller-Beissenhirtz H, Herget-Rosenthal S, et al. Grading symptoms in hyperleukocytocytic leukaemia: a clinical model for the role of different blast types and promyelocytes in the development of leukostasis syndrome. *Eur J Haematol.* 2005;74:501–510.

135. **How is AML diagnosed?**
When a cellular bone marrow aspirate shows blasts representing >20% of all nucleated WBCs. If erythroblasts comprise >50% of the nucleated bone marrow cells, erythroleukemia (M6) is present. If the marrow is cellular but blasts account for <20% of the nucleated RBCs, myelodysplasia is present. For acute megakaryoblastic leukemia (M7), at least 50% of the blasts should be of megarkaryocytic lineage (CD41, CD61).

136. **What are the subgroups of AML, and how has this changed?**
The original French-American-British (FAB) classification has been supplanted by the newer WHO schema. The WHO classification takes into account cytogenetics, in addition to therapy-related leukemia or leukemia arising from MDS. There are four main groups in the new classification: (1) AML with recurrent genetic abnormalities; (2) AML with MDS-related features; (3) therapy-related AML; and (4) AML not otherwise specified.
Walter RB, Othus M, Burnett AK, et al. Significance of FAB subclassification of "acute myeloid leukemia, NOS" in the 2008 WHO classification: analysis of 5848 newly diagnosed patients. *Blood.* 2013;121:2424–2431.

137. **What are the different risk groups in AML?**
At least 90% of patients with AML have cytogenetic abnormalities. Older adults have a worse prognosis. The age cut-off defining the older population varies through different studies between 55 and 60 years old. Prior myelodysplastic disorders or MPDs confer a worse prognosis.
The European Leukemia Net Classification has four groups:
1. Favorable
   a. Core binding factors (CBF) – t(8;21) RUNX1-RUNX1T1 or inv(16) or t(6;16) CBFB-MYH11
   b. Mutated NPM1 without FLT3-ITD (normal karyotype)
   c. Mutated CEBPA (normal karyotype)
2. Intermediate – 1
   a. Mutated NPM1 and FLT3-ITD (normal karyotype)
   b. Wild type NPM1 and FLT3-ITD (normal karyotype)
   c. Wild type NPM1 without NPM1 (normal karyotype)
3. Intermediate – 2
   a. Trisomy 8
   b. Trisomy 21
   c. Diploid karyotype
   d. −Y
4. Poor risk
   a. Del 5q
   b. Del 7q
   c. Inv(3p) or t(3;3) RPN1-EVI1
   d. Complex (over three aberrations)
   e. t(v;11)(v;q23) MLL rearranged
   f. t(6;9) DEK-NUP214

Mrózek K, Marcucci G, Nicolet DJ, et al. Prognostic significance of the European LeukemiaNet standardized system for reporting cytogenetic and molecular alterations in adults with acute myeloid leukemia. *J Clin Oncol.* 2012;30:4515–4523.

138. How can patients with normal karyotype be further subdivided?

Up to 50% of patients with normal karyotypes have identifiable genomic abnormalities. Mutant NPM1 (nucleophosmin) without FLT3-ITD and mutant CEBPA confer the best prognosis within this subgroup. Other genotypes (FLT3-ITD;MLL-PTD) confer a worse prognosis. IDH2 mutations appear to confer a better prognosis. ASXL1 and ASXL2 denote a worse prognosis. DNMT3A appears to have a worse prognosis as well.

Grossmann V, Schnittger S, Kohlmann A, et al. A novel hierarchical prognostic model of AML solely based on molecular mutations. *Blood.* 2012;120:2963–2972.

139. How is AML treated?

Little has changed in the past decades with regard to the treatment of AML. Standard induction chemotherapy with 7 + 3 (Ara-C × 7 days and anthracycline × 3 days) brings remissions in 70–80% of adults under the age of 60 and 40–50% in adults over the age of 60. Consolidation therapy is typically offered with two to three courses of either high-dose Ara-C (HDAC) or 5 + 2 (Ara-C × 5 days and anthracycline × 2 days).

Burnett AK, Russell NH, Hills RK, et al. A randomized comparison of daunorubicin 90 mg/m^2 vs 60 mg/m^2 in AML induction: results from the UK NCRI AML17 trial in 1206 patients. *Blood.* 2015;125:3878–3885.

140. Is there a role for growth factors in the treatment of AML?

No. A meta-analysis has failed to reveal any benefit or harm from G-CSF use after induction chemotherapy.

Wheatley K, Goldstone AH, Littlewood T, et al. Randomized placebo controlled trial of granulocyte colony stimulating factor as supportive care after induction chemotherapy in patients with acute myeloid leukemia: a study of the United Kingdom Medical Research Council Adult Leukaemia Working Party. *Br J Haematol.* 2009;146:54–63.

141. How does acute promyelocytic leukemia (APL) present?

With lower WBC counts than other AML subtypes and possibly a normal count when first examined. Careful attention to the morphologic appearance of the circulating WBCs discloses the presence of the hypergranular blasts or blasts with multiple Auer rods. Less frequently the blasts are hypogranular. A significant hemorrhagic diathesis may complicate either the presentation or the treatment of APL with standard AML chemotherapy. A picture resembling DIC is characteristic and may be accompanied by central nervous system (CNS) bleeding, which is sometimes fatal. Patients may require intensive support with platelets, fresh frozen plasma, and cryoprecipitate.

142. How is APL treated?

With induction chemotherapy with all-trans retinoic acid (ATRA) and an anthracycline. It should not be modified based on the presence of poor prognosis characteristics (e.g., secondary chromosome abnormalities, FLT3, CD56). Consolidation chemotherapy with two to three courses is considered standard. ATRA/ATO (arsenic trioxide) without concomitant conventional chemotherapy can be as effective.

Burnett AK, Russell NH, Hills RK, et al. Arsenic trioxide and all-trans retinoic acid treatment for acute promyelocytic leukaemia in all risk groups (AML17): results of a randomised, controlled, phase 3 trial. *Lancet Oncol.* 2015;16:1295–1305.

143. What is the APL differentiation syndrome?

Symptoms of dyspnea, unexplained fever, weight gain, peripheral edema, hypotension, acute renal failure, or congestive heart failure in patients treated with either ATRA or ATO. Prompt treatment with dexamethasone 10 mg IV twice daily should be started, but ATRA or ATO should be discontinued only in the severe cases.

Montesinos P, Bergua JM, Vellenga E, et al. Differentiation syndrome in patients with acute promyelocytic leukemia treated with all-trans retinoic acid and anthracycline chemotherapy: characteristics, outcome, and prognostic factors. *Blood.* 2009;113(4):775–783.

144. How are neutropenic infections treated?

The selection of initial antibiotic therapy must take into account the type, frequency of occurrence, and antibiotic susceptibility of the local hospital-acquired infections. Although as per guidelines patients with low-risk neutropenic infections can be managed with oral antibiotics, this requires vigilant observation and prompt access to appropriate medical care 24 hours per day, 7 days per week. In practice, unless strict criteria can be met, patients are treated as inpatients with broad coverage as per Infectious Diseases Society of America guidelines. Vancomycin is not generally recommended initially unless the hospital has a local flora of drug-resistant *Streptococci viridans*, clinically suspected serious catheter-related infection, or known colonization with methicillin-resistant *Staphylococcus aureus* (MRSA), or the patient has blood cultures with gram-positive cocci, hemodynamic instability, severe mucositis, fever > 40° C, or has had quinolone prophylaxis. If patients remain febrile after 5 days of broad-spectrum antibiotics, addition of antifungals is recommended.

Freifeld AG, Bow EJ, Sepkowitz KA, et al. Clinical practice guideline for the use of antimicrobial agents in neutropenic patients with cancer: 2010 update by the Infectious Diseases Society of America. *Clin Infect Dis*. 2011;52:e56–e93.

145. **What are the indications of removal of an indwelling cathether in patients with neutropenic fever?**
Evidence of a subcutaneous infection, septic emboli, hypotension associated with catheter, or a nonfunctioning catheter. Prompt cathether removal should also be strongly considered if there is documented bacteremia with *Bacillus* sp., *Pseudomonas aeruginosa*, *Stenotrophomonas maltophila*, *Corynebacterium jeikeium*, vancomycin-resistant *Enterococcus* (VRE), or fungemia due to *Candida*.

Mermel LA, Farr BM, Sheretz RJ, et al: Guidelines for the management of intravascular cathether-related infection. *Clin Infect Dis*. 2001;32:1249–1272.

146. **What is the galactomannan test?**
Measurement of an *Aspergillus* specific antigen (galactomannan, GM) that is released in the bloodstream by fungal hyphae during growth. The *Aspergillus* GM index correlates with survival, autopsy findings, and response outcome.

Maertens J, Buvé K, Theunissen K, et al. Galactomannan serves as surrogate endpoint for outcome of pulmonary invasive aspergillosis in neutropenic hematology patients. *Cancer*. 2009;115:355–362.

147. **What is the difference between galactomannan and the Fungitell assay?**
The Fungitell assay is positive in many fungal infections and is not specific for *Aspergillus*, but measures beta-D-glucan, a cell wall component of many fungi. The Fungitell assay is used for the diagnosis of invasive fungal infections but does not detect *Cryptococcus* and Zygomycetes (*Absidia*, *Mucor*, and *Rhizopus*).

Sulahian A, Porcher R, Bergeron A, et al. Use and limits of (1-3)-β-d-glucan assay (Fungitell), compared to galactomannan determination (Platelia Aspergillus), for diagnosis of invasive aspergillosis. *J Clin Microbiol*. 2014;52:2328–2333.

ACUTE LYMPHOBLASTIC LEUKEMIA (ALL)

148. **In what three main categories can ALL be subdivided according to the therapeutic implications?**
T cell, mature B cell, and B-cell precursor phenotypes.

149. **How does myeloid-associated antigen expression affect the prognosis or treatment of ALL?**
Not at all. Patients with myeloid-associated antigen expression should be treated with ALL protocols. Aberrant expression can be detected by flow cytometry and used to differentiate these cells from normal progenitors, thereby becoming useful in the detection of minimal residual disease.

150. **How is molecular remission defined?**
Disease below the detection of PCR (generally 1×10^4 cells or 1 blast in 10,000 normal cells).

151. **What are the indicators of a poor prognosis in adults with ALL?**
- In B-cell ALL, WBC count > 50,000/dL; in T-cell ALL, WBC count > 100,000/dL
- Extreme leukocytosis (>400,000/dL) increases the risk of leukostasis (CNS hemorrhage, pulmonary and neurologic complications) and requires leukapheresis.
- Age > 35
- T-cell or mature B-cell phenotype
- Delayed time to complete response (i.e., resistance to induction chemotherapy)

- Persistence of minimal resistant disease (MRD)
- IKZF1 deletions (Ikaros transcription factor)
- p210 fusion transcript (b3a2 and or b2a2), as opposed to p190 (which would be better)
- High-risk cytogenetics
  - t(9;22): Philadelphia chromosome
  - t (4;11) MLL translocation or other 11q23 translocation
  - Hypodiploidy (<45 chromosomes)
  - Balanced t(1;19)

DeBoer R, Mulkey F, Koval G, et al. Clinical impact of ABL1 kinase and IKZF1 mutations in adults with Ph+ ALL: CALGB10001 and 9665. *Haematologica*. 2015;100:392–399.

152. **How does testing for Philadelphia chromosome affect treatment of ALL?**
Adult patients with Ph+ chromosome ALL were considered the subgroup with worst outcome in the past. Since TKI (imatinib, dasatinib, nilotinib, ponatinib) were added to standard treatments the outcomes have changed significantly.

Chiaretti S, Vitale A, Elia L, et al. First results of the multicenter Total Therapy GIMEMA LAL 1509 Protocol for de novo adult Philadelphia chromosome positive ALL. *Blood*. 2014;124:797.

153. **How is ALL treated?**
There are several complex regimens that have been studied. Familiarity with the choice of protocol is the most important factor to consider when deciding upon a therapy.
- **Induction chemotherapy:** Options include CALGB roadmap, the Berlin-Frankfurt-Munster regimen, Hyper-CVAD, and GRAAL-2003. CNS prophylaxis is necessary and addition of asparaginase should be considered if Hyper-CVAD is chosen. Dexamethasone has been associated with better outcomes than prednisone.
- **Antibody conjugate protocols:** Under development.
- **After a complete response:** Choice of consolidation chemotherapy versus transplantation should be made on an individual basis.
- **Pediatric protocols:** Must be considered for **young patients.**

154. **What test should be sent if a patient has hematologic toxicity out of proportion to the expected side effects?**
Thiopurine methyltransferase. This enzyme catalyses *S*-methylation of thiopurines (mercaptopurine and thioguanine).

Relling MV, Pui CH, Cheng C, et al. Thiopurine methyltransferase in acute lymphoblastic leukemia. *Blood*. 2006;107:843–844.

155. **What is adoptive immunotherapy?**
Treatment using T cells expressing chimeric antigen receptors (CARs) or modified T-cell receptor (TCR) genes have been under development for the past years. CD19-directed CAR-T cells have shown very high remission rates in ALL.

Maude SL, Frey N, Shaw PA, et al. Chimeric antigen receptor T cells for sustained remissions in leukemia. *N Engl J Med*. 2014;371:1507–1517.

LYMPHOPROLIFERATIVE DISEASE

156. **What is the most common leukemia of adults?**
Chronic lymphocytic leukemia (CLL), a neoplastic growth of lymphocytes, most often B lymphocytes. Patients are often elderly with lymphadenopathy and splenomegaly. Most patients today are diagnosed only with an elevated WBC count, composed of lymphocytes with a normal morphologic appearance (Rai 0).

157. **List the diagnostic criteria for CLL.**
- Sustained lymphocyte count > 5×10^9/L for at least 3 months with "typical" morphologic features, but a lymphoproliferative bone marrow infiltration makes the diagnosis, *irrespective* of the lymphocyte count.
- B-cell immunophenotypes: Typically weak expression of membrane immunoglobulin, CD 20, expression of the T-cell antigen CD5.

Hallek M, Cheson B, Catovsky D, et al. Guidelines for the diagnosis and treatment of chronic lymphocytic leukemia: a report from the International Workshop on Chronic Lymphocytic Leukemia updating the National Cancer Institute-Working Group 1996 guidelines. *Blood*. 2008;111:5446–5456.

158. **What is monoclonal B-cell lymphocytosis (MBL)?**
Presence of a monoclonal B-cell population in numbers below 5000/mL with no other features of a lymphoproliferative disorder. Akin to MGUS and its relationship with multiple myeloma, CLL that requires treatment develops in patients with MBL at a rate of 1.1% per year.

Rawson AC, Bennett FL, O'Connor SJM. Monoclonal B cell lymphocytosis and chronic lymphocytic leukemia. *N Engl J Med.* 2008;359:575–583.

159. **What are the two currently used staging systems for CLL, and what other prognostic markers can be used to define prognosis?**
The Rai Staging System (Table 14.3) and the Binet Staging System (Table 14.4).

Table 14.3. Rai Staging System

STAGE	CLINICAL FEATURES	SURVIVAL (MO)
0	Lymphocytosis in blood and bone marrow only	>120
I	Lymphocytosis and enlarged lymph nodes	95
II	Lymphocytosis plus hepatomegaly, splenomegaly, or both	72
III	Lymphocytosis and anemia (hemoglobin < 110 g/L)	30
IV	Lymphocytosis and thrombocytopenia (platelets < 100×10^9/L)	30

Table 14.4. Binet Staging System

STAGE	CLINICAL FEATURES	SURVIVAL (MO)
A	Hemoglobin > 100 g/L; platelets > 100×10^9/L and < 3 areas involved[†]	> 120
B	Hemoglobin > 100 g/L; platelets > 100×10^9/L and > 3 areas involved	61
C	Hemoglobin < 100 g/L or platelets < 100×10^9/L or both (independent of the areas involved)	32

Patients who express a "germinal center" phenotype as defined by **absence of mutation** of the immunoglobulin heavy chain variable region genes (IgV_H genes) have a worse prognosis and more rapid disease course than patients with a post germinal center phenotype and presence of IgV_H gene mutation The presence of a **mutated** IgV_H denotes a **better** prognosis.

Two markers, ZAP-70 and CD38, correlate relatively well to the germinal center phenotype. However, their correlation is not absolute and testing of IgV_H in a laboratory that has standardized the procedure is preferred. Beta$_2$-microglobulin is a predictor of treatment-free survival when adjusted to the glomerular filtration rate. The percentage of smudge cells in the peripheral smear can also correlate with prognosis, although this is operator dependent. Smudge cells that are ≤ 30% denote a 10-year survival rate of 50% vs. 80% in patients with > 30% smudge cells (i.e., **fewer smudge cells are worse**).

Delgado J, Pratt G, Phillips N, et al. Beta2-microglobulin is a better predictor of treatment free survival in patients with chronic lymphocytic leukaemia if adjusted according to glomerular filtration rate. *Br J Haematol.* 2009;145:801–805.

Nowakowski GS, Hoyer JD, Shanafelt TD, et al. Percentage of smudge cells on routine bloods smear predicts survival in CLL. *J Clin Oncol.* 2009;27:1844–1849.

Weinberg JB, Volkheimer AD, Chen Y, et al. Clinical and molecular predictors of disease severity and survival in chronic lymphocytic leukemia. *Am J Hematol.* 2007;82:1063–1070.

160. **How are cytogenetics incorporated into the work-up for CLL?**
  - 17p deletion has the worse prognosis.
  - 11q deletions.
  - Normal karyotype, trisomy 12.
  - The best prognosis is associated with the 13q deletion (contrary to its effect in multiple myeloma). The cytogenetics findings may influence survival.

Bergmann M, Busch R, Eichhorst B, et al. Overall survival in patients with early stage CLL receiving treatment due to progressive disease: follow-up of the CLL1 Trial of the German CLL Study Group. *Blood.* 2013;122:412.

161. **What are the complications of CLL?**
   - Autoimmune phenomena: Warm antibody autoimmune hemolytic anemia, immune thrombocytopenia, neutropenia. *A DAT should be part of all initial work-up for CLL.*
   - Pure RBC aplasia.
   - Hypogammaglobulinemia: *Serum immunoglobulins should be part of all initial work-up for CLL.*
   - Richter syndrome: Transformation into a large cell lymphoma with poor prognosis.
   Rozman C, Montserrat E. Chronic lymphocytic leukemia. *N Engl J Med.* 1995;333:1052–1057.

162. **When is treatment started in CLL?**
   When one of the following is present:
   - Evidence of marrow failure (worsening anemia/thrombocytopenia)
   - Massive splenomegaly (>6 cm below costal margin) or progressive and symptomatic splenomegaly
   - Massive lymphadenopathy (>10 cm) or progressive and symptomatic lymphadenopathy
   - Progressive lymphocytosis with > 50% increase in 2 months or a lymphocyte doubling time of less than 6 months
   - Autoimmune anemia or thrombocytopenia that is poorly responsive to standard treatment (note that autoimmune hemolytic anemia or ITP is **not** an indication of treatment for CLL)
   Furthermore, at least one of the following must be present:
   - Unintentional weight loss (10% in previous 6 months)
   - Fatigue (Eastern Cooperative Oncology Group [ECOG] performance status [PS] 2)
   - Fevers > 100.5° F or 38° C
   - Night sweats of over 1 month in duration without signs of infection
   There is **no** benefit to early treatment prior to the patient becoming symptomatic. To date, prognostic markers (including p53 mutation, 17p, IgV$_H$, and ZAP-70) do **not** change this recommendation.

163. **What is the preferred treatment for CLL?**
   In short, there is none. Treatment should be tailored to the individual patient. Enrollment in a clinical trial or treatment as per National Comprehensive Cancer Network (NCCN) guidelines is recommended. FCR (fludarabine, cyclophosphamide, and rituximab) is considered one of the current standards of care by many authors. However, many patients cannot tolerate FCR. For patients > 65 without 17p–/TP53mut bendamustine/rituximab may be a good alternative. For more unfit patients ofatumumab- or obinutuzumab-based therapies are also appropriate. For patients requiring therapy with 17p–, ibrutinib is preferred. Alemtuzumab and idelalisib are also options.
   Available at: www.nccn.org. Accessed December 17, 2016.
   Goede V, Fischer K, Busch R, et al. Obinutuzumab plus chlorambucil in patients with CLL and coexisting conditions. *N Engl J Med.* 2014;370:1101–1110.

164. **Which lymphoproliferative disorder is associated with pancytopenia, splenomegaly, absence of lymphadenopathy, and circulating lymphoid cells with multiple projections?**
   Hairy cell leukemia (HCL). Although an uncommon malignancy (i.e., 2% of all leukemias), HCL receives a great deal of attention because of advances in treatment and the unusual infections observed in the course of the disease. HCL is an important consideration in the work-up of patients who present with pancytopenia. Some patients have presented with aplasia.

165. **How is HCL diagnosed?**
   Through bone marrow biopsy. Although often scanty, characteristic "hairy lymphs" may be observed. The biopsy may show a diffusely involved marrow with mononuclear cells situated in a network of fibrosis. Although hairy cells may be present in the marrow, the biopsy picture is one of profound hypocellularity. The hairy cell is a B lymphocyte with an immunophenotype consistent with a cell between a CLL-lymphocyte and a plasma cell. Hairy cells also possess the Tac antigen (CD25), a receptor for interleukin 2, usually seen on activated T cells. The distinctive cytochemical feature of the hairy cell is a tartrate-resistant acid phosphatase activity (TRAP). Monocytopenia is frequent. *BRAF* mutations are a disease-defining event in patients with classical HCL who do not express IGVH4-34.

Arcaini L, Zibellini S, Boveri E, et al. The BRAF V600E mutation in hairy cell leukemia and other mature B-cell neoplasms. *Blood*. 2015;119:188–191.

166. **How does the HCL variant differ from classic HCL?**
Patients are older, splenomegaly is less common, and the bone marrow is usually hypercellular with mild myelofibrosis. Circulating hairy cells resemble prolymphocytes and respond poorly to standard therapy. Instead of being strongly positive, CD103 is mildly positive or negative.

167. **How is HCL treated?**
With cladribine. Although initially given at a dose of 0.1 mg/kg/day as a continuous infusion for 7 days, recent trials have demonstrated the same efficacy with 0.14 mg/kg with 2-hour infusions daily × 5 days. Pentostatin and rituximab are possible alternatives.
For relapsed disease with activating *BRAF* mutations, vemurafenib can produce very high responses.
Tiacci E, Park JH, De Carolis L, et al. Targeting mutant BRAF in relapsed or refractory hairy-cell leukemia. *N Engl J Med*. 2015;373:1733–1747.

168. **Describe the manifestations of large granular lymphocyte (LGL) leukemia.**
Highly variable. LGLs can be divided as either T cells (CD3 positive and TCR rearrangement positive) or NK (natural killer) cells (CD3 negative, CD16 positive, and CD 56 positive). The leukemias can be indolent or aggressive. The aggressive variants are treated with ALL regimens while the indolent disease can be watched and treated with oral immunosuppressants after patients become symptomatic (methotrexate, cyclophosphamide, cyclosporine).
Dearden C. Large granular lymphocytic leukaemia pathogenesis and management. *Br J Haematol*. 2011;152:273–283.

HODGKIN AND NON-HODGKIN LYMPHOMAS

169. **What are the common presentations of Hodgkin lymphoma?**
Lymphadenopathy in the neck or axilla. Lymph nodes are nontender, rubbery, and discrete. Sometimes the nodes wax and wane in size until attention is sought. Important symptoms in the staging of Hodgkin lymphoma are fever, weight loss (>10% of body weight), and night sweats. Some patients are troubled by pruritus or flushing after drinking alcohol. Hodgkin lymphoma tends to originate in central lymph nodes, so that some patients present with mediastinal lymphadenopathy.

170. **How is Hodgkin lymphoma staged?**
See Table 14.5.

Table 14.5. Staging of Hodgkin Lymphoma

STAGE	SUBSTAGE	INVOLVEMENT
I	I	Single lymph node
	IE	Single extralymphatic organ
II	II	Lymph nodes on same side of diaphragm
	IIE	With localized extralymphatic site
III	III	Lymph nodes above and below diaphragm
	IIIE	With localized extralymphatic site
	IIIS	With isolated splenic site
	IIISE	With both extralymphatic and splenic sites
IV	IV	Disseminated or diffuse involvement of one or more extralymphatic sites
	IVA	Asymptomatic
	IVB	Fever, sweats, weight loss > 10% body weight

Bulky tumor: single mass 10 cm in largest diameter or mediastinal mass extending one third of the maximum transverse transthoracic diameter measured on a standard posteroanterior chest radiograph at the level of T5–T6.

171. How is early Hodgkin lymphoma staged?
See Table 14.6.

Table 14.6. Staging of Early Hodgkin Lymphoma	
Favorable	Stages I and II with ≤ 3 involved nodal areas, and age < 50 and M/T ratio < 0.33 and ESR < 50 mm/hr without B symptoms or ESR < 30 mm/hr with B symptoms
Unfavorable	Stage II > 4 nodal areas or age > 50 or M/T ratio ≥ 0.33 or ESR ≥ 50 mm/hr without B symptoms or ESR ≥ 30 mm/hr with B symptoms

B symptoms, fever, weight loss, night sweats; ESR, erythrocyte sedimentation rate; M/T, mediastinum/thorax.
From Aisenberg A. The staging and treatment of Hodgkin's disease. *N Engl J Med.* 1978;299:1228.

172. What are the Hasenclaver criteria?
A scoring system developed for advanced Hodgkin lymphoma.
The variables with an adverse prognostic impact are age > 45, male gender, stage IV, Hb < 10.5 g/dL, albumin < 4 g/dL, WBC count > 15 × normal, absolute lymphocyte count < 600/μL (or < 8% in the differential count).

Number of Risk Factors	% of Total	5-YR Freedom From Progression
0	7	84
1	22	77
2	29	67
3	23	60
4	12	51
≥5	7	42

Hasenclaver D, Diehl V. For the International Prognostic Factors Project on Advanced Hodgkin's Disease: A prognostic score to predict tumour control in advanced Hodgkin's Disease. *N Engl J Med.* 1998;339:1506–1514.

173. What is the initial work-up recommended for Hodgkin lymphoma?
- CBC, albumin, serum LDH, erythrocyte sedimentation rate (ESR), HBV, HCV, and HIV
- Computed tomography (CT) scan of neck/thorax/abdomen/pelvis or positron emission tomography (PET)/CT scan
- 2D (two-dimensional) echocardiogram to assess ejection fraction
- Pregnancy test in women of fertile age
- Bone marrow biopsy (unilateral) for patients with bone symptoms or stage III/IV disease and/or blood count abnormalities
- Dental care and thyroid function tests for patients who are candidates for neck radiation therapy
- Reproductive counseling to all patients of fertile age
Brusamolino E, Bacigalupo A, Barosi G, et al. Classical Hodgkin's lymphoma in adults: guidelines of the Italian Society of Hematology, the Italian Society of Experimental Hematology and the Italian Bone Marrow Transplantation on initial work-up, management and follow-up. *Haematologica.* 2009; 94:550–565.

174. What are the histologic subtypes of Hodgkin lymphoma?
In 2008 the WHO changed the name from Hodgkin disease to Hodgkin lymphoma and classified it as follows:
- Nodular lymphocyte predominant classic Hodgkin lymphoma
- Classic Hodgkin lymphoma which is subdivided into
  - Nodular sclerosis
  - Mixed cellularity
  - Lymphocyte-rich
  - Lymphocyte-depleted

175. What is the immunophenotype of Hodgkin lymphoma?
CD15, expressed in the Hodgkin/Reed Sternberg (H/RS) cells in 70–85%, and CD30 and fascin, positive in almost all cases. CD20 can be expressed in H/RS cells in 30–40% of cases with variable intensity.
Schnitzer B. Hodgkin lymphoma. *Hematol Oncol Clin North Am.* 2009;9:747–768.

176. **Which subtypes carry the worst prognosis?**
Lymphocyte depletion, associated with more advanced disease, retroperitoneal involvement, and presentation in older adults. Although staging generally determines the outlook, histologic subtype is also important. Nodular-sclerosing and lymphocyte-predominant subtypes tend to present with limited disease.

177. **What is the treatment for Hodgkin lymphoma?**
For early favorable Hodgkin lymphoma, the options are between two cycles of ABVD (doxorubicin, bleomycin, vinblastine, dacarbazine) and involved field radiation or ABVD for four to six cycles without radiation. The treatment standard for advanced Hodgkin lymphoma has been ABVD for six cycles. Stanford V is most likely equivalent to ABVD but the appropriate application of the radiation component is key. Radiation is usually added as consolidation in patients with bulky disease. In patients with high-risk disease, escalated BEACOPP (ES-BEACOPP [bleomycin, etoposide, doxorubicin, cyclophosphamide, vincristine, procarbazine, and prednisone]) has been shown to improve the overall survival of patients. However, patient selection is critical as ES-BEACOPP has been associated with increased secondary malignancies and infertility. It is in this regard that a risk-adapted approach using response PET after two cycles of chemotherapy has been proposed in order to tailor the chemotherapy to the specific patient.
    Meyer RM, Gospodarowicz MK, Connors JM, et al. ABVD alone versus radiation-based therapy in limited-stage Hodgkin's lymphoma. *N Engl J Med.* 2012;366:399–408.
    Radford J, Illidge T, Counsell N, et al. Results of a trial of PET-directed therapy for early-stage Hodgkin's lymphoma. *N Engl J Med.* 2015;372:1598–1607.

178. **In patients cured of Hodgkin disease, what are the late sequelae of therapy?**
Myelodysplasia, leukemia, and non-Hodgkin lymphoma, occurring 3–10 years after therapy. Certain complications of the radiation are also evident such as radiation pneumonitis pericarditis, pericardial effusions, and pericardial fibrosis. Coronary artery disease may be accelerated. Neurologic effects of irradiation include Lhermitte syndrome (paresthesia produced by flexion of the neck). Hypothyroidism is a frequent sequela of radiation therapy. Patients who received mantle radiation are at risk for breast cancer and in this group, breast MRI screening is recommended.
    Hodgson DC, Grunfeld E, Gunraj N, et al. A population-based study of follow-up care for Hodgkin lymphoma survivors: opportunities to improve surveillance for relapse and late effects. *Cancer.* 2010;116:3417–3425.

179. **How are non-Hodgkin lymphomas subdivided?**
As either B or T cells. B-cell non-Hodgkin lymphoma can be further subdivided into aggressive and indolent. Within the aggressive forms, the most common ones are Burkitt lymphoma, diffuse large B-cell lymphoma (DLBCL), and mantle cell lymphoma. Within the indolent categories the most common disorders are follicular lymphoma (FL), MALT (mucosa-associated lymphoid tissue), and marginal zone lymphomas. Within the non–B-cell lymphomas the most common ones are peripheral T-cell lymphomas, cutaneous T-cell lymphomas, angioimmunoblastic T-cell lymphomas, and NK-cell lymphomas.
    Tomita N, Tokunaka M, Nakamura N, et al. Clinicopathological features of lymphoma/leukemia patients carrying both BCL2 and MYC translocations. *Haematologica.* 2009;94:935–943.

180. **In Africa, Denis P. Burkitt described an aggressive neoplasm that bears his name. What are the salient features of this lymphoma?**
Burkitt lymphoma results from a proliferation of B lymphocytes with a striking appearance, presenting as round or oval cells with abundant basophilic cytoplasm-containing vacuoles that stain positively for fat. The tissue is replaced with a monotonous infiltrate of cells with interspersed macrophages, giving a "starry sky" appearance. When it presents as a leukemia, it is classified as L3 in the FAB scheme. These cells proliferate rapidly and have a potential doubling time of 24 hours, and Burkitt lymphoma is one of the few hematologic emergencies.
    The WHO classification describes two variants: classical and with plasmacytoid differentiation. Both express surface IgM, pan B-cell antigens (CD19, CD20, CD22, and CD79a. The plasmacytoid variant has monotypic cytoplasmic immunoglobulin. A defining feature of Burkitt lymphoma is the presence of a translocation between *c-myc* and the *IgH* gene (t(8;14) in 80% or *IgL* gene (t(2;8) or t(8;22) in the other 20% of cases.

181. **Distinguish the African and American forms of Burkitt lymphoma.**
In African Burkitt lymphoma, patients present with large extranodal tumors of the jaws, abdominal viscera (including kidney), and ovaries and retroperitoneum. In American Burkitt lymphoma, patients present with intra-abdominal tumors arising from the ileocecal region or mesenteric lymph nodes. Bilateral involvement of the breast can be seen in puberty or associated with lactation. In Africa,

the disease is associated with EBV, but this association is less common in American cases. Immunodeficiency-associated Burkitt lymphoma occurs mainly in patients with HIV, although it can also be seen in allograft recipients.

182. **What is the treatment for Burkitt lymphoma?**
Intensive chemotherapy regimens. Akin to ALL, it is important for the treating physician to choose a protocol he or she is comfortable with. Some examples are R CODOX-M/IVAC and R-HyperCVAD.

   Ribrag V, Koscielny S, Bosq J, et al. Rituximab and dose-dense chemotherapy for adults with Burkitt's lymphoma: a randomised, controlled, open-label, phase 3 trial. *Lancet*. 2016;387:2402–2411.

183. **In which patients with DLBCL should a lumbar puncture be performed?**
Those presenting with testicular, epidural, or sinus involvement.

184. **What is the revised International Prognostic Index (R-IPI)?**
The classical International Prognostic Index (IPI) risk factors, used to prognosticate the outcome of patients treated with modern chemotherapy. The risk factors can be remembered with the mnemonic APLES: Age > 60, PS > 2, elevated LDH, >1 Extranodal site, Stage III or IV.

Risk Group	No. of IPI Risk Factors	% of Patients	4-Year PFS	4-Year OS
Very good	0	10	94	94
Good	1–2	45	80	79
Poor	3–5	45	53	55

IPI, International Prognostic Index; PFS, progression-free survival; OS, overall survival.

   Sehn LH, Berry B, Chhanabhai M, et al. The revised International Prognostic Index (R-IPI) is a better predictor than the standard IPI for patients with diffuse large B-cell lymphoma treated with R-CHOP. *Blood*. 2007;109:1857–1861.

185. **What is the importance of the activated B-cell type in DLBCL?**
DLBCL can be subdivided into activated B cell (ABC) and germinal center (GC) types, depending on its cell of origin (COO). The ABC, typically CD10 negative, BCL6 negative, or BCL6 positive but MUM1 positive, is the least curable of DLBCL and is dependent on the constant activation of nuclear factor $\kappa\beta$, mediated in part by the cytoplasmic scaffolding protein CARD11.

   Visco C, Li Y, Xu-Monette ZY, et al. Comprehensive gene expression profiling and IHC studies support application of immunophenotypic algorithm for molecular subtype classification in DLBCL: International DLBCL R-CHOP Consortium Program Study. *Leukemia*. 2012;26:2103–2113.

186. **How is advanced DLBCL treated?**
Our preferred treatment approach outside a clinical trial is R-CHOP (rituximab, cyclophosphamide, doxorubicin, vincristine, prednisone) every 21 days with tumor lysis prophylaxis. If the patient presented with bulky disease we would consider consolidation with radiation. We reassess with imaging after 2–4 cycles. In patients who respond, we complete six cycles of therapy. In patients who have achieved remission and had a poor R-IPI score we would consider a consultation for consideration of autologous stem cell transplantation.

187. **What is a double-HIT lymphoma?**
Typically, cases with a *MYC* translocation in combination with either BCL2 or BCL6 with a poor prognosis and requiring more aggressive regimens (DA-R-EPOCH or R-HyperCVAD/MTX-AraC).

   Swerdlow SH. Diagnosis of "double hit" DLBCL and B-NHL, unclassifiable, with features intermediate between DLBCL and Burkitt lymphoma: when and how, FISH vs IHC. *Hematol Am Soc Hematol Educ Program*. 2014;2014:90–99.

188. **What are the typical characteristics of mantle cell lymphoma (MCL)?**
There are four cytologic variants of MCL: small cell, marginal zone, blastoid, and pleomorphic. Both blastoid (typically with skin involvement) and pleomorphic have a worse prognosis.

   MCL cells are usually CD10 negative, CD5 positive, and CD23 negative. They express IgM or IgD surface immunoglobulins and *cyclin D1 expression* (t(11;14)) can be shown in almost all cases. Gastrointestinal involvement is very frequent and endoscopies are recommended at diagnosis (80% involvement when biopsies from normal appearing mucosa are taken).

189. **What is the MIPI?**
The MCL International Prognostic Index that includes age > 60, performance status > 2, and elevated LDH and WBC count. The calculation of the index (akin to the Sokal score) needs a complex calculation and using available online aids or generation of a spreadsheet is recommended.
Available at: http://bloodref.com/lymphoid/lymphoma/mipi. Accessed December 17, 2016.
Hoster E, Klapper W, Hermine O, et al. Confirmation of the mantle-cell lymphoma International Prognostic Index in randomized trials of the European Mantle-Cell Lymphoma Network. *J Clin Oncol.* 2014;32:1338–1346.

190. **How is MCL treated?**
Off protocol, for transplant-eligible patients we would consider Maxi-CHOP alternative with R-high-dose ara-C followed by ASCT or HyperCVAD. For nontransplant candidates the options are between conventional chemoimmunotherapy (RCHOP, R CVP or BR) followed by rituximab maintenance versus lenalidomide, rituximab, bortezomib, or ibrutinib. Ibrutinib (Bruton tyrosine kinase) inhibitor and other B-cell receptor pathway modulators (PKC β; PI3K; SYK) have been tested and have a role in the relapsed or refractory setting. Caution: the treatment choice should be individualized according to the disease severity (it can be highly variable), comorbid conditions, and best evidence-based medicine at the time of diagnosis.
Abrahamsson A, Albertsson-Lindblad A, Brown PN, et al. Real world data on primary treatment for mantle cell lymphoma: a Nordic Lymphoma Group observational study. *Blood.* 2014;124:1288–1295.
Ruan J, Martin P, Shah B, et al. Lenalidomide plus rituximab as initial treatment for mantle-cell lymphoma. *N Engl J Med.* 2015;373:1835–1844.

191. **How are follicular lymphomas (FLs) graded?**
By the proportion of centroblasts per high-power field into grades I, II, and III.
FLs express CD19, CD20, CD22, and surface immunoglobulin. Translocation 14;18 leading to overexpression of the antiapoptotic protein BCL2 is a hallmark of this lymphoma.
The correct diagnosis of FL requires a complete excisional biopsy. A fine-needle aspiration is not adequate.

192. **When is treatment initiated in FL?**
Treatment recommendations differ. According to the GELF (French) criteria, patients ought to be followed if all of the following are present: maximum diameter of disease < 7 cm, fewer than three nodal sites, no systemic symptoms, spleen < 16 cm on CT, no significant effusions, no risk of local compressive symptoms, no circulating lymphoma cells, and no bone marrow compromise (Hb >10 g/dL, WBC count > 1.5 K/uL, and platelet count > 100 K/uL). On the other hand the BNLI (British) group recommends prompt treatment if any of the following are present: B symptoms (fever, night sweats, weight loss) or pruritus, rapid disease progression, bone marrow compromise (Hb < 10 g/dL, WBC count < 3 as opposed to 1.5, platelet count < 100), life-threatening organ involvement, renal infiltration, or bone lesions.

193. **How can FL be risk stratified?**
Traditionally, by the FLIPI1. Five adverse prognostic factors were identified: age > 60, Ann Arbor stage III or IV, Hb < 12 g/dL, >4 involved nodal areas, and serum LDH greater than the upper limit of normal.

Risk Group	5-Year Overall Survival Rate	10-Year Overall Survival Rate
Low risk (0–1 risk factors)	91%	71%
Intermediate risk (2 risk factors)	78%	51%
High risk (3 or more risk factors)	52%	36%

There has been an update with a new FLIPI2 used the following variable as adverse prognostic factors: elevated beta$_2$-microglobulin, largest lymph node > 6 cm, Hb < 12 g/dL, bone marrow involvement, and age > 60 years.

Risk Group	No. Risk Factors	Patients (%)	5-Year PFS (%)
Low	0	20	79.5
Intermediate	1–2	53	51.2
High	3–5	27	18.8

PSF, progression-free survival.

Federico M, Bellei M, Marcheselli L, et al. Follicular Lymphoma International Prognostic Index 2: a new prognostic index for follicular lymphoma developed by the international follicular lymphoma prognostic factor project. *J Clin Oncol.* 2009;27:4555–4562.

194. How is FL treated?

Individually, taking into account the prognosis, the symptoms, and the patient's priorities.

Treatments can be divided into watchful waiting, "soft" treatments (rituximab as single agent, R-chlorambucil, R-bendamustine, etc.), and "aggressive" treatments (R-CHOP, R-CVP, R-FCM, etc.). When choosing an aggressive regimen we would take into consideration the possibility of rituximab maintenance or radioimmunoconjugates consolidation.

PLASMA CELL DYSCRASIAS

195. How should the discovery of a monoclonal protein (M-protein) be worked up?

With a careful work-up for multiple myeloma (MM). Patients who have a small serum spike (<1.5 g/ dL), normal CBC, no proteinuria, and no lytic lesions, hypercalcemia, or renal dysfunction usually are followed with periodic serum protein electrophoresis. Patients meeting some of the criteria for MM but showing no progression with follow-up are described as having indolent or smoldering MM. Up to 5% of patients in their eighth decade have monoclonal gammopathy of undetermined significance (MGUS).

196. What is the differential diagnosis of an M-protein?

MGUS, MM, solitary plasmacytoma, AL amyloidosis, Waldenström macroglobulinemia (IgM), low-grade lymphoproliferative disorder, and others (cryoglobulinemia, polyneuropathies, etc.).

197. How is the diagnosis of smoldering MM (SMM) made? How does it differ from MGUS and MM?

MGUS can be differentiated from SMM by the lack of an M-spike greater than 3 g/dL, bone marrow plasma cells > 10%, and urinary M-protein < 500 mg/24 hours. The lack of myeloma-related organ or tissue impairment differentiates SMM from MM. MM is also diagnosed (in the absent of related organ damage) when there are > 60% clonal plasma cells in the bone marrow or there is > 1 focal lesions on MRI studies (at least 5 mm), or the uninvolved serum free light chain ratio is > 100 when the involved light chain is > 100 mg/L.

Rajkumar SV, Dimopoulos MA, Palumbo A, et al. International Myeloma Working Group updated criteria for the diagnosis of multiple myeloma. *Lancet Oncol.* 2014;15:e538–548.

198. What are the myeloma defining events (MDEs)?

Hypercalcemia, renal insufficiency attributable to MM, anemia (Hb < 10 g/dL), and lytic bone lesions (CRAB). Osteoporosis with compression fractures, symptomatic hyperviscocity, amyloidosis, recurrent bacterial infections (>2 in 12 months) and peripheral neuropathy alone are NOT considered MDEs.

199. What is the prognosis of MGUS and the predictors of malignant transformation?

The overall risk of malignant transformation in patients with MGUS is around 1% per year. A non-IgG M-protein, serum M-spike > 1.5 g/dL, and an abnormal serum free light chain denote a higher risk of transformation. Patients with none of these risk factors have a 5% chance of transformation at 20 years, whereas patients with 1, 2, and 3 risk factors have a 21%, 37%, and 58% chance of transformation at 20 years, respectively.

Rajkumar SV, Kyle RA, Thernau TM, et al. Serum free light chain is an independent risk factor for progression in monoclonal gammopathy of unknown significance. *Blood.* 2005;106: 812–817.

200. Which patients with MGUS should be referred to a hematologist?

Those with symptoms or physical signs of myeloma, lymphoproliferative disorders, or AL amyloidosis. Furthermore, patients with significant Bence Jones proteinuria (>500 mg/L) or non-IgG M-spike should also be considered for referral.

Bird J, Behrens J, Westin J, et al. UK Myeloma Forum (UKMF) and Nordic Myeloma Study Group (NMSG): guidelines for the investigation of newly detected M-proteins and the management of monoclonal gammopathy of undetermined significance (MGUS). *Brit J Haematol.* 2009;147:22–42.

201. **What are the prognostic factors in MM?**
   The international staging system (ISS) provides a simple and robust classification:
   - **Stage I:** Characterized by a beta$_2$-microglobulin less than 3.5 mg/L plus a serum albumin > 3.5 g/dL; median survival of 62 months
   - **Stage II:** Neither stage I or III; median survival of 44 months
   - **Stage III:** Defined by a beta$_2$-microglobulin > 5.5 mg/L; median survival of 29 months
   Furthermore, t(4;14), t(14;16), t(14;20), deletion 17p13, and deletion 13 have a poor prognosis, whereas t(11;14), t(6;14), or hyperdiploidy denotes a good prognosis.

202. **Is MM curable?**
   No. To date MM is not curable short of an allogeneic stem cell transplant, which is not an early option as it has high mortality and morbidity rates. With current therapies, the survival of myeloma patients is measured in years.

203. **How is MM treated?**
   Although a single standard therapy does not exist, patients are broadly divided in two groups: autologous stem cell transplant (ASCT) eligible and transplant ineligible. Newer approaches that are currently under investigation use maintenance therapies in order to attempt to delay the transplant. Patients with bone disease should receive bisphosphonates.

204. **Describe the clinical manifestations of Waldenström macroglobulinemia.**
   A B-cell disorder of proliferating plasmacytoid lymphocytes that produce an IgM M-protein. Patients frequently have hepatosplenomegaly, lymphadenopathy, and bone marrow involvement. The elderly are affected most often. Neurologic disease, including peripheral neuropathy and cerebellar dysfunction, is also seen. A prominent feature is retinopathy with large sausage-shaped, dilated retinal veins. Bleeding and purpura are also common. Of particular importance is the recognition of hyperviscosity syndrome, which also may occur in MM.
   Varettoni M, Arcaini L, Zibellini S, et al. Prevalence and clinical significance of the MYD88 (L265P) somatic mutation in Waldenstrom's macroglobulinemia and related lymphoid neoplasms. *Blood.* 2013;121:2522–2528.

205. **List the manifestations of the hyperviscosity syndrome.**
   - Global CNS dysfunction and stupor
   - Hypervolemia
   - Congestive heart failure
   - Retinopathy
   - Headache, vertigo, ataxia
   - Retinal hemorrhages
   - Stroke
   - Papilledema
   - Coagulopathy

206. **How is Waldenström macroglobulinemia treated?**
   The choice of treatment varies according to the severity of the disease and the comorbid conditions of the patient. Asymptomatic Waldenström macroglobulinemia should be observed and alkylators should be avoided in patients who are candidates for ASCT. Symptomatic hyperviscosity should be promptly relieved with plasmapheresis, and once the symptoms have resolved, treatment should be instituted. Careful monitoring for hyperviscosity flare (IgM flare) during the initial phase of treatment is needed and prompt pheresis should be readily available.

207. **How do patients with AL amyloidosis present?**
   With purpura from skin involvement, hepatosplenomegaly, macroglossia, orthostatic hypotension, congestive heart failure, malabsorption, nephrotic syndrome, peripheral neuropathy, and carpal tunnel syndrome. Of interest, the consequences of amyloid include an acquired factor X deficiency, resulting in a prolonged PT and PTT and functional hyposplenism. The latter results in the presence of Howell-Jolly bodies, even though the spleen is present.

208. **How is AL amyloidosis treated?**
   We prefer that such patients be treated under investigational protocols. Treatment of AL amyloid has followed that of MM, including melphalan/dexamethasone, thalidomide/dexamethasone, cyclophosphamide/dexamethasone, high-dose melphalan and ASCT, lenalidomide and bortezomib. Patients with cardiac involvement and autonomic dysfunction have poor prognosis, and brain

natriuretic peptide and troponin have been shown to be useful as prognosticators. Diuretics, salt restriction, and beta-blockers or calcium channel blockers can exacerbate the orthostasis, and midodrine might be of help in selected cases. Amiodarone prophylaxis is sometimes used in patients with nonsustained ventricular tachycardias.

Cordes S, Dispenzieri A, Lacy MQ, et al. Ten-year survival after autologous stem cell transplantation for immunoglobulin light chain amyloidosis. *Cancer.* 2012;118:6105–6109.

209. **What is hemophagocytic lymphohistiocytosis (HLH), and how is it diagnosed?**
A syndrome characterized by extreme immune activation, resulting in pathologic inflammation. Diagnosis is based on the criteria established by the HLH-2004 trial:
- A molecular diagnosis consistent with HLH (PRF1, UNC13D, STX11, RAB27A, LYST, and others) **or**
- Five of the following: fever, splenomegaly, cytopenias, hypertriglyceridemia (>265 mg/dL) and/or hypofibrinogenemia (>150 mg/dL), hemophagocytosis, low or absent NK activity, ferritin > 500 ng/mL, elevated soluble CD25 (IL-2 receptor alpha)
- A ferritin > 2000 ng/mL is concerning for HLH and > 10,000 ng/mL is highly suspicious.
Lehmberg K, McClain KL, Janka GE, et al. Determination of an appropriate cut-off value for ferritin in the diagnosis of HLH. *Pediatr Blood Cancer.* 2014;61:2101–2103.

HEMOSTASIS

210. **What are the four basic components of hemostasis?**
- Platelets
- Coagulation factors
- Antithrombotic/fibrinolytic system
- Endothelial cells

211. **How are disorders of platelets categorized?**
As quantitative or qualitative defects.

212. **What are the causes of quantitative defects of platelets?**
- Pseudothrombocytopenia
- Sequestration, usually due to splenomegaly.
- Increased consumption
- Increased destruction
- Secondary to bone marrow hypoproliferation
Thrombocytopenia is a decrease in platelet number, usually <150,000/μL.

213. **What is pseudothrombocytopenia?**
A falsely low platelet count that can occur with blood drawing errors, platelet satellites, or clumping. Platelet satellites occur when WBCs become coated with platelets. The in vitro clumping of platelets is usually caused by agglutination of the platelets by an autoantibody that reacts with the anticoagulant ethylene diamine tetraacetic acid (EDTA). Examination of the peripheral smear and redrawing the CBC in a citrated or heparinized tube will reveal the clumping and the true platelet count, respectively.

214. **What is ITP?**
Immune thrombocytopenic purpura, an autoimmune-mediated disorder in which platelets and megakaryocytes are targeted by platelet specific antibodies, with clearance occurring through the reticuloendothelial system.

215. **How is ITP diagnosed?**
By ruling out all other mechanisms of thrombocytopenia. A thorough history, with attention to medications and family history, is mandatory. Additional laboratory testing is dependent upon the appropriate clinical context (i.e., HIV testing in a patient with risk factors or bone marrow biopsy in an elderly patient with other cytopenias). The recommended initial work-up should include patient history, family history, physical examination, CBC and reticulocyte count, peripheral blood film, quantitative immunoglobulin level (in children), bone marrow examination in selected patients, blood group (Rh), DAT, *Helicobacter pylori* testing, and HIV and HCV testing. Tests that can have potential utility are glycoprotein-specific antibody, antiphospholipid antibodies, antithyroid antibodies and thyroid function, pregnancy test, antinuclear antibodies, and viral PCR for parvovirus and CMV. Only 40–60% of patients have detectable platelet autoantibodies, and testing is not recommended.

Provan D, Stasi R, Newland AC, et al. International consensus report on the investigation and management of primary immune thrombocytopenia. *Blood.* 2010;115:168–186.

216. **How is ITP treated?**

With corticosteroids with or without intravenous immunoglobulin (IVIG). One or two courses of high-dose dexamethasone (40 mg/day × 4 days) has a higher overall response than prednisone. If there is no improvement after 6–12 weeks or a relapse occurs, we consider adding further immunosuppression (rituximab, cyclosporine, mycophenolate). Both rituximab and splenectomy ought to be considered as second-line therapies because both have been associated with durable remissions. Thrombopoietin (TPO) receptor agonists are useful for patients with persistent severe thrombocytopenia after splenectomy and rituximab.

Wei Y, Xue-bin J, Wang Y, et al. High dose dexamethasone vs prednisone for treatment of adult immune thrombocytopenia: a prospective multicenter randomized trial. *Blood.* 2016;127:296–302.

217. **What is TPO, and how would this affect ITP treatment?**

TPO binds to the thrombopoietin receptor, inducing proliferation and differentiation of megakaryocytes, and increases the platelet count. Originally, the thrombocytopenia observed in ITP was thought to result from the peripheral destruction of platelets that outpaced the ability of the bone marrow to produce platelets. However, subsequent studies showed a relative deficiency in TPO levels in patients with ITP.

218. **What are some of the congenital causes of thrombocytopenia?**
- MYH9-associated disorders
- Bernard-Soulier syndrome
- Wiskott-Aldrich syndrome
- Congenital amegakaryocytic thrombocytopenia
- Thrombocytopenia and absent radii

Drachman JG. Inherited thrombocytopenia: when a low platelet count does not mean ITP. Blood 2004;103:390–398.

219. **What are the MYH9-associated disorders?**

Although previously known by a number of eponyms (May-Hegglin anomaly, Fechtner syndrome, Sebastian syndrome, or Epstein syndrome) these disorders are all linked by mutations in the *MYH9* gene, which codes for nonmuscle myosin heavy chain IIA (NMMHC-IIA). They are characterized by the presence of giant platelets on the peripheral blood smear, Döhle-like inclusions within neutrophils, an autosomal dominant pedigree, and a variable degree of sensorineural hearing loss. Recognition of the presence of giant platelets and the familial mode of transmission is important so that patients are not inappropriately diagnosed and treated for ITP.

220. **What are the factors involved in coagulation?**

During the course of the discovery and investigation of the coagulation cascade, a variety of labels and eponyms have been used.

Factor I: Fibrinogen
Factor II: Prothrombin
Factor III: Tissue factor
Factor IV: Calcium
Factor V: Proaccelerin or labile factor. Its deficiency was first characterized in 1943 by Paul Owren and was known as Owren disease or parahemophilia.
Factor VI: None. Factor VI was the original name for activated factor V but has since been discarded.
Factor VII: Stable factor, proconvertin, co-thromboplastin, serum prothrombin conversion accelerator
Factor VIII: Antihemophilic factor (AHF), thromboplastinogen
Factor IX: Christmas factor, plasma thromboplastin component
Factor X: Stuart-Prower factor
Factor XI: Plasma thromboplastin antecedent
Factor XII: Hageman factor
Factor XIII: Fibrin stabilizing factor, Laki-Lorand factor

Although not critical to the clotting cascade, the following factors are of occasional importance in the evaluation of a prolonged activated partial thromboplastin time (aPTT):

Prekallikrein: PK, Fletcher factor
High-molecular-weight kininogen: HMWK, Fitzgerald factor

221. **What is the prothrombin time (PT), and which factors are involved in it?**
PT measures the "extrinsic pathway" and the "common pathway." Within the extrinsic pathway alone are factor VII and tissue factor. The common pathway is composed of factors II, V, and X.

222. **What is the international normalized ratio (INR)?**
INR is a value valid only for patients who are on warfarin therapy, calculated from the ratio of the PT of the patient to a control, raised to the ISI, which is the international sensitivity index. Although the PT may have different values across laboratories, the INR is standardized to give a reproducible value across different laboratories. The ISI is different for each batch of thromboplastin, and each manufacturer compares their thromboplastin against a standardized sample.

$$INR = \left(PT_{patient}/PT_{control}\right)^{ISI}$$

223. **How do you work up an abnormal PT or aPTT?**
Initially with a thorough history and physical examination. In the history, attention must be paid to medications, concomitant medical conditions, previous surgical outcomes with respect to bleeding, use of alcohol, and any family history of bleeding disorders. For female patients, a detailed gynecologic history is crucial, with attention paid to the menstrual cycle. During the physical examination, the location of hemorrhagic stigmata can give a clue as to the underlying defect: mucocutaneous bleeding with von Willebrand disease (vWD) for platelet disorders; hemarthrosis for hemophilia. Finally, the abnormal test result must be compared with an old known value to establish whether this is a new or an old laboratory finding.

224. **Which laboratory tests should be performed next?**
A mixing study, but only after one makes sure that the sample with the abnormal results was not obtained from a line running an anticoagulant or from a patient who is being treated with an anticoagulant or due to some other preanalytic error.

225. **What is a mixing study?**
A procedure during which an aliquot of the patient's plasma is mixed 1:1 with normal plasma, and the PT or aPTT is repeated. If the repeat test gives a "normal" value, then the sample is said to have "corrected," usually implying a factor deficiency. However, if the time remains abnormal, even if the time has improved by a significant amount, then the test is said to have "not corrected," which indicates the presence of an inhibitor. *Note:* For an acquired factor VIII inhibitor, it is not uncommon for the aPTT to correct initially, but then on prolonged incubation, to prolong again.

226. **What are the causes of only an abnormal PT?**
- Congenital: factor VII deficiency
- Acquired
  - Liver dysfunction, causing a decrease in the vitamin K–dependent factors
  - Increased consumption (DIC)
  - Use of vitamin K antagonists
  - Very rare cases of acquired factor VII inhibitors

Note: Initially in liver disease and DIC, the PT will prolong. As the disease increases in severity, the aPTT will also begin to prolong.

227. **What are the causes of an abnormal aPTT?**
Congenital: Deficiencies in factor VIII, IX, XI, or XII; high-molecular-weight kininogen; or prekallikrein, which can be identified by an aPTT that corrects completely upon mixing.
If the repeat mix does not completely correct, an inhibitor is the likely cause of the abnormality. Commonly, this is due to the presence of heparin or a direct thrombin inhibitor. After the absence of such medication is determined, then the history will suggest which course to take next. If the patient has an acquired bleeding history, then a factor VIII inhibitor is likely. Otherwise, if the patient is asymptomatic or has a history of thrombosis, then a lupus anticoagulant (LA) is present. A shortened aPTT is usually due to an increase in an intrinsic pathway factor, most commonly factor VIII.

228. **What are the diseases caused by coagulation factor deficiencies?**
See Table 14.7.

Table 14.7. Coagulation Deficiencies

FACTOR DEFICIENCY	PREVALENCE	INHERITANCE	TREATMENT	NOTES
Fibrinogen	1:1,000,000	Recessive	Fibrinogen concentrates to obtain a level > 100 mg/dL	Higher incidence in consanguineous families
Factor II (prothrombin)	1:2,000,000	Recessive	FFP or prothrombin complex concentrates (PCC)	Complete deficiency (<1%) has not been described
Factor V	1:1,000,000	Recessive	FFP	Check factor VIII levels to make sure not combined deficiency
Factor VII	1:300,000	Recessive	PCC or rFVIIa	Need to evaluate for dietary or environmental variables
Factor VIII	1:5000 live male births	X-linked	Factor VIII concentrates	In women with low factor VIII levels, need to exclude vWD or combined factor V deficiency
Factor IX	1:30,000 live male births	X-linked	Factor IX concentrates	
Factor X	1:1,000,000	Recessive	PCC	Heterozygous factor X deficiency estimated at 1:500, but generally asymptomatic
Factor XI	Variable	Recessive	FFP	Although found in all racial groups, predominantly seen in Ashkenazi Jews
Factor XII	~1%	Recessive	None	Need to exclude LA as cause of deficiency; not considered to be a hemorrhagic state
Factor XIII	1:1,000,000	Recessive	FFP, cryoprecipitate, or factor XIII concentrates	Characterized by umbilical bleeding after birth

FFP, fresh frozen plasma; LA, lupus anticoagulant; rFVIIa, recombinant activated factor VII; vWD, von Willebrand disease.

Patients have been described with mild, moderate, or severe deficiencies of all known clotting factors, except for factor III (tissue factor) and factor IV (calcium).

229. What is the most common inherited hemorrhagic condition?
vWD. First described in 1926 by Professor Erik von Willebrand, who reported on a family with a severe bleeding phenotype that was eventually found to have a severe deficiency of von Willebrand factor (vWF). The index patient, a 14-year-old girl, bled to death after her fourth menses.

230. What does vWF do?
A protein vWF carrier for factor VIII, greatly prolonging half-life of factor VIII. vWF also binds to subendothelial collagen. In this capacity, vWF can then bind to its receptor on platelets, GPIb, to initiate adhesion of platelets to the damaged endothelium (primary hemostasis).

231. How is vWD diagnosed?
Through a thorough history and physical examination, with particular attention paid to mucocutaneous bleeding symptoms (epistaxes, gum bleeding). For women suspected of having vWD, a detailed menstrual history for menorrhagia is mandatory. The basic tests include assays for the total amount of von Willebrand factor antigen (vWF:Ag) and activity of the protein, the von Willebrand ristocetin cofactor assay (vWF:RCo), and multimer analysis. Additional tests include a ristocetin titration and collagen or factor VIII binding assays. Genetic testing is available in specialized centers.

Nichols WL, Rick ME, Ortel TL, et al. Clinical and laboratory diagnosis of von Willebrand disease: a synopsis of the 2008 NHLBI/NIH guidelines. *Am J Hematol.* 2009;84:366–370.

University of Sheffield: von Willebrand factor Variant Database (VWFdb), Available at: www.vwf .group.shef.ac.uk/vwd.html. Accessed November 1, 2016.

232. What are the different types of vWD?
Type 1, type 2 (which includes 2A, 2B, 2M, and 2N), and type 3. Type 1 is the most common and most difficult to diagnose, representing a quantitative deficiency of at least 50% of normal. A distinction must be made between type 1 vWD and merely "low vWF levels."

Type 2 vWD is characterized by qualitative defects. Type 2A is loss of the high-molecular-weight multimers of vWF, which is seen on multimer analysis. There is usually a discrepancy between the vWF:Ag and vWF:RCo, with the vWF:RCo being lower than the vWF:Ag. In **type 2B** a "gain of function" mutation in vWF causes inappropriate binding of vWF under normal conditions. Thrombocytopenia can occur and worsens as the vWF level increases. **Type 2M** is caused by mutations in the GPIb or collagen binding domain in vWF. Although vWF:Ag levels may be normal, the vWF:RCo is decreased, but the multimer assay should be normal, thus distinguishing it from type 2A. In **type 2N** mutations in the factor VIII binding domain of vWF abolish its carrier capacity. Factor VIII levels are then markedly decreased and can be confused with factor VIII deficiency. **Type 3** is the simplest to diagnose. It is defined as almost a complete absence of vWF antigen and activity. It is rare (i.e., 1:1,000,000) and is limited to compound heterozygotes or homozygosity as is seen in consanguinity.

233. What are the hemophilias?
Hemophilia A is factor VIII deficiency and hemophilia B is factor IX deficiency. Factor XI deficiency used to be called hemophilia C.

234. What is a lupus anticoagulant (LA)?
An autoantibody that binds plasma proteins, such as β_2-glycoprotein 1 (β_2-GP1), cardiolipin, or annexin V, that are bound to anionic phospholipids. Although the LA was originally described in 1952 in two patients with SLE who were noted to have a prolonged PT and bleeding symptoms, it was eventually observed that other lupus patients had prolonged aPTTs, and instead of bleeding, this prolonged aPTT was associated with thrombosis.

235. What is the antiphospholipid syndrome (aPS)?
Eventually, the constellation of a prolonged aPTT or the presence of other antiphospholipid antibodies (anticardiolipin antibodies, anti-β_2-GP1) occurring with vascular events, whether thrombosis or recurrent miscarriages. Anti-β_2-GP1 are central to the pathogenesis of APS and potentiate arterial and venous thrombosis. β_2-GP1 is associated with higher risk of thrombosis than anticardiolipin or antiprothrombin antibodies. In order to correctly diagnose aPS, there must be both the clinical and laboratory components present. The clinical requirements are documented thrombotic events or recurrent pregnancy losses. aPS is diagnosed when the laboratory investigation reveals:
1. Prolongation of a phospholipid dependent clotting assay (i.e., aPTT).
2. No aPTT correction with mixing studies.

3. Excess exogenous phospholipids can overcome the inhibition (e.g., platelet neutralization or hexagonal phase phospholipids).
4. The inhibitor is not directed toward a specific clotting factor.
5. Persistence of abnormality ≥ 12 weeks.
   Giannakopoulos B, Passam F, Ioannou, et al. How we diagnose the antiphospholipid syndrome. *Blood.* 2009;113:985–994.

236. What is an acquired factor VIII inhibitor?
A rare development of an autoantibody against a patient's factor VIII, also known as *acquired hemophilia,* occurring in pregnancy, patients with autoimmune disorders, or the elderly. Patients present with minor or even life-threatening hemorrhage, a newly prolonged aPTT that does not correct with mixing, and a low level of factor VIII.

237. What is a Bethesda titer, and why is it important?
The reciprocal of the dilution required to get 50% factor VIII activity. In other words, when the mixing study is performed, serial dilutions are made of the patient's sample (e.g., 1:2, 1:5, 1:10, 1:100, or even greater) in order to overcome the inhibitor. Therefore, if the patient's sample was diluted 1:64 and a factor VIII level of 50% was obtained, the Bethesda titer would be the reciprocal of this dilution (i.e., 64). The absolute value of the Bethesda titer is important, as levels < 5 can be overcome with increased doses of factor VIII. However, a Bethesda titer > 5 will not respond to factor VIII infusions and will require a bypassing agent.

238. What are bypassing agents?
Products that overcome or "bypass" the block in the intrinsic pathway caused by the factor VIII inhibitor. Currently two agents are available: recombinant factor VIIa (rFVIIa) and factor VIII inhibitor bypassing activity (FEIBA). rFVIIa given in pharmacologic doses leads to thrombin generation on the surface of activated platelets. FEIBA is a factor concentrate that is enriched in activated vitamin K–dependent factors.
   Kempton CL, White GC II. How we treat a hemophilia A patient with a factor VIII inhibitor. *Blood.* 2009;113:11–17.

239. What is DIC?
DIC in which all the coagulation factors are consumed and is described as follows: "the circulating plasma is transformed into circulating serum." It is characterized by a microangiopathic hemolytic anemia (as evidenced by the presence of RBC fragments, or schistocytes, on the peripheral blood smear), thrombocytopenia, a prolongation initially of the PT and then the aPTT, and signs of hemorrhage.
   Rodriquez-Erdmann F. Bleeding due to increased intravascular blood coagulation—hemorrhagic syndromes caused by consumption of blood-clotting factors (consumption-coagulopathies). *N Engl J Med.* 1965;273:1370–1378.

240. How can you distinguish among vitamin K deficiency, liver disease, and DIC?
In vitamin K deficiency, the vitamin K–dependent clotting factors (VKDCF) and factors II, VII, IX, and X, along with the anticoagulants protein C and protein S, will be diminished. With liver failure, the other coagulation factors in addition to the VKDCF will be decreased, such as fibrinogen, factor V, and factor XI. Furthermore, antithrombin levels will be low. However, in DIC there is widespread consumption of all coagulation factors, including factor VIII, which is not vitamin K dependent or made in the liver.

241. How is DIC scored?
In patients with an underlying disorder known to be associated with overt DIC a 5-step score can help predict mortality risk.
- Platelet count ($>100 \times 10^9$/L = 0; $< 100 \times 10^9$/L = 1; $< 50 \times 10^9$/L = 2)
- Elevated fibrin marker (e.g., D-dimer, fibrin degradation products) (no increase = 0; moderate increase = 2; strong increase = 3)
- Prolonged PT (<3 s = 0; >3 but <6 s = 1; >6 s = 2)
- Fibrinogen level (>1 g/L = 0; <1 g/L = 1)
   A score ≥ 5 is compatible with overt DIC. For each point in the score the odds ratio for mortality risk was 1.29 (compared to the APACHE II point of 1.07).
   Levi M, Toh CH, Thachil J, et al. Guidelines for the diagnosis and management of disseminated intravascular coagulation. *Br J Haematol.* 2009;145:24–33.

242. What are the naturally occurring anticoagulants?
Antithrombin, protein C, and protein S.

243. What is their mechanism of action?

Antithrombin, particularly when combined with unfractionated heparin, is stimulated to inactivate thrombin and factor Xa. The low-molecular-weight anticoagulants only activate antithrombin's anti-factor Xa activity. Protein C circulates in an inactive form. However, when thrombin combines with thrombomodulin on the intact endothelium, it activates protein C (APC). APC then combines with its cofactor, protein S, to inactive factor Va and factor VIIIa.

244. Is there a thrombotic risk with starting warfarin?

Yes, in select patients. Treatment with warfarin alone can increase the risk for thrombosis. Because protein C and protein S are vitamin K dependent, any deficiency in these anticoagulants, whether congenital or acquired, can be exacerbated with warfarin treatment, leading to potentially disastrous complications of warfarin-induced skin necrosis or gangrene of the limbs. These complications may be avoided by initially treating with an alternative anticoagulant, such as unfractionated heparin, LMWHs, fondaparinux, or direct thrombin inhibitors.

245. How are warfarin bleeding complications managed?

With vitamin K. When given intravenously (slow infusion) the effect of vitamin K starts at about 6 hours (FVII $t_{1/2}$6h). Plasma (FFP) or prothrombin complex concentrates (PCC), when available, are preferred. To raise vitamin K–dependent factors by 50% in a patient presenting with a supratherapeutic INR, a donor plasma volume equal to the patient's own would be needed (8–10 units of donor plasma), which is not feasible. Factor VIIa can be added in the case of severe hemorrhage such as intracranial bleeds.

Sarode R, Matevosyan K, Bhagat R, et al. Rapid warfarin reversal: 3-factor PCC and rFVIIa cocktail for ICH. *J Neurosurg.* 2012;116:491–497.

246. What is the thrombotic risk with heparin?

Surprisingly, use of heparin can create a markedly prothrombotic state, known as *heparin-induced thrombocytopenia* (HIT). In HIT, the unfractionated heparin combines with platelet factor 4 (PF4) and induces a conformational change, which in some people is immunogenic. The resultant IgG combines with the heparin/PF4 complex. This IgG/heparin/PF4 complex can then bind to the Fc_γRIIa on platelets, leading to platelet activation, thrombocytopenia, and thrombin generation. Despite treatment with an anticoagulant (heparin) that results in thrombocytopenia, the risks of HIT are not of hemorrhage but thrombosis. In fact, the risk for thrombosis is increased so greatly that it must be treated.

Arepally GM, Ortel TL. Heparin-induced thrombocytopenia. *N Engl J Med.* 2006;355:809–817.

247. How is HIT treated?

First, it must be recognized. Then, all heparin-containing products, including flushes and heparin-coated catheters, must be discontinued immediately. Subsequent use of LMWH is also contraindicated. A direct thrombin inhibitor is administered until the platelet count normalizes, at which point warfarin is initiated.

Linkins LA, Dans AL, Moores LK, et al. Treatment and prevention of heparin-induced thrombocytopenia: American College of Chest Physicians Evidence-Based Clinical Practice Guidelines (9th Edition). *Chest.* 2012;141:e495S–e530S.

248. What are the causes of activated protein C resistance (APCR)?

The most common cause of APCR is an inherited mutation in the FV gene, wherein a $G \rightarrow A$ substitution at nucleotide 1691 renders FVa resistant to inactivation by the activated protein C/S complex. This mutation is known as *factor V Leiden* (FVL), after Leiden, Netherlands, where it was discovered. Although ~95% of APCR is due to FVL, acquired cases of APCR can be due to elevated factor VIII levels, use of oral contraceptive therapy, lupus, or malignancy.

249. How long can ultrasound (US) abnormalities persist after deep vein thrombosis is treated with anticoagulation? Why is this important?

~80% persist at 3 months and 50% at 1 year after diagnosis. Because the US may not be able to determine whether the clot is new or old, it is NOT useful for determination of ipsilateral recurrent DVT.

Piovella F, Crippa L, Barone M, et al. Normalization rates of compression ultrasonography in patients with a first episode of deep vein thrombosis of the lower limbs: association with recurrence and new thrombosis. *Haematologica.* 2002;87:515–522.

250. **How do we diagnose a pulmonary embolism (PE) in pregnancy?**
Initially with bilateral lower extremity ultrasonography. Guidelines suggest ventilation-perfusion (V/Q scan) if the US scan is negative for deep venous thrombosis (DVT). It should be noted that multidetector CT has lower radiation than a V/Q scan.
The following are approximate fetal radiation doses:

Perfusion 200MBq: 0.2 to 0.6 mSv
Perfusion 40MBq: 0.11 to 0.2 mSv
Ventilation ^{99m}Tc aerosol: 0.1 to 0.3 mSv
Ventilation ^{81m}Kr 600MBq: 0.0001 mSv
CT: 0.13 mSV

Nijkeuter M, Geleijn J, De RA, et al. Diagnosing PE in pregnancy: rationalizing fetal radiation exposure in radiological procedures. *J Thromb Haemost.* 2004;2:1857–1858.

251. **What are the novel oral anticoagulants (NOACs)?**
Dabigatran (direct thrombin inhibitor) and rivaroxaban, apixaban, and edoxaban (direct factor Xa inhibitors) have been shown to be noninferior to warfarin. These agents may reduce major bleeding by 28% and may reduce intracranial and fatal hemorrhage when compared to warfarin by 50%.
Unlike warfarin, NOACs do not require routine laboratory monitoring.
Chai-Adisaksopha C, Crowther M, Isayama T, et al. The impact of bleeding complications in patients receiving target-specific oral anticoagulants. *Blood.* 2014;124:2450–2458.

252. **Can NOACs be reversed?**
Dabigatran can be reversed by idarucizumab, a humanized antibody. Other agents that are currently under study as reversal agents include PCC, activated PCC, and rVIIa. Ciraparantag, which binds via noncovalent bonding to several anticoagulants, is currently being studied with edoxaban. Andexanet alfa is a recombinant factor Xa which is inactive and can bind rivaroxaban, apixaban, betrixaban, and edoxaban.
Dzik WH. Reversal of oral factor Xa inhibitors by PCC: a re-appraisal. *J Thromb Haemost.* 2015;13:S187–S194.

WEBSITES

1. www.hematology.com.
2. www.bloodline.net.
3. www.nccn.org. National Comprehensive Cancer Network (NCCN) provides risk stratification and treatment guidelines for hematologic malignancies.

BIBLIOGRAPHY
1. Greer JP, Arder DA, Glader B, et al., eds. *Wintrobe's Clinical Hematology.* 13th ed. Philadelphia: Lippincott Williams & Wilkins; 2013.
2. Loscalzo J, Schafer AI, eds. *Thrombosis and Hemorrhage.* 3rd ed. Philadelphia: Lippincott Williams & Wilkins; 2002.

ONCOLOGY

*R. Anjali Kumbla, MD, Jeffrey M. Miller, MD, and
Teresa G. Hayes, MD, PhD*

CHAPTER 15

GENERAL ISSUES

1. **Define *carcinogenesis*.**
   The alteration of normal cells into malignant cells via a multistage evolution of genetic and epigenetic changes. The cells can escape the normal checkpoints of their host.

2. **What are the known gene categories that influence the mechanisms of neoplasia?**
   - Oncogenes
   - Tumor suppressor genes
   - Regulators of cell death (apoptosis)
   - Mutation control genes (includes mismatch repair genes)

3. **Describe the effects of oncogenes.**
   Oncogenes in humans and other animals have the capacity to transform normal cells into malignant ones. Mutations convert proto-oncogenes to oncogenes by amplification, translocation, and point mutation. These altered genes, acquired at conception or mutated during life, make the patient susceptible to cancer by altering or impairing several processes:
   - Production of nuclear transcription factors that control cell growth (e.g., *myc*)
   - Signal transduction within cells (e.g., *ras*)
   - Interaction of growth factors and their receptors (e.g., *her/neu*)
     More than 100 different oncogenes have been identified, but only some have been associated exclusively with human cancers.

4. **How do tumor suppressor genes affect carcinogenesis?**
   When functioning normally, tumor suppressor genes regulate the growth and division of cells. When mutations occur in both alleles of these genes, cellular regulatory function is lost and tumor growth can occur. Multiple tumor suppressor genes have been identified (e.g., *p53* and *rb*) and are found in many different types of cancers. These mutations are the basis of the inherited predispositions to cancers.

5. **How is cell death regulated?**
   Cell death genes are involved in the programmed death (**apoptosis**) of cells no longer needed by the body. Mutation in one of these genes (e.g., *bcl-2*) allows cells to live that should have died, causing excessive accumulation of cells. Activation of the **telomerase** gene, which controls cell senescence, is thought to cause cells to become immortal by turning off the normal aging process. Mutations in the telomerase gene are associated with diseases such as dyskeratosis congenita notable for bone marrow failure, nail dystrophy, leukoplakia, and abnormal skin pigmentation.

6. **What are mutation control genes?**
   Mismatch repair genes such as *hMSH2* and *hMLH1* that are responsible for ensuring the fidelity of the DNA duplication process. Microsatellite instability results from the faulty DNA editing process. Subsequently, the mutation rate increases and cancers occur.

7. **List common environmental causes of cancer.**
   - **Social agents:** Tobacco and alcohol
   - **Occupational exposure:** Arsenic, benzene, CCl_4, chromium, combustion byproducts (engine exhaust), and polycyclic hydrocarbons (coal byproducts)
   - **Ionizing radiation:** Ultraviolet B light (UVB), sunlight, mining, and others
   - **Dietary factors:** Aflatoxin B, high-fat diet, nitrates/nitrites (converted endogenously to nitrosamines), smoked foods, and diet low in fresh fruits and vegetables
   - **Foreign body reactants:** Asbestos fiber

- **Chronic inflammation:** Ulcerative colitis
- **Infectious agents:** Epstein-Barr virus (EBV), hepatitis B virus (HBV), hepatitis C virus (HCV), human immunodeficiency virus (HIV), human papillomavirus (HPV), human T-lymphotropic virus (HTLV), and *Helicobacter pylori*
- **Iatrogenic agents:** Cancer chemotherapeutic drugs, unopposed estrogens, childhood chest or neck radiation, and immune suppressants

8. Summarize dietary "protective" factors.
   Diets high in antioxidants and lycopene that include many fruits and vegetables (e.g., tomatoes and broccoli) are thought to protect against cancer development by scavenging for free radicals. Some vitamins may modify the effect of chemical carcinogenesis such as vitamin A (which promotes the differentiation of epithelial tissues), vitamin C (which blocks the formation of *N*-nitrosocarcinogens from nitrites and secondary amines), and vitamin E (which is a free radical scavenger). In general, these agents are more effective for cancer prevention when consumed in the diet rather than being taken in supplement form.

9. Which cancers tend to cluster in families?
   Breast, endometrial, colon, prostate, lung, melanoma, and stomach have an increased risk of development in first-degree relatives. This cluster may be due to hereditary factors, shared exposures to environmental carcinogens, chance associations, or a combination of all three.

10. Summarize the familial clustering of breast cancer.
    Mutation in a genetic locus (*BRCA1, BRCA2,* and several others) predisposes to the development of familial breast or ovarian cancer or both and occurs in approximately 10–15% of breast cancer cases.

KEY POINTS: FAMILIAL CANCER

1. Up to 15% of cancers are familial, due to inherited chromosomal alterations, and often occur in younger patients.
2. A careful family history is essential.
3. Screening of family members is indicated in autosomal dominant conditions.
4. Chemoprevention (e.g., tamoxifen for breast cancer) or prophylactic removal of the tissue at risk may be considered in high-risk families.

11. Describe the Lynch cancer family syndrome.
    Nonpolyposis colorectal cancer with an increased incidence of other cancers, including endometrial, ovarian, breast, stomach, small intestine, pancreatic, urinary tract, and biliary tract cancers, that is associated with an autosomal dominant pattern of predisposition. Mutations in the mismatch repair genes *hMLH1, hMSH2, hMSH6,* and *hPMS2* cause microsatellite instability and are associated with this syndrome.

12. What is Li-Fraumeni syndrome?
    A familial cancer syndrome with an autosomal dominant pattern of inheritance leading to a varied spectrum of malignancies beginning in childhood including sarcoma, leukemias, and cancers of the breast, brain, and adrenal glands. A mutation in *p53* tumor suppressor gene location on the short arm of chromosome 17 leads to the malignancy risk. *p53*, sometimes called the *guardian of the genome,* usually prevents damaged cells from duplicating themselves.

13. Describe the MEN 1 (multiple endocrine neoplasia type 1) syndrome.
    A defect in the *MEN1* gene on chromosome 11, associated with tumors of the parathyroid, pituitary (most commonly prolactinoma), and islet cells of the pancreas.

14. Summarize the two phenotypes of the MEN 2 syndrome.
    - **Type A:** medullary thyroid carcinoma, pheochromocytoma, and parathyroid hyperplasia
    - **Type B:** medullary thyroid carcinoma, pheochromocytoma, marfanoid habitus, and mucosal neuromas
    Germ-line point mutations of the *RET* proto-oncogene on chromosome 10 are responsible for both types of MEN 2.

15. **What are tumor markers?**

Enzymes, hormones, and oncofetal antigens that are associated with particular tumors. These markers are sometimes present on the cell surface or secreted by the malignant cells and can be detected in the bloodstream or by staining tissue samples. The markers reflect the presence of the tumor and sometimes also the quantity of the tumor or tumor burden. Tumor markers may not always be positive for a particular malignancy.

16. **How are tumor markers used?**

To follow the effects of therapy on tumor burden and in detecting recurrent disease after initial therapy. Some of the tumor markers, such as prostate-specific antigen (PSA) and alpha-fetoprotein (AFP), are highly sensitive and specific, strongly correlating with the presence of a particular type of cancer. Others, such as carcinoembryonic antigen (CEA and CA-125), are nonspecific and may be elevated in multiple conditions.

17. **Summarize the significance of CEA.**

High CEA can be found in a variety of cancers including lung cancer, colon cancer, breast cancer, and other adenocarcinomas. CEA is a glycoprotein of 200,000 Da that is found in gastrointestinal (GI) mucosal cells and pancreaticobiliary secretions. Elevations of CEA occur with breaks in the mucosal basement membrane by a tumor but can also occur in smokers and persons with cirrhosis, pancreatitis, inflammatory bowel disease, and rectal polyps. CEA is most useful in colorectal cancer and is used to monitor disease activity if the CEA level was elevated before treatment.

18. **Why is PSA important?**

PSA is a serine protease found only in the prostate that normally liquefies seminal gel. High levels of PSA, especially in patients with small-volume prostates, are a strong indicator of probable prostate cancer. Very elevated PSA levels (>100 ng/mL) correlate well with the presence of metastatic disease. The rate of rise of the PSA and the percentage of free PSA also can help to determine whether an elevated PSA level is due to benign or malignant causes. The serum level of PSA may be elevated in benign prostate disease, including benign prostatic hypertrophy (BPH) and prostatitis, as well as in prostate cancer.

19. **Discuss the role of AFP as a tumor marker.**

AFP is an α-globulin protein that is made by the yolk sac and liver of the human fetus. AFP is elevated in hepatocellular carcinoma (HCC) and certain germ cell neoplasms (nonseminomatous germ cell tumors [yolk sac and embryonal tumors]) and is a highly sensitive marker for disease activity in the proper clinical context. It can also be elevated in other nonmalignant conditions such as hepatitis.

20. **What is β-human chorionic gonadotropin (β-hCG)?**

A glycoprotein normally secreted by the trophoblastic epithelium of the placenta that is used as a sensitive and specific marker for germ cell tumors of the testes and ovary and extragonadal presentations of these tumors.

KEY POINTS: TUMOR MARKERS

1. Tumor markers are generally nonspecific and can be elevated in a variety of conditions.
2. Other than PSA, most tumor markers are not useful in screening for malignancies in the general population, and the usefulness of PSA is undergoing reevaluation.
3. Tumor markers are used to assist in diagnosis in patients suspected to have malignancy by clinical parameters.
4. CEA and CA-125 have clinical utility in patients diagnosed with colorectal and ovarian cancer, respectively, but only if the level was elevated before treatment of the cancer.
5. CA 19-9 can be highly elevated in cases of benign biliary tract obstruction.
6. PSA levels > 10 ng/mL have a 60% probability of prostate cancer; levels > 100 ng/mL correlate strongly with metastatic disease.

CEA, carcinoembryonic antigen; PSA, prostate-specific antigen.

21. **List the principles used in formulating combination chemotherapy regimens.**
    - Drugs used should have activity against the tumor.
    - Drugs should be selected with dissimilar toxicities.
    - Drugs with different mechanisms of action should be used.

- Several cycles of therapy, with adequate biologic effect, should be used before determining efficacy.
- Recovery of normal tissues should be allowed before starting the next cycle.

22. **What are the mechanisms of tumor resistance to chemotherapeutic agents?**
    - Intrinsic cellular or biochemical resistance
    - Impaired transport of the drug into the cell or active extrusion from the cell
    - Altered drug affinity for the target enzyme
    - Amplification of genes
    - Membrane alterations from overproduction of high-weight glycoproteins

23. **Summarize the toxic effects of chemotherapy.**
    See Table 15.1. Nausea and vomiting are the most common immediate effects and may vary in presence and degree with the type of drug. Some medications, such as cisplatin, are very emetogenic, whereas others, like fludarabine, are less likely to cause emesis. Many chemotherapy drugs cause myelosuppression. When myelosuppression occurs, leukopenia predisposes to acute and serious infections sometimes requiring primary prophylaxis with white blood cell growth colony stimulating factors; thrombocytopenia predisposes to bleeding; and anemia may worsen symptoms from other problems, such as chronic obstructive pulmonary disease and atherosclerotic cardiovascular disease requiring blood transfusion. Many, but not all, chemotherapy agents cause hair loss (alopecia). These agents are also known to cause hepatic and renal dysfunction depending on the clearance mechanisms.

Table 15.1. Toxicities of Chemotherapeutic Agents

DRUG	ACUTE TOXICITY	DELAYED TOXICITY
Bleomycin (Blenoxane)	Nausea/vomiting, fever, hypersensitivity reactions	Pneumonitis, pulmonary fibrosis,* rash and hyperpigmentation, stomatitis, alopecia, Raynaud phenomenon, cavitating granulomas
Carboplatin (Paraplatin)	Nausea/vomiting	Myelosuppression,* peripheral neuropathy (uncommon), hearing loss, hemolytic anemia, transient cortical blindness
Capecitabine (Xeloda)	Nausea, diarrhea, stomatitis	Hand-foot syndrome* (palmar-plantar erythrodysesthesia), hyperbilirubinemia
Chlorambucil (Leukeran)	Seizures, nausea/vomiting	Myelosuppression,* pulmonary infiltrates and fibrosis, leukemia, hepatic toxicity, sterility
Cisplatin (Platinol)	Nausea/vomiting, anaphylactic reaction	Renal damage,* ototoxicity, myelosuppression, hemolysis, $\downarrow$ Mg^{2+}/Ca^{2+}/K$^+$, peripheral neuropathy, Raynaud phenomenon
Cytarabine (ara-C)	Nausea/vomiting, diarrhea, anaphylaxis	Myelosuppression,* oral ulceration, conjunctivitis, hepatic damage, fever, pulmonary edema, neurotoxicity (high dose), rhabdomyolysis, pancreatitis with asparaginase
Dacarbazine (DTIC)	Nausea/vomiting, diarrhea, anaphylaxis, pain on administration	Myelosuppression,* cardiotoxicity,* alopecia, flulike syndrome, renal impairment, hepatic necrosis, facial flushing, paresthesias, photosensitivity, urticarial rash
Daunorubicin (Cerubidine)	Nausea/vomiting, diarrhea, red urine, severe local tissue necrosis on extravasation, transient ECG changes, anaphylactoid reaction	Myelosuppression,* cardiotoxicity,* alopecia, stomatitis, anorexia, diarrhea, fever and chills, dermatitis in previously irradiated areas, skin and nail pigmentation
Doxorubicin (Adriamycin)	Nausea/vomiting, red urine, severe local tissue necrosis on extravasation, diarrhea, fever, transient ECG changes, ventricular arrhythmia, anaphylactoid reaction	Myelosuppression,* cardiotoxicity,* alopecia, stomatitis, anorexia, conjunctivitis, acral pigmentation, dermatitis in previously irradiated areas, acral erythrodysesthesia, mucositis

Table 15.1. Toxicities of Chemotherapeutic Agents *(Continued)*

DRUG	ACUTE TOXICITY	DELAYED TOXICITY
Etoposide (VP16)	Nausea/vomiting, diarrhea, fever, hypotension, allergic reaction	**Myelosuppression,*** alopecia, peripheral neuropathy, mucositis and hepatic damage with high doses, leukemia
Floxuridine (FUDR)	Nausea/vomiting, diarrhea	**Oral and GI ulceration,*** myelosuppression,* alopecia, dermatitis, hepatic dysfunction with infusion
Fluorouracil (5-FU)	Nausea/vomiting, diarrhea, hypersensitivity, photosensitivity	**Oral and GI ulcers, myelosuppression,*** diarrhea, ataxia, arrhythmias, angina, hyperpigmentation, hand-foot syndrome, conjunctivitis
Gemcitabine (Gemzar)	Fatigue, nausea and vomiting	**Bone marrow depression,** especially thrombocytopenia; edema; pulmonary toxicity; anal pruritus
Ifosfamide (Ifex)	Nausea/vomiting, confusion, nephrotoxicity, metabolic acidosis, **cardiac toxicity with higher doses***	**Myelosuppression,* hemorrhagic cystitis,** alopecia, SIADH, neurotoxicity
Irinotecan (Camptosar)	Nausea and vomiting, diarrhea, fever	**Diarrhea, anorexia,** stomatitis, bone marrow depression, alopecia, abdominal cramping
Mechlorethamine (nitrogen mustard)	Nausea/vomiting, local reaction and phlebitis	**Myelosuppression,*** alopecia, diarrhea, oral ulcers, leukemia, amenorrhea, sterility
Methotrexate	Nausea/vomiting, diarrhea, fever, anaphylaxis, hepatic necrosis	**Oral/GI ulceration,* myelosuppression,*** hepatic toxicity, renal toxicity, **pulmonary infiltrates and fibrosis,*** osteoporosis, conjunctivitis, alopecia, depigmentation
Mitoxantrone (Novantrone)	Blue-green sclerae and pigment in urine, nausea/vomiting, stomatitis	**Myelosuppression,*** cardiotoxicity, alopecia, white hair, skin lesions, hepatic damage, renal failure
Paclitaxel (Taxol), docetaxel (Taxotere)	Hypersensitivity, hypotension, nausea, pain on extravasation	**Myelosuppression,*** alopecia, peripheral neuropathy, rash and edema (docetaxel)
Topotecan (Hycamtin)	Nausea/vomiting, diarrhea, headache	**Myelosuppression,*** alopecia, transient elevations in hepatic enzymes
Vinblastine (Velban)	Nausea/vomiting, local reaction and phlebitis with extravasation	**Myelosuppression,*** alopecia, stomatitis, loss of DTRs, jaw pain, muscle pain, paralytic ileus
Vincristine (Oncovin)	Local reaction with extravasation	**Peripheral neuropathy,*** alopecia, mild myelosuppression, constipation, paralytic ileus, jaw pain, SIADH
Vinorelbine (Navelbine)	Local reaction with extravasation	**Granulocytopenia,*** anemia, fatigue

*Dose-limiting effects.

CHF, chronic heart failure; DTRs, deep tendon reflexes; ECG, electrocardiographic; GI, gastrointestinal; SIADH, syndrome of inappropriate antidiuretic hormone.

Modified from Drugs of choice for cancer chemotherapy. *Med Lett Drugs Ther.* 2000;42:83–92.

24. **Which chemotherapeutic drugs are associated with cardiotoxicity?**

    Doxorubicin (Adriamycin) and other drugs of the anthracycline class, which cause a progressive loss of cardiac muscle cells via oxidative stress. In previously normal hearts, toxicity is dose related and does not become clinically important until a total dose of approximately 300 mg/m^2 of doxorubicin is administered. In patients with already compromised cardiac function, toxicity may occur at lower dosages. In the United States, dexrazoxane is the only approved medication to decrease incidence and severity of cardiomyopathy associated with doxorubicin toxicity in patients with metastatic breast cancer. Women with higher risk for cardiomyopathy may be medically managed with angiotensin-converting enzyme inhibitors and beta blockers while receiving therapy.

25. **How is doxorubicin-related cardiotoxicity monitored?**

    With cardiac radionuclide gated wall motion studies (multiple-gated acquisition scans [MUGA]) or echocardiograms measuring left ventricular ejection fraction.

26. **Distinguish between neoadjuvant therapy and adjuvant therapy.**

    Neoadjuvant therapy means treatment such as chemotherapy or hormones before definitive surgery or radiotherapy. Patients given neoadjuvant therapy often have large or fixed tumors, and the goal is to shrink these tumors to make subsequent surgical removal or radiation therapy easier and more complete. **Adjuvant therapy** is given after surgery. Adjuvant chemotherapy and radiotherapy are administered after an operation to eradicate possible micrometastatic disease and, therefore, prevent recurrence.

27. **What are radiation sensitizers?**

    Chemical agents that increase the sensitivity of cancer cells to radiation. This class of compounds includes drugs such as 5-fluorouracil (5-FU), platinum analogs, gemcitabine, and cetuximab. Radiation sensitizers likely have effects on the induction and repair of radiation-induced damage. They are most commonly used in rectal, head and neck, pancreatic, and anal cancers.

28. **Define tumor doubling time.**

    The time required for the tumor to double in volume. The doubling time varies greatly among types of cancer and, in a single cancer type, may vary among different individuals. Cancers with a slow doubling time include prostate cancer and colon cancer. Cancers with more rapid doubling times include lung cancer, cancers of the pancreas and esophagus, and certain types of lymphomas.

29. **What is the most common cause of cancer death in the United States today?**

    Lung cancer, for both men and women (Table 15.2).

Table 15.2. Leading Sites of New Cancer Cases and Deaths in the United States

MALE			FEMALE		
Estimated New Cases					
Prostate	217,730	25%	Breast	207,090	28%
Lung and bronchus	116,750	15%	Lung and bronchus	105,770	14%
Colon and rectum	72,090	9%	Colon and rectum	70,480	10%
Urinary bladder	52,760	7%	Uterine corpus	43,470	6%
Melanoma of the skin	38,870	5%	Thyroid	33,930	5%
Non-Hodgkin lymphoma	35,380	5%	Non-Hodgkin lymphoma	30,160	4%
Kidney and renal pelvis	35,370	5%	Melanoma of the skin	29,260	4%
Oral cavity and pharynx	25,420	3%	Kidney and renal pelvis	22,870	3%
Leukemia	24,690	3%	Ovary	21,880	3%
Pancreas	21,370	3%	Pancreas	21,770	3%
All sites	789,620	100%	All sites	739,940	100%
Estimated Deaths					
Lung and bronchus	86,220	29%	Lung and bronchus	71,080	26%

Table 15.2. Leading Sites of New Cancer Cases and Deaths in the United States *(Continued)*

MALE			FEMALE		
Prostate	32,050	11%	Breast	39,840	15%
Colon and rectum	26,580	9%	Colon and rectum	24,790	9%
Pancreas	18,770	6%	Pancreas	18,030	7%
Liver and intrahepatic bile duct	12,720	4%	Ovary	13,850	5%
Leukemia	12,660	4%	Non-Hodgkin lymphoma	9,500	4%
Esophagus	11,650	4%	Leukemia	9,180	3%
Non-Hodgkin lymphoma	10,710	4%	Uterine corpus	7,950	3%
Urinary bladder	10,410	3%	Liver and intrahepatic bile duct	6,190	2%
Kidney and renal pelvis	8,210	3%	Brain and other nervous system	5,720	2%
All sites	**299,200**	**100%**	**All sites**	**270,290**	**100%**

Excludes basal and squamous cell skin cancers and in situ carcinoma except urinary bladder. Estimates are rounded to the nearest 10.
Modified from Jemal A, Siegal R, Xu J, Ward R. Cancer Statistics, 2010. *CA Cancer J Clin.* 2010;60:277–300.

COMPLICATIONS OF CANCER

30. **What are the causes of anemia in patients with cancer?**
    - Anemia of chronic disease
    - Bone marrow suppression by chemotherapy
    - Marrow involvement by tumor
    - Hemolysis secondary to tumor-associated antibodies
    - Certain chemotherapeutic agents
    - Sepsis
    - Disseminated intravascular coagulation (DIC)
    - Paraneoplastic syndrome
    - Gastritis and GI bleeding from medications for pain control (such as nonsteroidal anti-inflammatory drugs [NSAIDs])
    - Decreased erythropoietin owing to renal effects due to chemotherapeutic agents such as cisplatin

31. **What are the predisposing factors for infection in patients with cancer?**
    - Defects in cellular and humoral immunity
    - Organ compromised due to tumor-related obstruction
    - Chemotherapy-related granulocytopenia
    - Disruption of mucosal (e.g., respiratory and alimentary tract) and integumental surfaces
    - Iatrogenic procedures or indwelling prosthetic devices
    - Hyposplenic or postsplenectomy states

32. **Discuss the sources of infection in patients with cancer.**
    The vast majority of infections originate from the patient's own endogenous flora. Sources of infection in neutropenic patients include the lungs, urinary tract, skin, upper aerodigestive tract (mouth, skin, teeth), central nervous system, rectum, perirectum, biopsy sites, and GI tract (appendicitis, cholecystitis, perforations). In investigating the cause of an infection, cultures should include blood, urine, sputum, and, if appropriate to the patient's clinical status, stool, pleural fluid, or peritoneal fluid.

33. **Which malignancies commonly spread to bone?**
    Lung, prostate, malignant melanoma, breast, thyroid, kidney, and multiple myeloma.

34. **Are metastatic bone lesions osteoblastic or osteolytic?**
Both. Renal cell carcinoma and multiple myeloma tend to be purely lytic; prostate carcinoma tends to be mostly blastic; and other bone lesions of metastatic carcinoma are mixed. Lytic bone lesions are often associated with hypercalcemia, unlike blastic metastases.

35. **To which bones does cancer most often metastasize?**
    - Spine
    - Ribs
    - Pelvis
    - Long bones (femurs, humeri)
    - Calvarium

36. **Characterize the pain associated with bone metastases.**
A dull, deep aching discomfort that is worse at night and may improve with physical activity.

37. **Which tumors metastasize to the lungs?**
Most types of tumors can metastasize to the lungs; therefore, the more common the tumor, the more common the lung metastases. Tumors that spread via the bloodstream, such as sarcomas, renal cell carcinoma, and colon cancer, tend to produce nodular lung lesions. GI cancers tend to metastasize locally first and to the liver before pulmonary involvement is seen. Those cancers that spread via lymphatic routes, such as breast, lung, pancreas, stomach, and liver, may manifest a pattern of lymphangitic spread.

38. **Discuss the symptoms of intracranial metastases.**
Headache occurs in up to 50% of patients with intracranial metastases and is classically described as occurring daily early in the morning, persistent, and associated with nausea and projectile vomiting. Other symptoms include focal signs such as unilateral weakness, numbness, seizures, visual disturbances, or cranial nerve abnormalities. Nonfocal complaints such as mental status changes or ataxia may occur.

39. **How are intracranial metastases diagnosed?**
By contrast-enhanced computed tomography (CT) with intravenous contrast agent or magnetic resonance imaging (MRI) with gadolinium of the brain.

40. **How are intracranial metastases treated?**
By decreasing intracranial pressure with steroids, followed by definitive therapy. Surgery is recommended for patients with single intracranial lesions if technically possible, whereas radiation therapy is generally administered for multiple lesions. Chemotherapy may also be used, but the results are not as reliable as the other modalities owing to the difficulty of chemotherapy agents penetrating the blood-brain barrier. Intrathecal chemotherapy may be considered for particular lymphomatous involvement but generally has not been as successful in carcinomas of the brain.

41. **What are the signs and symptoms of malignant pericardial effusion?**
Frequently similar to the symptoms of heart failure with dyspnea, peripheral edema, and an enlarged heart on chest radiograph. However, the dyspnea is often out of proportion to the degree of pulmonary congestion seen on the radiograph. Kussmaul sign, or jugulovenous distention with inspiration, and pulsus paradoxus of > 10 mm Hg with distant heart sounds are clues to the presence of a pericardial effusion.

42. **How is the diagnosis of malignant pericardial effusion confirmed?**
By echocardiogram or CT scan and by taking a sample of the pericardial fluid. Malignant effusions are usually exudative and are often hemorrhagic. Cytologic testing is helpful if positive but does not exclude cancer if negative as it may take multiple samplings before diagnosis is confirmed.

43. **Discuss the treatment of malignant pericardial effusion.**
Treatment depends on the patient's condition but should include drainage of the fluid for diagnostic as well as therapeutic reasons. A nonsurgical approach is preferred, with catheter drainage followed by sclerosis of the pericardium, sometimes with a sclerosing agent such as bleomycin or thiotepa. Other approaches include subxiphoid pericardiectomy, balloon pericardiectomy, pericardial window, and pericardial stripping for patients with prolonged life expectancy.

44. **What are the presenting symptoms and signs of spinal cord compression?**
Back pain in 95% of cancer patients. Other symptoms include lower extremity weakness, bowel or bladder incontinence, or increased deep tendon reflexes in the lower extremities. Once neurologic symptoms appear, the nerve damage may be irreversible; therefore, early recognition and diagnosis of cord compression are essential.

45. **How is spinal cord compression diagnosed?**
By MRI or myelography with CT, which will demonstrate blockage or pressure on the spinal canal or nerve roots.

46. **How is spinal cord compression treated?**
Initially by decreasing spinal cord swelling and pain with high-dose steroids and adequate pain medication. Definitive treatment with surgery or radiation therapy must be carried out emergently to prevent irreversible neurologic deterioration. Preservation of neurologic function is generally better with surgery. Radiation treatment is given to patients not eligible for surgical decompression.

47. **Which malignancies most commonly cause spinal cord compression?**
    - Lung
    - Breast
    - Prostate
    - Carcinoma of unknown primary
    - Lymphoma
    - Multiple myeloma

    The most common site of cord compression is the thoracic spine, followed by the lumbosacral spine and the cervical spine.

48. **Which tumors are associated with nonbacterial thrombotic endocarditis?**
Mucinous adenocarcinomas, most commonly of the lung, pancreas, stomach, or ovary. This paraneoplastic syndrome is also known as *marantic endocarditis* and has also been described in other types of cancers.

49. **How does nonbacterial thrombotic endocarditis present?**
Usually with the appearance of embolic peripheral or cerebral vascular events causing arterial insufficiency, encephalopathy, or focal neurologic defects. The emboli originate from sterile, verrucous, fibrin-platelet vegetations that accumulate on the heart valves, likely due to a hypercoagulable state from malignancy. Heart murmurs are not always present.

50. **How is nonbacterial thrombotic endocarditis diagnosed and treated?**
By transesophageal echocardiogram (TEE). However, echocardiograms may be negative, and the diagnosis is usually made postmortem. Treatment with anticoagulants or antiplatelet drugs has been tried with little success.

51. **What are the tumor-related causes of hypercalcemia?**
    - **Lytic bone metastases:** Release calcium into the bloodstream and are the most common cause of hypercalcemia in solid tumors with bony metastases.
    - **Humoral hypercalcemia of malignancy (HHM):** Occurs in patients without bony metastases. Cancers associated with this syndrome secrete a non-PTH (parathyroid hormone) substance with activity similar to PTH (parathyroid hormone–related protein [PTHrP]). HHM is associated most commonly with squamous cell cancers of the lung, esophagus, or head and neck but can also be found in renal cell carcinoma, transitional cell carcinoma of the bladder, and ovarian carcinoma.
    - **Osteoclast-activating factors:** Includes interleukin 1 (IL-1), IL-6, and tumor necrosis factor-α (TNF-α; lymphotoxin) that may cause hypercalcemia in plasma cell dyscrasias.
    - **Vitamin D metabolites:** Produced by some lymphomas and promote intestinal calcium absorption.

52. **What is tumor lysis syndrome?**
Electrolyte and metabolic disturbances such as hyperuricemia, hyperkalemia, hyperphosphatemia, and hypocalcemia that can result in renal failure, arrhythmias, and seizures. These disturbances occur when rapidly growing tumors are effectively treated with chemotherapy and breakdown products of dying tumor cells are released in large amounts into the bloodstream. The complication

is seen within hours to days after treatment of malignancies such as acute leukemia and high-grade lymphomas. Although rarely seen with solid tumors, tumor lysis syndrome has been described. Patients may occasionally present with tumor lysis syndrome even prior to treatment in the setting of bulky highly aggressive disease such as Burkitt lymphoma.

53. **How is tumor lysis syndrome treated?**
With allopurinol and supportive measures for renal failure such as vigorous hydration, dialysis if necessary, and appropriate treatment of electrolyte disorders. Rasburicase (recombinant urate oxidase) can be administered when uric acid levels are not lowered by standard approaches. Prophylactic treatment with aggressive hydration and allopurinol can prevent this serious complication and should always be given before chemotherapy in malignancies with high proliferative index.

54. **Which medications are commonly used for cancer pain?**
See also Chapter 19, Palliative Care.
   Pain medications are to be administered in a stepwise approach according to the intensity and pathophysiology of symptoms and individual requirements. For mild pain, the recommended baseline drugs are NSAIDs (if no renal issues). Patients with moderate to severe pain generally require an opioid agent such as codeine or oxycodone; severe pain requires a stronger opioid such as morphine and often longer-acting opioid medications.

55. **What are the neuromuscular complications of cancer?**
See Table 15.3.

Table 15.3. Neuromuscular Complications of Cancer*

SITE	PARANEOPLASTIC SYNDROME	AUTOANTIBODIES (ASSOCIATED CANCER)
Brain and cranial nerves	Paraneoplastic cerebellar degeneration	Anti-Yo (gyn, breast cancer) Anti-Hu, CV 2 (SCLC) Anti-Tr (HD) Anti-Ma (others)
	Opsoclonus-myoclonus	Anti-Hu (neuroblastoma) Anti-Ri (breast cancer)
	Carcinoma-associated retinopathy	Anti-recoverin, CV2 (SCLC) Anti-rod-bipolar cell (melanoma)
	Limbic encephalitis	Anti-Hu, CV2, amphiphysin (SCLC) Anti-Ma2 (testicular) Anti-VGKC (thymoma, SCLC)
	Encephalomyelitis	Anti-Hu, CV2, amphiphysin (SCLC)
Spinal cord	Myelitis Subacute motor neuronopathy Motor neuron disease/ALS Stiff-man syndrome	Anti-Hu (SCLC) Anti-Hu (SCLC) Anti-Hu (rarely) Anti-amphiphysin (breast, SCLC)
Peripheral nerves and dorsal root ganglia	Subacute or chronic sensorimotor neuropathy Acute polyradiculopathy (GBS) Neuropathy associated with plasma cell dyscrasias Brachial neuritis Mononeuritis multiplex Sensory neuronopathy Autonomic neuronopathy	Anti-Hu, CV2 (SCLC) Anti-MAG

Table 15.3. Neuromuscular Complications of Cancer* *(Continued)*

SITE	PARANEOPLASTIC SYNDROME	AUTOANTIBODIES (ASSOCIATED CANCER)
Neuromuscular junction	Lambert-Eaton myasthenic syndrome Myasthenia gravis	Anti-VGCC, anti-Sox1 (SCLC) Acetylcholine receptor Ab
Muscle	Dermatomyositis/polymyositis Acute necrotizing myopathy Carcinoid myopathy Neuromyopathy Neuromyotonia	Ab to potassium channels

*These syndromes frequently occur together as part of paraneoplastic encephalomyelitis/sensory neuronopathy with anti-Hu antibody.

Ab, antibody; ALS, amyotrophic lateral sclerosis; GBS, Guillain-Barré syndrome; gyn, gynecologic; HD, Hodgkin disease; MAG, myelin-associated glycoprotein; SCLC, small cell lung cancer; VGCC, voltage-gated calcium channel.

Data from Schiff D, Batchelor T, Wyn PY, et al. Neurologic emergencies in cancer patients. *Neurol Clin.* 1998;16:449–481; and Didelot A, Honnorat J. Update on paraneoplastic neurological syndromes. *Curr Opin Oncol.* 2009;21:566–572.

GASTROINTESTINAL AND LIVER CANCERS

56. **Who gets squamous cell carcinoma of the esophagus?**
Usually men aged 40–60 years. The incidence is increased and nearly equal in men and women, in China, Africa, Russia, Japan, Scotland, and the Caspian region of Iran. In the United States, African-American men living in urban areas are at increased risk.

57. **List the risk factors for squamous cell carcinoma of the esophagus.**
- Excessive alcohol and/or tobacco use.
- Native Bantu beer (southern Africa).
- Betel nut chewing (Asia).
- Chronic hot beverage ingestion.
- Caustic strictures (due to accidental or intentional ingestion): >30% of cases develop esophageal cancer.
- Tylosis (inherited disease with hyperkeratosis of palms and soles): >40% of cases develop esophageal cancer.
- Achalasia.
- Plummer-Vinson syndrome (presence of esophageal webs due to chronic iron-deficiency anemia).
- Nontropical sprue.
- Prior oral and pharyngeal cancer.
- Occupational exposure to asbestos, combustion products, and ionizing radiation.
- Decreased dietary intake of fruits and vegetables throughout adulthood.

58. **Discuss the incidence of adenocarcinoma of the esophagus.**
The incidence of esophageal adenocarcinoma has greatly increased since the 1970s. Adenocarcinoma of the esophagus is now more prevalent than squamous cell carcinoma in the United States and Western Europe, with most tumors located in the distal esophagus and esophagogastric junction.

59. **What are the risk factors for adenocarcinoma of the esophagus?**
- Obesity
- Chronic esophagitis
- Gastroesophageal reflux disease (GERD)
- Barrett esophagus

60. **How does esophageal cancer present?**
- Dysphagia (first with solids, then with liquids)
- Occult GI bleeding

- Choking
- Aspiration pneumonia
- Hoarseness
- Weight loss
- Cough
- Chest pain on swallowing
- Regurgitation
- Fever
- GERD

61. **How should esophageal cancer be treated?**
By surgical resection if possible. Fewer than half of patients appear to be operable at the time of presentation, and of these, only one half to two thirds have tumors that are completely resectable. Nonsurgical patients are treated with combined chemoradiotherapy or palliative measures if their performance status is too poor for active therapy. Some evidence indicates that survival in patients with adenocarcinoma of the esophagus is improved with preoperative combined chemotherapy and radiotherapy (CROSS [ChemoRadiotherapy for Oesophageal cancer followed by Surgery Study] trial).
> Van Hagen P, Hulsof MC, van Lanschot JJ, et al. Preoperative chemoradiotherapy for esophageal or junctional cancer. *N Engl J Med.* 2015;366:2074–2084.

62. **List the risk factors for gastric cancer.**
Precursor conditions
- Chronic atrophic gastritis and intestinal metaplasia
- Pernicious anemia
- Partial gastrectomy for benign disease
- *H. pylori* infection
- Ménétrier disease (rare acquired disease with massive gastric folds secreting excessive mucous)
- Gastric adenomatous polyps
- Barrett esophagus

Genetic and environmental factors
- Family history of gastric cancer
- Blood type A
- Hereditary nonpolyposis colon cancer (HNPCC) syndrome
- Low socioeconomic status
- Low consumption of fruits and vegetables
- Consumption of salted, smoked, or poorly preserved foods
- Cigarette smoking

63. **Discuss the role of gene mutations in gastric cancer.**
Allelic deletions of the *APC, E-cadherin (CDH1, p53),* and microsatellite instability genes have been reported in a significant proportion of gastric cancers, and the exact role of oncogenes and tumor suppressor genes is being elucidated. Additionally, *Her2/neu* testing in metastatic gastric cancer has been beneficial for treatment options in which targeted therapy with trastuzumab (*Her2/neu* blocking agent) improves progression-free survival. Differences between mutations associated with the intestinal and diffuse types of gastric cancers may account for their different natural histories.

64. **List the symptoms of gastric cancer at the time of diagnosis.**
- Weight loss: 61.6%
- Abdominal pain: 51.6%
- Nausea: 34.3%
- Anorexia: 32.0%
- Dysphagia: 26.1%
- Melena: 20.2%
- Early satiety: 17.5%
- Ulcer-type pain: 17.1%
- Lower extremity edema: 5.9%
> Fuchs CS, Mayer RJ. Gastric carcinoma. *N Engl J Med.* 1995;333:32–41.

65. **List the risk factors for pancreatic cancer.**
    - Smoking (two to three times increased risk)
    - Diet high in calories, fat, and protein and low in fruits and vegetables
    - Diabetes mellitus
    - Chronic pancreatitis
    - Surgery for peptic ulcer disease
    - Occupational exposure to 2-naphthylamine and petroleum products (>10 years increases risk to 5:1), dichlorodiphenyltrichloroethane (DDT)

66. **What hereditary syndromes increase the risk for pancreatic cancer?**
    - Familial pancreatic cancer
    - Hereditary pancreatitis
    - Familial adenomatous polyposis (FAP) syndrome
    - Familial atypical multiple mole melanoma syndrome (hereditary dysplastic nevus syndrome)
    - *BRCA2* gene
    - Peutz-Jeghers syndrome

67. **Do gender and ethnicity affect the risk for pancreatic cancer?**
    Yes. Males > females; African Americans > whites.

68. **List the symptoms and signs of pancreatic cancer based on tumor location.**
    See Table 15.4.

Table 15.4. Signs and Symptoms of Cancer of the Pancreatic Head and Body or Tail

SIGNS AND SYMPTOMS	Frequency of Occurrence by Pancreatic Site (%)	
	HEAD	BODY/TAIL
Weight loss	92	100
Jaundice	82	7
Pain	72	87
Anorexia	64	33
Nausea	45	43
Vomiting	37	37
Weakness	35	43
Palpable liver	83	–
Palpable gallbladder	29	–
Tenderness	26	27
Ascites	19	20

Adapted from Moossa AR, Schimpff SC, Robson MC. Tumors of the pancreas. In Moossa AR, Schimpff SC, Robson MC, editors. *Comprehensive Textbook of Oncology*. 2nd ed. Baltimore: Williams & Wilkins; 1991, p 964.

69. **Describe the diagnostic and staging evaluation for patients suspected of having pancreatic cancer.**
    Endoscopic ultrasound (EUS) and helical CT are useful diagnostic modalities for suspected carcinoma of the pancreas that allow accurate depiction of local tumor extent, involvement of adjacent vascular structures, and distant metastases. Gadolinium-enhanced MRI is available but is not commonly used to assess pancreatic cancer. Endoscopic retrograde cholangiopancreatography (ERCP) has a higher complication rate and should be reserved for patients in need of endoscopic stenting, for nondiagnostic findings on standard evaluation, or when tissue diagnosis is needed and cannot be obtained by EUS. A high level of CA 19-9 is specific for pancreatic cancer only if the bilirubin is not elevated, because biliary tract obstruction can cause extremely high levels of CA 19-9. See Table 15.5.

Table 15.5. Diagnostic Evaluation for Pancreatic Cancer

TEST	DIAGNOSTIC YIELD IN VARIOUS SERIES (%)
CA 19-9 level > 200 U/mL	97
CT scan of abdomen	74–94
ERCP	91–94
EUS	94
Angiography	88–90
Ultrasound of abdomen	69–90
MRI of abdomen	Not applicable

CT, computed tomography; ERCP, endoscopic retrograde cholangiopancreatography; EUS, endoscopic ultrasound; MRI, magnetic resonance imaging.

70. **How is the diagnosis of pancreatic cancer confirmed and the extent of metastatic disease evaluated?**
    By CT or EUS-guided fine-needle aspirate. Additional staging includes routine laboratory studies, chest radiograph, and other tests as directed by the history and physical examination. If there is bone pain or elevated alkaline phosphatase, bone scan should be done.

71. **What is the most important risk factor for HCC?**
    See also Chapter 7, Gastroenterology.
    Cirrhosis. Macronodular cirrhosis is found in 85% of patients with HCC. In the United States, alcohol use is an important cause of cirrhosis. Chronic infection with HBV or HCV leading to cirrhosis is the major etiologic agent for HCC worldwide. Nonalcoholic steatohepatitis can also lead to cirrhosis and possible increased risk of HCC.

72. **List the common presenting features of primary tumors of the liver.**
    - **Asthenia:** 85–90%
    - **Hepatomegaly:** 50–100%
    - **Abdominal pain:** 50–70%
    - **Jaundice:** 45–80%
    - **Fever:** 10%

73. **List the unusual ways in which HCC may present.**
    - Hemoptysis secondary to pulmonary metastases
    - Rib mass secondary to bony metastasis
    - Encephalitis-like picture secondary to brain metastasis or liver failure
    - Heart failure secondary to cardiac metastasis and thrombosis of the inferior vena cava
    - Priapism secondary to soft tissue metastasis
    - Bone pain and pathologic fractures secondary to bony metastases

74. **What are the systemic manifestations of HCC?**
    - **Endocrine:** Erythrocytosis and hypercalcemia
    - **Nonendocrine:** Hypoglycemia, porphyria cutanea tarda, cryofibrinogenemia, osteoporosis, hyperlipidemia, dysfibrinogenemia, and AFP synthesis
      Margolis S, Horncy C. Systemic manifestations of hepatoma. *Medicine.* 1972;51:381–390.

75. **Which environmental factors are thought to be related to the development of colon cancer?**
    Increased risk
    - Diet high in fat and red meat
    - Physical inactivity and central obesity
    Decreased risk
    - Diet high in fresh fruits and vegetables
    - Regular use of NSAIDs, especially aspirin

76. **What genetic syndromes are associated with colon cancer?**
    - FAP
    - Gardner syndrome
    - Lynch syndrome (HNPCC)

    These all are autosomal dominant syndromes. The first two account for < 1% of all colorectal cancers, and the last for 6–15%.

77. **What is FAP?**
    A syndrome characterized by the occurrence of thousands of adenomatous polyps throughout the large bowel. If left untreated, cancer will develop in all patients with this syndrome, usually before the age of 40. If FAP syndrome is confirmed, total proctocolectomy should be done, because cancer surveillance is not possible among the thousands of polyps present. FAP is associated with mutations of the adenomatous polyposis coli (APC) tumor suppressor gene.

78. **What is Gardner syndrome?**
    A syndrome related to mutations of the APC gene leading to colonic polyps and associated with other extraintestinal disorders such as osteomas, dental abnormalities, desmoid tumors, retinal pigment epithelial abnormalities, adrenal adenomas, and nasal angiofibromas.

79. **What is Lynch syndrome?**
    The most common hereditary colon cancer syndrome that is also associated with extracolonic cancers such as endometrial, ovarian, pancreatic, gastric, renal, hepatic, and small bowel cancer.

80. **What are the presenting signs and symptoms of colon cancer?**
    Ascending colon
    - Fatigue, lethargy, dyspnea (due to anemia related to chronic blood loss)
    - Positive fecal occult blood testing (FOBT) during screening

    Transverse colon
    - Abdominal cramping and pain
    - Bowel perforation

    Rectosigmoid colon
    - Tenesmus
    - Decreased stool caliber
    - Hematochezia

81. **What are the uses and limitations for CEA level testing?**
    CEA is an antigen produced by many colorectal cancers and should not be used for cancer screening because it is nonspecific and not sensitive enough to pick up early cancers. CEA has also been found to be elevated in cancers of the stomach, pancreas, breast, ovary, and lung and with various nonmalignant conditions such as alcoholic liver disease, inflammatory bowel disease, heavy cigarette smoking, chronic bronchitis, and pancreatitis. If elevated before cancer surgery, CEA should return to normal within 1 month after surgery. A subsequent rise in CEA will be strongly indicative of recurrent cancer. CEA can also be used as a marker for response to chemotherapy.

82. **When should CEA testing be done?**
    Preoperatively in patients undergoing resection for colon cancer. If elevated, it should be retested 30–45 days after complete resection of the cancer. National Comprehensive Cancer Network (NCCN) guidelines recommend obtaining a postoperative CEA every 3–6 months for 2 years, then every 6 months for a total of 5 years.

    National Comprehensive Cancer Network: Available at www.nccn.org. Accessed September 25, 2016.

83. **List the two roles of chemotherapy in the treatment of colon cancer.**
    Treatment of metastatic disease and adjuvant therapy.

84. **Which agents are commonly used for treatment of metastatic disease?**
    5-FU, leucovorin, capecitabine, irinotecan (CPT-11), and oxaliplatin, alone or in combination, plus targeted agents such as bevacizumab, cetuximab, panitumumab, and regorafenib. Use of these chemotherapy regimens has significantly prolonged survival in patients with metastatic colorectal cancer.

85. **How is chemotherapy used as an adjuvant treatment for colon cancer?**
As standard postoperative therapy for stage III patients. In stage II disease, adjuvant treatment is sometimes given to patients at high risk for recurrence, as judged by pathologic features of the resected specimens. In clinical studies, patients who were treated with adjuvant chemotherapy after curative-intent resections of stage III colon cancer were found to have reduced recurrence rate and death rate compared with untreated control subjects.

   Sargent D, Sobrero A, Grothey A, et al. Evidence for cure by adjuvant therapy in colon cancer: observations based on individual patient data from 20,898 patients on 18 randomized trials. *J Clin Oncol.* 2009;27:872–877.

86. **How is therapy for rectal cancer different from that for colon cancer?**
Both utilize the TNM (tumor, node, metastasis) staging, but the two entities are treated differently because of the locations. In stages II and III rectal adenocarcinoma, patients are often treated with neoadjuvant concurrent chemotherapy and radiation to optimize surgical outcomes. Additionally, rectal adenocarcinoma has higher rates of local recurrence and the addition of neoadjuvant therapy has decreased these risks. Both colon and rectal cancers may require adjuvant chemotherapy based on initial staging and nodal status.

87. **How are metastatic colon and rectal cancers treated?**
With chemotherapy (first-line 5-FU based therapy). Patients with metastatic rectal cancer may benefit from palliative radiation to the rectum if symptomatic (hematochezia, pain). Palliative colonic radiation is not used often unless a large mass is present and may have significant risk of adverse effects because the bowel floats whereas the rectum is fixed.

88. **What is the typical histologic diagnosis of anal cancer?**
Squamous cell carcinoma but rarely may be adenocarcinoma. Rectal cancer is typically adenocarcinoma but rarely may be squamous type.

89. **What are risk factors for anal cancer?**
HPV infection, HIV infection, chronic immunosuppression (solid organ transplantation, autoimmune disease), tobacco use.

90. **How is anal cancer treated?**
Concurrent chemotherapy and radiation has emerged as the effective therapy in anal cancer in an effort to preserve the anal sphincter. In the past, abdominoperineal resection (APR) was preferred and left patients with colostomy. Then, the Nigro protocol (Wayne State University) was developed in which patients received chemotherapy with 5-FU and mitomycin with an intermediate dose of radiation therapy (RT). Patients were seen to have cure without need to have an APR, which was reserved for residual tumor.

   National Comprehensive Cancer Network Clinical Practice Guidelines: Available at www.nccn.org. Accessed October 1, 2016.

GENITOURINARY CANCERS

91. **What tests are available for the diagnosis and staging of prostate cancer? How do their results correlate with the stage?**
See Table 15.6.

92. **What is the long-term survival rate of patients with prostate cancer?**
100% disease-specific survival at 5 years for patients with a localized or regionally advanced stage of prostate cancer. Twenty-nine percent of patients with distant metastases at the time of diagnosis will be alive after 5 years.

   Surveillance, End Results and Survival Program: SEER Cancer Statistics Review 2006–2012. Available at: http://seer.cancer.gov/statfacts/html/prost.html. Accessed September 25, 2016.

93. **Summarize the effects and mechanisms of the various androgen-deprivation therapies for prostate cancer.**
See Fig. 15.1.

Table 15.6. Diagnostic Evaluation and Staging of Prostate Cancer

| PROSTATE STAGE | HISTOLOGY OF BIOPSY SPECIMEN | URINARY SYMPTOMS | Noninvasive Assessment of Metastatic Disease | | | | SURGICAL LN SAMPLING |
			SAP	PSA	BONE SCAN	PELVIC CT SCAN	
I	Incidental histologic finding in ≤ 5% of resected tissue, well differentiated			Often ↑	—	—	Usually not performed
II	Incidental histologic finding in > 5% of resected tissue, or tumor not well differentiated, or palpable nodule confined to prostate			Often ↑	—	—	+ in 8–25% (indicating stage IV disease)
III	Extends through prostate capsule	Present	N	Usually ↑	—	—	+ in 40–50% (indicating stage IV disease)
IV	Invades other organs or metastatic	Present	Often	Usually ↑	±	±	+ in 95% of patients with elevated SAP

↑, elevated; −, negative; +, positive; BPH, benign prostatic hypertrophy; CT, computed tomography; LN, lymph node; PSA, prostate-specific antigen; SAP, serum alkaline phosphatase.

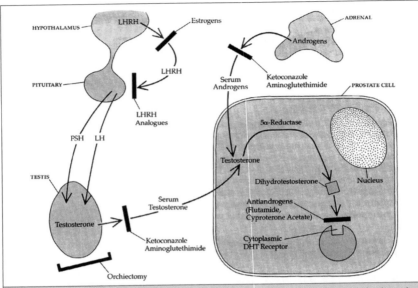

Fig. 15.1. Androgen deprivation, which prevents the trophic influence of testosterone on the prostate in advanced prostate carcinoma, can be affected in a variety of ways. Estrogens such as diethylstilbestrol inhibit the release of luteinizing hormone–releasing hormone (LHRH) from the hypothalamus, thus diminishing the release of follicle-stimulating hormone (FSH) and luteinizing hormone (LH) from the anterior pituitary and reducing the signal that stimulates testosterone production by the testes. LHRH analogs such as leuprolide initially stimulate but ultimately inhibit the release of FSH and LH from the anterior pituitary and thus have an estrogen-like effect. The testes, which produce most of the testosterone, can be removed by orchiectomy. Ketoconazole and aminoglutethimide inhibit a variety of steroid synthetic pathways, including those that produce androgens in the testes and adrenal glands. In the prostate cells, testosterone is converted into dihydrotestosterone (DHT) by the enzyme 5α-reductase. Antiandrogens such as bicalutamide, cyproterone acetate, and certain progestational agents block the binding of DHT to its cytoplasmic receptor. *(From Rubenstein E, Federman DD, editors.* Scientific American Medicine. *New York: Scientific American; 1993, p 12[IXA]:8, used with permission.)*

94. **What does Gleason score predict about a prostate cancer?**
    How aggressive a prostate cancer is likely to be, based on its appearance on light microscopy. The pathologist assigns a number from 1 to 5 to the two most common patterns of differentiation in the specimen. A score of 1 represents well differentiated and 5 the most poorly differentiated pattern. The sum of the two numbers is Gleason score. Values of 2–4 represent the least aggressive cancers; scores of 5–7 are intermediate in their behavior; 8–10 are the most aggressive.

95. **What is appropriate therapy for stage I prostate cancer?**
    - Watchful waiting for patients who would not benefit from definitive treatment but receive symptom relief through palliative care
    - Active surveillance including close monitoring of serum PSA, digital rectal examination, and prostate biopsy with subsequent treatment if indicated (Note that some physicians use the terms *watchful waiting* and *active surveillance* interchangeably.)
    - Radical prostatectomy
    - External-beam radiation therapy
    - Brachytherapy
    - Transurethral resection of the prostate (TURP) if needed for symptoms of BPH

96. **List the appropriate therapy options for stage II prostate cancer.**
    - Radical prostatectomy
    - External-beam radiation therapy
    - Brachytherapy
    - Watchful waiting for selected patients
    - Active surveillance for selected patients

97. List the appropriate therapy options for stage III prostate cancer.
    - Radiation therapy ± hormonal therapy
    - Radical prostatectomy with pelvic lymphadenectomy ± hormonal therapy
    - Watchful waiting for selected patients

98. What is appropriate therapy for stage IV prostate cancer?
    - TURP or radiation therapy for urinary obstruction
    - Endocrine manipulation or close observation for asymptomatic patients
    - Hormonal therapy for symptomatic disease
    - Palliative radiation therapy for localized symptoms
    - Chemotherapy for disease refractory to hormonal therapy

99. List the environmental risk factors for the development of bladder cancer.
    - **Occupational hazards:** Workers in dye industry, hairdressers, painters, and leather workers
    - **Geographic factors** (causing chronic bladder irritation): Endemic schistosomiasis
    - **Self-ingested toxins:** Tobacco, phenacetin, and possibly artificial sweeteners
    - **Alkylating agents:** Cyclophosphamide
    - **Previous cancers:** Especially those of the urothelial tract

100. What is the classic triad of symptoms of renal cell cancer and the frequency of occurrence?
    - Gross hematuria: 59%
    - Abdominal mass: 45%
    - Pain: 41%

    All three symptoms, however, are present in only 9% of patients with renal cell cancer. Renal cell tumors are often diagnosed on scans incidentally when evaluating for other conditions such as back pain.

101. List other symptoms of renal cell cancer and their frequency.
    - Weight loss: 28%
    - Anemia: 21%
    - Tumor calcification on radiograph: 13%
    - Symptoms from metastases: 10%
    - Fever: 7%
    - Asymptomatic when diagnosed: 7%
    - Hypercalcemia: 3%
    - Acute varicocele: 2%

    Skinner DG, Colvin RB, Vermillion CD, et al. Diagnosis and management of renal cell carcinoma: a clinical and pathologic study of 309 cases. *Cancer.* 1971;28:1165–1177.

102. Why is renal cell cancer called *the internist's tumor*?
    Because of the varied and unusual presentations that may obscure the true diagnosis. Many of these signs and symptoms are the result of paraneoplastic syndromes and include hypercalcemia, hypertension, hepatopathy without liver metastases, enteropathy, heart failure, cachexia, erythrocytosis, immune complex glomerulonephritis, amyloidosis, and a polymyalgia rheumatica (PMR) type syndrome.

103. What determines the prognosis for renal cell cancer?
    The stage and grade of the tumor.

104. What are the molecular alterations associated with the different histologic types of renal cell carcinoma?
    - **Clear cell:** von Hippel–Lindau gene (*VHL*)
    - **Papillary type 1:** hereditary papillary renal carcinoma (HPRC): *Met* oncogene
    - **Papillary type 2:** hereditary leiomyomatosis renal cell cancer (HLRCC): *FH* (fumarate hydratase gene)
    - **Chromophobe RCC/oncocytoma:** Birt-Hogg-Dube (BHD) syndrome: *BHD* (folliculin gene)

105. Give the 5-year survival rates for the four stages of renal cell cancer.
    - **Stage I** (confined to the renal parenchyma, ≤7 cm in greatest dimension): 88–95%
    - **Stage II** (confined to the renal parenchyma, >7 cm in greatest dimension): 67–88%
    - **Stage III** (involves the renal vein, inferior vena cava, or regional lymph nodes): 40–59%
    - **Stage IV** (invades beyond Gerota fascia or distant metastases): 2–20%

106. **What treatments are available for advanced stage renal cell cancer? How effective are they?**

Once renal cell carcinoma is widespread, there are few curative therapies, but there are several agents that can delay progression or induce partial remissions. Biologic response modifiers such as interferon and IL-2 induce long-term remissions in a minority of patients but with significant possibility for adverse events including death. Targeted agents such as sunitinib, sorafenib, temsirolimus, everolimus, and bevacizumab can significantly prolong progression-free survival in many patients. New advances in immunotherapy with PD-1 (programmed death 1) inhibition (nivolumab) are improving overall survival.

107. **How often does testicular cancer occur in the United States?**

Approximately 1% of all cancers in U.S. males. The majority of these are men 29–35 years of age, with 8700 new cases annually. The incidence of testicular cancer is higher in patients with cryptorchidism, Klinefelter syndrome, and testicular feminization syndrome.

  Siegel RL, Miller KD, Jemal A. Cancer statistics, 2016. *CA Cancer J Clin.* 2016;66:7–30.

108. **What causes testicular cancer?**

The cause is unknown, but age, genetic influences, repeated infection, radiation, and possible endocrine abnormalities have been suggested. Almost all tumors show an increased copy number of the short arm of chromosome 12 (12p), either as an isochromosome (an abnormal chromosome with two identical arms) or as tandem duplications. When 12p is present in multiple copies, the prognosis is poor.

109. **What are the presenting features of testicular cancer?**

Frequently as a painless scrotal mass, although pain is noted in ~25% of reported cases. When the tumor has already spread (5–15%), symptoms of metastases to the lungs and liver are demonstrated.

110. **Which pathologic types are most commonly seen among testicular cancers?**

Tumors of one histologic type
- Seminoma (germinoma)
  - Typical (35%)
  - Anaplastic (4%)
  - Spermatocytic (1%)
- Embryonal carcinoma (20%)
- Teratoma (10%)
- Choriocarcinoma (1%)

Tumors of mixed histologic type
- Embryonal carcinoma and teratoma (teratocarcinoma) (24%)
- Other combinations (5%)

111. **What are the stages of testicular cancer?**
- **Stage I:** no lymph node involvement or distant metastases, normal tumor markers
- **Stage II:** regional lymph node metastasis, with or without elevated tumor markers
- **Stage III:** distant metastasis to nonregional lymph nodes, lungs, or other sites, with or without elevated tumor markers.
- There is no stage IV in testicular cancer.

112. **What tumor markers are associated with testicular cancer?**
- Serum lactic dehydrogenase (LDH)
- AFP
- β-hCG

113. **What determines survival rate in testicular cancer?**

The response to therapy. Survival rate is not determined on the basis of stage. In patients who respond to therapy, the survival rate curves plateau at ~90%.

114. **How should stage I testicular cancer be treated?**

With transinguinal orchiectomy.

115. **How is pure seminoma treated after orchiectomy?**

Limited-stage cases are treated with radiation to the retroperitoneal nodes or close observation followed by radiation if there is relapse. Disseminated disease is treated with combination chemotherapy.

116. **How are nonseminomatous tumors treated after orchiectomy?**
With retroperitoneal lymphadenectomy. If nodes are positive, patients may be treated with two to four cycles of adjuvant chemotherapy.

117. **Describe the treatment for stage III disease.**
With bulky mediastinal or retroperitoneal masses, three to four courses of chemotherapy are given, followed by resection of any residual disease.

118. **How are patients followed for recurrent disease?**
With tumor markers. Many patients with germ cell tumors will have elevated levels of the tumor markers AFP or β-hCG or both. AFP is not elevated in pure seminoma. AFP and β-hCG should return to normal levels after treatment and can be monitored subsequently for evidence of recurrent disease. These markers are very sensitive for the presence of disease, although normal values do not rule out malignancy.

119. **Describe the extragonadal germ cell syndrome.**
The occurrence of germ cell tumors in the mediastinum, retroperitoneum, or pineal gland in relatively young males, with elevated β-hCG or AFP and marked elevation of LDH. Patients often respond to treatment with chemotherapy developed for testicular cancer. A careful search for an occult testicular primary tumor must be carried out, because the testis is a relative sanctuary from the effects of chemotherapy. Ultrasound evaluation is useful in this setting.

LUNG CANCER

120. **Describe the extent of lung cancer spread that can influence the presenting signs and symptoms.**
    - Central or endobronchial growth of the primary tumor
    - Peripheral growth of the primary tumor
    - Regional spread of the tumor in the thorax by contiguity or by metastasis to regional lymph nodes
    - Distant metastases or systemic effects

121. **List symptoms secondary to central or endobronchial growth of the primary tumor.**
    - Cough
    - Dyspnea from obstruction
    - Wheezing and stridor
    - Pneumonitis from obstruction with fever and productive cough
    - Hemoptysis

122. **Which symptoms may be secondary to peripheral growth of the primary tumor?**
    - Pain from pleural or chest wall involvement
    - Dyspnea from restriction
    - Lung abscess syndrome from tumor cavitation
    - Cough

123. **List symptoms related to regional spread of the tumor in the thorax by contiguity or by metastasis to regional lymph nodes.**
    - Tracheal obstruction
    - Recurrent laryngeal nerve paralysis with hoarseness
    - Sympathetic nerve paralysis with Horner syndrome
    - Superior vena cava (SVC) syndrome due to vascular obstruction
    - Lymphatic obstruction with pleural effusion
    - Esophageal compression with dysphagia
    - Phrenic nerve paralysis with elevation of the hemidiaphragm and dyspnea
    - C8 and T1 nerve compression with ulnar pain and Pancoast syndrome
    - Pericardial and cardiac extension with resultant tamponade, arrhythmia, or cardiac failure
    - Lymphangitic spread through the lungs with hypoxemia and dyspnea

124. Which symptoms may be due to distant metastases or systemic effects?
    - Bone pain
    - Painful lymphadenopathy
    - Hypercalcemia
    - Hemiparesis
    - Weight loss
    - Fatigue
    - Malaise
      Cohen MH. Signs and symptoms of bronchogenic carcinoma. In: Straus MJ, ed. *Lung Cancer: Clinical Diagnosis and Treatment.* 2nd ed. New York: Grune & Stratton; 1983: 97–111.

125. What are the types of lung cancer?
    - Small cell lung cancer (SCLC)
    - Non–small cell lung cancer (NSCLC): Adenocarcinoma, squamous cell carcinoma, large cell carcinoma, adenosquamous lung carcinoma

126. What are the accepted and proposed risk factors for lung cancer?
    - **Cigarette smoking:** Causes 85% of lung cancers in men. In women, lung cancer has surpassed breast cancer as the leading cause of cancer death. Passive smoking also increases the risk of lung cancer, causing 25% of the lung cancers in nonsmokers.
    - **Radon exposure:** Increases the risk of lung cancer, especially in smokers, who have a 10-fold higher risk. An estimated 25% of lung cancer in nonsmokers and 5% in smokers are attributed to radon daughter exposure in the home.
    - **Marijuana smoking:** Increases the risk of lung cancer in smokers.
    - **Other agents:** Bischloromethyl ether, arsenic, nickel, ionizing radiation, asbestos, and chromates.
    - **Radiation therapy**
    - **Pulmonary fibrosis**
    - **HIV infection and acquired immunodeficiency syndrome (AIDS):** Increases the risk of multiple cancers, including lung cancer.
      Patel P, Hanson DL, Sullivan PS, et al. Incidence of types of cancer among HIV-infected persons compared with the general population in the United States, 1992–2003. *Ann Intern Med.* 2008;148:728–736.

127. Which chromosomal defects are associated with lung cancer?
    Deletion of 3p (usually 3p14–23) occurring in virtually all cases (93%) of SCLC, in 100% of bronchial carcinoids, and 25% of NSCLC. A *ras* family oncogene is mutated in ~20% of NSCLC but not in SCLC. A mutation of the epidermal growth factor receptor (EGFR) is frequently found in Asian female nonsmokers with bronchoalveolar lung cancer (lepidic) and lung adenocarcinoma and responsive to tyrosine kinase inhibitors such as erlotinib, gefitinib, and afatinib. Gene rearrangement in the anaplastic lymphoma kinase (ALK) is another target in 4% of NSCLC that can be treated with crizotinib and alectinib. ROS1, a tyrosine kinase, is another driver oncogene similar to ALK that is positive in 1–2% of NSCLC and responsive to crizotinib.

128. Which tests are used for the evaluation of suspected lung cancer?
    Chest radiograph and sputum cytologic test. If the expectorated sputum cytologic finding is negative, bronchoscopy with biopsy, percutaneous biopsy, or thoracoscopy may be done. Preoperative evaluation includes CT scanning of the chest and upper abdomen to evaluate for mediastinal and hilar nodes and for liver and adrenal metastases. Pulmonary function tests, mediastinoscopy, and positron-emission tomography (PET) scan should be performed if surgical resection of NSCLC is considered. (SCLC is treated with radiation and chemotherapy, not surgery.) In SCLC and advanced-stage NSCLC, screening for the presence of brain metastases is recommended, using CT or MRI with contrast. Elevated alkaline phosphatase with normal liver CT suggests bony metastasis, which can be demonstrated by bone scan or PET scan.

129. Which paraneoplastic syndromes are associated with lung cancer?
    See Table 15.7.

Table 15.7. Paraneoplastic Syndromes in Lung Cancer

1. Systemic Symptoms
Anorexia-cachexia (31%)
Fever (21%)
Suppressed immunity

2. Endocrine Symptoms (12%)
Ectopic PTH: hypercalcemia (NSCLC)
SIADH (SCLC)
Ectopic secretion of ACTH: Cushing syndrome

3. Skeletal Symptoms
Clubbing (29%)
Hypertrophic pulmonary osteoarthropathy:
    periostitis (1–10%) (adenocarcinoma)

4. Coagulation-Thrombosis
Migratory thrombophlebitis, Trousseau syndrome:
    venous thrombosis, nonbacterial thrombotic
    endocarditis: arterial emboli; DIC: hemorrhage

5. Neurologic-Myopathic Symptoms
Lambert-Eaton syndrome (SCLC)
Peripheral neuropathy
Subacute cerebellar degeneration
Cortical degeneration
Polymyositis
Retinal blindness

6. Cutaneous Symptoms
Dermatomyositis
Acanthosis nigricans

7. Hematologic Symptoms (8%)
Anemia
Granulocytosis
Leukoerythroblastosis

8. Renal Symptoms (1%)
Nephrotic syndrome
Glomerulonephritis

ACTH, adrenocorticotropic hormone; DIC, disseminated intravascular coagulation; NSCLC, non–small cell lung cancer; PTH, parathyroid hormone; SCLC, small cell lung cancer; SIADH, syndrome of inappropriate antidiuretic hormone.

Data from Cohen MH. Signs and symptoms of bronchogenic carcinoma. In Straus MJ, editor. *Lung Cancer: Clinical Diagnosis and Treatment.* New York: Grune & Stratton; 1977, pp 85–94.

130. How is NSCLC treated?
     With surgery as a potential cure if the patient is a candidate for resection. Resection should be performed if the patient is medically fit and there is no evidence of the following:
     - Distant metastases
     - Malignant pleural effusion
     - SVC obstruction
     - Involvement of supraclavicular, cervical, or contralateral mediastinal nodes
     - Recurrent laryngeal nerve paralysis
     - Involvement of the mediastinum, tracheal wall, or main bronchus < 2 cm from the carina
     - Small cell carcinoma histologic appearance

131. How is stage IIIA (large tumor or mediastinal node involvement) NSCLC treated?
     Neoadjuvant chemotherapy (given before surgery) may improve survival. If patients are unable to undergo surgery or the tumor is locally advanced but inoperable, combined chemotherapy and radiotherapy are indicated. In higher-stage disease, systemic chemotherapy or palliative care is an option, depending on the performance status of the patient.

132. How is stage IV NSCLC treated?
     With the advent of targeted agents of EGFR, ALK, and ROS1 mutations, these therapies are first-line treatment for patients who have a positive mutation. The mutations are mutually exclusive; thus, if one is positive, there is no utility in testing the other two. After failure of targeted agents, chemotherapy may be discussed. Immunotherapy with the PD-1 checkpoint inhibitors, nivolumab, and pembrolizumab has been approved after failure of chemotherapeutic agents.

133. How is SCLC staged?
     - Limited stage: Involves cancer on one side of the chest in one radiation port field. Lymph nodes may be involved but must also be in same port.
     - Extensive stage: Includes cancer spread throughout the lung, contralateral side, multiple lymph nodes outside the port, or distant disease (bone, brain, liver).

134. Which treatment modalities are used to manage SCLC?
     Chemotherapy (using combinations of drugs such as etoposide, cisplatin, carboplatin, or CPT-11) and radiotherapy are used concurrently or sequentially. These therapies in limited-stage disease have resulted in complete remission rates of 40–60%, median survival of 16–24 months, and 5-year

survival rates of 5–10%. Prophylactic radiotherapy to the brain is recommended for patients with limited-stage disease who achieve a complete response to therapy. Because of early hematogenous spread, surgery is not generally an option for patients with SCLC.

135. **How effective is the treatment of advanced stage (IV) SCLC?**
Generally fairly good for short-term survival. Patients with advanced-stage SCLC often have good partial responses to chemotherapy, but the responses are not durable. Median survival for patients with extensive disease who respond to treatment is 6–12 months. However, this is a significant improvement compared with the survival of untreated patients, which is measured in weeks.

136. **What is the SVC syndrome? What is its significance in lung cancer?**
Symptoms resulting from blood flow obstruction in the SVC due to thrombosis within the vessel or external compression of the vein by tumor (Fig. 15.2). The obstruction generally occurs when there is a lesion in the right upper lobe. Lung cancer, especially SCLC, accounts for up to 80% of cases. Lymphoma and other mediastinal malignancies account for the remaining 20% of SVC syndrome caused by neoplastic disease. Other causes of SVC syndrome include catheter thrombosis and sclerosis of the mediastinum.

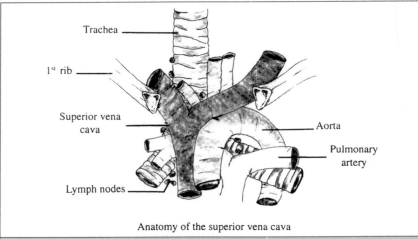

Anatomy of the superior vena cava

Fig. 15.2. Anatomy of the superior vena cava. *(From Wood ME, Bunn PA Jr. Hematology/Oncology Secrets. Philadelphia: Hanley & Belfus; 1994, p 240.)*

137. **What are the presenting signs and symptoms of SVC syndrome?**
- Dyspnea
- Face and arm edema
- Sense of fullness in the head
- Cough
- Prominent veins over the neck and chest
- Failure of hand veins to collapse when the arms are lifted above the head

138. **Why are the symptoms of SVC syndrome often not more significant?**
Because collateral circulation develops around the obstruction. Although obstruction of the vena cava has been considered a life-threatening oncologic emergency, only rarely does it progress to cause laryngeal edema, seizures, coma, and death.

139. **How is SVC syndrome treated?**
With radiotherapy or stent placement. Patients with SVC syndrome should not be given intravenous medications in the upper extremities owing to obstruction of the venous circulation.

KEY POINTS: LUNG CANCER

1. The most common cause of cancer death in the United States for both men and women is lung cancer.
2. Eighty-five percent of lung cancer is caused by smoking; these deaths are entirely preventable.
3. Lung cancer is rarely curable unless it is diagnosed in a very early stage.
4. Patients should be counseled at every physician's visit to quit all forms of tobacco use.

HEAD AND NECK CANCER

140. **What are the presenting symptoms of head and neck cancer?**
See Table 15.8.

Table 15.8. Presenting Symptoms of Head and Neck Cancer

SITE	SYMPTOMS
Oral cavity: lips, buccal mucosa, alveolar ridge, retromolar trigone, floor of mouth, hard palate, anterior two thirds of tongue	Mass, ulcer, leukoplakia, erythroplasia, bleeding, pain, loose teeth, earache, trismus, halitosis
Larynx: supraglottic (false cords, arytenoid), glottic (true vocal cords), subglottic	Hoarseness, bleeding, sore throat, thyroid cartilage pain
Pharynx: nasopharynx, oropharynx, soft palate, uvula, tonsil, base of tongue, hypopharynx, piriform sinus	Sore throat, earache, epistaxis, nasal voice, dysphagia, masses, hearing loss, blood-streaked saliva
Maxillary sinus	Sinusitis, epistaxis, headache
All sites	Bleeding (oral or nasal), neck nodes, pain at site of tumor or referred pain

141. **What are the two major risk factors for squamous cell cancer of the head and neck area?**
Tobacco is the most significant contributing factor to the development of head and neck cancers. Nine of 10 patients with cancer in this area are smokers. Snuff dipping and tobacco chewing are important causes of oral cancer. Smokers have an increased mortality rate related to head and neck cancer once it has been diagnosed, showing a twofold increase in mortality rate over nonsmokers.
      Alcohol is also strongly correlated with the development of head and neck cancer. About half of patients with head and neck cancer have cirrhosis, and three quarters drink alcohol excessively.

142. **What other risk factors have been identified?**
- **Viral exposure:** HPV, EBV, and herpes simplex (HSV) type 1
- **Occupation:** woodworkers and nickel compound exposure
- **Syphilis:** glossitis
- **Other:** poor dental hygiene

143. **Describe the evaluation and initial staging of patients with head and neck cancer.**
Triple endoscopy of upper and lower airway and upper aerodigestive tract, with biopsy of any suspicious lesions. Measurement and biopsy, if indicated, of any cervical or supraclavicular nodes should be performed. A **CT scan** of the head/neck and chest or a **PET scan** help to determine the extent of disease.

144. **What are the most common sites of metastases of head and neck cancer?**
Local lymph nodes in the neck, followed by lung metastases. Bone metastases occur in up to 15% of patients. Brain metastases are rare and are seen mainly in patients with nasopharyngeal cancer. Depending on tobacco and alcohol history, a second cancer of the head and neck, esophagus, or lung may occur in up to 20% of patients at some time in the course of their disease, especially if they continue to smoke and drink. Head and neck cancer rarely metastasizes to the abdomen.

145. **What is the most appropriate treatment of head and neck cancer?**
Primarily surgery for early-stage cancer, sometimes involving radical neck node dissection and postoperative radiotherapy. Radiation therapy is used for locations not amenable to surgery or if

surgery would be too disfiguring. In more advanced stages, head and neck cancers are treated with **multimodality therapy,** using chemotherapy or targeted agents in combination with radiotherapy. For cancer of the larynx, vocal cord preservation with chemotherapy and radiotherapy is preferred whenever possible. Cessation of smoking and alcohol consumption is essential to decrease the occurrence of second primary cancers in the head and neck region. Metastatic disease is treated initially with chemotherapy alone, and radiation may be considered for local palliation.

146. **Which chemotherapeutic agents are used in the treatment of squamous cell cancers of the head and neck? How effective are they?**
5-FU infusions with cisplatin or carboplatin, taxanes, and methotrexate, singly and in combination. Tumors may also respond to treatment with cetuximab, a monoclonal antibody against EGFR. Response rates for these agents vary depending on the agent, schedule, tumor type/location, previous treatment, and patient performance status. Combination chemotherapy regimens usually show higher initial response rates but have yet to show an increase in survival rates. Induction chemotherapy prior the concomitant chemoradiotherapy has not proved to improve overall survival but can be considered in bulky disease to help fit into one radiation port.

BREAST CANCER

See also Chapter 2, General Medicine and Ambulatory Care, for screening guidelines.

147. **How do you identify women at high risk for breast cancer?**
Initially by family history of breast or ovarian cancer. These patients have a high incidence of mutations in the *BRCA1* and *BRCA2* genes on chromosomes 17 and 13, respectively. In families with these mutations, generally over half of the female relatives have breast or ovarian cancer that is usually multifocal and has early age of onset. Patients with these gene mutations have a cumulative lifetime risk of developing breast cancer ranging up to 87%.

148. **What factors other than *BRCA* mutations significantly increase a woman's risk of breast cancer?**
    - Age > 40 years
    - Previous cancer in one breast
    - Breast cancer in a first- or second-degree family member
    - History of multiple breast biopsies
    - Parity: nulliparous, or first pregnancy after age 31 years
    - Lobular carcinoma in situ
    - Gene mutations: *BRCA1*, *BRCA2*, *p53*, Peutz-Jeghers syndrome, others
    - Radiation exposure to chest wall during childhood or adolescence

149. **What factors also increase a woman's risk for breast cancer?**
    - Early menarche or late menopause
    - Hormone replacement therapy (HRT) with estrogen and progesterone
    - Long-term use of estrogen therapy
    - History of cancer of the ovary, uterus, or colon
    - Alcohol use
    - Obesity
    - Lack of physical activity
    - Diethylstilbestrol (DES) exposure in utero
    National Cancer Center: Breast cancer risk assessment tool. Available at: www.cancer.gov/bcrisktool/. Accessed September 25, 2016.

150. **What can women do to reduce their risk of breast cancer?**
Prophylactic tamoxifen, raloxifene, exemestane, and anastrozole may reduce the occurrence of new breast cancers in women at high risk owing to a previous personal history of breast cancer, first-degree family members with breast cancer, and other factors, but there is an increased risk of thromboembolism and uterine cancer. Prophylactic mastectomy may also be selected by women who are known to carry the *BRCA1* or *BRCA2* gene mutations, which may reduce the incidence of breast cancer by about 90%.
    Visyanathan K, Chlebowski RT, Hurley P, et al. American Society of Clinical Oncology Clinical Practice Guideline update on the use of pharmacologic interventions including tamoxifen, raloxifene, and aromatase inhibition for breast cancer risk reduction. *J Clin Oncol.* 2009;24:3235–3258.

151. **What are the poor prognostic factors in primary breast cancer?**
   - Estrogen or progesterone receptors negative
   - Fixed axillary nodes
   - Positive *HER2/neu* status
   - Distant metastasis
   - Premenopausal patient
   - Large tumor size
   - Nuclear grade 3 (poor)
   - Positive axillary nodes
   - Local skin involvement

152. **What are the surgical options for treatment of localized breast cancer?**
   Modified radical mastectomy versus breast conservation surgery (lumpectomy) followed by radiation therapy. In both types of surgery, axillary node staging with sentinel node biopsy or axillary node dissection is performed. Lumpectomy followed by radiotherapy is used if complete excision is possible and radiation therapy can be delivered to the tumor bed. Modified radical mastectomy is performed if tumor mass is large relative to breast size, the cancer is multifocal, or radiation therapy is not technically feasible.

153. **What are the overall treatment guidelines for locally advanced breast cancer?**
   If the tumor is large or has unfavorable prognostic characteristics on the preliminary biopsy, preoperative (neoadjuvant) chemotherapy may be administered, followed by surgery. After the operation, adjuvant therapy with chemotherapy, hormone therapy, or trastuzumab or combination therapy may be given to help eradicate any possible micrometastases in the circulation. The types of agents chosen will depend on tumor characteristics that include estrogen and progesterone receptor status and *Her2/neu* status. Patient-specific factors such as menopausal category, age, and comorbid conditions are also important in the choice of adjuvant therapy. Local radiation therapy is administered to patients whose tumors are at high risk for local recurrence.

154. **When is radiation therapy given to the chest wall and regional lymph nodes after breast cancer surgery?**
   For patients identified at high risk for recurrence by:
   - Lumpectomy as procedure for initial treatment
   - Four or more axillary nodes positive for cancer
   - Extracapsular nodal extension
   - Large (>5 cm) primary tumor
   - Positive or very close tumor resection margin

155. **How is adjuvant therapy used in the management of breast cancer?**
   See Table 15.9.

Table 15.9. Current Recommendations for the Use of Adjuvant Systemic Therapy in Breast Cancer

	PREMENOPAUSAL	POSTMENOPAUSAL
Node Negative*†‡		
ER and PR negative	Chemotherapy	Chemotherapy
ER or PR positive	Chemotherapy + TAM, ± ovarian ablation or LHRH agonist	Endocrine therapy§ ± chemotherapy
Node Positive‡‖		
ER and PR negative	Chemotherapy	Chemotherapy
ER or PR positive	Chemotherapy + TAM, ± ovarian ablation or LHRH agonist	Endocrine therapy§ ± chemotherapy

*Adjuvant therapy is not recommended for tumors < 0.5 cm or well-differentiated tumors < 1 cm.

†Adjuvant therapy is recommended for all tumors > 1 cm and for tumors 0.5–1.0 cm with poor prognosis features: poorly differentiated, high nuclear grade, lymphovascular invasion, high S-phase fraction.

‡Patients with *Her2/neu*-positive tumors require ≤ 1 year of adjuvant trastuzumab in addition to chemotherapy and/or endocrine therapy.

§Endocrine therapy may consist of an aromatase inhibitor for 5 years or tamoxifen for 2–3 years followed by an aromatase inhibitor for a total of ≥ 5 years.

‖Adjuvant therapy is recommended for all patients.

ER, estrogen receptor; LHRH, luteinizing hormone–releasing hormone; PR, progesterone receptor; TAM, tamoxifen.

156. **How is stage IV breast cancer treated?**
With either systemic chemotherapy or hormone therapy, depending on hormone receptor status, location of metastases, and patient characteristics, reserving surgery and radiotherapy for local control. Trastuzumab, an antibody against the *Her2/neu* receptor, may be added for patients whose tumors are *Her2/neu*-positive.

157. **Discuss the role of aromatase inhibitors in adjuvant therapy for breast cancer.**
In postmenopausal women with hormone-positive breast cancers, aromatase inhibitors such as anastrozole may be more effective than tamoxifen, and the addition of letrozole after 2 to 3 years of adjuvant tamoxifen may offer additional benefit.

158. **Which chemotherapy agents are used in the treatment of metastatic breast cancer?**
Paclitaxel, docetaxel, doxorubicin, epirubicin, vinorelbine, cyclophosphamide, methotrexate, fluorouracil, and capecitabine. These agents are used singly or in combination in the treatment of advanced or metastatic breast cancer. If the tumor overexpresses the *Her2/neu* oncogene, trastuzumab, pertuzumab, TDM-1, or lapatinib may be added to improve the effectiveness of chemotherapy.

159. **How effective are chemotherapy agents in the treatment of metastatic breast cancer?**
Overall induction response rates range from 55–65%. Median survival times are 14–18 months. The survival rates depend more on the site of the metastatic disease than on the treatment, with visceral disease faring more poorly than bony or soft tissue metastases. Most patients receive more than one treatment regimen, because the median time to failure of most programs is about 6 months.

160. **What other drugs may be used to treat metastatic breast cancer?**
Hormonal agents such as tamoxifen, anastrozole, letrozole, exemestane, or luteinizing hormone–releasing hormone (LHRH) agonists (in premenopausal women) can be used for bony or soft tissue metastases in patients with estrogen or progesterone receptor–positive breast cancer and can be effective palliation lasting many months. Exemestane in combination with everolimus has been shown to be effective with improved progression-free survival but has significant toxicity such as stomatitis, pneumonitis, and hypertriglyceridemia. Newer drugs in breast cancer such as palbociclib and a cell cycle cyclin-dependent kinase inhibitor (CDK4/6) are effective as well but have significant side effects of neutropenia and diarrhea that must be closely monitored while on therapy.

GYNECOLOGIC CANCERS

See Chapter 2, General Medicine and Ambulatory Care, for screening guidelines.

161. **What should be done if invasive cancer is found on cervical biopsy?**
Metastatic work-up to determine the extent of disease. For early-stage disease, treatment options include radiation therapy or surgery with postoperative radiation therapy plus chemotherapy. For locally advanced disease, the treatment is radiation therapy combined with chemotherapy. Once the cancer is metastatic, it is treated with chemotherapy. Radiation therapy may be used to palliate local symptoms or distant metastases.

162. **Which studies are used in the staging of carcinoma of the cervix?**
- Pelvic examination.
- Biochemical profile.
- Chest radiograph.
- CT scan or MRI (MRI is preferred).
- Lymphangiograms may be useful in selected cases.
- Cystoscopy and proctosigmoidoscopy for advanced disease.

163. **What are the 5-year survival rates, relative to stage, for carcinoma of the cervix?**
See Table 15.10.

Table 15.10. Five-Year Survival Rates for Cervical Cancer Relative to Stage

STAGE	DESCRIPTION	5-YEAR SURVIVAL RATE (%)
I	Tumor strictly confined to the cervix.	89–100
II	Tumor extends beyond the uterus but not to the pelvic wall. The tumor involves the vagina but not the lower third.	67
III	Tumor extends to the pelvic wall, and/or involves the lower third of the vagina, and/or causes hydronephrosis or nonfunctioning kidney.	53
IV	Tumor extends beyond the true pelvis, or has involved the bladder or rectal mucosa, or has distant metastases.	5–24

164. **How is stage I carcinoma of the cervix treated?**
   - **IA:** total or modified radical hysterectomy, conization, or intracavitary radiation.
   - **IB:** external-beam pelvic irradiation combined with two or more intracavitary radiation applications; radical hysterectomy with bilateral pelvic lymphadenectomy ± postoperative total pelvic irradiation plus chemotherapy; or radiation therapy plus chemotherapy with cisplatin or cisplatin/5-FU for patients with bulky tumors.

165. **Summarize the treatment of stage II carcinoma of the cervix.**
   - **IIA:** same as stage IB.
   - **IIB:** radiation therapy plus chemotherapy: intracavitary radiation and external-beam pelvic irradiation combined with cisplatin or cisplatin/fluorouracil.

166. **How is stage III carcinoma of the cervix treated?**
   The same as stage IIB.

167. **Summarize the treatment of stage IV carcinoma of the cervix.**
   - **IVA:** same as stage IIB and stage III.
   - **IVB:** chemotherapy with agents such as cisplatin, paclitaxel, ifosfamide-cisplatin, or irinotecan. Radiotherapy may be used for palliation.
   National Cancer Institute: Cervical Cancer Treatment (PDQ®)-Health Professional Version. Available at https://www.cancer.gov/types/cervical/hp/cervical-treatment-pdq. Accessed September 25, 2016.

168. **Name the risk factors for carcinoma of the endometrium.**
   - Infertility
   - Obesity
   - Failure of ovulation
   - Dysfunctional bleeding
   - Prolonged estrogen use
   - Diabetes mellitus
   - Hypertension
   - Polycystic ovary syndrome (PCOS)
   - Familial cancer syndrome (Lynch)
   - Tamoxifen use

169. **What are the 5-year survival rates for the various grades and stages of endometrial cancer?**
   See Table 15.11.

170. **List the risk factors for ovarian cancer.**
   - Nulliparity or low parity
   - Presence of basal cell nevus syndrome
   - Family history of ovarian cancer or ovarian cancer syndromes, including *BRCA1* and *BRCA2* mutations

Table 15.11. Five-Year Survival Rates for Grades and Stages of Endometrial Cancer

GRADE/STAGE	DESCRIPTION	5-YEAR SURVIVAL RATE (%)
Grade		
I	Differentiated	81
II	Intermediate	74
III	Undifferentiated	50
Stage		
I	Tumor confined to the corpus	92
II	Tumor involves the corpus and cervix	78
III	Tumor extends outside the corpus but not outside the true pelvis (may involve the vaginal wall or parametrium but not the bladder or rectum)	42
IV	Tumor involves the bladder or rectum, extends outside the pelvis, or has distant metastases	14

- Gonadal dysgenesis (46,XY type)
- History of breast, endometrial, or colon cancer
- Asbestos exposure
- Presence of Peutz-Jeghers syndrome

171. Discuss the appropriate use of the CA-125 antigen.
CA-125 serum tumor marker, an antigenic determinant detected by radioimmunoassay, is elevated in 80% of epithelial ovarian cancers. Because it is high in only half of patients with stage I cancers and is increased in a significant proportion of healthy women and women with benign disease, it is not a sensitive or specific test and should not be used for screening in women with average risk for ovarian cancer. In high-risk patients or in patients suspected of having an ovarian cancer, it can be used in conjunction with bimanual rectovaginal pelvic examination and transvaginal ultrasonography. When the CA-125 value is elevated before treatment in a patient with an established diagnosis of ovarian cancer, it is useful as a marker of disease recurrence after surgical resection.

172. List the neurologic paraneoplastic syndromes associated with ovarian cancer.
- Peripheral neuropathy
- Organic brain syndrome
- Acute myelogenous leukemia–like syndrome
- Cerebellar ataxia (anti-Yo paraneoplastic cerebellar degeneration)
- Cancer-associated retinopathy
- Opsoclonus myoclonus

173. What other paraneoplastic syndromes may be associated with ovarian cancer?
- Cross-matching of blood antigens
- Cushing syndrome
- Hypercalcemia
- Thrombophlebitis
- Dermatomyositis
- Palmar fasciitis and polyarthritis

174. What are the 5-year survival rates for the various stages of carcinoma of the ovary?
- **I:** growth limited to the ovaries: 84%
- **II:** growth involving one or both ovaries with pelvic extension: 63%
- **III:** tumor involving ovaries with peritoneal implants outside the pelvis and/or positive retroperitoneal or inguinal nodes: 29%
- **IV:** distant metastases: 17%

175. Describe the treatment for advanced-stage ovarian cancer.

Patients with stage III epithelial ovarian cancers are first treated with surgery, consisting of total abdominal hysterectomy and bilateral salpingo-oophorectomy with omentectomy and debulking of as much gross tumor as possible. This is followed by intravenous chemotherapy with cisplatin or carboplatin combined with paclitaxel or cyclophosphamide. Patients with stage IV disease are given combination chemotherapy. The survival benefit of surgical debulking in patients with stage IV extra-abdominal disease is not yet known.

MISCELLANEOUS TOPICS

176. Which cancers are associated with AIDS and are AIDS-defining conditions?
- Kaposi sarcoma (decreasing incidence)
- Non-Hodgkin lymphoma including primary central nervous system lymphoma (most frequent)
- Cervical cancer

177. What are other AIDS-related cancers?

Hodgkin disease and cancers of the lung, oral cavity, cervix, and anus.

178. What phenotype is most highly associated with the development of melanoma?

Fair skin, reddish hair, and freckles. Melanoma families have been described in which > 25% of the kindred are affected, with a vertical distribution of disease. There is an early age of onset, from the third to fourth decades. The incidence of multiple primary melanomas is increased, as is the presence of atypical nevi (B-K moles or familial atypical multiple melanoma with melanocyte dysplasia). However, there is a superior overall survival, possibly related to earlier detection. Ocular melanoma is also seen in this group of patients. The gene for the dysplastic nevus syndrome/familial melanoma is located on chromosome 1.

179. What is a key driver mutation in melanoma?

BRAF V600E mutation (a part of the MAPK [mitogen-activated protein kinase] pathway) for which there are targeted therapies with BRAF inhibitors such as vemurafenib and dabrafenib. Additionally, there is a MEK mutation for which there are MEK inhibitors such as cobimetinib and selimetinib.

180. Where does melanoma metastasize?

To anywhere in the body, including lungs, liver, bowels, and bones. Melanoma is one of the few cancers that can cross the placenta and spread to a developing fetus. Bowel metastases can cause obstruction and bleeding, and lesions appear on barium dye studies as ulcerated with a central crater and a surrounding heaped-up border, causing the barium to pool in a "target" configuration.

181. What is immunotherapy?

Treatments that utilize the patient's own immune system to control the tumor. T-cell downregulation via the tumor is part of its escape mechanism and allows the tumor to proliferate without attack from our immune system. Cytotoxic T-lymphocyte associated protein 4 (CTLA-4) acts as a negative regulator of T-cell activation. Inhibition of CTLA-4 with ipilumumab was studied in melanoma with good outcomes. Further research yielded discovery of programmed cell death (PD-1) proteins that bind PD-ligand 1 (PD-L1). The PD-1 and PD-L1 interact directly with the tumor cell allowing for inhibition of apoptosis of tumor cell and T cell exhaustion. Drugs that target PD-1 and PD-L1 include nivolumab and pembrolizumab. Immunotherapy targeting these two entities leads to increased T-cell activation and immune response with good tumor response. These therapies are being tested widely throughout hematologic and oncologic malignancies.

WEBSITES

1. National Cancer Database: www.facs.org/cancer/ncdb/index.html
2. National Guideline Clearinghouse: www.guideline.gov/
3. PDQ Cancer Information Summaries: www.cancer.gov/

BIBLIOGRAPHY
1. American Joint Committee on Cancer. *Cancer Staging Manual.* 7th ed. New York: Springer-Verlag; 2010.
2. Casciato DA, Territo DA, eds. *Manual of Clinical Oncology.* 7th ed. Boston: Little Brown; 2012.
3. Devita T Jr, Lawrence T, Rosenberg SA, eds. *Cancer Principles and Practice of Oncology.* 8th ed. Philadelphia: Lippincott Williams & Wilkins; 2008.
4. Kufe DW, Frei E, Holland JF, eds. *Holland-Frei Cancer Medicine.* 8th ed. Shelton, CT: People's Medical Publishing House; 2010.

ENDOCRINOLOGY

CHAPTER 16

Susan E. Spratt, MD, and Whitney W. Woodmansee, MD

In diabetes the thirst is greater for the fluid dries the body.... For the thirst there is need of a powerful remedy, for in kind it is the greatest of all sufferings, and when a fluid is drunk, it stimulates the discharge of urine.

Aretaeus of Cappadocia
2nd-Century Greek Physician
From *Therapeutics of Chronic Diseases II*, Chapter II, pp 485–486

DIABETES MELLITUS AND GLYCEMIC DISORDERS

1. List the three main categories of diabetes mellitus (DM).
   - **Type 1:** Previously called *insulin-dependent DM* or *juvenile-onset DM*
   - **Type 2:** Previously called *non–insulin-dependent DM* or *adult-onset DM*
   - **Gestational diabetes mellitus** (GDM): Diabetes diagnosed in pregnancy

2. Describe type 1 DM.
   Type 1 DM is generally due to autoimmune destruction of the pancreatic beta cells, leading to absolute insulin deficiency, and accounts for approximately 5–10% of patients with DM. Although typically diagnosed in patients before age 30, it can present at any age owing to variability in the rate of beta-cell destruction.

3. What autoimmune diseases are associated with type 1 DM?
   - Adrenal insufficiency
   - Hyperthyroidism
   - Hypothyroidism
   - Celiac sprue
   - Pernicious anemia

4. What autoimmune diseases should be considered when a patient with type 1 DM presents with iron deficiency?
   Celiac sprue and pernicious anemia.

5. What are the major characteristics of type 2 DM?
   Insulin resistance and relative insulin deficiency. Most patients are obese with predominantly abdominal accumulation of fat. Type 2 DM is usually diagnosed in adults, but increasing numbers of children and adolescents are now diagnosed with type 2 DM as childhood obesity rates increase. These patients are not prone to developing ketoacidosis except in association with stress from another illness.

6. Compare and contrast the general features of type 1 and type 2 DM.
   See Table 16.1.

7. Which pregnant women should be screened for GDM at the first prenatal visit?
   Those who have
   - Obesity
   - Prior history of GDM
   - Given birth to a baby weighing over 9 lb
   - Polycystic ovary syndrome (PCOS)
   - Glycosuria
   - Family history of type 2 DM
   - Inclusion in high-risk racial/ethnic group
   - Physical inactivity
   - Hypertension
   - High-density lipoprotein (HDL) cholesterol less than 35 mg/dL

431

Table 16.1. Characteristics of Diabetes Mellitus

TYPE 1 DIABETES MELLITUS	TYPE 2 DIABETES MELLITUS
5% of diagnosed cases	95% of diagnosed cases
Usually presents at a younger age but can occur at any age	Typically presents at age > 40 yr
Normal weight or thin but may be seen with obesity	Obese
Usually no family history	Strong family history
Autoimmune markers may be positive (anti-GAD and anti-islet cell antibodies)	Not autoimmune in nature
Insulin-sensitive	Insulin-resistant
Requires insulin for treatment	Often managed with diet or oral agents but frequently eventually requires insulin

GAD, glutamic acid decarboxylase.

- Hemoglobin A_{1c} (A_{1c}) over 5.7%
- Clinical signs or symptoms concerning for insulin resistance
  All other women can be screened for GDM between weeks 24 and 28 of gestation with a 75-g oral glucose tolerance test (OGTT). (See Question 9.)

8. What is GDM?
   Diabetes diagnosed during pregnancy that is not clearly overt diabetes. Glucose tolerance usually returns to normal after delivery, but women with GDM should be screened for diabetes 6–12 weeks postpartum and routinely approximately every 3 years because 50–100% of women with GDM will develop diabetes over their lifetime.
   Bellamy L, Casas JP, Hingorani AD, et al. Type 2 diabetes mellitus after gestational diabetes: a systematic review and meta-analysis. *Lancet.* 2009;373:1773–1779.

9. What are the diagnostic criteria for GDM using 75-g oral glucose solution?
   A glucose value exceeding one of the following values:
   - Fasting glucose ≥ 92 mg/dL
   - 1-hour glucose ≥ 180 mg/dL
   - 2-hour glucose ≥ 153 mg/dL
   A two-step strategy for GDM screening is also acceptable which initially uses a 50-g oral glucose solution. If blood glucose (BG) ≥ 140 mg/dL, then a 100-g OGTT is performed.

10. What are the complications of GDM?
    - Preeclampasia
    - Polyhydramnios
    - Fetal macrosomia
    - Birth trauma
    - Cesarean section
    - Perinatal death and morbidity

11. Describe other specific types of DM.

DM Type	Cause
Maturity-onset diabetes of the young	Genetic defect in beta-cell function
Insulin receptor/action dysfunction	Genetic defect in insulin receptor
Exocrine pancreas disease	Hemochromatosis, neoplasm, cystic fibrosis
Endocrinopathies	Cushing syndrome, acromegaly, somatostatinoma, glucagonoma
Drug-induced	Pentamidine, glucocorticoids, interferon-α
Infection-induced	Viral infection (Coxsackie, enterovirus, hepatitis C)
Rare genetic disorders	Wolfram syndrome (diabetes insipidus, diabetes mellitus, optic atrophy, deafness)

12. **What criteria are used to diagnose DM?**
   One of the following:
   - Symptoms of diabetes (polyuria, polydipsia, and unexplained weight loss) plus casual plasma glucose concentration ≥ 200 mg/dL (11.1 mmol/L). "Casual" is defined as any time of day without regard to last meal.
   - Fasting plasma glucose ≥ 126 mg/dL (7.0 mmol/L). "Fasting" is defined as no caloric intake for at least 8 hours.
   - Two-hour plasma glucose > 200 mg/dL with OGTT using a 75-g glucose challenge
   - A_{1c} ≥ 6.5%

13. **Is a single reading of any of these values sufficient to diagnose DM?**
   No. In the absence of unequivocal hyperglycemia with acute metabolic decompensation, any abnormal value should be confirmed by repeat testing on a different day.

14. **What is the role of A_{1c} in the diagnosis of DM?**
   To estimate average blood glucose control in patients with diagnosed DM and, more recently, for initial diagnosis of DM with confirmatory testing.

15. **What is prediabetes?**
   A condition in which the glucose values are too high to be considered normal but do not fit the criteria for the diagnosis of DM. Categories that may define prediabetes include impaired glucose tolerance (IGT), impaired fasting glucose (IFG), and abnormal A_{1c} (5.7–6.4%).

16. **Define IGT and IFG.**
   - **IGT:** A 2-hour postload glucose of 140–199 mg/dL (7.8–11.1 mmol/L), using the OGTT
   - **IFG:** A fasting plasma glucose of 100–125 mg/dL (5.6–6.9 mmol/L)
   IGT and IFG are associated with the metabolic syndrome and a high risk of developing DM and cardiovascular disease.

17. **List the diagnostic criteria for the metabolic syndrome.**
   - Prediabetes or diabetes (hyperinsulinemia)
   - Abdominal (central) obesity
   - Hypertension
   - Atherosclerosis
   - PCOS
   - Waist circumference ≥ 102 cm in men and ≥ 88 cm in women
   - Triglycerides (TG) ≥ 150 mg/dL or history of drug treatment for the condition
   - Systolic BP ≥ 130 mm Hg or diastolic BP ≥ 85 mm Hg
   - HDL cholesterol < 40 mg/dL in men and < 50 mg/dL in women
   - Fasting glucose ≥ 100 mg/dL
   Metabolic syndrome is diagnosed if three of the preceding criteria are present.
   Grundy SM, Cleerman JI, Daniels SR, et al. Diagnosis and management of the metabolic syndrome: an American Heart Association/National Heart and Blood Institute Scientific Statement. *Circulation.* 2005;112:2735–2752.

KEY POINTS: CRITERIA FOR CONDITIONS ASSOCIATED WITH METABOLIC SYNDROME

1. Atherogenic dyslipidemia (elevated TG, apolipoprotein B, small density LDL, and low HDL)
2. Prothrombotic state (impaired fibrinolysis, elevated plasminogen activator inhibitor-1)
3. Proinflammatory state (elevated high-sensitivity C-reactive protein and inflammatory cytokines)
4. Polycystic ovary syndrome
5. Vascular dysregulation (microalbuminuria and chronic kidney disease)
6. Insulin resistance
7. Abnormal body fat distribution

HDL, high-density liroprotein; LDL, low-density lipoprotein; TG, triglycerides.

---

18. **Describe the pathophysiology of diabetic ketoacidosis (DKA).**
   An increase in counterregulatory hormones (catecholamines, cortisol, glucagon, and growth hormone) accompanied by insulin deficiency. All of these hormonal factors contribute to increased hepatic and

renal glucose production and decreased peripheral glucose utilization. These hormonal changes also serve to enhance lipolysis and ketogenesis as well as glycogenolysis and gluconeogenesis and serve to worsen hyperglycemia and acidosis. Insulin is required to block glycogenolysis and gluconeogenesis. Lipolysis leads to increased free fatty acid synthesis for ultimate conversion by the liver to ketones. This state is associated with increased production and decreased utilization of glucose and ketones. Glucosuria leads to osmotic diuresis and dehydration that is associated with reduced renal function and worsening acidosis.

19. **List the clinical features of DKA.**
   - Polydipsia
   - Polyphagia
   - Polyuria
   - Severe dehydration
   - Altered mental status (including coma)
   - Gastrointestinal (GI) distress (nausea, vomiting, abdominal pain)
   - Weight loss
   - Hyperventilation
   - Weakness

20. **What physical examination findings are associated with DKA?**
   - Dehydration
   - Poor skin turgor
   - Rapid shallow breathing (initially) followed in late DKA by Kussmaul breathing (deep, gasping breath)
   - Mental status changes (wide range)
   - Hypotension
   - Tachycardia
   - Musty (fruity) breath
   - Hyporeflexia
   - Hypothermia
     Findings will vary with the severity of DKA. Untreated DKA can progress to coma, shock, and death.

21. **Summarize the laboratory data associated with DKA.**
   Plasma glucose > 250 mg/dL, arterial pH < 7.3, serum bicarbonate < 18 mEq/L, positive serum and urine ketones, and elevated anion gap (>10–12). Although these laboratory results are diagnostic for DKA and may vary with severity, one may see other abnormalities, including elevated blood urea nitrogen and creatinine with dehydration, leukocytosis, low serum sodium, and elevated serum potassium due to extracellular shifting caused by insulin deficiency.

22. **How is DKA managed?**
   With fluid resuscitation, insulin therapy, and careful monitoring and correction of electrolyte imbalances. Any precipitating factors should be identified when possible. The most common precipitating factor is infection. The hospitalized patient should have appropriate bacterial cultures (e.g., blood, urine) and antibiotic therapy if infection is suspected.

23. **What factors other than infection may precipitate DKA?**
   Myocardial infarction, stroke, pancreatitis, trauma, alcohol abuse, or medications (particularly inadequate insulin therapy).

24. **Should patients with DKA be hospitalized?**
   Almost always. Hospitalization depends on the severity of DKA, and very mild DKA in experienced patients with type 1 DM can be managed in the outpatient setting. Most patients, however, require hospitalization for intravenous (IV) fluid management, insulin (IV insulin infusion is the treatment of choice), and correction of electrolytes (sodium, potassium, phosphate, bicarbonate).

25. **What principle should be kept in mind when patients are transitioned from IV to subcutaneous (SC) insulin?**
   That SC insulin must be given before discontinuing IV insulin (usually 1–2 hours to allow for adequate plasma insulin levels) to avoid return of hyperglycemia and DKA.

26. **What is hyperglycemic hyperosmolar nonketotic syndrome (HHNS)?**
Severe hyperglycemia with profound dehydration and some degree of alteration in mental status (50%). Typically, patients have type 2 DM and mild renal impairment. The plasma glucose is frequently very elevated (>600 mg/dL). Ketosis is usually only very mild or absent. Plasma hyperosmolarity (>340 mOsm/L) is one hallmark of this condition.

27. **How is HHNS treated?**
With aggressive fluid replacement, insulin, and correction of electrolyte disturbances. As with DKA, a search for the precipitating factor is warranted.

28. **What are the recommended A_{1c} goals for nonpregnant adult diabetics?**
Generally <7%, but a goal of <6.5% may be considered for those individuals who can achieve this goal without significant hypoglycemia or adverse effects. Such patients include those with lifestyle or metformin treatment for type 2 DM, long life expectancy, or significant cardiovascular disease. Older patients with multiple comorbid conditions, limited life expectancy, or advanced complications of their diabetes may best be managed with $A_{1c} < 8\%$.
American Diabetes Association. Glycemic targets. *Diabetes Care.* 2017;40:S48–S56.

29. **What diseases or conditions reduce the accuracy of A_{1c}?**
- Hemolysis (from artificial cardiac valves and transjugular intrahepatic portosystemic shunts [TIPS])
- Transfusion
- Dialysis
- Hemoglobinopathies such as sickle cell disease and thalassemia

30. **How should one screen for diabetic nephropathy?**
With an annual urine spot albumin-to-creatinine ratio to detect microalbuminuria. Microalbuminuria is defined as 30–299 μg albumin/mg creatinine and must be confirmed on repeated examinations. Clinical albuminuria is defined as ≥ 300 μg albumin/mg creatinine. Any abnormal results should be repeated over a several-month period. Patients with type 1 DM should begin microalbuminuria screening when they have had DM for longer than 5 years; patients with type 2 DM should begin screening at the time of diagnosis.

31. **Summarize the screening recommendations for diabetic retinopathy.**
Patients with type 1 DM should receive a comprehensive dilated eye examination within 3–5 years of diagnosis and annually thereafter. Patients with type 2 DM should receive a comprehensive dilated examination at the time of diagnosis and annually. The eye-care specialist may determine altered timing of follow-up examinations.

32. **How are patients screened for diabetic neuropathy?**
With monofilament sensory testing of the foot for loss of protective sensation (LOPS). A detailed foot examination that includes vibratory and pin sensation, vascular assessment, and physical examination for foot deformities (Charcot changes, bunions, hammer toes, tinea, and onychomycosis) should be done yearly. Foot inspection for foot ulcers should be done at every visit. Patient education about foot care should be given at least annually.

33. **Who is at risk for diabetes foot ulcer?**
Those with:
- History of prior foot ulcer
- History of previous amputation
- Presence of foot deformities
- Presence of callus
- Peripheral vascular disease
- Renal replacement therapy (dialysis)
- Tobacco abuse

34. **When should an ankle brachial index (ABI) be performed?**
In patients with symptoms (claudication) or signs (absent pedal pulses) of peripheral arterial disease. (See also Chapter 5, Vascular Medicine.)

35. Identify the noninsulin agents available for the treatment of type 2 DM. See Table 16.2.

Table 16.2. Available Noninsulin Agents for the Treatment of Type 2 Diabetes Mellitus

CLASS	MEDICATIONS	ACTIONS	COMMON SIDE EFFECTS
Sulfonylureas	Glyburide	↑ insulin secretion	Hypoglycemia, dizziness, GI upset, weight gain
	Glipizide		
	Glimepiride		
Meglitinides	Repaglinide	↑ insulin secretion	Hypoglycemia, GI upset, weight gain
	Nateglinide		Requires frequent dosing
Biguanides	Metformin	↓ glucose production in liver, ↓ vitamin B_{12}	Anorexia, diarrhea, GI upset, lactic acidosis (rare), contraindicated if eGFR < 30 mL/min/1.73 m^2
Thiazolidinediones	Pioglitazone	↑ insulin sensitivity	Weight gain, heart failure, bone fracture, hypoglycemia if used with insulin
	Rosiglitazone		
α-Glucosidase inhibitor	Acarbose	↓ intestinal carbohydrate	Flatulence, diarrhea, GI distress, frequent dosing schedule
	Miglitol		
DPP-IV inhibitors	Sitagliptin	↑ insulin secretion	Angiodemia, ? pancreatitis, heart failure
	Saxiglitpin	↓ glucagon secretion	
	Linagliptin		
	Alogliptin		
GLP-1 agonists	Exenatide	↑ insulin secretion	Injectable, nausea, weight loss, GI upset, tachycardia, ? pancreatitis, C-cell hyperplasia
	Liraglutide		
	Albiglutide		
	Lixisenatide Dulaglutide		
GLT-2 inhibitors	Canagliflozin	Blocks glucose resorption by kidney	UTI, polyuria, volume depletion
	Dapagliflozin	↑ LDL-C	
	Empaglifozin		
Amylinomimetics	Pramlintide	↓ glucagon secretion	Injectible, GI upset, frequent dosing, hypoglycemia with insulin
		↓ gastric emptying	

*Only for use in patients whose glucose is uncontrolled with any other medicine.

CHF, congestive heart failure; Cr, creatinine; DPP, dipeptidyl peptidase; eGFR, estimated glomerular filtration rate; GI, gastrointestinal; GLP, glucagon-like peptide; LDL-C, low-density lipoprotein cholesterol; SGLT, sodium-glucose cotransporter; UTI, urinary tract infection.

Adapted from American Diabetes Association: Standards of medical care in diabetes 2017. *Diabetes Care.* 2017;40:S1–S135.

36. **What vitamin deficiency is associated with the use of metformin?**
Vitamin B_{12}.

37. **Describe the different types of insulin.**
See Table 16.3.

Table 16.3. Types of Insulin*

INSULIN TYPE	TIME OF ONSET	PEAK	DURATION OF ONSET
Rapid-Acting			
Lispro	<30 min	30–90 min	3–5 hr
Aspart	<15 min	1–3 hr	3–5 hr
Glulisine	12–30 min	1.6–1.8 hr	3–4 hr
Short-Acting			
Regular	0.5–1 hr	2–4 hr	6–12 hr
Intermediate-Acting			
NPH	1–2 hr	4–14 hr	10–24 hr
Lente	1–3 hr	6–16 hr	12–24 hr
Long-acting			
Glargine U-100	3 hr	No real peak	20–24 hr
Glargine U-300	3 hr	No real peak	24–37 hr
Detemir (Levemir)	1–3 hr	Small peak at 6–8 hr	12–24 hr
Degludec	1 hr	9 hr	24 hr
Regular U-500	1 hr	4–8 hr	12–24 hr (dose dependent)
Mixtures			
70% NPH/30% regular	30 min	4–8 hr	16–24 hr
50% NPH/50% regular	30 min	7–12 hr	16–24 hr
75% NPL/25% lispro	<30 min	Lispro 30–90 min Protamine 2–4 hr	6–12 hr
70% NPA/25% aspart	<15 min	1–4 hr	12–24 hr

*These values are highly variable among individual patients. Even in a given person, these values vary depending on the site and depth of injection, skin temperature, and exercise. *Note:* Insulin glargine cannot be mixed with other insulins owing to the low pH of its diluent. Rapid-acting insulins can be mixed with NPH, Lente, and Ultralente.
NPA, neutral protamine aspart; NPH, neutral protamine hagedorn; NPL, neutral protamine lispro.

38. **Where is insulin cleared?**
Mainly in the liver. Approximately 50% of insulin is cleared via first pass through the liver. Once insulin is in the periphery, 30% is cleared by the kidney. IV insulin has an extremely short half-life regardless of the type of insulin used (e.g., regular or lispro). As soon as the insulin IV infusion is discontinued, it is generally cleared quickly (i.e., within 5 minutes) from the circulation.

39. **What are the indications for an insulin pump?**
Need for flexibility in insulin dosing and meal timing in motivated patients. Both continuous subcutaneous insulin infusion (CSII) administered through an insulin pump and multiple daily insulin injections can effectively control blood glucose. Some patients and physicians prefer the use of an insulin pump, which requires extensive patient education, meticulous monitoring, and supervision by a health care provider who is comfortable with this mode of insulin delivery.

40. **What are incretin hormones and which drugs are based on them?**
Hormones produced in the GI tract when food is eaten that enhance the action of insulin. Their existence was postulated when it was noted that a glucose challenge given IV required more insulin to achieve glycemic control than a glucose challenge given orally. Incretin hormones include glucagon-like peptide-1 (GLP-1) and amylin. Drugs that have been manufactured to take advantage of these incretin hormones include exenatide and liraglutide (GLP-1 agonist), symlin (amylin agonist), and dipeptidyl peptidase (DPP) IV inhibitors, which block the degradation of GLP-1.

41. **List the chronic complications of DM.**
Microvascular
- Neuropathy: Painful paresthesias, autonomic neuropathy
- Retinopathy: Nonproliferative and proliferative retinopathy, blindness
- Nephropathy: Microalbuminuria, chronic kidney disease, end-stage renal disease

Macrovascular
- Cardiovascular: Hypertension, dysplipidemia, coronary artery disease
- Peripheral arterial disease: Claudication, nonhealing ulcers, amputations, stroke

42. **What is important to know about diabetes in pregnancy?**
Patients with diabetes should plan all pregnancies. A_{1c} should be < 7% before pregnancy is attempted. Medications such as angiotensin-converting enzyme (ACE) inhibitors, angiotensin receptor blockers (ARBs), statins, fibrates, and certain antidepressant medications should be discontinued. Diabetes health care maintenance screening, including thyroid, urine albumin, and retinal examination should be up to date. Patients with retinopathy should have a dilated eye examination every trimester. Women should take 1000 μg of folate daily before conception and during pregnancy. Once pregnant, glucose levels are much more stringent. Fasting glucose should be < 90 mg/dL, and 2-hour postmeal blood glucose should be < 120 mg/dL. Patients should perform fingerstick test for glucose six times per day.
  The Guideline Development Group. Management of diabetes from preconception to the postnatal period: summary of NICE guidance. *BMJ.* 2008;336:714–717.

43. **What are the symptoms of hypoglycemia?**
See Table 16.4. Symptoms can be divided into two categories: **catecholamine mediated** (due to excess secretion of epinephrine) and **neuroglycopenic** (due to cerebral dysfunction). Patients with DM typically develop symptoms of hypoglycemia when blood glucose values fall below 50–60 mg/dL, but severity of symptoms can vary with the individual. In addition, some fasting individuals (particularly women) without DM can be completely asymptomatic with glucose values approximately 50 mg/dL.

Table 16.4. Symptoms of Hypoglycemia

ADRENERGIC	NEUROGLYCOPENIC
Sweating	Dizziness
Tachycardia	Headache
Tremor	Decreased cognition, confusion
Anxiety	Clouded vision
Hunger	Seizures
	Coma

44. **How is hypoglycemia treated?**
If profound hypoglycemia is likely and the patient is unable to speak or swallow, intramuscular (IM) glucagon or IV glucose should be administered. Patients who are unable to communicate or swallow on their own should not be force-fed juice or sugar. Patients who are awake and able to swallow can consume 15 g of rapid-acting carbohydrate in the form of 4 ounces of juice or soda, or glucose tablets. Ice cream, cake, or candy bars should not be used to treat hypoglycemia because fat delays absorption of glucose. Glucose should be rechecked in 15–30 minutes. Patients should not drive or operate heavy machinery until blood glucose is normal. Patients on insulin pumps should suspend insulin delivery for 15–30 minutes.

45. Describe hypoglycemia-associated autonomic failure.

A syndrome of inappropriate response to hypoglycemia that occurs in patients with DM. Under normal physiologic conditions, hypoglycemia induces a reduction in insulin levels and an enhancement of glucagon and epinephrine secretion, both of which serve to defend against continued hypoglycemia. Patients with type 1 DM and many patients with type 2 DM have defective glucose counterregulation. Because they cannot reduce exogenous insulin levels and have impaired glucagon and epinephrine responses to hypoglycemia, they become prone to severe iatrogenic hypoglycemia. In addition, they frequently have attenuated sympathoadrenal responses to hypoglycemia. Hypoglycemia-associated autonomic failure is induced by hypoglycemia and reversed by avoidance of hypoglycemia.

46. What is hypoglycemic unawareness?

Hypoglycemia that is unnoticed by the patient because it is not associated with any adrenergic symptoms. These patients may have exceedingly low glucose levels without symptoms and may rapidly progress to confusion, seizures, or coma without warning.

47. What is the diagnostic approach to hypoglycemia in patients without diabetes?

Confirmation of hypoglycemia through the Whipple triad: presence of symptoms consistent with hypoglycemia (e.g., sweating, hunger, palpitations, and weakness), documented low plasma glucose at the time of symptoms, and relief of symptoms when the plasma glucose concentration is raised to normal levels. Hypoglycemia in the fasting state is typically more clinically concerning than reactive (postprandial) hypoglycemia. Although the exact criteria are debated, glucose levels of < 50 mg/dL in men and < 40 mg/dL in women are generally accepted as indicative of hypoglycemia.

48. Summarize the differential diagnosis of adult hypoglycemia not related to diabetes.

- **Drug-induced or factitious hypoglycemia:** Related to exposure to exogenous insulin, oral antidiabetic agents such as sulfonylureas, ethanol (inhibits gluconeogenesis), salicylates, sulfon-amides, pentamidine, monoamine oxidase (MAO) inhibitors, and quinine
- **Critical illness:** Including liver and renal failure
- **Adrenal insufficiency:** Due to lack of the counterregulatory hormone cortisol
- **Insulinoma:** Tumor of the pancreatic beta cells that produces too much insulin
- **Non–beta-cell tumors:** Include mesenchymal tumors, such as fibrosarcoma, mesothelioma, and leiomyosarcoma, that produce insulinlike growth factor-1 (IGF-1) or IGF-2
- **Insulin or insulin receptor autoantibodies:** Rare

49. How do you distinguish between endogenous and exogenous hyperinsulinemia?

By insulin and C-peptide levels. Insulin and its cleavage product C-peptide are secreted by the pancreatic beta cell in equimolar amounts. If a patient is getting exogenous insulin, insulin levels will be high and C-peptide levels low. Both values are elevated in patients with surreptitious sulfonylurea use because these drugs stimulate release of endogenous insulin and C-peptide. Sulfonylurea blood levels can also help rule out drug-induced hypoglycemia in this setting.

50. Identify the hereditary syndrome associated with pancreatic tumors. (See also Chapter 7, Gastroenterology.).

Multiple endocrine neoplasia syndrome type 1 (MEN-1). MEN syndromes are characterized by neoplastic transformation in multiple endocrine glands. MEN-1 is now known to be caused by a mutation in the tumor suppressor *MEN1* gene, whose product is named "menin."

51. What tumors or hyperplasia are associated with MEN-1?

- Pituitary: Prolactinoma (most common)
- Parathyroid: Hyperplasia
- Pancreas: Gastrinoma (most common), insulinoma

52. What are MEN-2A and MEN-2B?

MEN-2A includes neoplasms of the thyroid (medullary thyroid carcinoma), parathyroid (primary hyperparathyroidism), and adrenal gland (pheochromocytoma). MEN-2B includes medullary thyroid carcinoma, pheochromocytoma, and mucosal neuromas. MEN-2A and MEN-2B are due to activating mutations of the *RET* proto-oncogene

OBESITY

53. How is obesity currently defined?.
Excessive body fat determined by body mass index (BMI). The BMI is calculated by dividing weight in kilograms by height in meters squared: (weight in kg)/(height in m)^2. BMI categories are defined as follows:
- **BMI < 25 kg/m^2:** Normal
- **BMI 25–29.9 kg/m^2:** Overweight
- **BMI > 30 kg/m^2:** Obesity
  - Class I: BMI 30–34.9 kg/m^2
  - Class II: BMI 35–39.9 kg/m^2
  - Class III: BMI > 40 kg/m^2: extreme/severe/massive obesity

54. Is waist circumference significant for diagnosing obesity?
Yes. Waist circumference can also be used to diagnose obesity. Health risks of obesity are correlated with visceral (abdominal) adiposity. People with larger waist sizes have increased risks of obesity-related disorders such as hypertension, cardiovascular disease, and diabetes. Waist circumference is determined by placing a tape measure horizontally around the abdomen at the level of the iliac crest. Measurements should be taken at the end of a normal expiration. The tape measure should be snug but not compress the skin. Increased risk of obesity-related disease occurs in men with a waist circumference ≥ 40 inches (102 cm) and women with a waist circumference ≥ 35 inches (88 cm).

55. List the health risks associated with obesity.
- DM type 2
- Hypertension
- Hyperlipidemia
- Cardiovascular disease
- Cerebral vascular disease
- Osteoarthritis
- Nonalcoholic fatty liver disease
- Obstructive sleep apnea
- Gallbladder disease
- Cancers of endometrium, breast, colon, and prostate
- Psychological complications (depression, poor self-esteem, discrimination)

56. How common is obesity?
Increasingly common. Obesity is now thought to be one of the leading health disorders in the United States whose prevalence continues to increase dramatically. Current estimates suggest one third of the U.S. population is obese (BMI > 30). The growth in obesity appears to be stabilizing in more recent estimates. The prevalence is higher in ethnic minorities and has been increasing in children and adolescents (youth obesity prevalence approaches 17%). Obesity is more prevalent in women than men and is higher in middle-aged and older adults compared to younger adults.
    Centers for Disease and Prevention. Adult Obesity Facts. Available at: www.cdc.gov/obesity/data/adult. Accessed March 27, 2017.

57. What causes people to gain weight?
Unequal energy balance caused by increased caloric intake or decreased energy expenditure relative to caloric intake. Weight maintenance occurs when people consume as many calories as they expend per day. Other additional factors such as hormonal alterations and medications may contribute to weight gain in some people.

58. List the three components of total daily energy expenditure (EE).
- Basal metabolic rate (~65% of total daily EE)
- Energy of physical activity (30% of average person's daily EE)
- Thermic effect of food (energy cost of digesting food, which accounts for 5% of daily EE)

59. What factors control energy homeostasis?
Complex interactions between the brain and neural factors that control appetite and satiety, nutrient metabolism, and hormonal systems. Much research is currently being conducted in the neural mechanisms that regulate feeding and energy balance. The brain regulates energy homeostasis by integrating signals from long-term energy stores (adipose tissue) with short-term meal-related cues from food and the gut. Satiety and energy balance are regulated through an extremely complex

interaction between hypothalamic neural circuits and gut-related hormones. Most evidence suggests that obese people do not have major alterations in their basal metabolic rates. In fact, because total EE is linearly related to BMI, obese people actually require more calories for weight maintenance than lean people. Obesity likely develops as a multifactorial process involving genetic predisposition as well as environmental and behavioral factors.

Apovian CM, Aronne LJ, Bessesen DH, et al. Pharmacological management of obesity: an Endocrine Society clinical practice guideline. *J Clin Endocrinol Metab.* 2015;100:342–362.

Morton GJ, Meek TH, Schwartz MW. Neurobiology of food intake in health and disease. *Nat Rev Neurosci.* 2014;15:367–378.

60. Who should be treated for obesity?

All obese people should be instructed about proper diet and exercise to prevent obesity-related complications. People with more severe obesity or those who already have obesity-related complications should be treated more aggressively, including medications and surgery if indicated. Obesity medications should be considered in people with BMI ≥ 30 or ≥ 27 if associated with comorbid conditions, and bariatric surgery should be considered in people with BMI ≥ 40 or ≥ 35 with comorbid conditions.

61. Describe the general lifestyle approach to treatment of obesity.

Individualized treatment is important and the patient's goals must be discussed. Readiness to change lifestyle should be assessed. A reduction in caloric/energy intake is the main requirement for weight loss. Greater weight loss is typically noted when the reduction in energy intake is associated with a concomitant increase in EE (i.e., exercise). Frequently, patients desire a rapid, substantial weight loss. Unfortunately, this goal is usually not healthy or attainable in the patient's desired time frame. Because 1 lb of fat stores approximately 3500 kcal, in order to lose 1 lb of weight/week, the person must decrease caloric intake by roughly 500 kcal/day. This regimen is often extremely difficult to follow. Consequently, a more moderate approach is to restrict caloric intake (250–500 kcal reduction from basal intake) and increase EE (30 minutes of moderate physical activity most days of the week). Generally, people should aim to get 150 or more minutes of moderate exercise per week (divided in three to five sessions/week).

62. When should pharmacotherapy be considered for the treatment of obesity?

In patients with a BMI ≥ 30, a BMI ≥ 27 with comorbid conditions, or minimal response after 6 months of lifestyle modifications. Typically, the first approach is diet and exercise with behavioral modifications followed by the addition of pharmacotherapy.

Garvey WT, Mechanick JI, Brett EM, et al. American Association of Clinical Endocrinologists and American College of Endocrinology Comprehensive Clinical Practice Guidelines for Medical Care of Patients with Obesity. *Endocr Pract.* 2016;22:842–884.

63. What medications are U.S. Food and Drug Administration (FDA) approved for the treatment of obesity as of 2017?

- Phentermine: Approved for short-term use
- Orlistat
- Naltrexone extended release (ER)/bupropion ER
- Locaserin
- Phentermine/topiramate ER
- Liraglutide 3 mg

Apovian CM, Aronne LJ, Bessesen DH, et al. Pharmacologic management of obesity: an Endocrine Society clinical practice guideline. *J Clin Endocrinol Metab.* 2015;100:342–362.

64. Describe the mechanism of action for each weight loss medication listed previously. See package inserts for full prescribing information.

Medication	Route/Maximum Dosing	Mechanism of Action	Effect
Phentermine*	15–37.5 mg daily (capsule)	Norepinephrine agonist	Appetite suppressant
Orlistat*	120 mg TID	Pancreatic lipase inhibitor,	Blocks fat absorption
Naltrexone ER/ bupropion ER*	2 tabs 8/90 mg BID	Opioid receptor antagonist + DA/NE reuptake inhibitor	Appetite suppressant
Lorcaserin*	10 mg BID (immediate release)	5-HT 2C agonist	Appetite suppressant

Medication	Route/Maximum Dosing	Mechanism of Action	Effect
Phentermine/ topiramate ER*	Recommended 7.5/46 mg/ day, maximum dose 15/92 mg/day	Norepinephrine agonist + neurostabilizer	Appetite suppressant
Liraglutide*	Subcutaneous injection, maximum dose 3 mg/day	GLP-1 receptor agonist	Appetite suppressant

*Oral; + subcutaneous injection.
BID, twice a day; DA, dopamine; ER, extended release; GLP, glucagon-like peptide; 5-HT, 5-hydroxytryptamine (serotonin); NE, norepinephrine; TID, three times daily .

65. **Describe the most common side effects of the weight loss medications.**
See package inserts for full prescribing information including contraindications.

Medication	Common Side Effects
Phentermine	Increased blood pressure, heart rate, insomnia, anxiety/agitation, dry mouth, headache, tremor, GI disturbance, sexual dysfunction
Orlistat	GI disturbance (diarrhea, fecal incontinence), decreased absorption of fat-soluble vitamins
Naltrexone ER/bupropion ER	Nausea, vomiting, constipation, headache, dizziness
Lorcaserin	Headache, nausea, dizziness, fatigue, constipation, dry mouth; use with caution in patients on SSRI, SNRI, MAOI, or triptans
Phentermine/topiramate ER	Phentermine (as preceding) Insomnia, dry mouth, constipation, dizziness, parasthesias
Liraglutide, 3 mg	Nausea, vomiting, pancreatitis; black box warning for thyroid C-cell tumors; contraindicated in patients with personal or family history of medullary thyroid carcinoma or MEN-2

ER, extended release; GI, gastrointestinal; MAOI, monoamine oxidase inhibitors; MEN-2, multiple endocrine neoplasia syndrome type 2; SNRI, serotonin-norepinephrine reuptake inhibitor; SSRI, selective serotonin reuptake inhibitor.

66. **How effective are medications in treating obesity?**
In general, medications require chronic use for effectiveness and can be expected to produce a 5–10% weight loss in most people when used in combination with lifestyle interventions. Obesity medications should be discontinued if the patient has < 5% weight loss.

67. **What medications are associated with weight loss in patients with type 2 diabetes?**
Metformin, exenatide, liraglutide, and pramlitide.

68. **Summarize the role of surgery in the treatment of obesity.**
Surgery is generally reserved for people with severe obesity (BMI > 40) but can be considered in patients with BMI ≥ 35 with comorbid conditions. Frequently people have failed other forms of therapy before electing to proceed with bariatric surgery. There are a number of procedures available, and the most frequently performed procedures are the vertical banded gastroplasty and Roux-en-Y gastric bypass.

PITUITARY GLAND

69. **Summarize the general functions of the pituitary gland.**
The pituitary gland is the "master gland" of the endocrine system and is involved in many body functions, including growth and development, metabolism, and reproduction. These functions are regulated by the secretion of hormones that interact at specific target organ sites.

70. **Describe the anterior pituitary gland.**
The anterior pituitary or adenohypophysis, which composes 80% of the entire gland, is derived embryologically from Rathke pouch and is oral ectoderm in origin. Anterior pituitary hormones are synthesized in the pituitary by specific cell types and are regulated by hypothalamic and target organ factors.

71. List the six major hormones secreted by the anterior pituitary.
    - **Somatotropin** (growth hormone [GH])
    - **Prolactin**
    - **Corticotropin** (adrenocorticotropic hormone [ACTH])
    - **Thyrotropin** (thyroid-stimulating hormone [TSH])
    - **Luteinizing hormone** (LH)
    - **Follicle-stimulating hormone** (FSH)

72. How is secretion of these hormones regulated?

    By positive- and negative-feedback mechanisms. Most hormones are stimulated by a hypothalamic hormone and inhibited by a target organ hormone. The one exception is prolactin, which is under tonic inhibitory control by hypothalamic dopamine neurons. A schematic diagram is presented in Fig. 16.1 (Table 16.5).

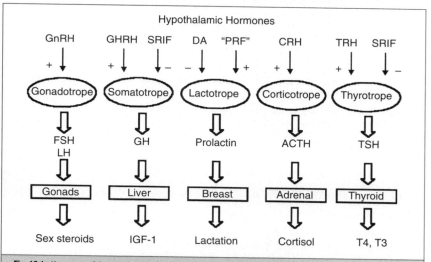

Fig. 16.1. Hormones of the anterior pituitary gland. CRH, corticotropin-releasing hormone; GHRH, growth hormone–releasing hormone; GnRH, gonadotropin-releasing hormone; PRF, prolactin-releasing factor; SRIF, somatostatin; TRH, thyrotropin-releasing hormone.

Table 16.5. Hormones of the Anterior Pituitary Gland

PITUITARY CELL TYPE	HORMONE	HYPOTHALAMIC FACTOR
Corticotrope	Corticotropin (ACTH)	CRH stimulates
Thyrotrope	Thyrotropin (TSH)	TRH stimulates and SRIF inhibits
Gonadotrope	LH FSH	GnRH
Somatotrope	GH	GHRH stimulates and SRIF inhibits
Lactotrope	Prolactin	Dopamine inhibits prolactin-releasing factors (e.g., TRH, suckling)

ACTH, adrenocorticotropic hormone; CRH, corticotropin-releasing hormone; FSH, follicle-stimulating hormone; GH, growth hormone; GHRH, growth hormone–releasing hormone; GnRH, gonadotropin-releasing hormone; LH, luteinizing hormone; SRIF, somatostatin; TRH, thyrotropin-releasing hormone; TSH, thyroid-stimulating hormone.

73. Describe the posterior pituitary. What hormones does it secrete?

    The posterior pituitary or neurohypophysis is an extension of the floor of the third ventricle of the brain and originates from cells of the central nervous system. Posterior pituitary hormones include oxytocin include arginine vasopressin (AVP) which is also known as antidiuretic hormone (ADH). These hormones are synthesized in the cell bodies of hypothalmic neurons and stored in the axons that terminate in the posterior pituitary.

74. **Describe the general approach to hormonal evaluation of a patient with pituitary disease.**

A detailed history regarding anterior and posterior pituitary function and hormonal hyper- or hypofunction of each hormonal axis will help identify the extent of the disease. Specific questions to assess hormone function related to each specific pituitary disorder include:

- **Diabetes insipidus** (deficient ADH/AVP): Presence of polyuria, polydipsia, or nighttime polydipsia
- **Hypothyroidism** (secondary): Fatigue, constipation, cold intolerance, dry skin, weight gain
- **Hyperthyroidism** (TSH adenoma): Anxiety, insomnia, palpitations, tremor, heat intolerance, increased bowel frequency, weight loss; very rare
- **Adrenal insufficiency** (secondary): Fatigue, dizziness, nausea, weight loss
- **Cushing disease** (excessive ACTH): Weight gain, purple striae, easy bruising, hirsutism, DM, osteoporosis, hypertension, depression
- **Prolactinoma:** Galactorrhea, amenorrhea or male hypogonadism, infertility, headache
- **Acromegaly** (excessive GH): Increased size of hands, head, and feet; hypertension; sweating; snoring; colon polyps; carpal tunnel syndrome; and fatigue (due to sleep apnea)
- **GH deficiency:** Impaired linear growth/short stature (prepuberty), central adiposity, fatigue, impaired exercise capacity

75. **What symptoms should be closely evaluated in patients with pituitary tumors?**

Headaches, visual loss, ophthalmoplegia, and cranial nerve abnormalities, which may indicate mass effects of the tumor and pituitary hormonal dysfunction, either hyper- or hypofunction. Posterior pituitary dysfunction is rarely a consequence of a pituitary tumor but can be seen in patients with pituitary trauma, surgery, or disorders of the pituitary stalk.

KEY POINTS: MECHANISMS BY WHICH PITUITARY TUMORS CAUSE PROBLEMS

1. Mass effect: tumors apply pressure to surrounding structures causing functional disruption that may lead to:
   - Headaches (most common)
   - Visual loss or visual field defects (bitemporal hemianopia)
   - Cranial nerve dysfunction (most commonly cranial nerves II, III, IV, and VI)
   - Anterior pituitary hormone deficiencies
2. Endocrine hyperfunction: due to excessive secretion of a particular anterior pituitary hormone by the tumor

76. **What physical examination findings suggest pituitary disease?**

- Abnormal visual field testing by confrontation
- Enlarged hands and feet, skin tags, and macroglossia (acromegaly)
- Cranial nerve palsies
- Purple striae, moon facies, hirsutism, proximal muscle wasting, supraclavicular and dorsocervical fat accumulation (Cushing disease)
- Loss of body hair, gynecomastia (hypogonadism)
- Delayed deep tendon reflexes, coarse hair or hair loss, nonpitting edema (hypothyroidism)

77. **What causes acromegaly?**

An oversecretion of GH. Ninety-nine percent are caused by a GH-secreting pituitary adenoma, either a pure somatotrope (produces solely GH) or a mammosomatotrope (producing prolactin and GH). Rare causes of acromegaly include a pituitary or hypothalamic gangliocytoma, growth hormone–releasing hormone (GHRH)–secreting tumor found in a bronchial or GI carcinoid tumor, pancreatic islet cell tumor, adrenal adenoma, or small cell carcinoma.

78. **How does acromegaly present clinically?**

As gigantism if the tumor occurs in childhood before the closure of the epiphyses. Children with acromegaly can grow to heights much higher than genetic potential. When a GH-producing tumor is present in association with deficiency in gonadal hormones, epiphyses can remain open for even longer, allowing even higher growth heights to be obtained. GH and IGF-1 levels can be high during adolescence but in patients without abnormal GH levels, GH suppresses with glucose challenge. Adult patients frequently present late in the disease with large tumors (macroadenomas in 85%) owing to the very slow development of the clinical features. Acromegaly often goes unrecognized by the patient, his or her family, and the physician because the physical changes occur so slowly. Such patients can present with soft tissue hypertrophy; headache; arthritis/carpal tunnel syndrome; increased size of hands, head, and feet; organomegaly, including cardiomegaly with congestive heart failure; and obstructive sleep apnea.

79. **What physical examination findings suggest acromegaly?**
Soft tissue changes (large doughy hands), frontal bossing, widening spaces in teeth, skin tags, organomegaly, large body size, signs of hyperprolactinemia (gynecomastia, galactorrhea), hypogonadism, and visual field deficits. Patients may also have diaphoresis and thick heel pads.

80. **How is acromegaly diagnosed?**
By clinical features, laboratory evaluation, and magnetic resonance imaging (MRI) of the pituitary. Diagnostic laboratory abnormalities include elevated GH with failure to suppress with oral glucose administration and an elevated IGF-1 (somatomedin-C). Patients may also have insulin resistance or DM, hyperprolactinemia due to stalk compression, hypogonadism, and hypercalciuria/nephrolithiasis. Mortality rates are increased for these patients as is the risk of colon polyps and cancer. Elevated phosphorus levels can also be seen.

81. **Explain the goal for treatment of acromegaly.**
To normalize anterior pituitary function and GH secretion. Mortality rates return to baseline levels if the GH is normalized (normal GH, normal IGF-1, and normal GH suppression [<1 μg/L or <0.4 μg/L if using ultrasensitive GH assay] following oral glucose).

82. **How can this goal be achieved?**
Through transsphenoidal surgical resection. Medical treatment after resection is often required because many tumors are too large at presentation to be completely excised by surgery. In such cases, somatostatin analogs are indicated for medical therapy to control GH secretion. GH cells have somatostatin receptors, and treatment with somatostatin analogs (octreotide, lanreotide, and pasireotide) has been shown to decrease GH levels and induce tumor shrinkage. GH receptor antagonist pegvisomant is also approved for medical therapy. Although less effective, dopamine agonists such as bromocriptine and cabergoline may also control GH levels, particularly in patients who also secrete prolactin. Finally, radiation therapy can be offered to patients who fail surgical and medical interventions. Radiation therapy can result in partial or complete hypopituitarism.

   Katznelson L, Laws ER Jr, Melmed S, et al. Acromegaly: an endocrine society clinical practice guideline. *J Clin Endocrinol Metab.* 2014;99:3933–3951.

83. **Prolactinomas are the most common type of pituitary tumor. In general, how do they present?**
With hypogonadism, but the clinical picture of hyperprolactinemia is variable, depending on age, sex, duration of hyperprolactinemia, and tumor size. Hypogonadism is due to prolactin inhibition of gonadotropin-releasing hormone (GnRH) neurons and leads to suppression of the hypothalamic-pituitary-gonadal axis. Women of reproductive age present earlier with amenorrhea and galactorrhea. Men and postmenopausal women usually present later in the disease course with mass effect such as headache and visual deficits.

84. **List the clinical features of hyperprolactinemia.**
   - Galactorrhea
   - Amenorrhea/menstrual irregularities
   - Infertility
   - Hirsutism
   - Gynecomastia and erectile dysfunction in men
   - Growth arrest/delayed puberty
   - Mass lesions/visual field defects (primarily in men and postmenopausal women)
   - Osteopenia (due to hypogonadism)

85. **What is the differential diagnosis of hyperprolactinemia?**

If values > 200 ng/mL:
- Prolactinoma
- Renal failure
- Pregnancy (normal physiologic cause of hyperprolactinemia)

If values < 100 ng/mL:
- Prolactinoma
- Pregnancy
- Renal failure
- Drugs (see Question 86)
- Stalk effect from other pituitary adenomas or hypothalmic/sellar masses (craniopharyngioma, meningioma, metastatic disease)
- Infiltrative disorders (sarcoidosis, tuberculosis)
- Neurogenic disorder (chest wall lesion, suckling; do not measure prolactin after a breast examination)
- Estrogen use
- Primary hypothyroidism (thyrotropin-releasing hormone [TRH] also stimulates prolactin secretion)
- Idiopathic disease

86. **What medications are associated with hyperprolactinemia?**
- Antipsychotics (chlorpromazine, clomipramine, fluphenazine, prochlorperazine, thioridazine, haloperidol, respiradone, olanzapine)
- GI agents (metoclopromide, cimetidine)
- Selective serotonin reuptake inhibitors (SSRIs [fluoxetine])
- Tricyclic antidepressants (TCAs [imipramine])
- Antihypertensive medication (reserpine, methyldopa, verapamil)
- Alcohol
- Morphine
- Cocaine

87. **What are the treatment options for hyperprolactinemia?**

Treatment depends on the cause. When due to a medication, it is obviously best to stop the offending agent if possible. If unable to discontinue medical therapy, though, such as in patients with schizophrenia or severe mental illness, replace sex hormone (estrogen or testosterone) if not contraindicated. Unlike other hyperfunctioning pituitary adenomas, medical therapy with dopamine agonists (preferably cabergoline due to better tolerability and efficacy) is the treatment of choice for prolactinomas. Oral contraceptives can be used to restore normal menstrual cycles and protect against bone loss in female patients who have mild elevations in prolactin in the absence of a visible pituitary tumor. Surgery is not typically the treatment of choice for prolactinomas owing to a high recurrence rate (especially for macroadenomas) but can be considered in invasive tumors or tumors resistant to medication. Radiation can always be considered in patients who fail other modalities.

88. **How do dopamine agonists work?**

By inhibiting prolactin secretion and causing tumor shrinkage. Examples include bromocriptine and cabergoline. All must be started at low doses and titrated upward very slowly to avoid side effects. The most common side effects include nausea, vomiting, and orthostatic hypotension. Cabergoline appears to be the best tolerated and is most efficacious.

89. **What cardiac side effects are associated with dopamine agonists?**

Valvular heart disease and heart failure. Careful cardiac examination and screening echocardiogram are recommended periodically.

90. **What is the "stalk effect"?**

Compression of the pituitary stalk by large non–prolactin-secreting tumors, thus interrupting the tonic inhibitory effect of dopamine (or prolactin-inhibiting factor) on the pituitary. The result is elevation of prolactin levels ≤ 200 ng/mL.

91. **What is pituitary apoplexy?**

The syndrome of sudden headache, visual change, ophthalmoplegia, and altered mental status caused by the acute hemorrhage or infarction of the pituitary gland. Most cases are due to pituitary hemorrhage of a previously undiagnosed pituitary adenoma (65%) but can also be caused by Sheehan syndrome, conditions that increase bleeding (such as anticoagulation), or intracranial pressure. Patient presentation may range from asymptomatic to symptoms of severe retro-orbital headache, visual defects, meningeal signs, altered sensorium, seizure, or coma depending on the extent of the lesion. Clinical symptoms and signs plus computed tomography (CT) scan or MRI of the pituitary aid in the diagnosis. This condition can be life threatening if unrecognized.

92. **How is pituitary apoplexy treated?**
    With stress doses of glucocorticoids (for cerebral edema and presumed adrenal insufficiency) and neurosurgical decompression. Hormonal deficiencies after apoplexy are the rule, and panhypopituitarism is common. Hypogonadism occurs in nearly 100%, GH deficiency in 88%, hyperprolactinemia in 67%, adrenal insufficiency in 66%, hypothyroidism in 42%, and DI in 3%.

93. **What is Sheehan syndrome?**
    Pituitary apoplexy after obstetric hemorrhage.

94. **What is a thyrotropinoma?**
    A tumor of the TSH-producing cells. This rare tumor occurs in approximately 1 in a million people, producing a clinical syndrome of hyperthyroidism that is indistinguishable clinically from other more common causes (e.g., Graves disease, toxic nodular goiter). Thyrotropinomas are differentiated from primary hyperthyroidism by an inappropriately normal or elevated TSH in the setting of elevated thyroid hormone levels, because TSH is secreted as a dimer peptide composed of the TSH beta and alpha subunits; alpha subunit levels are typically elevated. Patients have an elevated molar ratio of alpha subunit/TSH > 1.

95. **How is a thyrotropinoma diagnosed?**
    By pituitary MRI and laboratory results. If not seen on MRI, octreotide scanning may be used for tumor localization, because these tumors display somatostatin receptors.

96. **What causes hypopituitarism?**
    - Mass lesions from tumors (pituitary adenoma, craniopharyngiomas, metastatic lesions)
    - Iatrogenic causes (pituitary surgery, radiation)
    - Infiltrative disease (hemochromatosis, lymphoma, sarcoid, histiocytosis X)
    - Pituitary infarction (Sheehan syndrome, after coronary artery bypass grafting, trauma)
    - Pituitary apoplexy
    - Genetic disease (transcription factor mutations)
    - Empty sella syndrome (typically secondary)
    - Hypothalamic dysfunction (mass lesions, infiltrative diseases, radiation, trauma, infection)
    - Autoimmune lymphocytic hypophysitis
    - Immune-mediated medication-induced hypophysitis (i.e., ipilimumab)
    - Miscellaneous (abscess/infection; aneurysm)
    Hypopituitarism can be partial or complete (panhypopituitarism).

97. **How do patients with hypopituitarism present?**
    With signs and symptoms of hormonal deficiency. Evaluation is aimed at documenting deficiency and may include stimulation testing.

98. **How is hypopituitarism treated?**
    With correction of the hormonal deficiency. Replacement options exist for each hormonal axis (thyroid, adrenal, gonadal, and GH) except prolactin and are as follows:
    - **Thyroid:** Levothyroxine to achieve free T_4 (thyroxine) in normal range. Note that TSH cannot be used to guide therapy in pituitary insufficiency.
    - **Adrenal:** Glucocorticoids (hydrocortisone or prednisone). Patients with adrenal insufficiency need to be educated about stress-dose steroids for acute illness, and all patients should wear medical alert jewelry.
    - **Gonadal:**
        - Men: Testosterone
        - Women: Estrogen/progesterone administered as oral contraceptives or low-dose estrogen/progesterone therapy. Generally, estrogen/progesterone therapy is no longer recommended for long-term use in postmenopausal women.
    - **Growth hormone:** Human recombinant GH

99. **What are the goals of surgical management of pituitary adenomas?**
To correct hyperfunctioning/oversecretion of endocrine hormones (except in the case of prolactinoma in which medical treatment should be tried first), prevent or treat panhypopituitarism, prevent tumor recurrences, treat mass effect symptoms, and obtain definitive pathologic diagnosis. Urgent surgical resection is indicated in cases of pituitary apoplexy or tumors with significant mass effect (i.e., visual loss).

100. **What is lymphocytic hypophysitis?**
A lymphocytic infiltration of the pituitary gland that often occurs after pregnancy and causes panhypopituitarism. Patients present with headache, visual field disturbances, weakness, and fatigue. Lymphocytic hypophysitis can be fatal if not recognized.

101. **What is diabetes insipidus (DI)? How is it treated?**
An inability to concentrate urine owing to insufficient AVP release or activity. Large amounts of dilute urine are excreted inappropriately in the setting of hyperosmolality and hypernatremia.

102. **What are the two types of DI?**
Central (neurogenic) DI and nephrogenic DI. **Central DI** is due to impaired or inadequate secretion of AVP from the posterior pituitary. Central DI can be partial or complete and is typically an acquired condition related to trauma or infiltrative disease of the hypothalamus/posterior pituitary. **Nephrogenic DI** is due to AVP resistance and can be acquired owing to hypercalcemia or hypokalemia, may be drug-induced (lithium), or can be congenital.

103. **How do patients with DI present?**
With polyuria (typically large volumes with osmolality < 200 mOsm/kg), polydipsia, and hypernatremia if the patients do not have an intact thirst mechanism or do not drink water. Diagnosis is confirmed by performing a water deprivation test.

104. **How is a water deprivation test performed?**
A patient suspected of having DI is asked to fast without drinking any liquids from a time point deemed safe by the physician. The patient is carefully monitored in the outpatient clinic or inpatient setting. Weight, urine output, BP, and pulse are monitored hourly. Serum and urine osmolality and serum sodium are checked every 2 hours. Once serum osmolality or serum osmolality is over normal, desmopressin (DDAVP) is administered and serum and urine osmolality and serum sodium are monitored at 30 minutes and 1 hour after injection of DDAVP. If serum osmolality is above normal and urine osmolality < 600 mOsm/kg, a diagnosis of DI is made. Patients who maintain normal serum osmolality and are able to concentrate urine osmolality over 600 mOsm/kg and who have decreased urine output with time should be considered for primary polydipsia. Patients who are able to concentrate urine and decrease urine output after DDAVP have central DI and those who do not have nephrogenic DI.

105. **How is DI treated?**
With AVP replacement in the form of DDAVP, a synthetic AVP agonist. There are no good therapies for nephrogenic DI, but treatment is usually aimed at volume contraction using thiazide diuretics, salt depletion, or prostaglandin synthesis inhibitors. These agents decrease renal blood flow by volume contraction and decrease urine output by reducing glomerular filtration rates.

106. **Outline the perioperative management of pituitary adenomas.**
Preoperative assessment: Perform a detailed neurologic examination, including assessment for mass effect of tumor and pituitary hormonal deficiency or excess. Replace hormonal deficiencies as needed. Adrenal and thyroid hormone replacement is particularly important preoperatively.
Acute perioperative assessment: In the inpatient setting, monitor for potential neurologic complications such as meningitis, cerebrospinal fluid (CSF) leak, and visual loss. Assess for endocrine complications including DI, syndrome of inappropriate secretion of antidiuretic hormone (SIADH), and acute adrenal insufficiency.
Long-term management: Evaluate patients clinically and with pituitary function assessments at short- and long-term intervals after surgery. Continue long-term monitoring of pituitary function and observation for potential tumor recurrences. The pituitary MRI is repeated at 3 months, then annually for a period of time (~5 years). Extend imaging intervals if the patient remains without tumor recurrence or progression.
Woodmansee WW, Carmichael J, Kelly D, et al. American Association of Clinical Endocrinologists and American College of Endocrinology Disease State Clinical Review: postoperative management following pituitary surgery. *Endocr Pract.* 2015;21:832–838.

ADRENAL GLANDS

107. List the hormones secreted by the adrenal glands.
See Table 16.6.

Table 16.6. Adrenal Hormones

HORMONE	SYNTHESIS	SYNDROMES
Cortisol	Synthesized from cholesterol in the adrenal cortex (zona fasciculata, zona reticularis)	Hyperfunction: Cushing syndrome Hypofunction: adrenal insufficiency
Aldosterone	Synthesized from cholesterol in the adrenal cortex (zona glomerulosa)	Hyperfunction: hyperaldosteronism Hypofunction: adrenal insufficiency
Androgens/sex steroids	Synthesized from cholesterol in the adrenal cortex (zona fasciculata, zona reticularis)	Hyperfunction: hirsutism/virilization Hypofunction: no clear syndrome
Catecholamines (norepinephrine, epinephrine)	Synthesized in the adrenal medulla	Hyperfunction: pheochromocytoma Hypofunction: hypotension

108. Differentiate Cushing syndrome from Cushing disease.
Cushing syndrome refers to hypercortisolemia and its associated signs and symptoms due to any cause. **Cushing disease** refers specifically to hypercortisolemia due to ACTH overproduction by a pituitary adenoma. The most common cause of Cushing syndrome is iatrogenic owing to exogenous steroid treatment for a variety of conditions (rheumatologic, organ transplant, and reactive airway disease). If one excludes iatrogenic hypercortisolemia, the most common cause of Cushing syndrome is Cushing disease, which accounts for approximately two thirds of all cases.

109. What are the signs and symptoms of Cushing disease?
* Atrophic, thin skin with easy bruising and purple striae on abdomen, axillae, hips, and thighs
* Weight gain or central obesity
* Dorsocervical (buffalo hump) and supraclavicular fat accumulation
* Moon facies
* Menstrual irregularities
* Hirsutism
* Diabetes or insulin resistance
* Muscle weakness
* Hypertension
* Increased susceptibility to infection
* Frequent fungal infections
* Osteoporosis or osteopenia
* Psychiatric symptoms such as depression, mood changes, and even psychosis
* Hypercoagulable state

110. List the sequence of steps involved in evaluating a patient for Cushing syndrome.
* **Step 1:** Screen for and document hypercortisolemia with a 24-hour urine cortisol or dexameth-asone suppression test (DST).
* **Step 2:** Measure ACTH to differentiate between ACTH-dependent and ACTH-independent causes.
* **Step 3:** Distinguish pituitary Cushing disease from ectopic ACTH secretion with a pituitary MRI or inferior petrosal sinus sampling (IPSS).
* **Step 4:** Surgically resect the tumor once identified.

111. When should one screen for Cushing syndrome?
In the presence of multiple clinical features of Cushing syndrome or worsening symptoms suggestive of Cushing syndrome such as weight gain, an abnormal fat distribution, proximal muscle weakness, large (>1-cm-wide) purple striae, and new cognitive/depression complaints. Young people with nontraumatic bone fractures, cutaneous atrophy, or hypertension and patients with incidental adrenal

adenomas also should be screened. Note, though, that the symptoms associated with Cushing syndrome, such as weight gain, hypertension, diabetes, osteoporosis, and depression, are common.

112. How should one screen for Cushing syndrome?
With the low-dose (1-mg) overnight DST, 24-hour urine free cortisol levels, or late-evening salivary cortisol levels.
> Nieman LK, Biller BM, Findling JW, et al. The diagnosis of Cushing's syndrome: an Endocrine Society Clinical Practice Guideline. *J Clin Endocrinol Metab.* 2008;93:1526–1540.

113. How is the low-dose DST performed?
Give 1 mg of dexamethasone at 11 PM and measure cortisol at 8 AM the following morning. If the patient does not have Cushing syndrome, the 8 AM cortisol is suppressed to < 1.8 µg/dL if a sensitive assay is used.

114. How is the 24-hour urine free cortisol test done?
By collecting urine over 24 hours to measure free cortisol. To ensure an accurate result, the urine collection should be confirmed with a complete and simultaneous urine creatinine excretion. Urinary cortisol should be normal in patients without Cushing syndrome. Up to three collections may be needed for diagnosis if the first tests are normal and there is a high index of suspicion.

115. What is the late-evening salivary cortisol test?
Measurement of cortisol levels in salivary samples collected by the patient at home late at night (11 PM). Some clinicians advocate this test because it is easy to perform and salivary and plasma cortisol levels are highly correlated. Normal cortisol levels should be low, confirming normal diurnal variation. Cushing patients have abnormally high late-night levels. Normal ranges are assay-dependent and must be validated for each laboratory. Although helpful as an initial screening test, particularly in patients with episodic hypercortisolemia, many endocrinologists still use the DST or 24-hour urine free cortisol test as first-line modalities.

116. Once hypercortisolemia has been documented, what is the next step in evaluating a patient with Cushing syndrome?
Measurement of ACTH. If the ACTH > 10 pg/mL, the patient most likely has an ACTH-dependent cause of Cushing syndrome. In addition, an ACTH value > 10 pg/mL after peripheral corticotropin-releasing hormone (CRH) administration suggests ACTH dependency.

After ruling out ingestion of exogenous steroids, the next step is to differentiate between ACTH-dependent (80%) and ACTH-independent (20%) disease. ACTH-dependent disease is associated with pituitary adenoma (80%), ectopic ACTH (20%), and CRH hypersecretion (rare). ACTH-independent disease is associated with adrenal adenoma (40–50%), adrenal carcinoma (40–50%), nodular dysplasia (rare), and McCune-Albright syndrome (rare).

117. Once ACTH-dependent Cushing syndrome has been confirmed, what is the final step in making the biochemical diagnosis?
A high-dose (8-mg) DST to differentiate between a corticotrope adenoma and an ectopic ACTH-secreting tumor. Patients with a pituitary source of ACTH retain suppressibility of cortisol to high-dose dexamethasone, whereas patients with ectopic ACTH tumors do not.

118. How is the dexamethasone test confirmed?
With IPSS. This test takes advantage of the concentration gradient between pituitary venous drainage via the inferior petrosal sinus (IPS—central) and peripheral venous values of ACTH to further determine whether an ACTH-producing corticotropic adenoma is present in the pituitary; the inclusion of CRH stimulation adds greater sensitivity to the test.

119. Explain how the IPSS is done.
Samples of ACTH and cortisol are obtained simultaneously from the IPS (central) and from a peripheral site (e.g., inferior vena cava [IVC]). In patients with Cushing disease, the central/peripheral ratio (C/P = IPS/IVC ratio) of ACTH > 2. In patients with ectopic ACTH, the ratio < 2 and selective venous sampling (e.g., of the pulmonary, pancreatic, or intestinal beds) may localize the ectopic tumor.

120. How does the administration of CRH increase diagnostic accuracy during IPSS?
By eliciting an ACTH response in the few patients with pituitary tumor who did not have a diagnostic C/P gradient in the basal samples. All patients with Cushing disease have had a C/P ratio > 3 after CRH, whereas patients with ectopic ACTH or adrenal disease have had C/P ratios < 3 after CRH.

121. **What is the most significant limitation of IPSS with or without CRH?**
Because IPSS has not been extensively performed in normal subjects, correct interpretation of the results requires accurate catheter placement and that the patient be hypercortisolemic at the time of the study in order to suppress the response of normal corticotropes to CRH. See Fig. 16.2. If results indicate an ectopic source, a CT or MRI of the chest is usually performed first because most are due to small cell carcinoma or bronchial or thymic carcinoid tumors. IPSS should be performed in tertiary-care centers that perform this invasive test often.

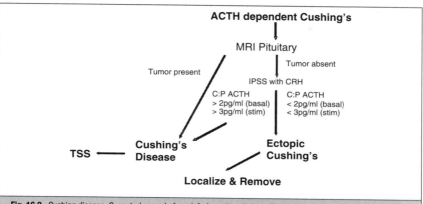

Fig. 16.2. Cushing disease. C, central, sample from inferior petrosal sinus; P, peripheral, inferior vena cava; TSS, transsphenoidal surgery.

122. **What is the treatment of choice for Cushing disease?**
Transphenoidal pituitary tumor resection by an experienced neurosurgeon. Note that if the tumor is successfully resected, the patient will have adrenal insufficiency postoperatively and will need treatment with glucocorticoid replacement until the remaining nontumor corticotropes begin to function again. Patients should know that it may take months, even up to a year, to taper off the glucocorticoid replacement therapy.

123. **What treatment options are available for treating hypercortisolism in Cushing disease if surgery fails?**

- Repeat transsphenoidal surgery
- Medical therapy
- Steroidogenesis inhibitors
  - Ketoconazole
  - Metyrapone
  - Mitotane (adrenolytic, approved for adrenocortical carcinoma)
  - Etomidate (ICU only)
- Pituitary tumor targeted therapies
  - Cabergoline: dopamine agonist
  - Pasireotide*: somatostatin analog
- Mifepristone*: cortisol receptor antagonist
- Radiation
- Bilateral adrenalectomy (only corrects hypercortisolism, does not treat tumor)
*FDA approved.
ICU, intensive care unit.

Nieman LK, Biller BM, Findling JW, et al. Treatment of Cushing's syndrome: an Endocrine Society Clinical Practice Guideline. *J Clin Endocrinol Metab.* 2015;100:2807–2831.

124. What is pseudo-Cushing syndrome?
A clinical state characterized by mild overactivity of the hypothalamic-pituitary-adrenal axis that is not associated with true Cushing syndrome (hypercortisolemia) typically seen in a variety of psychiatric states (depression, anxiety), alcoholism, uncontrolled diabetes, and severe obesity. The dexamethasone-CRH stimulation test can be used to help distinguish this disorder from true Cushing syndrome. Alternatively, an elevated midnight plasma cortisol level rules out pseudo-Cushing because, unlike patients with true Cushing syndrome, patients with pseudo-Cushing retain the diurnal rhythm of cortisol secretion.

125. Explain how the dexamethasone-CRH stimulation test is done.
Patients take 0.5 mg of dexamethasone every 6 hours for 8 doses starting at noon. At 8 AM (after the eighth dose of dexamethasone), IV CRH (human recombinant CRH [Acthrel]) is given at a dose of 1 µg/kg, and cortisol is measured 15 minutes later. A cortisol value > 1.4 mg/dL indicates Cushing syndrome.

126. What is Nelson syndrome?
Symptoms of a mass effect of corticotrope hyperplasia or adenoma in patients after bilateral adrenalectomy. Nelson syndrome occurs in up to 30% of patients after bilateral adrenalectomy and patients often present with headache, visual field deficits, ophthalmoplegia, and hyperpigmentation owing to high levels of ACTH (with resultant high levels of melanocyte-stimulating hormone). Pituitary tumor resection followed by pituitary radiation can prevent Nelson syndrome in someone who has had bilateral adrenalectomy.

127. Define adrenal insufficiency.
Insufficient release of adrenal hormone, typically from the adrenal cortex, including cortisol and aldosterone.

128. What causes adrenal insufficiency?
The causes can be divided into two categories: primary and central. **Primary adrenal insufficiency** (Addison disease) is due to adrenal gland dysfunction. **Central adrenal insufficiency** includes both secondary (pituitary) and tertiary (hypothalamic) causes.

129. List the causes of primary adrenal insufficiency.
Autoimmune destruction (70–80%), tuberculosis (20%), adrenal destruction by bilateral hemorrhage or infarction, tumor, infections (other than tuberculosis), surgery, radiation, drugs, amyloidosis, sarcoidosis, hyporesponsiveness to ACTH, and congenital abnormalities.

130. List the causes of central adrenal insufficiency.
Withdrawal of exogenous steroids (common), treatment and cure of Cushing syndrome, pituitary adenoma/infarction, other causes of panhypopituitarism, pituitary or brain irradiation, and hypothalamic abnormalities (rare).

131. What are the major symptoms and signs of Addison disease?
See Table 16.7.

Table 16.7. Clinical Presentation of Primary Adrenal Insufficiency (Addison Disease)

SYMPTOMS	SIGNS
Weakness, fatigue	Hyperkalemia (mild)
Anorexia, weight loss	Hyponatremia
Dizziness	Orthostatic hypotension
GI upset: nausea, vomiting, diarrhea abdominal pain	Hyperpigmentation (buccal mucosa, skinfolds, extensor surfaces, new scars)
Salt craving	Vitiligo Adrenal calcifications on CT scan

CT, computed tomography; GI, gastrointestinal.

132. How do Addison disease and central adrenal insufficiency differ in their presentation?
Primary adrenal insufficiency (Addison disease) is caused by failure or destruction of the adrenal glands, leading to underproduction of glucocorticoids and mineralocorticoids and an increase in ACTH production by the pituitary. **Central** adrenal insufficiency is caused by deficient production of

ACTH, leading to underproduction of glucocorticoids. The manifestations are the same as those of Addison disease with the following exceptions:

- Hyperpigmentation is not seen in central disease. Patients do not have hypersecretion of melanocyte-stimulating hormone (a product of the propiomelanocortin gene, like ACTH) that is responsible for the hyperpigmentation.
- Electrolyte abnormalities (hyponatremia, hyperkalemia) are not typically present in central disease because the aldosterone system is largely intact.
- Central disease may involve other manifestations of hypopituitarism.
- Hypoglycemia is more commonly seen with central disease owing to the presence of combined ACTH and GH deficiency.

133. **What test do most clinicians use to assess adrenal insufficiency?**
An ACTH stimulation test. In the classic test, a baseline cortisol is drawn and 250 μg of IV synthetic ACTH is given. Blood samples for cortisol are collected at 30 and 60 minutes. A normal response is a stimulated cortisol value of > 18 μg/dL. A normal response rules out primary adrenal insufficiency. Patients with acute central adrenal insufficiency (i.e., pituitary apoplexy or head trauma) may respond to synthetic ACTH because the adrenal glands have not had sufficient time to become atrophic and unresponsive to ACTH. Lack of a normal response indicates decreased adrenal reserve but does not differentiate between primary and central adrenal insufficiency.

134. **How do you distinguish between primary and central adrenal insufficiency?**
By ACTH level which is high in primary adrenal insufficiency and low or normal in central. More recently, clinicians have considered the 250-μg ACTH test less accurate in detecting patients with mild secondary adrenal insufficiency (because it is a supraphysiologic dose) and have recommended a 1-μg ACTH stimulation test. The test is performed the same way as the higher-dose test but requires dilution of the ACTH. ACTH (Cortrosyn) is available only in a 250-μg vial and must be diluted for this low-dose test. Therefore, careful attention must be given to ensure proper administration of the drug to avoid a high false-positive rate.

135. **Summarize the differences in treatment of primary and central adrenal insufficiency.**
Patients with primary adrenal insufficiency (Addison disease) typically require replacement of both glucocorticoid (prednisone or hydrocortisone) and mineralocorticoid (fludrocortisone) hormones, whereas patients with central adrenal insufficiency typically need only glucocorticoids. Patients with central disease do not usually require mineralocorticoids because aldosterone secretion is largely unaffected. All patients should be instructed to increase steroid replacement during times of illness and should wear medical alert jewelry. The goal of treatment is to ameliorate the signs and symptoms of adrenal insufficiency without causing Cushing syndrome due to excessive exogenous glucocorticoid replacement. Always use the lowest possible doses that control symptoms to avoid side effects.

136. **What is the gold standard test to assess adequacy of the hypothalamic-pituitary-adrenal axis?**
The insulin tolerance test (ITT). The principle of the test is to induce hypoglycemia (plasma glucose < 40 mg/dL) with IV insulin, which acts as a major stressor to stimulate production of ACTH, cortisol, and GH. The ITT can be dangerous and requires close monitoring.

137. **What are other tests that can be used to diagnose central adrenal insufficiency?**
Metyrapone stimulation test. Metyrapone can be given orally at 11 PM to suppress cortisol synthesis. If the pituitary adrenal axis is intact, morning measurements of ACTH and 11-deoxycortisol, the precursor to cortisol, will rise to > 75 pg/mL and 7 μg/dL, respectively, if there is no secondary adrenal insufficiency. Metyrapone is not commercially available but can be obtained by contacting the manufacturer or the distributors (www.metopirone.us).

138. **Why is it important to rule out adrenal insufficiency in pituitary patients with central hypothyroidism?**
Because patients with central hypothyroidism metabolize cortisol more slowly than euthyroid patients. Thyroid hormone replacement increases cortisol metabolism and can precipitate adrenal crisis in a patient with undiagnosed central adrenal insufficiency. Adrenal insufficiency should be detected and treated before starting thyroid hormone replacement.

139. **What is the "classic triad" of symptoms of pheochromocytoma?**
Episodic headache, diaphoresis, and tachycardia with or without hypertension. The hypertension may be paroxysmal. Other symptoms may include anxiety/psychiatric disturbances, tremor,

pallor, visual changes (blurred vision), weight loss, polyuria, polydipsia, hyperglycemia, dilated cardiomyopathy, and arrhythmias. Most patients have two of the three symptoms of the classic triad. If the patient is hypertensive and has the classic triad of symptoms, the sensitivity and specificity for pheochromocytoma are both > 90%.

140. **What other diagnoses should be considered in the diagnosis of pheochromocytoma?**
Anxiety/panic attacks, alcoholism (or alcohol withdrawal), sympathomimetic drugs (cocaine, amphetamines, phencyclidine, epinephrine, phenylephrine, and terbutaline), combined ingestion of MAO inhibitors and tyramine-containing food, hyperthyroidism, menopause, hypoglycemia, and abrupt discontinuation of short-acting sympathetic antagonists (e.g., clonidine).

141. **What is the "rule of 10" for pheochromocytomas?**
   - 10% are extra-adrenal
   - 10% are bilateral
   - 10% are familial
   - 10% are malignant

142. **How do you evaluate a patient with suspected pheochromocytoma?**
By making a biochemical diagnosis before embarking on radiographic imaging. Confirming the presence of excess catecholamines is crucial because people can have incidental adrenal tumors that do not hypersecrete catecholamines.

143. **Describe the main screening tests for pheochromocytoma.**
Although preferences may vary by institution, 24-hour urine catecholamines and metanephrines measurements are available in most laboratories. Plasma-free normetanephrine and metanephrine levels are also useful.

144. **Under what conditions is the 24-hour urine test performed?**
Usually when the patient is symptomatic because catecholamine hypersecretion may be episodic. If possible, testing should be performed after discontinuing medications. TCAs and antipsychotics are most likely to interfere with the measurement. Caffeine, alcohol, acetaminophen, decongestants, and tobacco should be avoided during testing. Cocaine, appetite suppression drugs, and other sympathomimetics should also be discontinued.

145. **After the biochemical diagnosis is made, how is the tumor localized?**
By using CT or MRI (first of the adrenals, then of the chest, abdomen, and pelvis). If the tumor cannot be localized with standard imaging, perform a ^{123}I-metaiodobenzylguanidine (MIBG) scan to localize functional catecholamine-rich tissue.
   Lenders JW, Duh QY, Eisenhofer G, et al. Pheochromocytoma and paraganglioma: an Endocrine Society Clinical Practice Guideline. *J Clin Endocrinol Metab.* 2014;99:1915–1942.

146. **What is the treatment of choice for patients with pheochromocytomas?**
Surgery after tumor localization. All patients must be preoperatively treated with alpha-adrenergic (phenoxybenzamine) and beta-adrenergic (atenolol) blockade to avoid stress-induced catecholamine excess and hypertensive crisis during surgery. Dose should be titrated to cause orthostatic hypotension. If only beta-adrenergic blockade is provided, the patient may develop peripheral vasoconstriction and an exacerbation of hypertension.

147. **What is an adrenal incidentaloma?**
Previously unsuspected adrenal mass that is detected in approximately 1% of all abdominal CT scans. These tumors fall into three categories: nonfunctioning mass, hyperfunctioning mass, and pseudoadrenal mass. Because approximately 10% are hormonally active and < 3% are adrenocortical carcinomas, it is important to assess hormonal hyperfunction and malignant potential.

148. **How do you evaluate an adrenal incidentaloma?**
Although there are numerous approaches, evaluations should be individualized. A careful history and physical examination may detect signs and symptoms of hormone excess. Screening for Cushing syndrome (1-mg overnight DST) and pheochromocytoma (24-hour urine metanephrines/catecholamines or plasma metanephrines) is helpful. If the patient is hypertensive or has low potassium, tests for hyperaldosteronism are indicated. Plasma aldosterone concentration (PAC) and plasma renin activity (PRA) may be used to test for an aldosterone-secreting tumor, looking for a PAC/PRA ratio > 25. The search for androgen-secreting tumors is necessary only if symptoms are present

(hirsutism, virilization, or menstrual irregularities [women]). Nonfunctioning tumors < 4 cm are typically observed for growth. Functional tumors or tumors > 4 cm (or growing) are typically removed by surgery.
> Zeiger MA, Thompson GB, Duh QY, et al. The American Association of Clinical Endocrinologists and American Association of Endocrine Surgeons medical guidelines for the management of adrenal incidentalomas. *Endocr Pract*. 2009;(Suppl 1):1–20.

149. **What is primary hyperaldosteronism?**
Excessive production of aldosterone independent of the renin-angiotensin system, found in approximately 0.5–2% of the population. The differential diagnosis includes solitary aldosterone-producing adenoma (65%), bilateral or unilateral adrenal hyperplasia, adrenal carcinoma, and glucocorticoid-remediable aldosteronism.

150. **How do patients with primary hyperaldosteronism present?**
With hypertension, hypokalemia (weakness, muscle cramping, paresthesias, headaches), low magnesium levels, and metabolic alkalosis.

151. **How should patients with primary hyperaldosteronism be evaluated initially?**
With a morning ambulatory plasma aldosterone level and PRA in the absence of drugs that alter the renin-aldosterone axis (spironolactone, eplerenone, or high-dose amiloride). A PAC to PRA ratio of ≥ 20 and a PAC of ≥ 15 ng/dL makes the diagnosis of hyperaldosteronism likely.

152. **How is the diagnosis of primary hyperaldosteronism confirmed?**
With a high 24-hour urine aldosterone level in the presence of normokalemia and adequate volume status or inadequate suppression of aldosterone levels using the saline suppression or salt-loading test. As always, biochemical diagnosis should precede diagnostic imaging. Treatment depends on the cause but usually includes surgery except in cases of adrenal hyperplasia or glucocorticoid-remediable hyperaldosteronism. Renal vein sampling can lateralize the aldosterone source before surgery.

153. **How should adrenal vein sampling be performed?**
With cortisol and aldosterone levels measured in the vena cava and right and left adrenal vein before and after Cortrosyn stimulation. An experienced interventional radiologist should collect the samples. Cortisol concentration in the adrenal veins should be 10 times higher than peripheral (vena cava) measurements. Cortisol concentration should be slightly higher in the right over the left adrenal vein. Aldosterone measurements should be adjusted for this difference.

THYROID GLAND

154. **Diagram the hypothalamic-pituitary-thyroid axis.**
See Fig. 16.3.

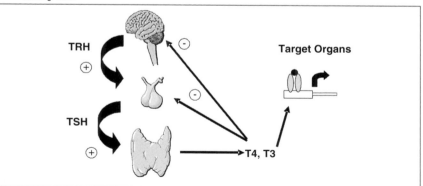

Fig. 16.3. Hypothalamic-pituitary-thyroid axis. Thyrotropin-releasing hormone (TRH) is made in the hypothalamus and stimulates the pituitary thyrotropes to release thyroid-stimulating hormone (TSH; thyrotropin), which acts at the level of the thyroid gland and directs release of two hormones, T_4 (thyroxine) and T_3 (triiodothyronine). These two hormones circulate in the blood bound to protein, primarily thyroid-binding globulin. It has been thought that most of the actions of thyroid hormone are mediated by the binding of T_3 to nuclear hormone receptors and the altering of gene transcription (either positively or negatively) of the thyroid hormone–responsive gene in target tissues. The axis is regulated as a classic negative feedback system as shown.

155. Describe the laboratory findings in hyperthyroidism and hypothyroidism.
See Table 16.8.

Table 16.8. Laboratory Testing in Thyroid Disease

LABORATORY TEST	HYPERTHYROIDISM	HYPOTHYROIDISM
TSH	Low or undetectable	High
Free T_4	High	Low
Total T_4	High	Low
Free T_3 (not often accurate)	High	Low
Total T_3	High	Low
T_3 resin uptake*	Usually high if no TBG abnormality	Usually low if no TBG abnormality

*Inverse measure of thyroid hormone binding sites on TBG.
T_3, triiodothyronine; T_4, thyroxine; TBG, thyroid-binding globulin; TSH, thyroid-stimulating hormone.

156. How does pregnancy affect thyroid disease?
Pregnant women with hypothyroidism treated with thyroid hormone require approximately 30–50% more thyroid hormone than they did before pregnancy. Initially, thyroid hormone doses are increased by 30% at the time pregnancy test is positive. The thyroid hormone dose increase can by calculated by multiplying the current dose by 1.3 or by adding two extra pills per week. The dose would not be changed for women on thyroid hormone suppression therapy for thyroid cancer or who are already taking excessive thyroid hormone. Thyroid hormone levels should be measured at the diagnosis of pregnancy and every 4 weeks during pregnancy. Women can restart their prepregnancy dose the day of delivery. TSH levels should be checked 6 weeks postpartum.

157. Distinguish between subclinical and overt thyroid disease.
Thyroid disease occurs along a continuum. At either end is hyperthyroidism or hypothyroidism. Milder forms of thyroid dysfunction are often referred to as **subclinical** disease, meaning below the limit of detection by clinical evaluation. **Overt** disease refers to hyperthyroidism or hypothyroidism with classic clinical signs and symptoms, abnormal TSH, and abnormal hormone levels.

158. Discuss the significance of subclinical thyroid disease.
Subclinical disease was originally thought to be a laboratory diagnosis in which patients had an abnormal TSH and normal thyroid hormone levels and were "asymptomatic." We now know that subclinical disease is often associated with subtle clinical signs and symptoms and that it represents an early, mild form of thyroid disease.

Garber JR, Cobin RH, Gharib H, et al. Clinical practice guidelines for hypothyroidism in adults: cosponsored by the American Association of Clinical Endocrinologists and the American Thyroid Association. *Thyroid.* 2012;22:1200–1235.

LeFevre ML. Screening for thyroid dysfunction: U.S. Preventive Services Task Force Recommendation Statement. *Ann Intern Med.* 2015;162:641–650.

159. Should subclinical hypothyroidism be treated in nonpregnant adults?
Maybe. Although these milder forms of thyroid dysfunction have been shown to be associated with abnormal physiology (particularly subclinical hypothyroidism), treatment is currently quite controversial. For nonpregnant adults, decisions to treat asymptomatic TSH < 10.0 mU/L should be individualized. In particular, older adults do not appear to benefit from thyroid replacement in subclinical disease.

Stott DJ, Rodondi N, Kearney PM, et al. Thyroid hormone therapy for older adults with subclinical hypothyroidism. *N Engl J Med.* 2017;376(26):2534–2544.

160. What about pregnant women?
If the TSH is > 2.5 mU/L, thyroid peroxidase (TPO) antibodies should be measured. Thyroid replacement therapy is indicated for TPO antibody-positive women with TSH level greater than the pregnancy-specific reference range and considered for those antibody-positive women with TSH > 2.5 mU/L but below the upper limit of the pregnancy-specific range.

Alexander EK, Pearce EN, Brent GA, et al. Guidelines of the American Thyroid Association for the Diagnosis and Management of Thyroid Disease During Pregnancy and the Postpartum. *Thyroid.* 2017;27:315–389.

161. How should subclinical hyperthyroidism be treated?
If TSH < 0.1 mU/mL is confirmed on repeat testing, treatment should be considered, particularly if the patient has concomitant osteoporosis or atrial fibrillation.

162. How common is thyroid disease?
Relatively common, affecting more women than men. Subclinical thyroid disease is more common than overt disease. The prevalence of hypothyroidism increases with age in both men and women. In fact, more than 20% of women older than 60 years have hypothyroidism. General overall prevalence rates are as follows.
- **Hyperthyroidism:** 1.2% (0.5% overt and 0.7% subclinical)
- **Hypothyroidism:** 4.6% (0.3% overt and 4.3% subclinical)

Canaris GJ, Manowitz MR, Mayor G, et al. The Colorado thyroid disease prevalence study. *Arch Intern Med.* 2000;160:526–534.

Hollowell JG, Staehling NW, Flanders WD, et al. Serum TSH, T(4), and thyroid antibodies in the United States population (1988–1994): National Health and Nutrition Examination Survey (NHANES III). *J Clin Endocrinol Metab.* 2002;87:489–499.

KEY POINTS: THYROID-STIMULATING HORMONE

1. The best initial screening test for evaluation of thyroid status is the TSH level.
2. TSH is the most sensitive measure of thyroid function in the majority of patients.
3. The one exception is patients with pituitary/hypothalamic dysfunction, in whom TSH cannot be used to reliably to assess thyroid function.

TSH, thyroid-stimulating hormone.

163. How do you evaluate a patient with hyperthyroidism?
By history, physical examination, and thyroid function tests including TSH, T_4, and triiodothyronine (T_3). Thyroid function tests usually show a low or undetectable TSH, high or normal T_4, and high or normal T_3. Normal T_4 and T_3 in the presence of low or undetectable TSH typically suggest subclinical hyperthyroidism except in the patient with pituitary dysfunction. The TSH is not a reliable indicator of hyperthyroidism in patients with pituitary dysfunction.

164. Describe the presentation of patients with hyperthyroidism.
See Table 16.9.

Table 16.9. Clinical Presentation of Hyperthyroidism

SYMPTOM	SIGNS
Lethargy, fatigue	Tremor
Anxiety/palpitations	Tachycardia, atrial arrhythmias, hypertension
Hyperactivity	Hyperdynamic precordium (often), congestive heart failure (rare)
Increased defecation	Agitation (mental status alterations if severe or in elderly patients)
Weight loss	Goiter
Sleep disturbance/insomnia	Increased deep tendon reflexes
Heat intolerance	Warm, moist, soft skin
Menstrual irregularities in women	Proximal muscle weakness
Erectile dysfunction in men	Ophthalmopathy: lid lag, stare (Graves disease: proptosis, diplopia, color vision changes, optic neuropathy, chemosis, eye irritation, extraocular muscle dysfunction)
Infertility	Brittle nails
Increased appetite	Edema (Graves disease: pretibial myxedema)
Poor exercise capacity, dyspnea	

165. **What disorders lead to hyperthyroidism?**
    - Graves disease
    - Autonomously functioning nodule(s)
    - Inflammation and destruction of all or part of the gland with resultant release of stored hormone (thyroiditis)
    - Exogenous thyroid hormone source outside the thyroid (pituitary tumor, dermoid ovarian tumor)

166. **How does the thyroid ^{123}I scan help differentiate among the different causes of hyperthyroidism?**
    By demonstrating the pattern and degree of ^{123}I uptake by the thyroid gland. See Table 16.10.

Table 16.10. Causes of Hyperthyroidism

ETIOLOGY	^{123}I SCAN PATTERN	RAIU	PATHOGENESIS
Common Causes			
Graves disease	Homogeneous	High (can be high normal)	Stimulating TSH receptor antibody
Multinodular goiter	Patchy	Moderate	Autonomous thyroid function
Solitary toxic nodule	Suppressed gland with one area of high uptake	Normal gland with suppressed uptake, high nodule uptake	Autonomous thyroid function
Thyroiditis	Homogeneous	Low	Release of preformed hormone
Silent Subacute Drug-induced Radiation-induced			
Exogenous thyroid	Homogeneous	Low	Excess thyroid hormone in drug or food
Less Common Causes			
Hashitoxicosis	Patchy	Moderate	Release of preformed hormone
Iodine (Jod-Basedow)	Homogeneous	Low	Iodine excess
Hyperemesis gravidarum	Do not scan due to pregnant state	Would expect high	Circulating hCG
Lithium	Variable	High	Variable
Rare Causes			
TSH-producing pituitary adenoma	Homogeneous	High but can be normal	Excess TSH production from tumor
Pituitary resistance to thyroid hormone	Homogeneous	High but can be normal	Excess TSH production from impaired feedback
Choriocarcinoma Trophoblastic disease	Homogeneous	High	Circulating hCG cross-reacts with TSH receptor
Struma ovarii (teratoma)	Homogeneous	Low	Ovarian teratoma
Metastatic thyroid cancer	Homogeneous	Low	Foci of functional autonomous tissue
Thyroid adenoma Infarction	Homogeneous	Low	Release of preformed hormone

hCG, human chorionic gonadotropin; RAIU, radioactive iodine uptake; TSH, thyroid-stimulating hormone.

167. **Summarize the treatment approach to hyperthyroidism.**
Treatment is based on the cause of the hyperthyroidism. The most common causes are overly zealous replacement of thyroid hormone, Graves disease, hyperfunctioning nodular disease, and thyroiditis. Overreplacement is easily treated by titrating down the thyroid hormone dose. All hyperthyroid patients benefit from beta blockers to treat the hyperadrenergic state.

168. **What is Graves disease?**
An autoimmune disease in which patients develop antibodies that mimic TSH by binding to its receptor on thyroid cells to stimulate thyroid hormone production. Graves disease is the most common cause of endogenous hyperthyroidism.

169. **How is Graves disease treated?**
With ^{131}I radioiodine ablation or antithyroid drugs (ATDs). Surgery can be performed to remove the Graves gland, but most patients prefer the nonsurgical options.

170. **How are ATDs used in Graves patients?**
As primary treatment or short-term management in preparation for ^{131}I radioablation. If the second approach is chosen, the ATD must be discontinued 7–10 days prior to the ^{131}I ablation so that it will not inhibit iodine uptake into the gland. ATDs should be titrated to normalize the TSH and T_4 (total or free T_4). Because normalization of TSH lags behind normalization of the T_4 level (by ~4–6 weeks), both laboratory tests must be monitored initially to avoid induction of hypothyroidism. Patients are typically treated with an ATD for 12–18 months, then tapered off to determine whether they have remained in remission. Relapse rates are high (50–60%) within the first year and are highest in patients with large goiters and more severe hyperthyroidism.

171. **Compare the two available ATDs.**
Both ATDs, propylthiouracil (PTU) and methimazole (Tapazole), inhibit T_4 and T_3 synthesis by the thyroid gland and are effective for treating hyperthyroidism. PTU has been associated with acute hepatic injury and should only be used in patients unable to tolerate other therapies or in pregnant women during or just before the first trimester. Methimazole is more convenient than PTU owing to its once-daily dosing.

172. **Summarize the side effects of ATDs.**
    - Rash (most common)
    - Abnormal taste
    - Agranulocytosis (0.2–0.5%)
    - Mild elevated transaminases
    - Fulminant hepatitis (rare)
    - Vasculitis (fever, arthralgias)
    Side effects can occur at any time and at any dose, although higher doses are associated with higher risk of adverse effects. Patients should be warned to stop the medication if they experience sore throat, fever, or joint pain.

173. **How does one manage pregnant patients previously treated for Graves disease?**
Pregnant women with a past or present history of Graves disease should have thyrotropin receptor (TR) antibodies measured at 20–24 weeks' gestation for a maternal serum determination to determine whether the fetus has a risk for fetal or neonatal Graves or goiter.

174. **How is hyperthyroidism treated during pregnancy?**
With PTU during the first trimester and methimazole starting in the second trimester. ^{131}I treatment should not be used in patients who are pregnant or nursing. Surgery can be attempted during the second trimester if necessary. PTU is preferred for treating pregnant patients because methimazole has been associated with a rare congenital scalp defect known as *aplasia cutis*.

Alexander EK, Pearce EN, Brent GA, et al. Guidelines of the American Thyroid Association for the Diagnosis and Management of Thyroid Disease During Pregnancy and the Postpartum. *Thyroid*. 2017;27:315–389.

175. **What is thyroid storm?**
A dramatic, life-threatening exacerbation of hyperthyroidism (thyrotoxicosis), associated with a 20% mortality rate if untreated. Thyroid storm is diagnosed clinically based on the severity of hyperthyroidism.

176. **Describe the presentation of thyroid storm.**
Severe signs and symptoms of hyperthyroidism including severe tachycardia, cardiac arrhythmias (tachycardia), heart failure, GI disturbances (hepatitis, jaundice), and mental status changes.

177. **How is thyroid storm treated?**
With general supportive care (often in the intensive care unit) and initiation of the following medications:
- Antithyroid medication (PTU) to block thyroid hormone synthesis and peripheral conversion of T_4 to T_3.
- Beta blockers (propranolol or IV esmolol) to inhibit the adrenergic system.
- Saturated solution of potassium iodide or other iodine-rich compounds to block the release of preformed thyroid hormones.
- Glucocorticoids may also be part of the initial management because thyroid hormones increase metabolism of endogenous cortisol and steroids can inhibit conversion of T_4 to T_3.

178. **How is solitary or multinodular disease treated?**
With ^{131}I ablation or surgery, particularly if the gland is large and the patient has compressive symptoms. ATDs can be used to render patients euthyroid but typically are not recommended for long-term use because they do not treat the underlying pathophysiology of the disease. The hyperthyroidism invariably returns if the ATD is discontinued.

179. **Describe the treatment of thyroiditis.**
With beta blockers until the usually transient thryoiditis resolves. Some patients with painful or subacute thyroiditis can be treated with steroids if the pain is particularly severe.
Ross DS, Burch HB, Cooper DS, et al. 2016 American Thyroid Association Guidelines for Diagnosis and Management of Hyperthyroidism and Other Causes of Thyrotoxicosis. *Thyroid.* 2016;26:1343–1421.

180. **What is T_3 toxicosis?**
Hyperthyroidism that is due primarily to high T_3 levels. Such patients have a low or undetectable TSH, normal T_4, and elevated T_3. If subclinical hyperthyroidism is suspected, a T_3 level should be measured to rule out T_3 toxicosis. The differential diagnosis, evaluation, and treatment are otherwise the same as for patients with hyperthyroidism due to any cause.

181. **How do you confirm a diagnosis of hypothyroidism?**
By history, physical examination, and thyroid function tests that show elevated TSH, low or normal T_4, and low or normal T_3. Normal hormone levels in the presence of an elevated TSH suggest subclinical hypothyroidism. TSH is a more sensitive marker of thyroid disease than circulating hormone levels and even if the T_4 or T_3 laboratory measurement is normal, the thyroid hormone level may not be physiologically "normal" for that particular patient if the TSH is elevated. Measurement of thyroid antibodies is not routinely indicated in the evaluation of primary hypothyroidism but can identify Hashimoto thyroiditis.

182. **When should thyroid autoantibodies be measured?**
The presence of TPO antibodies can be helpful in predicting which patients with subclinical hypothyroidism may progress over time to overt disease. TR antibodies should be monitored in patients with well-differentiated thyroid cancer to assess the reliability of thyroglobulin (Tg) as a tumor marker.

183. **How do hypothyroid patients present clinically?**
See Table 16.11.

184. **What are the pathologic types of hypothyroidism?**
Primary, secondary, tertiary, and peripheral (generalized) resistance to thyroid hormone.

185. **Explain the mechanisms of primary hypothyroidism.**
Any pathologic process intrinsic to the thyroid gland, leading to defective production of thyroid hormone or destruction of the gland.

186. **What are the causes of primary hypothyroidism?**
- Thyroiditis (Hashimoto, silent, painful/subacute, postpartum, and drug-induced)
- "Burnt-out" Graves disease

Table 16.11. Clinical Presentation of Hypothyroidism

SYMPTOMS	SIGNS
Lethargy, fatigue	Goiter
Dry skin	Dry skin (common in dry climates)
Hair loss, brittle hair, brittle nails	Coarse hair, alopecia, brittle nails
Decreased energy	Delayed relaxation phase of deep tendon reflexes
Constipation	Periorbital edema, edema
Weight gain (not usually > 50 lb)	Deepened voice
Hoarseness	Hypothermia
Cold intolerance	Lipid abnormalities (elevated cholesterol, LDL)
Menstrual irregularities in women	Elevated transaminases, creatinine phosphokinase
Erectile dysfunction in men	Reduced respiratory effort
Infertility	Proximal muscle weakness
Children: precocious or delayed puberty, abnormal growth/cognition	Bradycardia, hypertension, cardiomegaly
Depression, cognitive dysfunction	Neuropathy
Poor exercise capacity, dyspnea Muscle pain, joint stiffness	
Chest pain/angina	
Paresthesias	

LDL, low-density lipoprotein.

- Thyroid ablation from any cause (radiation, radioactive iodine, surgical resection, and metastatic tumor/neoplasia)
- Thyroid hormone biosynthetic defects
- Iodine deficiency
- Thyroid agenesis or dysgenesis

187. **What is the most common cause of primary hypothyroidism?**
Hashimoto thyroiditis.

188. **How does secondary hypothyroidism develop?**
When there is a deficiency of TSH from the pituitary (central hypothyroidism), most frequently found in patients with pituitary tumors or pituitary damage (e.g., radiation, surgery).

189. **Name the major cause of tertiary hypothyroidism.**
A deficiency of TRH from the hypothalamus (central hypothyroidism).

190. **What is peripheral (generalized) resistance to thyroid hormone?**
A rare genetic cause of hypothyroidism in which patients have generalized tissue resistance to thyroid hormone due to mutations in the thyroid hormone beta receptor gene. There is also a form that seems to cause primarily pituitary resistance to thyroid hormone. Unlike patients with generalized resistance, these patients present with symptoms of tissue hyperthyroidism and high T_4 and T_3 levels accompanied by an elevated or "inappropriately" normal TSH.

191. **How should hypothyroidism be treated?**
With levothyroxine (T_4). The goal is to reverse the clinical syndrome by restoring the TSH and hormone levels to the normal range. A typical replacement dose is 1.6 µg/kg/day in young healthy patients. Elderly patients often require lower doses. The best approach is to "start low, go slow." When initiating therapy, measure the TSH every 4–6 weeks with dose adjustments until the goal TSH is reached. More frequent measurements are not useful because the half-life of the drug is 7 days and the TSH should be measured in a state of equilibrium. Once the patient is on a stable dose, the TSH can be monitored annually unless there are changes in the patient's clinical status. Supplement with T_3 is generally not recommended.

Garber JR, RH Cobin, H Gharib, et al. Clinical Practice Guidelines for Hypothyroidism in Adults: Cosponsored by the American Association of Clinical Endocrinologists and the American Thyroid Association. *Thyroid.* 2012;22:1–36.

Jonklass J, Bianco AC, Bauer AJ, et al. Guidelines for the treatment of hypothyroidism. *Thyroid.* 2014;24:1670–1751.

192. **How does iodide affect thyroid gland function?**
Through multiple inhibitory effects on thyroid function, including decreased iodide transport, decreased iodide organification, and decreased thyroid hormone secretion.

193. **Describe the Wolff-Chaikoff effect.**
The normal transient inhibitory effect of an iodide load on thyroid function causing hypothyroidism or decreased thyroid hormone production. Most patients "escape" from these inhibitory effects within 2–4 weeks after iodide exposure.

194. **What is the Jod-Basedow phenomenon?**
Iodide-induced thyrotoxicosis. This phenomenon typically occurs in elderly patients with underlying nodular thyroid disease after they receive an iodide load such as radiographic contrast agent. In iodide-deficient countries, the Jod-Basedow phenomenon can occur after reintroduction of iodide in patients with goiter.

195. **Describe postpartum thyroiditis.**
An inflammation of the thyroid that can cause both hyperthyroidism and hypothyroidism, occurring in approximately 5–9% of women after pregnancy. Women with type 1 DM have a higher frequency (25%). Pathologic examination reveals an inflammatory process that is indistinguishable from lymphocytic thyroiditis (Hashimoto disease). In fact, women with positive antithyroid antibodies are at much higher risk of developing postpartum thyroiditis and permanent thyroid dysfunction.

196. **What are the phases of postpartum thyroiditis?**
- **Hyperthyroidism** (lasting 1–3 months)
- **Hypothyroidism** (lasting 4–8 months)
- **Euthyroid state**
Only 25–30% of women develop permanent hypothyroidism, and the clinician should assess whether a woman has returned to a euthyroid phase before prescribing unnecessary lifelong therapy with thyroid hormone. Treatment is based on phase of presentation.

197. **How common are thyroid nodules?**
Very common and prevalence depends on method of detection. The prevalence of a thyroid nodule is approximately 10% if detected by thyroid palpation and 50% if detected by ultrasound. The prevalence is known to increase with age.

198. **List the risk factors for malignancy in a thyroid nodule.**
- Family history of thyroid cancer
- Age < 20 or > 60 years
- Rapid growth of a preexisting nodule
- Large, painful, or firm nodule
- Invasive and compressive symptoms
- Lymphadenopathy
- Fixation of nodule to adjacent structures
- Vocal cord paresis
- History of head and neck irradiation
Any nodule ≥ 1–1.5 cm should be evaluated with fine-needle aspiration (FNA) in a clinically euthyroid patient.

199. **What is the most cost-effective method for evaluating a thyroid nodule?**
TSH and FNA biopsy (FNAB). Radioiodide (RAI) thyroid scan is recommended only in patients with a low TSH to detect hyperthyroidism. FNAB is recommended for nodules detected on ultrasound and normal or high TSH. Newer guidelines for FNAB have been developed that incorporate thyroid nodule characteristics and size on ultrasound into the decision regarding which nodules require biopsy.

200. List the types of thyroid cancer.
- Well-differentiated: papillary (85%), follicular (10%)
- Medullary thyroid cancer (3%): May be associated with multiple endocrine neoplasia type 2A (MEN-2A)
- Anaplastic (1%): Undifferentiated and most aggressive form
- Primary thyroid lymphoma (1%)

201. How should differentiated thyroid cancer be treated?
Usually with thyroidectomy. In higher risk patients, RAI therapy can be used while TSH is elevated. Thyroid hormone withdrawal for 4 weeks can raise the TSH naturally or patients can receive synthetic recombinant human TSH (rhTSH). RAI has been shown to reduce the risk of cancer recurrence in selected patients. Some centers use RAI to facilitate monitoring, but other centers are moving away from this practice due to the risks of RAI, including the rare increase in secondary malignancy, sialadenitis, and tear duct dysfunction. Patients are treated with thyroid hormone to keep the TSH suppressed. The level of TSH suppression is determined by the aggressiveness of the disease (initial stage), risk of recurrence, and time elapsed from initial diagnosis. This therapy has been shown to decrease cancer recurrence and mortality rate and to facilitate monitoring for residual/recurrent cancer.

202. Describe the typical follow-up for patients with differentiated thyroid cancer.
Serial physical examinations, Tg measurements both on thyroid hormone suppression therapy and after TSH stimulation, diagnostic whole-body ^{131}I scans (WBSs), and thyroid ultrasound. Previously, TSH stimulation was achieved by induction of hypothyroidism after withdrawal of thyroid hormone. Because an elevated TSH is required to stimulate ^{131}I uptake into thyroid cells, patients typically discontinue thyroid hormone replacement a number of weeks before the WBS and Tg test. As expected, hypothyroidism is uncomfortable for most patients, and some patients experience very severe symptoms and refuse or delay these cancer-monitoring procedures. See Question 203 for a discussion of the use of rhTSH.

> Haugen BR, Alexander EK, Bible KC, et al. 2015 American Thyroid Association management guidelines for adult patients with thyroid nodules and differentiated thyroid cancer: The American Thyroid Association Guidelines Task Force on Thyroid Nodules and Differentiated Thyroid Cancer. *Thyroid.* 2016;26:1–133.

203. What other option for monitoring is available?
Fortunately, the development of rhTSH provides a tool whereby TSH levels can be elevated without the need for the patient to become hypothyroid. This discovery has revolutionized care of patients with thyroid cancer. Although rhTSH is currently approved by the FDA for diagnostic monitoring of differentiated thyroid cancer and remnant ablation, the overall goal is to have no evidence of disease based on negative imaging studies and undetectable Tg levels.

> Woodmansee WW, Haugen BR. A review of the potential uses for recombinant human TSH in patients with thyroid cancer and nodular goiter. *Clin Endocrinol.* 2004;61:163–173.

204. What is Tg?
A normal protein produced by benign and malignant thyroid cells. Elevated levels of TSH can stimulate Tg production. Patients who have had thyroidectomy and ^{131}I remnant ablation should not have any residual cells to make Tg; thus, Tg can be used as a tumor marker to determine whether there are residual thyroid cells present.

205. What are the limits of Tg measurement?
Tg level in patients with anti-Tg antibodies cannot be measured accurately. Patients who have been treated only with surgery and not ^{131}I therapy will have some residual Tg production. Dedifferentiated thyroid cancer may not produce Tg.

206. How do you determine the initial degree of thyroid hormone suppression needed after thyroid cancer treatment?
By the disease risk. Low-risk patients have no metastases, no residual tumor, no local tumor invasion, nonaggressive disease, and no ^{131}I uptake outside the thyroid bed (if given) and should have TSH suppression to 0.1–0.5 mU/L. All other (intermediate- and high-risk) patients should have TSH suppression to < 0.1 mU/L. Patients with heart disease and elderly patients may also require a higher TSH goal. Long-term suppression goals will vary for the individual patient.

REPRODUCTIVE ENDOCRINOLOGY

207. **Define erectile dysfunction (ED).**
The inability to obtain and maintain an erection sufficient for sexual intercourse. ED is usually multifactorial in cause, and most men have at least some psychogenic factors that contribute to the disorder (i.e., performance anxiety can exacerbate underlying organic cause).

208. **List the six main categories of ED.**
   - **Hormonal:** Hypogonadism (primary or secondary), hyperprolactinemia (with resultant hypogonadism), hyperthyroidism or hypothyroidism, diabetes, adrenal insufficiency, and Cushing syndrome
   - **Pharmacologic:** Many causative medications such as antihypertensives (clonidine, beta blockers, vasodilators, thiazide diuretics, spironolactone); antidepressants (SSRIs, TCAs); antipsychotics; anxiolytics; histamine 2 (H_2) antagonists; phenytoin; carbamazepine; ketoconazole; metoclopramide; digoxin; alcohol; and illicit drugs (marijuana, cocaine, and heroin)
   - **Systemic disease:** Any severe illness that leads to hypogonadotropic hypogonadism
   - **Vascular:** Diabetes, peripheral arterial disease, venous dysfunction
   - **Neurologic:** Alzheimer disease, Parkinson disease, spinal cord injury, neuropathy, stroke
   - **Psychogenic:** Uncommon in isolation but contributes to most cases owing to other causes and should be considered a diagnosis of exclusion

209. **Describe the typical evaluation of a patient with ED.**
   - Detailed history including alcohol and illicit drug use, timing of symptom onset (gradual vs. sudden), satisfaction with current sexual partner, occurrence of nocturnal erections, previous surgeries, and current medical illnesses
   - Review of medications
   - Physical examination with particular attention to lower extremity vasculature, genitals, and findings of hypogonadism
   - Endocrine laboratory testing (TSH, prolactin, and total testosterone [morning or fasting])
   - Systemic disease testing (urinalysis, lipid panel, complete chemisty panel, A_{1c}, and complete blood count)
   - Nocturnal penile tumescence testing if assessment of erectile function is needed

210. **What are the most important steps in the management of ED?**
Identifying and treating organic causes and discontinuing any offending medications, if possible.

211. **What are the potential treatment options for men with ED?**
   - Correction of any hormonal abnormality, such as testosterone replacement for hypogonadism, correction of thyroid dysfunction, maximal glycemic control in diabetes, and treatment of hyperprolactinemia with dopamine agonist
   - Treatment of any underlying systemic disorders, including depression, but note that although SSRIs can cause ED, SSRIs may help to prevent premature ejaculation
   - Medical therapy
   - Mechanical devices including rings and vacuum pump device that may be cumbersome to some patients but have minimal side effects
   - Surgical interventions, typically used as a last resort and include revascularization, removal of venous shunts, and penile implants
   - Supportive counseling and couples therapy

212. **What medical therapies are available for ED?**
   - Alpha$_2$-adrenergic receptor blocker: Yohimbine (oral).
   - Phosphodiesterase-5 inhibitors: Sildenafil, vardenafil, tadalafil, and avanafil. All four are administered orally, but none should be used in combination with nitrates.
   - Intracavernosal injections of vasodilating medications: Alprostadil (prostaglandin E_1), and papaverine.
   - Transurethral alprostadil suppositories.

213. **List the three etiologic categories of gynecomastia.**
Idiopathic, physiologic, and pathologic.

214. List the physiologic changes that occur throughout the life cycle that may lead to gynecomastia.

Life Stage	Physiologic Change
Newborn	Fetal exposure to maternal estrogens during pregnancy
Puberty	Increased estrogen-to-androgen ratio
Older age	Combined effect of decreasing testosterone and increased estrogen due to peripheral aromatization of androgens to estrogens in adipose tissue, but the exact mechanism is unclear

215. What causes pathologic gynecomastia?

Usually, estrogen excess from either overproduction or peripheral aromatization including:
- Drugs that increase estrogen activity or production or reduce testosterone activity or production.
- Tumors that increase human chorionic gonadotropin (hCG) or estrogen production, such as testicular tumors (Leydig cell, Sertoli cell, germ cell, and granulosa cell), choriocarcinomas, and adrenal tumors. Male breast cancer is an uncommon cause.
- Decreased androgens or androgen resistance as found in hypogonadism due to any cause such as Klinefelter syndrome (male with extra X chromosome) and Kallmann syndrome (hypogonadotropic hypogonadism with absent sense of smell).
- Increased activity of enzyme that catalyzes estrogen production (aromatase) that is found in obesity, hyperthyroidism, and certain genetic mutations.
- Displacement of estrogens from sex hormone–binding globulin.
- Other illnesses such as end-stage liver disease, renal disease, human immunodeficiency virus (HIV) infection, familial syndromes, and starvation refeeding.

216. How does one begin to evaluate the causes of amenorrhea?

First, determine whether amenorrhea is primary (the patient has never had menses) or secondary (cessation of menses after she has started). Next, rule out pregnancy as a cause of amenorrhea. After pregnancy is ruled out, consider the following four broad categories of amenorrhea:
- Anatomic/outflow tract defect
- Ovarian failure
- Hypogonadotropic hypogonadism (pituitary or hypothalamic failure)
- Chronic anovulation

KEY POINTS: REPRODUCTIVE ENDOCRINOLOGY

1. The most common presentation of hypogonadism in men is erectile dysfunction and decreased libido.
2. The most common presentation of hypogonadism in women is amenorrhea and infertility.

217. Give examples of anatomic/outflow tract defects.
- Imperforate hymen
- Asherman syndrome (amenorrhea due to uterine adhesions)
- Müllerian agenesis
- Sexual differentiation disorders

218. What are the causes of primary ovarian failure?
- Genetic alterations (Turner syndrome with XO genotype)
- Autoimmune destruction
- LH or FSH receptor or postreceptor defects
- Physical insults (radiation, chemotherapy, viral infection, oophorectomy)
  Levels of FSH and LH are generally high in these disorders (hypergonadotropic hypogonadism).

219. List the causes of hypogonadotropic hypogonadism.
- **Hypothalmic dysfunction:** Induced by exercise or eating disorders
- **Pituitary dysfunction:** Tumors, hypopituitarism

- **Androgen excess:** Adrenal tumors, PCOS, tumors with high human choriogonadotropin, congenital adrenal hyperplasia
- **Thyroid dysfunction:** Hyperthyroidism, hypothyroidism
- **Systemic illness:** Liver disease, renal disease
- **Obesity**
- **Adrenal dysfunction**
  Levels of FSH and LH are generally low in these disorders.

220. Describe PCOS.

Also known as Stein-Leventhal syndrome, PCOS is characterized by (1) oligo- or anovulation, (2) hyperandrogenism, and (3) polycystic ovaries. Patients can be diagnosed with PCOS if they have at least two of the three classic features and other causes have been excluded.

221. How do women with PCOS typically present?

With menstrual dysfunction, hirsutism, and insulin resistance. Long-term consequences of PCOS include increased risk of developing type 2 DM, hyperlipidemia, and endometrial cancer.

222. Describe the management of PCOS.

Correction of the underlying metabolic disorder and addressing cosmetic concerns related to hirsutism. Weight loss and treatment of insulin resistance with thiazolidinediones or metformin are recommended. Oral contraceptives are used to regulate menstrual cycles and suppress hyperandrogenism. Because most patients have impaired ovulation, fertility must also be addressed. Most women can be treated with the ovulation-induction drug clomiphene citrate, either alone or in combination with insulin-sensitizing medication. Hirsutism is treated by suppressing androgen production with oral contraceptives, androgen receptor blockers, or 5-alpha-reductase inhibitors and appropriate cosmetic treatments.

223. Summarize the traditional rationale behind hormonal treatment of menopausal women.

Menopause represents the time in a woman's life that cyclic ovarian function ceases. Hormone replacement therapy (HRT), which consists of combined estrogen and progesterone in women with an intact uterus and estrogen only for women without a uterus, has been controversial. Previously, HRT was frequently recommended to women at the time of menopause and continued indefinitely because HRT was considered of clinical benefit to women by ameliorating vasomotor symptoms (hot flashes), improving lipids, and decreasing risk of cardiovascular disease, osteoporosis, and dementia.

224. How have the recommendations of HRT changed in current practice?

HRT is now mainly used for the short-term treatment of menopausal vasomotor symptoms, using the lowest effective dose based on the findings of the Women's Health Initiative (WHI). The WHI and subgroup studies showed that HRT was associated with an increased risk of breast cancer, thromboembolic diseases, and cardiovascular disease (coronary artery disease and stroke) and a reduced risk of colon cancer and osteoporosis. Although the absolute risk of these disorders is small, HRT is no longer recommended for disease prevention. HRT is currently only recommended in symptomatic menopausal women at the lowest doses and for the shortest duration required to control menopausal symptoms.

Moyer VA. Menopausal hormone therapy for the primary prevention of chronic conditions: U.S. Preventive Services Task Force Recommendation Statement. *Ann Intern Med.* 2013;158:47–54.

PARATHYROID HORMONE, CALCIUM, AND BONE DISORDERS

225. Identify the principal organs responsible for maintaining serum calcium in the normal range.

- **Bone:** storage of calcium
- **Kidney:** excretion of calcium
- **Intestine:** absorption of calcium

226. List the three main hormones involved in calcium regulation.

- **Parathyroid hormone (PTH):** increases serum calcium levels
- **Vitamin D:** increases serum calcium levels
- **Calcitonin:** decreases serum calcium levels

227. List the mechanisms by which PTH increases serum calcium levels.
- Increases bone resorption
- Increases 1,25-(OH)$_2$ vitamin D production
- Increases renal calcium retention
- Increases renal phosphate excretion
  PTH is synthesized and secreted by the parathyroid gland in response to low calcium levels.

228. Describe how vitamin D works to increase serum calcium levels.
- Increases bone resorption
- Increases renal calcium and phosphate retention
- Enhances intestinal calcium absorption
  The most active form is 1,25-(OH)$_2$ vitamin D, which is synthesized in the kidney by conversion of 25-(OH) vitamin D by 1-alpha-hydroxylase.

229. How does calcitonin work to decrease serum calcium levels?
By promoting calcium deposition in bone and inhibiting osteoclastic bone resorption. Calcitonin is synthesized by thyroidal C cells.

KEY POINTS: CALCIUM HOMEOSTASIS

1. Calcium homeostasis is tightly regulated to keep calcium in a very narrow physiologic range.
2. The three organs involved in calcium homeostasis are the bone (storage), kidney (excretion), and intestine (absorption).
3. The three hormones involved in calcium homeostasis are parathyroid hormone, vitamin D, and calcitonin.
4. Parathyroid hormone and vitamin D work to increase calcium levels.
5. Calcitonin works to decrease calcium levels.

---

230. List the signs and symptoms of hyper- and hypocalcemia.
See Table 16.12.

Table 16.12. Clinical Presentation of Calcium Disorders*

Hypercalcemia		Hypocalcemia	
SYMPTOMS	**SIGNS**	**SYMPTOMS**	**SIGNS**
CNS: cognitive impairment (variable), weakness	Dehydration (patient may have hypotension, if severe)	Perioral and peripheral paresthesias (initially)	Chvostek sign
GI symptoms: N/V, reflux, constipation	Hypertension	Carpal-pedal spasm	Trousseau sign
Renal: impaired function, polyuria, polydipsia, nephrocalcinosis	Arrhythmias (shortened QT interval)	Irritability	Bradycardia/arrhythmias, prolonged QT interval
Osteopenia		Tetany	Hypotension
Pancreatitis		Seizures	Laryngospasm
		Congestive heart failure (rare)	Bronchospasm

CNS, central nervous system; GI, gastrointestinal; N/V, nausea and vomiting.
*All signs and symptoms are a function of severity of calcium abnormality, acuteness of onset, and central patient's underlying medical status (often more severe in elderly patients).

231. Identify the two most common causes of hypercalcemia.
Primary hyperparathyroidism (55%) and hypercalcemia of malignancy (35%).

232. Describe how you would distinguish between the two.

Hypercalcemia diagnosed on an outpatient basis is usually due to primary hyperparathyroidism, whereas malignancy is the most common cause in hospitalized patients. The PTH level distinguishes between hypercalcemia of malignancy (undetectable PTH with high levels of PTH-related peptide) and primary hyperparathyroidism (high PTH levels). When faced with an elevated calcium, always check PTH before embarking on an expensive evaluation. High or normal PTH levels confirm the diagnosis of hyperparathyroidism. PTH values < 20 pg/L suggest another cause of hypercalcemia.

233. What are the uncommon causes of hypercalcemia?
- Thyrotoxicosis
- Granulomatous disease (sarcoidosis, tuberculosis, histoplasmosis, coccidioidomycosis)
- Drug-induced (thiazides, lithium, vitamins A and D intoxication, aluminum toxicity in renal failure)
- Immobilization
- Renal insufficiency with tertiary hyperparathyroidism
- Total parenteral nutrition

234. List the rare causes of hypercalcemia.
- Adrenal insufficiency
- Pheochromocytosis
- Pancreatic islet-cell tumors
- Familial hypocalciuric hypercalcemia (FHH)
- Milk alkali syndrome

235. What is FHH?

A very rare autosomal dominant genetic disorder that has nearly 100% penetrance due to an inactivating germ-line mutation in the calcium-sensing receptor. In this disorder, parathyroid cells are insensitive to inhibition by calcium. Renal tubule cells are also insensitive to calcium.

236. Summarize the clinical characteristics of FHH.

FHH is generally a benign disorder that results in alteration of the calcium "set point." Patients have lifelong moderately elevated calcium, normal to slightly elevated intact PTH, and normal to low calcium excretion. The fractional excretion of calcium (which normalizes calcium excretion for glomerular filtration rate) is usually low. Most patients have a ratio of calcium clearance (C_{Ca}) to creatinine clearance (C_{Cr}) < 0.01. This ratio is calculated by the following equation:

$$C_{Ca} : C_{Cr} = [U_{Ca} \times S_{Cr}] / [S_{Ca} \times U_{Cr}]$$

where U_{Ca} = urinary calcium, U_{Cr} = urinary creatinine, S_{Ca} = serum calcium, and S_{Cr} = serum creatinine. Owing to the abnormal calcium sensor, patients have "relative hypocalciuria" (unusually normal for the degree of hypercalcemia). An estimate of free serum calcium not bound by albumin should be used in this calculation by multiplying total calcium by 0.6.

237. How does one diagnose primary hyperparathyroidism?

By elevated levels of calcium and PTH. Primary hyperparathyroidism is usually due to a single parathyroid adenoma. FHH can be excluded with a 24-hour urine for calcium and family history.

238. How is primary hyperparathyroidism treated?

With surgery for patients < 50 years old with identified complications of hypercalcemia. However, some patients do not present with classic signs and symptoms and are believed to have a mild form of the disease that has been termed *asymptomatic hyperparathyroidism*. Many of these patients have mild elevations in calcium and complain of mild cognitive symptoms or symptoms of depression that are not always clearly related to the disease. Because a large number of patients are "asymptomatic" and may be observed, a list of indications for surgery has been developed. See Table 16.13.

Bilezikian JP, Brandi ML, Eastell R, et al. Guidelines for the management of asymptomatic primary hyperparathyroidism: summary statement from the Fourth International Workshop. *J Clin Endocrinol Metab.* 2014;99:3561–3569.

Table 16.13. Indications for Surgery in Primary Hyperparathyroidism

MEASUREMENT	INDICATION FOR SURGERY
Serum calcium	1 mg/dL above upper limit of normal
Creatinine clearance	<60 mL/min if hypercalcemic
Radiograph, US, or CT	Nephrolithiasis or nephrocalcinosis
24-hour urine for calcium	>400 mg/dL and increased stone risk by biochemical stone risk analysis
Bone mineral density	T score (DXA): ≤2.5 at lumbar spine, total hip, femoral neck, or distal one-third radius or vertebral fracture by radiograph, CT, MRI, or VFA
Age	<50 yr

CT, computed tomography; DXA, dual-energy x-ray absorptiometry; MRI, magnetic resonance imaging; US, ultrasound; VFA, vertebral fracture assessment.
Bilezikian JP, Brandi ML, Eastell R, et al. Guidelines for the management of asymptomatic primary hyperparathyroidism: summary statement from the Fourth International Workshop. *J Clin Endocrinol Metab.* 2014;99:3561–3569.

239. **Why is it necessary to distinguish FHH from primary hyperparathyroidism?**
To avoid unnecessary parathyroidectomy. FHH cannot be surgically cured.

240. **What is Fracture Risk Assessment Tool (FRAX)?**
A calculation that assesses a patient's 10-year fracture risk by entering clinical data regarding risk factors for fracture and femoral neck BMD measurement. Patients who have a 10-year fracture risk > 3% in the hip or 20% in other areas should be treated or considered for antiosteoporosis, antifracture medication. The calculation can be accessed at https://shef.ac.uk/FRAX.

241. **Identify the risk factors for fractures according to FRAX.**
See Table 16.14.

Table 16.14. Risk Factors for Fractures

- Advanced age
- Previous low-trauma fracture
- Long-term glucocorticoid use
- Low body weight (<58 kg)
- Family history of hip fracture
- Tobacco use
- Excess alcohol use
- Chronic disease states; e.g., diabetes mellitus, androgen deficiency, inflammatory bowel disease, hyperthyroidism, hypercortisolism

From Ferri F. *Ferri's Clinical Advisor.* St. Louis, MO: Elsevier; 2018; 925–927.e5, used with permission

242. **What is osteopenia?**
A bone density that is lower than normal but not low enough for classification as osteoporosis. Osteopenia is diagnosed with the bone density in the one-third radius, total lumbar spine, total hip, or femoral neck is between 1 and 2.5 standard deviations below peak normal, as defined as the average bone density in a population of the same gender and race at age 30.

243. **List the causes of secondary osteoporosis.**
- **Medications:** glucocorticoids (most common), thyroid hormone when excessively replaced, anticonvulsants, heparin, isoniazid, loop diuretics, cyclosporine, proton pump inhibitors, GnRH agonists and antagonists, and transplant antirejection medications
- **Endocrine:** DM type 1, hyperthyroidism, vitamin D deficiency, male hypogonadism, Cushing syndrome, hyperparathyroidism, hyperprolactinemia, amenorrhea, estrogen deficiency, and osteomalacia
- **GI:** gastrectomy/malabsorption syndromes, celiac disease, inflammatory bowel disease, malnutrition, liver disease, chronic pancreatitis, hemochromatosis, and gastric bypass surgeries
- **Malignancy:** multiple myeloma, metastatic carcinoma, leukemia, mastocytosis, and lymphoma
- **Hematologic:** sickle cell anemia and thalassemia

- **Renal disease:** idiopathic hypercalciuria, hypophosphatasia, homocystinuria
- **Connective tissue disorders:** rheumatoid arthritis, osteogenesis imperfecta
- **Miscellaneous:** poor nutrition, alcohol use, tobacco use, immobilization, anorexia nervosa, sarcoidosis, and amyloidosis

244. List the treatment options for patients with osteoporosis. Which agents have been shown both to increase bone mineral density and to reduce fractures? See Table 16.15.

Table 16.15. Medications Currently Available for the Treatment of Osteoporosis

MEDICATION	MECHANISM OF ACTION	INCREASES BMD DATA AVAILABLE	REDUCES FRACTURES DATA AVAILABLE	FDA APPROVED INDICATION
Bisphosphonates				
Alendronate	Antiresorptive	Yes	Hip: yes Spine: yes	Prevention: yes Treatment: yes
Risedronate	Antiresorptive	Yes	Hip: yes Spine: yes	Prevention: yes Treatment: yes
Zoledronate	Antiresorptive	Yes	Hip: yes Spine: yes	Prevention: yes Treatment: yes
Ibandronate	Antiresorptive	Yes	Hip: not significant Spine: yes	Prevention: yes Treatment: yes
Recombinant PTH				
Teriparatide (human)	Anabolic	Yes	Hip: uncertain Spine: yes	Prevention: no Treatment: yes
Miscellaneous				
Raloxifene	Antiresorptive	Yes	Hip: not significant Spine: yes	Prevention: yes Treatment: yes
Denosumab	Antiresorptive	Yes	Hip: yes Spine: yes	
Estrogen agonists			Hip: yes Spine: yes	Prevention: yes Treatment: no
Calcitonin	Antiresorptive	Yes	Hip: not significant Spine: yes	Prevention: no Treatment: yes

BMD, bone mineral density; FDA, U.S. Food and Drug Administration; PTH, parathyroid hormone.
Not significant: indicates effect on hip has been examined but no significant differences found. Trial may have been underpowered to detect differences. Hip data may have been combined in all nonvertebral fractures.
Uncertain: results variable or data insufficient to determine or trial is under way.

245. How do you decide which treatment options to use for a specific patient?

246. What are the contraindications to teriparatide therapy?
- Past or present history of radiation therapy
- Bone cancer
- Paget disease
- Elevated PTH
- Vitamin D deficiency
- Past or present hypercalcemia

247. What is Paget disease?
A disorder of abnormal bone remodeling that can affect one or more skeletal sites. Initially, the disorder begins with abnormal bone resorption followed by compensatory bone formation, resulting in disorganized bone remodeling that predisposes the affected region to deformity

and fracture. The exact cause is unknown. Patients may be asymptomatic with elevated serum alkaline phosphatase levels noted on routine serum chemistries or present with bone pain and deformity.

248. How is Paget disease diagnosed?
With bone scan and confirmatory plain radiographs of areas showing increased uptake.

249. Summarize the management of Paget disease.
Bisphosphonates are used for patients with progressive bone pain, planned surgery at an active bone site, and disease at bone sites that are at high risk for future complications such as skull, spine, weight-bearing bones, or bones near joints.

250. How are the causes of hypocalcemia classified?
As related to hypoparathyroidism or nonhypoparathyroidism. **Hypoparathyroidism** causes can be divided into PTH deficiency (e.g., surgical, autoimmune, congenital aplasia, radiation-induced, and infiltrative diseases) or PTH resistance (PTH antibodies, pseudohypoparathyroidism, and magnesium deficiency). **Nonhypoparathyroidism** causes include vitamin D deficiency or resistance (dietary deficiency, lack of sunlight, liver and renal disease), accelerated bone mineralization (hungry bone syndrome after parathyroidectomy), drugs (anticalcemic, antineoplastic), and acute complexing/sequestration of calcium (rhabdomyolysis, tumor lysis syndrome, pancreatitis, phosphate infusions, blood transfusions).

251. How should hypocalcemia be treated?
Treatment depends on the severity and duration of symptoms. Patients with acute hypocalcemia should be hospitalized with telemetry monitoring and given IV calcium in addition to magnesium, if indicated. Patients with chronic hypocalcemic disorders are managed with oral calcium and vitamin D supplementation. *Note:* Never give calcium with phosphate.

WEBSITES

1. American Association of Clinical Endocrinologists: www.aace.com
2. American Diabetes Association: www.diabetes.org
3. American Society for Bone and Mineral Research: www.asbmr.org
4. American Thyroid Association: www.thyroid.org
5. National Osteoporosis Foundation: www.nof.org
6. Pituitary Society: www.pituitarysociety.org
7. The Endocrine Society: www.endocrine.org

BIBLIOGRAPHY

1. Braverman LE, Cooper DS, eds. *Werner and Ingbar's Thyroid. A Fundamental and Clinical Text.* 10th ed. Philadelphia: Lippincott Williams & Wilkins; 2010.
2. Dickey J. Diabetes. In: Dickey J, ed. *The Eye Beaters, Blood, Victory, Madness, Buckhead, and Mercy.* Garden City, NY: Doubleday; 1970.
3. Rosen CJ, ed. *Primer on the Metabolic Bone Diseases and Disorders of Mineral Metabolism.* 8th ed. Ames, Iowa: Wiley-Blackwell; 2013.
4. Melmed S, Polonsky KS, Larson PR, et al., eds. *Williams Textbook of Endocrinology.* 13th ed. Philadelphia: Elsevier; 2016.
5. Wierman ME, ed. *Diseases of the Pituitary: Diagnosis and Treatment.* Totowa, NJ: Humana Press; 1997.

CHAPTER 17

NEUROLOGY

David B. Sommer, MD, MPH

My hand moves because certain forces—electric, magnetic, or whatever 'nerve-force' may prove to be—are impressed on it by my brain. This nerve-force, stored in the brain, would probably be traceable, if Science were complete, to chemical forces supplied to the brain by the blood, and ultimately derived from the food I eat and the air I breathe.

Lewis Carroll (1832–1898)
from *Sylvie and Bruno, 1890*

OVERVIEW AND APPROACH TO THE PATIENT

1. **What is localization?**
   The process of determining which part(s) of the nervous system are malfunctioning in order to produce the patient's signs or symptoms. Localization is key to the neurologic evaluation and often plays an important role in neurology teaching rounds. After the history and physical examination are presented, a discussion begins to "localize the lesion." A differential diagnosis of pathologic processes is discussed after localization. By formulating a case in terms of localization, you're starting to think like a neurologist!
   Pathologic processes can be:
   - **Focal:** Explained by a single lesion (e.g., peroneal neuropathy, right thalamic stroke)
   - **Diffuse:** Affecting a specific level(s) of the neuraxis symmetrically (e.g., polyneuropathy)
   - **Multifocal:** Explained by multiple lesions (e.g., multiple sclerosis [MS])
   Neurologists often refer to *levels* of the nervous system or *neuraxis.* In broad terms these levers are cerebral cortex, subcortical brain, cerebellum, brainstem, spinal cord, nerve roots, plexus, peripheral nerves, neuromuscular junction (NMJ), and skeletal muscle.

2. **How is the neurologic lesion localized?**
   By evaluating the symptoms and examination findings and considering if this fits with dysfunction at each level of the neuraxis. Neurologists pride themselves on being "old school." Case formulation and localization are typically based on a thorough history and physical examination. Ancillary studies such as laboratory results, computed tomography (CT), or magnetic resonance imaging (MRI) should not be considered during the initial localization evaluation because many laboratory or imaging results are coincidental and not causal of the patient's problem. Localization requires knowledge of functional neuroanatomy. You'll find it helpful to carry a neuroanatomy reference on your neurology rotation.
   Examples of good localizing formulations:
   Mr. Weaker is a 75-year-old man presenting with subacute progressive difficulty getting up from a chair. On examination he has nonfatiguable proximal symmetrical weakness of bilateral upper and lower extremities with normal sensory function, reflexes, cranial nerve function, and mental status. The examination findings would suggest this is a diffuse process affecting skeletal muscles (i.e., a myopathy).
   Ms. Understood is a 48-year-old woman with acute onset of expressive aphasia and upper-motor-neuron pattern weakness affecting the right face and arm. These findings localize to the left cerebral hemisphere (cortical and subcortical brain).

3. **What are the components of the neurologic examination?**
   See Table 17.1.

Table 17.1. The Neurologic Examination

COMPONENT TESTED	FUNCTION ASSESSED	MANEUVER OR OBSERVATION
Mental status	Level of arousal	Alert, drowsy, stuporous, or comatose
	Attention and concentration	Attentive, neglectful, or easily distracted
	Language	Name objects, repeat sentences, comprehend directions
	Memory	Remember short lists of words
	Calculation, abstraction, and sequencing	Perform simple calculations
	Affect	Appropriate, shows full range
	Thought processes and content	Assess for presence of hallucinations and delusions, insight, judgment, and appropriateness
Cranial nerves	I	Identify scent (such as common spice)
	II	Visual acuity, visual fields by confrontation testing and pupillary responses
	III, IV, and VI	Extraocular movements
	V	Facial sensation to light touch
	VII	Facial movements (eyebrow raising, grimace, smiling)
	VIII	Hearing (whisper test), observe presence of nystagmus
	IX and X	Palatal movement
	XI	Trapezius and sternocleidomastoid strength (shoulder shrug)
	XII	Tongue movement or deviation
Motor	Bulk and appearance	Atrophy, hypertrophy, and fasciculation
	Tone	Increased with spasticity, rigidity, or geggenhalten* or decreased with flaccidity
	Strength	Graded as: 5—full strength 4—weak but can move against some resistance 3—can move against gravity but not resistance 2—cannot move against gravity 1—muscle contracts or twitches but limb does not move
	Pattern of abnormalities noted	Symmetrical vs. asymmetrical Proximal vs. distal Central or upper motor neuron pattern
Sensory	Sensations	Pinprick, temperature, vibration, proprioception
	Pattern of abnormalities noted	Proximal vs. distal
Reflexes	Deep tendon (biceps, brachioradialis, triceps, patellar, ankle)	Graded as: 0—absent 1—reduced 2—normal 3—hyperreflexic 4—sustained clonus
	Plantar response	Babinski (positive with upgoing great toe and fanning of other toes)

Table 17.1. The Neurologic Examination *(Continued)*

COMPONENT TESTED	FUNCTION ASSESSED	MANEUVER OR OBSERVATION
Coordination		Finger to nose, heel to shin, rapid movement
Gait		Ability to get up without assistance or using arm support Posture (stooped, upright) Base width (between insides of feet) Stride length Arm swing present or absent Symmetry Weakness

*Geggenhalten: increased resistance to movement that is overcome when distracted.

4. **How is a neurologic examination performed if the patient is comatose?**
   The key parts of the examination for a comatose patient are:
   - **Responsiveness,** with assessment of severity of brain injury by Glasgow Coma Scale (Table 17.2):
     - Response to painful stimuli in unrestrained limbs
     - Ability to track objects with eyes
     - Response to threatening stimulus with blink
     - Ability to follow commands ("look up," "blink")
     - Ability to answer yes/no questions
   - **Cranial nerves:**
     - Pupillary responses to light
     - Extraocular movements (EOMs)
     - Oculocephalic reflex ("doll's eyes") if EOMs absent or abnormal
     - Cold caloric testing if "doll's eyes" abnormal or not present
   - **Motor testing:**
     - Tone
     - Strength, even if able to assess only withdrawal and movement against gravity
   - **Sensory testing:**
     - Compare stimuli responses on right and left side of the body (although limited)

Table 17.2. Glasgow Coma Scale

	Observed Response		
POINTS	EYE OPENING	VOCAL RESPONSE	MOTOR RESPONSE
1	None	None	None
2	To pain	Grunts	Extends to pain
3	To voice	Utters inappropriate words	Abnormal flexion to pain
4	Spontaneously	Confused or disoriented	Withdrawal from pain
5	—	Oriented and appropriate	Purposeful or localizes
6	—	—	Follows commands

Scoring: Add the points as indicated in the left column, based on the observed response.
- ≥13: Mild brain injury
- 9–12: Moderate brain injury
- ≤8: Severe brain injury

The minimum score is 3 and maximum score is 15.
Adapted from Teasdale G, Jennett B. Assessment of coma and impaired consciousness. A practical scale. *Lancet* 1974;2:81–84.

- **Reflexes:**
  - Deep tendon
  - Plantar responses

5. **How should the patient be approached if the examiner thinks the patient is "faking" or imagining her or his symptoms?**
Carefully. The term *functional* is used to describe neurologic phenomena or symptoms that occur when the basic structure and function of relevant primary neurologic symptoms are intact. Examination findings are often inconsistent and incompatible with classically localizable disorders. The pathophysiology of functional neurologic disorders is poorly understood, and patients with functional symptoms are among the most challenging patients to care for. The vast majority of patients with functional neurologic problems are not voluntarily producing their symptoms. A careful neurologic examination is important, but the presence of a functional disorder often makes this examination difficult. Relevant portions of the examination should be repeated and consistent and inconsistent findings between the examinations documented. Examining the patient in different positions and during distracting maneuvers and casually observing the patient apart from the formal examination may all provide useful information. Honestly tell patients that their symptoms are difficult to explain given our understanding of neurology but that you believe their symptoms are real—not feigned or imagined. Suggesting that the symptoms will likely improve may be helpful.

KEY POINTS: APPROACH TO THE PATIENT

- Localization of pathologic process is key to neurologic assessment.
- Many elements of the neurologic examination can be performed even if the patient is comatose or unable to cooperate with the examination.
- Inconsistent symptoms and examination findings may suggest a functional neurologic disorder.

NEUROLOGIC TESTS AND PROCEDURES

6. **When are an electromyogram (EMG) and nerve conduction study (NCS) helpful?**
During the evaluation of possible neuropathies (focal or diffuse), radiculopathies, plexopathies, myopathies, motor neuron disease, or NMJ disorders. Sometimes NCS and EMG are referred to collectively as *EMG*. When ordering an EMG be sure to list the diagnoses being considered so that the most appropriate studies can be done. EMG is more sensitive in conditions that have been present for at least a couple of weeks, though sometimes an acute study is indicated such as in suspected Guillain-Barré syndrome (GBS). See Table 17.3.

Table 17.3. Clinical Syndromes in Which Electromyography and Nerve Conduction Studies Are Used for Diagnosis*

Myopathy	
Polyneuropathy	Differentiation between axonal and demyelinating neuropathies
Neuromuscular junction disease	Assessment of large sensory and motor fibers (may be normal in small fiber sensory neuropathy)
Focal compression neuropathies	Focal root, plexus, or nerve lesions

*Both electromyography and nerve conduction studies are generally required for appropriate diagnosis.

7. **How are EMG and NCS done?**
   - **Sensory NCS:** Electrically stimulate a nerve and record a response at a distant point on the same nerve.
   - **Motor NCS:** Electrically stimulate a nerve at different points and record an electrical response over a target muscle belly.
   - **EMG:** Place a needle electrode into various muscle bellies to observe electrical activity with rest and activation (no electrical stimulus is applied).

Specialized studies such as repetitive stimulation to evaluate the NMJ may be performed in special cases.

8. **When is an electroencephalogram (EEG) helpful?**
   - To evaluate for a seizure disorder (by seeing abnormal interictal activity)
   - To look for subclinical seizure activity in altered states of consciousness
   - To determine whether episodes of altered consciousness/behavior are in fact seizures with a prolonged EEG

9. **Is EEG sensitive to diagnose seizures?**
   No. An interictal EEG is frequently normal despite a definite history of seizures. Thus a normal EEG does not rule out a seizure disorder. Sleep-deprived recording, repeated EEG, and prolonged recording increase sensitivity. An EEG recorded during a seizure is sensitive, so a normal EEG during an observed seizure is diagnostic of nonepileptic events.

10. **How is an EEG done?**
    By placing multiple electrodes on a patient's scalp and recording electrical activity generated by the brain. From an electrician's standpoint, this is a fairly unsatisfactory way to record brain activity, given the significant amount of electrical insulation between cortex and scalp. Nonetheless, it is impractical in most clinical circumstances to remove the skull, and surface (scalp) EEG can still be quite clinically useful. In special situations, such as evaluation for epilepsy surgery, electrode arrays can be surgically placed directly on the surface of the brain for monitoring.

11. **When should one order a polysomnogram (PSG) or sleep study?**
    When evaluating sleep disorders such as sleep apnea, sleep behavior disorders, nonrestorative sleep (suspect sleep, breathing, or movement disorder), and morning headache (suspect sleep apnea).

12. **What is monitored during PSG?**
    Respirations (airflow), oxygen saturation, respiratory muscle movement, cardiac rhythm, limb movement, and limited EEG are monitored overnight in a sleep laboratory. Video is typically recorded as well.

13. **What are the advantages of CT scanning over MRI for imaging the brain?**
    Availability and ease of performance. A scan can be accomplished in less than a minute. There are no major safety issues (screening for implants, metal, etc.) to be addressed prior to scanning. CT is very good at showing acute bleeding, calcification, and processes involving bone.

14. **What is the advantage of MRI over CT for imaging the brain?**
    Provision of a more detailed picture of the brain tissue. MRI is more sensitive for both acute and chronic ischemic changes and those associated with demyelinating disease. Acute ischemia can be seen using diffusion-weighted imaging as areas of restricted diffusion.

15. **When is contrast helpful with CT and MRI?**
    When looking for breakdown of the blood-brain barrier such as in acute inflammation and when trying to characterize masses. Contrast does not add much to the evaluation of acute stroke unless given to obtain CT angiography.

16. **What modalities are available to image the cerebrovascular system?**
    - MR angiogram (MRA):
      - Done without contrast, sensitive though less specific than CTA
      - Most sensitive modality for cervical artery dissection if fat-saturated images are done (need to request specifically).
      - MR venogram can be done to look at the venous system.
    - CT angiogram (CTA):
      - Obtained quickly
      - Provides good quality images
      - Exposes patient to iodinated contrast agent and increased ionizing radiation
      - CT venogram can be done to look at venous outflow.
    - Ultrasound:
      - Easily obtained with less cost than CTA/MRA
      - Provides hemodynamic information
      - Detailed analysis limited to accessible portions of the extracranial carotid arteries
      - Transcranial Doppler—useful in specialized applications but not widely used

- Conventional catheter angiography:
  - Provides most detailed images of medium-sized and small arteries
  - Provides best characterization of collateral flow patterns as each carotid and vertebral artery can be selectively injected with contrast agent
  - Allows for potential of interventional procedures such as thrombectomy, thrombolysis, angioplasty, and coiling of aneurysms
  - Most invasive

17. **How are evoked potentials (EPs) recorded, and when are they helpful?**
By averaging EEG recordings during hundreds of stimuli—changing visual patterns for visual evoked responses, clicking stimuli for brainstem auditory evoked responses, and electric shocks for somatosensory evoked responses. EPs are the only objective physiologic test that evaluates an entire pathway from sensory organ to cerebral cortex and are particularly useful when evaluating for optic neuritis and dorsal column disease.

KEY POINTS: NEUROLOGIC TESTS AND PROCEDURES

- Always include clinical information and differential diagnosis when ordering any neurologic test; protocols may be altered to give the most useful information.
- Interictal EEG is not sensitive for seizures. Ictal EEG is sensitive for seizures.

NEUROLOGIC SYMPTOMS

ALTERED MENTAL STATUS

See also Chapter 18, Geriatrics.

18. **What is the most common cause of altered mental status in the hospitalized patient?**
Delirium, also called *toxic/metabolic encephalopathy*. Encephalopathy is diffuse cortical brain dysfunction. Delirium in the hospitalized patient is most often due to an underlying medical process such as infection, renal failure, hepatic failure, hypercarbia, or hypoxia. Physiologic stress, sleep deprivation, and medication effects can also contribute. Baseline mild cognitive impairment (sometimes previously undiagnosed) or dementia is a risk factor for delirium.

19. **What is the appropriate initial evaluation for a patient with altered mental status?**
   - Review of current medications
   - If hospitalized, review of home medications that were not continued in the hospital, possibly resulting in a withdrawal syndrome
   - Review of current and past alcohol and nonprescription drug use
   - Laboratory tests: complete blood count (CBC), serum chemistries, hepatic enzymes, ammonia, thyroid function tests, urinalysis
   - Chest radiograph
   - Serum and urine drug screens (if indicated)
   - Urine and blood cultures
   - Oxygen saturation

20. **When is a brain CT scan or MRI indicated for evaluation of delirium?**
Whenever the cause of delirium is unclear after the initial evaluation or a structural process such as hemorrhage, mass lesion, ischemic stroke, or hydrocephalus is suspected. A dramatic abrupt change in neurologic status without clear explanation indicates urgent imaging.

21. **When is a lumbar puncture (LP) indicated for evaluation of altered mental status?**
When the initial evaluation suggests infection or inflammation of the brain, vasculitis affecting the brain, or neoplasm that may have spread to cerebrospinal fluid (CSF). In the setting of encephalopathy, LP should be performed only **after** either CT or MRI, because the presence of a mass lesion could cause a pressure gradient with risk of cerebral herniation if the lumbar CSF space is decompressed through an LP.

22. What tests should be done on the CSF?
    - Cell counts on tubes 1 and 4
    - Protein
    - Glucose
    - Gram stain
    - India ink preparation and cryptococcal antigen testing (if cryptococcal meningitis suspected)
    - Cytologic test, if malignancy suspected
    - Oligoclonal bands and IgG index/IgG synthesis rate (if MS or other immune disorder suspected)
    - Specific assays and antibodies for any suspected infections (e.g., Lyme disease, Venereal Disease Research Laboratory [VDRL] test)
    - Viral polymerase chain reactions (PCR) (if indicated)

23. How can an EEG aid in diagnosis of altered mental status?
    - Rule out ongoing seizure activity (complex partial status epilepticus)

KEY POINTS: ALTERED MENTAL STATUS

- Delirium is the most common cause of altered mental status in the hospitalized patient.
- Evaluation for underlying medical illness and drug effects is imperative.

    - Confirm presence of diffuse cortical dysfunction (manifested as diffuse slowing of the background frequency)
      A normal EEG in the setting of altered mental status is surprising and indicates either subcortical or psychiatric pathology.

APHASIA

24. What is aphasia?
    A deficit in language function. Aphasia is important to recognize because of its localizing value as a focal deficit. Aphasia should be distinguished from global encephalopathy, but assessment becomes difficult when both are present. The aphasic patient will typically appear more frustrated than confused.

25. What are the types of aphasia?
    See Table 17.4.

Table 17.4. Types of Aphasias and Their Characteristics

APHASIA TYPE	Speech Function Affected				LOCALIZATION
	Fluency	Naming	Repetition	Comprehension	
Broca	+	+	+	−	Left posterior inferior frontal gyrus
Wernicke	+	−	+	+	Left posterior superior temporal gyrus
Transcortical motor	+	+	−	−	Left frontal lobe
Transcortical sensory	−	+	−	+	Left temporal-parietal-occipital junction
Conductive	−	+	+	−	Arcuate fasciculus
Global	+	+	+	+	Large left hemispherical

+, impaired; −, spared.

26. **How does one assess for aphasia?**
By assessing object naming. Patients with mild to moderate global encephalopathy will have no difficulty naming objects, but aphasic patients will. To detect mild deficits, ask the patient to name objects that are rarely named (driver's license, stethoscope). Listen for paraphasic errors (wrong word that sounds like or is topically related to desired word) and fluency or dysfluency.

27. **What causes aphasia?**
Any process that causes focal cerebral dysfunction such as stroke, tumor, MS, seizure, or migraine in specific areas of the dominant cerebral hemisphere (or subcortical structures that connect these). The most common cause of aphasia is stroke.

28. **Are reading and writing affected in aphasia?**
Yes. Aphasia is a language problem, not a speech problem. Typically, reading and writing are affected in proportion to the ability to comprehend and produce spoken language.

29. **Is slurred speech aphasia?**
No. Although some patients with aphasia may also have slurred speech or dysarthria, slurred speech is usually not aphasia. Slurred speech can be produced by a focal process such as facial or bulbar weakness or can be a manifestation of a global encephalopathy. Dysarthria in isolation is a nonspecific symptom with many potential causes.

KEY POINTS: APHASIA

- All patients with altered speech or consciousness should be assessed for aphasia.
- Aphasia has localizing value whereas encephalopathy and dysarthria do not.

VISUAL COMPLAINTS

30. **What questions should be asked to localize a visual disturbance?**
    - Is one (monocular) or are both (binocular) eyes affected?
    - Is the disturbance transient or fixed?
    - Was onset of the disturbance gradual or abrupt?
    - If binocular, is one part of the visual field involved?
    - Are other phenomena present such as flashing lights and zigzag lines?

31. **What is the most common cause of transient and evolving visual disturbances?**
Migraine. Migraine activity frequently produces vision disturbances, typically evolving over minutes with binocular symptoms. Headache need not be present.

32. **What is the differential diagnosis for monocular vision loss?**
    - Glaucoma
    - Retinal detachment
    - Retinal artery occlusion
    - Ischemic optic neuropathy (e.g., giant cell arteritis or vasculitis)
    - Optic neuritis

33. **Where does a monocular visual disturbance localize?**
Anterior to the optic chiasm—either within the eye itself or the optic nerve.

34. **How does optic neuritis present?**
As the relatively abrupt (hours to days) onset of vision loss or blurring. Optic neuritis is usually monocular but can be binocular and sometimes is associated with pain, particularly with eye movement. Peripheral color perception, particularly for red, is reduced. An associated relative afferent pupillary defect (less constriction of both pupils when light is shone in the affected eye than when light is shone in the unaffected eye) may also be present.

35. **How is optic neuritis treated?**
Usually with high-dose intravenous (IV) steroids (i.e., 1 g methylprednisolone daily × 3 days followed by an oral steroid taper.). Steroids have been shown to improve short-term outcomes, but long-term outcomes were not improved in the Optic Neuritis Treatment Trial.

36. Do patients with optic neuritis have MS?

Possibly. Optic neuritis can be the presenting symptom in MS. In the cohort from the Optic Neuritis Treatment Trial, the risk of subsequent diagnosis of MS depended heavily on whether there were MS-like abnormalities on initial MRI. The majority of patients with abnormal MRIs went on to be diagnosed with MS (versus about one fourth of the patients with normal MRIs).

Beck RW, Clear PA, Anderson MM Jr, et al. A randomized, controlled trial of corticosteroids in the treatment of acute optic neuritis. The Optic Neuritis Study Group. *N Engl J Med.* 1992;326:582–581.

37. What is the significance of transient ischemic monocular vision loss?

May suggest increased risk of stroke. Although this symptom carries less subsequent risk of stroke than a transient ischemic attack (TIA) involving a cerebral hemisphere, these patients should undergo appropriate evaluation and treatment if significant carotid stenoses are found (see Chapter 5, Vascular Medicine). The arterial supply for the eye derives from the internal carotid artery (ICA). A common cause for retinal artery occlusion is atheroembolism from plaques in the ICA. Sometimes, cholesterol emboli can be seen as bright yellow spots in the vessels on funduscopic examination and are called *Hollenhorst plaques.*

Benavente O, Eliasziw M, Streifler JY, et al. Prognosis after transient monocular blindness associated with carotid-artery stenosis. *N Engl J Med.* 2001;345:1084–1090.

38. What is the localization of a homonymous field deficit?

A left or right field cut localizes posterior to the optic chiasm. The farther posterior the defect is, the more congruent it will be in the two eyes. A lesion to the optic radiation in the temporal lobe (Meyer loop) will produce a contralateral superior quadrantanopia—a "pie in the sky" deficit.

39. What is the localization for binocular diplopia?

To the structures affecting eye alignment. Binocular diplopia (diplopia that resolves with closure of either eye) results from ocular misalignment. Asking historical questions about whether the double images are horizontally displaced, vertically displaced, or skewed and whether the diplopia consistently worsens in a particular direction of gaze can help localize which eye movement(s) are involved. A careful examination of eye movements to look for dysconjugate gaze is a must.

40. What is the differential diagnosis of binocular diplopia?

- Orbital abnormality that restricts eye movement (e.g., orbital pseudotumor)
- Myopathy of extraocular muscles (e.g., in thyroid disease)
- NMJ disorder such as myasthenia gravis
- Cranial neuropathy of cranial nerve III, IV, or VI—compressive, traumatic, microvascular
- Brainstem lesion

If the diplopia is inconsistent, worsens in evenings, or intermittent ptosis is present, then myasthenia gravis is likely.

KEY POINTS: VISUAL COMPLAINTS

- Monocular problems localize to the eye or optic nerve.
- Bilateral disturbances that evolve are typically due to migraine.

DIZZINESS AND VERTIGO

41. If a patient tells you he feels "dizzy," what does he mean?

Hard to know. The most important step in taking the history from a dizzy patient is to figure out what is meant by "dizziness." Patients may use the term, "dizzy," to refer to:

- **Vertigo:** The perception of translational or rotational movement in the absence of stimulus. A vertiginous patient should be able to identify the direction of movement.
- **Presyncope:** A feeling of "lightheadedness" that is experienced in the setting of global cerebral hypoperfusion. The presyncopal patient, as implied by the term, often feels "about to pass out." Others experience "blood rushing to the head," tinnitus, or "blacking out."
- **Disequilibrium:** A term for feelings of dizziness or unsteadiness that cannot be accurately described as vertiginous or presyncopal. Disequilibrium can occur in ataxia, gait apraxia, postural instability, or anxiety. Patients will usually describe a feeling of the ground moving beneath them, being unsure of their footing, or "floating about" without a specific direction.

42. What is the localization of vertigo?

To the vestibular apparatus, the vestibulocochlear nerve (cranial nerve VIII), the brainstem, or the cerebellum. The key clinical differential localization of vertigo is whether it is peripheral (i.e., due to vestibular or nerve dysfunction) or central (i.e., localizing to the brainstem or cerebellum).

Peripheral vertigo is typically accompanied by lateralized horizontal or rotational nystagmus and the absence of other brainstem or cerebellar findings. A positive Dix-Hallpike maneuver is relatively specific for benign positional vertigo (BPV) (see Chapter 18, Geriatrics). Peripheral vertigo can be severe and associated with emesis and inability to walk unassisted at onset.

Central vertigo is often accompanied by other brainstem findings (cranial nerve deficits, crossed sensory or motor findings) or cerebellar findings. Vertical nystagmus is suggestive of a central cause.

43. What is benign (paroxysmal) positional vertigo (BPV/BPPV)?

Brief intense periods of vertigo, often accompanied by nausea, provoked by movement of the head. Classically produced by extending the neck and twisting the head as if to look on a high shelf or rotating the head while supine (e.g., looking under a cabinet or rolling over in bed). BPV is thought to be caused by precipitated crystals in the endolymph of the semicircular canals displacing hair cells. Cannolith repositioning procedures (e.g., the Epley manuever) can be remarkably effective at ameliorating symptoms (see Chapter 2, General Medicine and Ambulatory Care).

44. What are vestibulitis and vestibular neuronitis?

Idiopathic dysfunctions of vestibular function. In **vestibulitis,** the patient primarily experiences vertigo. In **vestibular neuronitis,** hearing loss or tinnitus or both are felt in addition to vertigo. Although the name implies an infectious or inflammatory cause and a viral cause is often suspected, an "-itis" has not been confirmed. Symptoms are not provoked by head movement and are less paroxysmal than in BPV. Vestibular neuronitis is sometimes treated empirically with oral corticosteroids.

45. What is Meniere disease?

An inner ear disorder with symptoms of episodic vertigo, tinnitus, and sensorineural hearing loss. Hearing loss is typically progressive. Endolymphatic hydrops (excess hydrostatic pressure in the vestibular system) is associated with Meniere, disease, though the pathophysiology is incompletely understood. Diuretics are sometimes used for treatment.

46. Will meclizine help vertigo?

Maybe. Meclizine and other anticholinergics are somewhat helpful for symptomatic relief of most cases of peripheral vertigo.

47. Can a migraine have vertigo symptoms?

Yes. Migraine can produce both episodic and chronic vertigo or dysequilibirum and motion sensitivity. Anticholinergics are typically not helpful, but migraine abortive and prophylactic medications may help.

48. What are the causes of presyncope?

- Vagal response to pain, gut distention, micturition, defecation, or anxiety producing hypotension and bradycardia
- Hypoglycemia
- Cardiac dysrhythmia
- Heart failure
- Hypoxia or hypercarbia
- Volume depletion

49. What is the appropriate evaluation of disequilibrium?

Nonspecific disequilibrium is difficult to evaluate. A careful neurologic examination including analysis of gait is imperative. Loss of proprioceptive function in the setting of a sensory neuropathy often leads to a mild gait ataxia and disequilibrium. Midline cerebellar dysfunction, whether toxic or degenerative, is another cause of disequilibrium. Parkinsonian conditions often lead to a loss of postural reflexes. These can be assessed by standing behind the patient and pulling firmly backward (after warning the patient and instructing him/her to step back as needed to maintain balance). An electronystagmogram (ENG) can be ordered to quantify vestibular function.

- Peripheral vertigo is characterized by the presence of lateralized horizontal or rotational nystagmus and the lack of other brainstem or cerebellar findings.
- Cannolith repositioning maneuvers are the most effective treatment for benign positional vertigo.

HEADACHE

See also Chapter 2, General Medicine and Ambulatory Care.

50. **How are headaches classified?**
As primary or secondary. **Primary headaches** are *not* associated with any identifiable structural factor or precipitant. Migraine and tension headache are the most common primary headaches. **Secondary headaches** are associated with underlying disorders such as trauma, vasculitis, medications, infection, hypertension, and tumor. The International Headache Society maintains a web-based version of their official classification of headache disorders with criteria and accompanying ICD-10 codes.
    The International Headache Society. *The International Classification of Headache Disorders,* 3rd ed. Available at www.ihs-classification.org. Accessed December 5, 2016.

51. **What are migraine headaches?**
Episodic primary headaches that can be preceded or accompanied by premonitory symptoms and auras. Migraines without aura are more common. Auras include specific neurologic deficits or disturbances such as visual, sensory, motor, or speech symptoms. When auras present as focal neurologic deficits, the headache can be mistaken for stroke. Premonitory symptoms include nausea, vomiting, photophobia (light sensitivity and avoidance), or phonophobia (sound sensitivity and avoidance). Patients typically feel better lying down in a quiet place. Migraines can occur without the headache and present only with neurologic symptoms.

52. **What drugs can be used to treat migraine acutely?**
    - Nonsteroidal anti-inflammatory drugs (NSAIDs)
    - 5-Hydroxytryptamine (5-HT) agonists (triptans)
    - Ergotamine
    - Magnesium
    - Dopamine antagonists (e.g., metoclopramide)
    - Opiates (treatment of last resort)
    Ask patients what has worked in the past. Patients should be assessed for any contraindications to particular medications before administration.

53. **What are the contraindications to triptan/ergotamine use for migraine?**
    - Uncontrolled hypertension
    - Pregnancy
    - Coronary artery disease
    - Vasospastic angina (variant or Prinzmetal angina)
    - Stroke
    - Familial hemiplegic migraine
    - Basilar migraine

54. **What drugs can be used daily to reduce frequency migraine?**
    - Propranolol
    - Amitriptyline
    - Valproic acid
    - Verapamil
    - Topirimate
    - Purified butterbur root extract
    - Zonisamide

55. **Describe a tension headache.**
Typically bilateral with a pressing or tightening ("bandlike") quality and no associated migranous features. Tension headache is the most common type of headache. The pathophysiology of tension headache is not understood, nor is the role of cranial muscle tension (from which the headache name is derived) confirmed.

56. **What is a cluster headache?**

A unilateral orbital, frontal, or temporal headache usually associated with ipsilateral conjunctival injection, lacrimation, rhinorrhea, facial sweating, miosis, or ptosis. Pain is severe and stabbing. Cluster headaches occur most commonly in men aged 20–40 years. High-flow oxygen can be an effective treatment.

57. **What is rebound headache?**

Also known as *medication-overuse headache* (MOH). The symptoms occur when medication doses wear off after habitual use of many of the types of medications used to treat headaches including triptans, ergotamine, butalbital combinations, and other analgesics. Treatment must include discontinuing the inciting medication. A long-acting NSAID can be used as a bridging therapy.

KEY POINTS: HEADACHE

- Medication overuse (rebound) headache should be considered in all chronic headache patients.
- Several medications can be effective at reducing episodic migraine frequency and severity.

WEAKNESS

58. **How can one distinguish peripheral from central facial weakness?**
    - If one side of forehead is weak and eye closure is weak, cause is peripheral.
    - If the forehead is spared, cause is more likely to be central.
    - If subtle ipsilateral limb weakness is present, then central cause is likely.
    - If taste is affected on ipsilateral two thirds of tongue, cause is likely peripheral.

59. **What is Bell palsy? What work-up is indicated?**

Idiopathic facial nerve dysfunction, typically sudden in onset and unilateral. Work-up includes imaging (preferably MRI) if any atypical features or examination findings implicating localization other than cranial nerve VII and Lyme antibody in endemic areas.

60. **What is the treatment for Bell palsy?**

Oral corticosteroids and eye protection. In a randomized, controlled trial, oral steroids were shown to be effective, whereas acyclovir did not improve outcome. Eye protection is needed because these patients frequently cannot close their eyes fully and can develop scleral damage. Applying a gel lubricant approved for eye use at night and taping the eye closed is inexpensive and effective. Ophthalmologic follow-up should be arranged.

    Sullivan FM, Swan IR, Donnan PT, et al. Early treatment with prednisolone or acyclovir in Bell's palsy. *N Engl J Med*. 2007;357:1598–1607.

61. **How can one tell whether the patient has a neurologic disorder causing perceived weakness?**

By muscle strength testing (see Table 17.1). To the neurologist, true weakness is an inability to generate normal force with voluntary skeletal muscle despite maximal effort. Weakness can localize to muscle, NMJ, lower motor neurons (anterior horn cell to NMJ), or upper motor neurons (motor cortex to anterior horn cell). True motor weakness has a characteristic feel on muscle strength testing with a steady but diminished resistance to movement of the limb. Functional or subjective weakness is characterized by inconsistent resistance that suddenly drops out or "gives way." Giveway weakness can be due to a variety of causes including pain (guarding), poor sensory processing, or poor effort.

62. **Describe patterns of muscle weakness and localization.**
    - **Symmetrical:** Diffuse process
    - **Asymmetrical:** Focal structural problem
    - **Distal:** Neuropathy
    - **Proximal:** Myopathy
    - **Extensors weaker than flexors in upper extremities and flexors weaker than extensors in lower extremities:** Upper motor neuron lesion (upper motor neuron pattern)

KEY POINTS: WEAKNESS

- Weakness should be described in terms of distribution and severity.
- Pattern of weakness can aid in localization.
- Giveway weakness can have multiple causes and does not always indicate poor effort.

NUMBNESS

63. Differentiate anesthesia, paresthesia, and dysesthesia.
    - **Anesthesia:** Lack of ability to detect sensory stimuli
    - **Paresthesia:** Perception of sensory phenomena (e.g., tingling) in the absence of stimuli
    - **Dysesthesia:** Experience of abnormal or unpleasant sensations with normal stimulus
    Patients may use the word "numbness" to describe any of these sensory abnormalities.

64. Can an organic process cause subjective numbness without an objective sensory deficit?
    Yes. The more central the lesion, the more likely there is to be a discrepancy between reported symptoms of numbness and ability to detect stimuli on a sensory examination. Infarcts to the thalamus can produce contralateral hemibody numbness with a normal sensory examination.

ATAXIA

65. What is ataxia?
    A deficit in coordination of voluntary movements leading to irregular deviations from the intended movement. Ataxia can affect the extremities, speech, or postural reflexes. During finger pointing tasks, intention tremor, which is a regular oscillation about the intended path, can be mistaken for ataxia.

66. What is the location of lesions that cause ataxia?
    The cerebellum or sensory systems. Strokes, degenerative diseases, and inflammatory or demyelinating diseases affecting the cerebellum or cerebellar outflow can cause ataxia. In a number of genetically determined ataxias such as Friedreich ataxia and some spinocerebellar ataxias (SCA), sensory deficits are prominent.

67. Name some causes of ataxia.
    - Intoxication with alcohol, medications, or other substances
    - Chronic alcohol use
    - Cerebellar or brainstem stroke
    - Neurosyphilis
    - Vitamin B_{12} deficiency
    - Human immunodeficiency virus (HIV)–associated myelopathy
    - Paraneoplastic syndromes
    - Multiple system atrophy
    - Progressive supranuclear palsy
    - MS
    - Postinfectious cerebellitis (usually in children)
    - Multiple genetic disorders

GAIT DYSFUNCTION

68. Differentiate between an ataxic gait and an apraxic gait.
    Both gait **ataxia** and **apraxia** are commonly associated with subjective balance difficulty and falls, though they look different clinically and have different localization. Gait ataxia is a cerebellar or sensory problem and is characterized by a wide-based gait and difficulty standing with the feet together. (A Romberg sign is present if the patient can stand with feet together and eyes open but cannot maintain balance with eye closure.)
    Gait apraxia is a motor planning deficit and, thus, has a cerebral localization. Patients with gait apraxia have a hard time getting started with walking and may have a "magnetic" or shuffling gait. Gait apraxia is commonly seen in dementia, subcortical vascular disease, and normal-pressure hydrocephalus (NPH).

69. When should one consider NPH?
    In any patient with gait apraxia. NPH classically presents with the triad of gait dysfunction, urinary incontinence, and cognitive difficulties. Not all elements must be present to consider the diagnosis.

70. How is NPH diagnosed?
    By brain imaging (CT or MRI) with appropriate clinical findings. The radiologic hallmark of NPH is ventriculomegaly out of proportion to cerebral atrophy. Ventriculomegaly that results from cerebral

atrophy is known as *ex vacuo hydrocephalus*. Sometimes the degree of ventriculomegaly is suspicious but not overwhelming. In these cases response to a high-volume LP or temporary drain can be assessed to help predict response to shunting.

71. How is NPH treated?
With drainage of CSF, typically through placement of a ventriculoperitoneal (VP) shunt.

72. Do unsteady patients sway, rock, and swing their arms a lot to improve balance?
Usually not. Exaggerated movements of the arms or swaying and rocking movements of the trunk (especially when superimposed on a narrow-based gait) should raise suspicion of a functional overlay to a gait problem.

KEY POINTS: NUMBNESS, ATAXIA, AND GAIT DYSFUNCTION

- Ataxia is caused by a cerebellar or sensory problem. Alcohol abuse and sensory neuropathy are the most common causes of ataxia.
- Gait apraxia is characterized by short steps and hesitations. This finding should prompt an evaluation for NPH.

DEMENTIA

73. What is dementia?
A chronic impairment in memory and at least one other cognitive domain (e.g., executive function, language, motor planning) of sufficient severity to impair performance of activities of daily living. Impairments of memory and other cognitive functions of insufficient severity of dementia are diagnosed as **mild cognitive impairment (MCI)**. Obtaining collateral history from friends or family about function is important. Quantify cognition with a standard screening instrument such as the Montreal Cognitive Assessment (MoCA).
MoCA Montreal Cognitive Assessment. Available at www.mocatest.org. Accessed October 1, 2016.

74. Should dementia be diagnosed in the hospitalized patient?
Not ideally. Delirium may be present and adversely affect performance. Dementia can be suspected in a previously undiagnosed confused patient, but cognitive testing should be done after discharge and recovery from any acute illness.

75. What is the most common dementia syndrome?
Alzheimer disease (AD). Pathologically AD is characterized by the presence of beta-amyloid plaques and neurofibrillary tangles. Hippocampal neurons are preferentially involved. AD is insidious in onset and progressive. Patients often lack insight into deficits, and current medical therapies (cholinesterase inhibitors and memantine) are only marginally effective.

76. What are other common causes of dementia?
- Vascular dementia (VaD)
- Frontotemporal dementia (FTD)
- Dementia with Lewy bodies (DLB)
- Dementia associated with Parkinson disease (PD)
- Alcohol-related dementia (Korsakoff)

77. Describe the clinical features of FTD.
Behavioral abnormalities without obvious impairment in memory. The most common presentation is a lack of insight and social awareness leading to inappropriate social interactions. Patients can appear apathetic or disinhibited. As the disease progresses, more global impairment becomes obvious. Initially, FTD is sometimes mistaken for primary psychiatric disease.

78. Describe DLB.
Relatively simultaneous development of cognitive impairment and parkinsonian motor features. The cognitive impairment in DLB waxes and wanes and formed visual hallucinations appear early.

79. **Describe the characteristics of VaD.**

   Previously called *multi-infarct dementia,* VaD can result from symptomatic or individually asymptomatic strokes due to large-vessel infarction, hemorrhage, or small-vessel cerebrovascular disease due to atherosclerosis or amyloid angiopathy. Clinically, patients present with slowed thinking, executive dysfunction, and sometimes slowed movements. A step-wise progression is often mentioned in texts but overrated. VaD and Alzheimer dementia may be present in the same patient.

80. **Is there a recommended work-up for dementia?**

   Yes. Some form of neuroimaging (CT or MRI) is recommended to evaluate for structural causes, including NPH and vascular disease. CBC, serum chemistries including liver function tests (LFTs), thyroid panel, vitamin B_{12} levels, and clinical screening for depression are indicated routinely. Specific testing for syphilis with fluorescent treponemal antibody absorption test (FTA-Abs) is not indicated unless there is suspicion of neurosyphilis. LP, genetic testing, EEG, and testing for Creutzfeld-Jakob disease are not routinely indicated but should be performed if clinical suspicion exists for a specific atypical cause.

KEY POINTS: DEMENTIA

- Dementia should be diagnosed outside the setting of acute hospitalization and medical illness.
- CT or MRI of the brain, thyroid-stimulating hormone (TSH), vitamin B_{12}, CBC, comprehensive metabolic panel, and depression screening should be done in all suspected cases of dementia.

STROKE AND CEREBROVASCULAR DISEASE

81. **What is a stroke?**

   An acute, focal, cerebrovascular event leading to brain infarction or hemorrhage. Most strokes are ischemic (not getting blood to part of the brain).

82. **What is a TIA?**

   A transient episode of neurologic dysfunction caused by focal brain, spinal cord, or retinal ischemia without acute infarction. Although historically TIAs were defined as ischemic neurologic events that lasted <24 hours, the advent of diffusion-weighted MRI allows detection of stroke within this period and has led to a new tissue-based definition. If one can see infarction on an MRI, a stroke has occurred—not a TIA, even if the neurologic symptoms have resolved.

83. **Name some possible mechanisms of ischemic stroke.**
   - In-vessel thrombosis
   - Embolism from cerebral artery, aortic arch, or heart
   - Hypoperfusion ("watershed stroke")

84. **What cardiac conditions contribute to a cardiac source of the embolus or thrombosis?**
   - Atrial fibrillation (AF)
   - Ischemic or nonischemic cardiomyopathy with hypokinesis
   - Atrial septal defect: venous thrombosis
   - Patent foramen ovale (PFO): venous thrombosis
   - Mechanical prosthetic valves
   - Atrial myxoma
   - Bacterial endocarditis

85. **Which tests should be ordered immediately in suspected acute stroke?**
   - CT brain (MRI brain if available immediately)
   - Carotid ultrasound or CTA if large anterior circulation stroke suspected (evaluate for ICA or middle cerebral artery [MCA] occlusion)
   - Glucose, CBC, basic metabolic panel, coagulation studies
   - Electrocardiogram (ECG), baseline troponin
     Only the glucose and CT results are absolutely necessary before making a decision about IV thrombolysis. Waiting for other results should not delay therapy.

86. **Is there a standard rating scale for acute stroke severity?**
Yes. The National Institutes of Health Stroke Scale (NIHSS) should be recorded in all acute stroke cases. The scale is available online and in multiple smartphone apps that automate scoring and guide administration. NIH Stroke Scale, Revised 10/1/2003. Available at www.ninds.nih.gov/doctors/NIH_Stroke_Scal e.pdf. Accessed October 1, 2016.

87. **What are the indications and contraindications for IV thrombolysis with recombinant tissue plasminogen activator (r-tPA) in acute ischemic stroke?**
See Table 17.5. Despite the expansion of eligibility to 4.5 hours, it is imperative to remember that the potential benefit from thrombolysis decreases with each passing minute. Therapy should be administered as soon as possible—time is brain! The 2018 guidelines [reference new guidelines as in note below] emphasize that most contraindications are relative and risks must be weighed against potential benefits in all cases.

Table 17.5. Determinants of Use of Thrombolytic Therapy in Ischemic Stroke

PRESENCE OF	ABSENCE OF
• Neurologic deficits that would create disability • Symptoms started < 3 hr 4.5 h before planned treatment* • Systolic BP < 185 mm Hg and diastolic BP < 110 mm Hg • PT in the normal range if heparin received in previous 48 hr • Blood glucose concentration > 50 mg/dL	• Findings suggestive of SAH • History of head trauma in previous 3 months • History of prior stroke in previous 3 months (relative contraindication) • Gastrointestinal or urinary tract hemorrhage in previous 21 days • Major surgery in previous 14 days • Arterial puncture at a noncompressible site in previous 7 days • Previous ICH • Known platelet count < 100,000/mm^3 • Active bleeding, acute trauma, or fracture on examination • Use of oral anticoagulant, or if taking anticoagulant, INR < 1.7

*The window for treatment initiation can be extended to 4.5 hours if the patient is < 80 years old, has no use of anticoagulants, has NIH Stroke Scale score > 25, and no history of stroke and diabetes.
2018 Guidelines for the Early Management of Patients With Acute Ischemic Stroke: A Guideline for Healthcare Professionals From the American Heart Association/American Stroke Association.
Powers WJ, Rabinstein AA, Ackerson T, et al. American Heart Association Stroke Council.
Stroke. 2018;49(3):e46–e110. http://doi:10.1161/STR.0000000000000158. Epub 2018 Jan 24.

88. **Does IV thrombolysis in acute stroke improve outcomes? By how much?**
Yes. Various studies have shown an absolute increase in probability of a good functional recovery of approximately 15%. The number needed to treat (NNT) to create one extra favorable outcome is six acute strokes.

89. **What is the bleeding risk with r-tPA?**
The risk is 5% to 7% for symptomatic intracerebral hemorrhage. Risk of fatal hemorrhage is about 2%. The more severe the stroke, the higher the risk. Patients without stroke (i.e., patients with presentations mimicking stroke who got r-tPA but ended up not having a stroke) have the lowest risk of hemorrhage. The improved odds of favorable outcome already take into account the bleeding risk.

90. **When is mechanical extraction of thrombus with an intravascular catheter-based clot retrieval device considered for treatment of acute ischemic stroke?**
   • Causative occlusion of ICA or proximal MCA (M1)
   • Good functional status before stroke (modified Rankin 0 or 1)
   • NIHSS score at least 6
   • Large area of infarct not evident on CT (ASPECTS [Alberta Stroke Program Early CT Score] at least 6)
   • Treatment initiated within 6 hours

All eligible patients should receive IV r-tPA even if thrombus retrieval is being considered. There are emerging data and standards for treatment with mechanical thrombectomy for strokes meeting above criteria and in the 6hr–24hr timeframe. All cases in which above criteria are met except for time >6 but <24 hours should be discussed with a comprehensive stroke center.

2018 Guidelines for the Early Management of Patients With Acute Ischemic Stroke: A Guideline for Healthcare Professionals From the American Heart Association/American Stroke Association.

Powers WJ, Rabinstein AA, Ackerson T, et al; American Heart Association Stroke Council. *Stroke*. 2018;49(3):e46–e110. http://doi:10.1161/STR.0000000000000158. Epub 2018 Jan 24.

91. Should blood pressure (BP) be tightly controlled to normal levels for patients with acute ischemic stroke?

No. For thrombolysis patients, BP must be maintained below 185/110 mm Hg, and in nonthrombolysis patients BP must be maintained below 220/120 mm Hg, but excessive lowering of BP should be avoided. Reduction of BP to "normal" levels in the setting of acute stroke worsens functional recovery. Systemic hypertension is a physiologic response to cerebral ischemia and maximizes penumbral perfusion. In the first few days after stroke, antihypertensives should thus be used judiciously. Control of hypertension is, of course, an important part of secondary stroke prevention and should be achieved in follow-up. If patients have completely resolved deficits, then permissive hypertension is not necessary.

92. What additional work-up is indicated in acute ischemic stroke or TIA?

- **MRI of brain** (not needed if stroke is clearly visible on CT)
- **Lipid panel, hypercoagulability laboratory test** if cryptogenic stroke in young patient (especially if patent foramen ovale present)
- **Carotid artery imaging** (duplex ultrasound, MRA, or CTA) if not already obtained at presentation
- **Transthoracic echocardiogram (TTE)** with "bubble study" to assess for intra-atrial shunt
- **Transesophageal echocardiogram** if cardioembolic stroke and TTE unrevealing
- **Cardiac monitoring for paroxysmal AF**—at a minimum 24 hours telemetry, 30-day monitor should be considered in cryptogenic embolic stroke
- **Assessments by physical, occupational, and speech therapy** if new deficits present

93. What is the role of antiplatelet therapy in secondary stroke prevention?

All patients who have had stroke or TIA should be on antiplatelet therapy unless there is clear contraindication (e.g., history of problematic bleeding, severe thrombocytopenia). Aspirin (81 mg daily), clopidogrel (75 mg daily), aspirin + dipyridamole, and cilostazol are all good options supported by evidence. Dual antiplatelet therapy is not generally recommended but may be considered in particularly high-risk patients.

94. What is the role of warfarin or novel oral anticoagulants (NOACs) in secondary stroke prevention?

To reduce the risk of stroke in patients with persistent or paroxysmal AF. Relative risk is reduced by two thirds. Warfarin should thus be strongly considered in all patients with stroke and AF. Warfarin is also indicated in patients with mechanical heart valves. In patients with noncardioembolic stroke warfarin has not shown benefit over antiplatelet therapy in multiple randomized trials. Dabigatran, rivaroxaban, and apixaban are acceptable alternatives to warfarin for stroke prevention in nonvalvular AF.

95. What is the role of statins in secondary stroke prevention?

High-quality randomized clinical trial evidence showed that high-dose statin therapy (atorvastatin 80 mg/day) reduced recurrent stroke risk in patients with low-density lipoprotein (LDL) levels of at least 100 mg/dL. Withholding statins for 3 days after acute stroke in patients who had already been taking statins was associated with poorer outcomes. Many experts feel that all stroke patients should be on statin therapy indefinitely unless there is clear contraindication.

Aggressive Reduction in Cholesterol Levels (SPARCL) Investigators. High-dose atorvastatin after stroke or transient ischemic attack. *N Engl J Med*. 2006;355:549–559.

96. What behavioral risk factors should be assessed and addressed in stroke?

Smoking, cocaine use, sedentary lifestyle, medication, and dietary recommendation adherence.

97. What are the common causes and location of hemorrhagic stroke?
See Table 17.6.

Table 17.6. Causes and Locations of Hemorrhagic Stroke

CAUSE	STROKE LOCATION
Hypertension	Thalami, basal ganglia, pons, or cerebellum
Ruptured intracranial aneurysm	Subarachnoid
Amyloid angiopathy	Lobar
Neoplasm	Lobar
Vascular malformation	Lobar

98. How does one work up and treat nontraumatic subarachnoid hemorrhage (SAH)?
Initially with CTA or MRA to evaluate for a cerebral aneurysm. If an aneurysm is discovered, urgent intervention to secure the aneurysm via surgical clipping or intravascular coiling is typically indicated. Patients with aneurysmal SAH must be monitored closely for the development of delayed cerebral vasospasm 3 to 14 days after hemorrhage, which can cause delayed ischemic stroke. Nimodipine has been shown to improve outcomes and is typically given to SAH patients. SAH patients must also be monitored for the development of hydrocephalus. Care is typically in a neurologic intensive care unit (ICU).

99. How does one work up and treat parenchymal intracranial hemorrhage (ICH)?
Unless the hemorrhage is in a classic location for hypertensive hemorrhage (see Table 17.6) and the patient has a clear history of uncontrolled hypertension, both immediate and delayed (4–8 weeks) contrasted imaging by CT or MRI is indicated to evaluate for the presence of underlying defect that may have caused the bleed. Some form of angiography to look for vascular malformations should be considered. Any coagulopathy (iatrogenic or intrinsic) should be reversed promptly and anticoagulant and antiplatelet agents should be held. BP should be managed typically to maintain a systolic pressure of 120–140 mm Hg. Trials of procoagulant administration in absence of coagulopathy have failed to show improvement in outcomes.

100. When does one need to consult a neurosurgeon in ICH?
For:
- Symptomatic subdural hematoma
- Posterior fossa hemorrhage causing mass effect on brainstem
- Intraventricular hemorrhage with hydrocephalus
Surgical evacuation is not indicated in most cases of ICH.

KEY POINTS: STROKE

- A noncontrast CT brain and blood glucose are the only test results absolutely necessary before deciding whether to administer r-tPA in acute stroke.
- Acute stroke patients with NIHSS score of at least 6 and anterior circulation symptoms should receive urgent CTA to look for occlusion of the ICA or proximal MCA, as they may be candidates for intravascular stent clot retrieval.
- All patients with probable acute stroke meeting criteria for IV r-tPA administration should be advised to receive the drug.

CT, computed tomography; CTA, CT angiogram; ICA, internal carotid artery; IV, intravenous; MCA, middle cerebral artery; NIHSS, National Institutes of Health Stroke Scale; r-tPA, recombinant tissue plasminogen activator.

SEIZURES AND EPILEPSY

101. What is a seizure?
An abnormal, rhythmic, synchronous firing of a group of neurons. Seizures can manifest as both positive (e.g., rhythmic shaking, hallucinations, or lip smacking) and negative (e.g., lack of

responsiveness or inability to move) neurologic phenomena. A generalized tonic-clonic seizure has a typical appearance with generalized muscle contractions, followed by synchronous convulsions, followed by a postictal period of slowly improving lethargy and confusion. Partial seizures, however, can look like just about anything in terms of neurologic symptoms depending on what area of brain is involved. Seizures are typically stereotyped (i.e., the same from one episode to another) within a given patient.

102. **How are seizures and seizure disorders classified?**
The classification of seizures is a work in progress. The International League Against Epilepsy is the official classifier and maintains up-to-date recommendations on line.
Types of seizures are classified as:
- **Generalized:** Rapidly involving both cerebral hemispheres, includes tonic-clonic, absence, and myoclonic
- **Focal:** Originating within one hemisphere, may spread to the contralateral hemisphere. The historical categories of "simple partial" and "complex partial" are no longer officially recognized. Instead, focal seizures are further characterized as with or without:
  - Impairment of consciousness or awareness
  - Motor or autonomic components
  - Evolution to bilateral convulsive seizure (formerly "secondary generalization")
- **Epileptic spasms**
- **Unknown**
Causes of seizures are classified as:
- Genetic
- Structural/metabolic
- Unknown
    International League Against Epilepsy. Available at: www.ilae.org [accessed 01.10.16].
    Scheffer IE, Berkovic S, Capovilla G, Connolly MB, French J, Guilhoto L, et al. ILAE classification of the epilepsies: position paper of the ILAE commission for classification and terminology. *Epilepsia.* 201;58:512–521. http://doi:10.1111/epi.13709.

103. **What is the work-up for a first seizure in an adult?**
- **History:** Focus on provocative factors such as substance use or withdrawal, recent infection, head trauma, strokes, or prior brain surgery
- **Laboratory data:** Serum electrolytes, CBC, urinalysis, toxicology screen
- **Neuroimaging:** Preferably MRI with contrast
- **EEG:** Preferably within 24 hours of the event

104. **When does driving need to be restricted?**
Whenever a patient has had a sudden unprovoked impairment in consciousness that would impair operation of a motor vehicle such as seizure, syncope, or event of unclear cause. Legal requirements about length of time event-free before returning to driving and physician reporting vary state by state, though 6 months is typical.
    Epilepsy Foundation. State driving laws database. Available at http://www.epilepsy.com/driving-laws [accessed 01.10.16].

105. **When should one start a seizure medication?**
Most neurologists adhere to a "two-strikes-you're-out" policy for unprovoked seizures. If EEG findings are suggestive of a seizure disorder or there is a clear structural problem that correlates with localization of seizure onset, then it may be reasonable to start an antiepileptic drug (AED) after the first seizure.

106. **When should one add a second seizure medication or switch seizure medications?**
If a patient continues to have seizures on a given antiseizure regimen or cannot tolerate the initial medication. Generally, the dose and plasma level of each AED should be maximized before adding another AED or switching AEDs. If lack of efficacy rather than intolerability is the issue, then typically a second AED is added, and then, if the add-on AED provides good control, the first AED can be tapered to see whether control is maintained. For each subsequent AED regimen that fails to provide good seizure control, the odds of achieving good control with a subsequent change diminishes.

107. Which AED should one start?

Whichever one your particular attending neurologist thinks is best for the patient! Many AEDs are available (in 2018, 24 unique AEDs, not including the benzodiazapines and many different extended-release or alternative formulations), and there is a paucity of conclusive head-to-head data to guide selection. Some childhood epilepsies have been found to respond well to specific AEDs (e.g., ethosuxamide for absence epilepsy). In adults, pragmatics often guide drug selection. Phenytoin is still commonly used because it is inexpensive, available IV and orally, and levels can be easily followed. Lamotrigine is well tolerated but must be titrated up slowly to avoid severe rash. Levetiracetam has gained wide use as a first-line drug because of its wide therapeutic window (eliminating need for level monitoring), ability to start at full dose, lack of hepatic metabolism, and lack of drug-drug interactions but can cause behavioral side effects.

108. Define status epilepticus.

Continuous seizure activity or intermittent seizure activity without regaining normal consciousness between spells lasting >5 minutes. Status epilepticus is a neurologic emergency. Most seizures are self-limited and last less than 2 minutes. A seizure that has stopped does not need to be treated with IV lorazepam.

109. How should status epilepticus be initially managed?

- Protect airway, give supplemental oxygen, ensure IV access.
- Measure stat fingerstick glucose; give IV thiamine then glucose if hypoglycemic.
- Give IV lorazepam 2 mg followed by 2 mg every 5 minutes if ongoing seizure activity.
- Load IV fosphenytoin 20 mg/kg.
- If seizures are still ongoing despite initial treatment with lorazepam and fosphenytoin, patient should be transferred to ICU with continuous EEG monitoring.

KEY POINTS: SEIZURES AND EPILEPSY

- Most seizures are self-limited and resolve within 2 minutes. A seizure that has stopped does not require emergent treatment with a benzodiazepine.
- Status epilepticus is constant or repeated seizure activity lasting more than 5 minutes without intercurrent normal consciousness. This is a medical emergency.

MULTIPLE SCLEROSIS

110. What causes MS?

The short answer is, "we don't know," although MS is clearly an immune-mediated disease causing multifocal inflammation in the central nervous system. Genetic risk factors for MS have been identified, and an association with geographic latitude and vitamin D deficiency has been demonstrated, but the cause remains incompletely understood.

111. How does MS present clinically?

Typically with a fairly acute onset of focal numbness or weakness. Optic neuritis is another common symptomatic presentation, as is binocular diplopia due to an internuclear ophthalmoplegia (INO). The diagnosis is typically made by MRI findings in the appropriate clinical setting.

Relapsing-remitting MS (RRMS) is the most common form. MS can also be primarily progressive (PPMS) and secondarily progressive (SPMS). SPMS begins as RRMS then becomes inexorably progressive.

112. Are there typical MRI findings in MS?

Yes, and include fairly well circumscribed areas of increased signal in the white matter of the brain and spinal cord. There is a predilection for areas adjacent to the corpus callosum. The prototypical lesion is a perpendicularly oriented pericallosal "Dawson's finger" best seen on sagittal T2 or fluid-attenuated inversion-recovery (FLAIR) images. Contrast-enhancing lesions indicate active inflammation.

113. Are there accepted diagnostic criteria for MS?

Yes, the McDonald criteria that were first issued in 2001 and revised in 2005 then again in 2010. The classic description of MS as a process with lesions separated by time and space (i.e., anatomically distinct) still basically holds true, but the new criteria allow for the use of MRI findings to satisfy these requirements.

Polman CH, Reingold SC, Banwell B, et al. Diagnostic criteria for multiple sclerosis: 2010 Revisions to the McDonald criteria. *Ann Neurol.* 2011;69:292–302.

114. **What treatments are available for MS?**

High-dose corticosteroids are typically used for acute exacerbations. Traditionally 1 g of methylprednisolone is given IV daily in single or divided doses for 3–5 days. Low-dose oral steroids (e.g., prednisone 60 mg daily) are ineffective, though doses equivalent to 1000–1250 mg of prednisone orally, if tolerated, can be effective. Most patients are maintained on one of several immune-modulating therapies in hopes of reducing relapse rate and progression of disability. These include multiple preparations of interferon given by intramuscular or subcutaneous injection every other day to weekly or glatiramer acetate given daily or three times weekly by injection. Three oral medications with different mechanisms of action—dimethyl fumarate, teriflunomide, and fingolimod—are available as daily therapies. For refractory cases of RRMS, monthly IV infusions of natalizumab and a single-course of IV alemtuzumab × 5 days with a booster course at 1 year are options. There are risks, including rare cases of progressive multifocal leukoencephalopathy (PML), associated with many of these therapies. There are no proven effective therapies for SPMS and PPMS.

KEY POINTS: MULTIPLE SCLEROSIS

- MS is an immune-mediated inflammatory disorder of the CNS presenting with lesions disseminated in time and space.
- Multiple disease-modifying therapies are available for RRMS.

CNS, central nervous system; MS, multiple sclerosis; RRMS, relapsing-remitting multiple sclerosis.

MOVEMENT DISORDERS

115. **What is the classification of movement disorders?**
- Hyperkinetic (causing excess involuntary movement): Tremor, dystonia, myoclonus, tics, stereotypies, and chorea
- Hypokinetic (causing paucity of movement or difficulty initiating movement): Parkinsonian disorders

116. **Define tremor and list the most common types.**

Tremor is a regular rhythmic oscillatory movement. **Essential tremor (ET)** is the most common movement disorder. It is a **postural and action tremor** that is typically bilateral and can affect head, voice, trunk, and legs to varying degrees. It is frequently familial. Tone and speed of movement are not affected. A **parkinsonian tremor** is a **resting tremor** that is typically most prominent when attention is focused on other cognitive or motor tasks. Other causes of tremor include **medication-induced tremor** and **psychogenic tremor**.

117. **How is ET treated?**

Initially with propranolol or primidone. Medications that may be exacerbating tremor should be removed if possible. Second-line medications include topirimate, gabapentin, and benzodiazepines. For disabling, medically refractory ET, deep brain stimulation of the ventral intermediate (VIM) nucleus of the thalamus can be a highly effective intervention.

118. **What is the difference between parkinsonism and PD?**

Parkinsonism is a clinical phenotype consisting of bradykinesia and rigidity. Resting tremor can be part of parkinsonism but is not necessarily present. Postural instability may also be present. "Bradykinesia" refers not just to a slowness of movements but to difficulty initiating movements with a characteristic diminishing amplitude to repetitive movements. Parkinsonian rigidity worsens when the patient is distracted. Parkinsonism can be caused by neuroleptic exposure (drug-induced and tardive parkinsonism), cerebrovascular disease, and other neurodegenerative conditions. **PD** is an idiopathic neurodegenerative disorder producing parkinsonism as its cardinal manifestation. The pathologic hallmark of PD is the presence of Lewy bodies, which are abnormal aggregates of alpha-synuclein.

119. **How is PD treated?**
Chiefly by providing pharmacologic stimulation of dopaminergic pathways in the brain. Degeneration of dopaminergic nigrostriatal neurons is a pathologic hallmark of PD, and administration of exogenous dopamine (in the form of carbodopa/levodopa) or dopamine agonists partially ameliorates symptoms of the disease. Drugs that inhibit dopamine metabolism are also used. Anticholinergics are sometimes used for the amelioration of tremor, and amantadine can also provide symptomatic benefit. No drug therapy has been conclusively shown to alter the rate of progression of PD. Rehabilitation and maintenance of physical activity are vitally important components to PD treatment. Deep brain stimulation can be beneficial in carefully selected candidates.

120. **Describe chorea and myoclonus.**
Chorea is a flowing "dancelike" hyperkinetic movement that is characteristic of Huntington disease. Chorea can also be seen in other neurodegenerative disorders and in tardive dyskinesia.
   Myoclonus is defined by very short, jerky involuntary contractions. Myoclonus is most often symptomatic of a metabolic derangement but can also be seen after anoxic brain injury, in several genetic disorders, and in neurodegenerative disease. Asterixis or sudden brief interruptions in normal muscle tone is a related phenomenon.

KEY POINTS: MOVEMENT DISORDERS

- Parkinsonism is a clinical constellation of bradykinesia and rigidity that can have many causes. Parkinson disease is a neurodegenerative disorder, pathologically defined by Lewy bodies, that is the most common cause of parkinsonism.
- Essential tremor is the most common cause of tremor.

NEUROMUSCULAR DISORDERS

121. **Classify the most common causes of myopathy.**
   - **Rheumatic diseases:** Polymyositis, dermatomyositis, polymyalgia rheumatica, Sjögren syndrome, vasculitis
   - **Endocrine disorders:** Hypothyroidism, hyperthyroidism, Cushing disease, adrenal insufficiency, hyperaldosteronism
   - **Electrolyte disorders:** Hypokalemia
   - **Malabsorption:** Celiac sprue, vitamin D deficiency, vitamin E deficiency
   - **Medications:** Glucocorticoids, lipid-lowering drugs (statins and fibrates), colchicines, chloroquine, phenothiazines, nucleoside reverse transcriptase inhibitors (NRTIs), d-penicillamine
   - **Toxic exposure:** Alcohol, cocaine
   - **Infections:** HIV, other viral infections
   - **Genetic disorders:** Muscular dystrophies, mitochondrial disorders
   - **Paraneoplastic syndromes**

122. **How is myopathy diagnosed?**
By clinical evaluation, EMG, and muscle biopsy, if necessary. Clinically, myopathy typically presents as symmetrical proximal weakness. Blood levels of muscle enzymes (creatine kinase and aldolase) should be obtained. They are typically elevated in inflammatory myopathies but normal in metabolic myopathies. EMG may show "myopathic" low-amplitude complex motor units. Muscle biopsy can be very helpful when the cause of myopathy is not otherwise apparent and is useful in confirming the diagnosis of an inflammatory myopathy.

123. **How does myasthenia gravis (MG) present, and how is it diagnosed?**
Frequently, with intermittent diplopia, ptosis, or both. Generalized fatigable weakness may or may not be present. When generalized, MG can cause limb girdle, bulbar, and respiratory weakness and can be a medical emergency. MG is an autoimmune disorder in which antibodies to the acetylcholine (ACh) receptors of the NMJ impair neuromuscular transmission. Commercial blood tests are available for acetylcholinesterase receptor (AChR) antibodies and for muscle-specific kinase (MuSK) antibodies. These antibodies are specific but not sensitive, especially when symptoms are limited to eyes. Repetitive nerve stimulation studies (a specialized NCS) is highly specific. Single-fiber EMG is more sensitive but more difficult to perform and less widely available.

124. How is MG treated?

By administration of the peripheral cholinesterase inhibitor pyridostigmine and by immunosuppression. In purely ocular MG or in very mild cases, monotherapy with pyridostigmine may be appropriate, but in patients with generalized myasthenia, some form of immunosuppressive therapy is indicated to control the underlying disease. Prednisone is highly effective, though steroid-sparing treatment with azathioprine, mycophenolate mofetil, or other immunosuppressive therapies is commonly used to avoid long-term complications of prednisone therapy. In severe myasthenic exacerbations, plasma exchange provides the most rapid clinical improvement in symptoms. IV immunoglobulin (IVIG) is also an effective therapy, but response is less rapid.

125. Are there other disorders of the NMJ?

Yes. The Lambert-Eaton myasthenic syndrome (LEMS) is an autoimmune or paraneoplastic disorder in which ACh release is inhibited by antibodies to the presynaptic voltage-gated calcium channel. LEMS produces proximal weakness and autonomic dysfunction. About 50% of cases are associated with small cell lung cancer. Botulism, whether from infection or iatrogenic, is another presynaptic disorder. Genetic disorders creating congenital myasthenic syndromes also exist.

126. Describe the clinical features of polyneuropathy.

Neuropathies present with sensory and motor dysfunction. Most polyneuropathies affect nerves symmetrically in a length-dependent fashion such that the toes and feet are most affected. Sometimes burning pain is present.

127. What are some common causes of neuropathy?

- **Abnormal glucose metabolism:** Prediabetes and diabetes
- **Toxins and drugs:** Chronic alcohol exposure, chemotherapeutic agents (taxanes, platin-based drugs, bevacizumab)
- **Infection:** HIV, Lyme disease, neurosyphilis, hepatitis virus
- **Endocrine disorders:** Hypothyroidism
- **Deficiencies:** Vitamin B_{12}, copper
- **Rheumatic disorders:** Rheumatoid arthritis, Sjögren syndrome, vasculitis
- **Paraproteinemias**

  Washington University. Neuromuscular Disease Center. Available at http://neuromuscular.wustl.edu/ [accessed 01.10.16].

128. What are the features of an unusual neuropathy?

Most neuropathies are chronic and insidious in onset. The acute presentation of neuropathy should raise a red flag for toxic, inflammatory, or immune causes. Most neuropathies have widespread symmetrical involvement. The acute presentation of multiple isolated neuropathies (mononeuritis multiplex) should raise a red flag for vasculitic processes.

129. What is the routine work-up for polyneuropathy?

NCSs and EMG are helpful and can differentiate between predominantly axonal and demyelinating neuropathies. Recommended laboratory tests for all patients with neuropathy include thyroid function tests, vitamin B_{12} levels (with methylmalonic acid [MMA] and homocysteine, or both, if indicated), fasting glucose, and serum protein electrophoresis. In selected patients, testing for autoimmune and inflammatory disorders should be considered. LP for analysis of CSF protein and serum testing for specific antibodies (e.g., myelin-associated glycoprotein [MAG], GQ1b) may be helpful in the work-up of demyelinating neuropathies.

130. How does Guillain-Barré syndrome (GBS) present?

As rapidly (several hours to a few days) progressive weakness usually beginning in the lower extremities. GBS is often preceded or accompanied by paresthesias and sensory loss. Areflexia is the norm. In severe cases, bulbar weakness, autonomic dysfunction, and respiratory weakness can be life-threatening without aggressive supportive care. There is characteristic elevation of protein in the CSF without presence of white blood cells—"cytoalbuminologic dissociation." Some cases are postinfectious or vaccine related.

131. How is GBS treated?

With plasmapheresis and IVIG. Cardiac and respiratory monitoring is necessary acutely while symptoms are still progressing. Most patients make a good functional recovery, but it can take many months.

KEY POINTS: NEUROMUSCULAR DISORDERS

- Most neuropathy is insidious, symmetrical, and distally predominant.
- Prediabetes and diabetes are the most common causes of neuropathy.
- Rapidly progressive weakness and loss of reflexes should raise concern for Guillain-Barré syndrome. The presentation need not be "ascending."
- Fluctuating diplopia should raise concern for myasthenia gravis.

SLEEP DISORDERS

132. How are sleep disorders classified?
     - Insomnia
     - Sleep-related breathing disorders
     - Hypersomnia
     - Circadian rhythm disorders
     - Parasomnias
     - Sleep-related movement disorders

133. How common is sleep apnea?
     Prevalence is estimated at 3–7% of the general population. Key symptoms include excessive daytime sleepiness, loud snoring, and witnessed apneas. Obesity is a significant risk factor though not necessary.

134. Does continuous positive airway pressure (CPAP) help sleep apnea?
     Yes. Multiple randomized trials have demonstrated improvement in sleep parameters including oxygen desaturation, number of apneas, and daytime sleepiness with CPAP compared with sham CPAP. Some patients have a difficult time tolerating CPAP apparatus, and it is worth trying various commercially available masks to enhance tolerability. Whereas many experts believe that CPAP improves cardiovascular outcomes and mortality rate, this has not been proved prospectively.

135. What is rapid eye movement behavioral disorder (RBD)?
     Loss of normal muscle atonia during rapid eye movement (REM) sleep accompanied by complex motor behaviors. Patients enact dreams and can engage in behavior that is harmful to self and others. Clonazepam is highly effective anecdotally (though this has not been demonstrated in a randomized trial) and is the treatment of choice. RBD can be the harbinger of a neurodegenerative disorder—especially PD.

136. How is narcolepsy diagnosed?
     With an overnight PSG followed by a multiple sleep latency test, a test consisting of multiple naps. Intrusive REM sleep during naps in the absence of another significant sleep disorder documented by PSG is basically diagnostic of narcolepsy. CSF hypocretin levels are sometimes measured; low levels are felt to be specific but not sensitive. Narcolepsy should be suspected in the setting of excessive daytime sleepiness accompanied by a history of cataplexy (brief loss of muscle tone during wakefulness often precipitated by emotional trigger) or sleep paralysis (inability to move or speak upon awakening from sleep).

137. What is the most common cause of excessive daytime somnolence?
     "Voluntary" sleep deprivation. Life situations and choices cause people to get inadequate sleep.

NEOPLASTIC AND PARANEOPLASTIC DISEASE

138. What are the most common intracranial malignancies?
     Metastatic disease, usually lung, breast, or melanoma. Primary brain malignancy rarely metastasizes outside the CNS; however, systemic malignancies often metastasize to the brain.

139. How are primary brain tumors classified?
     Primarily by cell type of origin (astrocytomia, ependymoma, lymphoma, etc.) and further classified by histologic and molecular features (e.g., SHH-activated and TP53-mutant medulloblastoma). Glioblastoma is the most common adult-onset primary brain tumor.

Louis DN, Perry A, Reifenberger G, et al. The 2016 World Health Organization Classification of Tumors of the Central Nervous System: a summary. *Acta Neuropathol.* 2016;131:803–820.

140. **How are glioblastomas and other primary brain tumors treated?**
Typically with resection of as much of the mass is technically possible followed by radiation therapy and possibly chemotherapy depending on the tumor subtype.

141. **Do meningiomas need to be treated?**
Usually not. Meningiomas are common benign neoplasms of the dura that are usually incidental finds during imaging for unrelated symptoms.

Meningiomas may need to be resected if they are causing symptoms via significant mass effect or have atypical features by imaging (e.g., causing edema in adjacent tissue).

142. **What are paraneoplastic syndromes?**
Disorders caused by an autoimmune reaction to malignancy. Important paraneoplastic syndromes include Lambert-Eaton myasthenic syndrome (usually associated with small cell lung cancer), paraneoplastic limbic encephalitis, cerebellitis, and sensory neuropathy. Sometimes paraneoplastic neurologic syndromes can occur before the primary malignancy can be diagnosed. Serum and CSF assays for some paraneoplastic antibodies are commercially available.

WEBSITES

1. American Academy of Neurology: www.aan.org—visit the Practice Guidelines Pages for evidence-based reviews and recommendations.
2. National Institute of Neurological Disorders and Stroke: www.ninds.nih.gov.

BIBLIOGRAPHY

1. Ropper AH, Samuels MA, Klein JP. *Adam's and Victor's Principals of Neurology.* 10th ed. New York: McGraw-Hill Education; 2014.

CHAPTER 18

GERIATRICS

John Meuleman, MD, and Henrique Elias Kallas, MD, CMD

It's like walking ten miles, a step at a time, living and breathing, one day at a time, one week at a time. Before you know it, you're a hundred years old. The body doesn't function, of course. You know, some young girls gave me a seat on the bus. I was flattered.

Abe Goldstein,
From Ellis N: *If I live to be 100.*
Available at: www.ifilivetobe100.com

1. **What changes in organ function occur in advanced age?**
   See Table 18.1.

Table 18.1. Changes in Organ Systems With Aging and Their Consequences

SYSTEM	AGING-RELATED CHANGE	CONSEQUENCE OF THIS CHANGE
Skin	Xerosis (dry skin)	Frequent, diffuse pruritus
Cardiovascular	Decreased LV compliance and relaxation	Elevated LV end-diastolic pressures, greatly increased prevalence of heart failure
Renal	With loss of muscle mass, decreased creatinine clearance not reflected in commensurate increase in serum creatinine	Underdiagnosis of renal insufficiency with concomitant overdosage of certain medications
	Decreased maximum urine osmolarity	Inappropriately high urine outputs in hypovolemic states increasing propensity for dehydration
Pulmonary	Decreased forced vital capacity and forced expiratory volume, increased A-a oxygen gradient	Propensity for hypoxia in the setting of pneumonia or other pulmonary insults
	Decreased cough reflex	Propensity for aspiration
Skeletal muscle	Sarcopenia (aging-related loss of muscle mass)	Weakness
Vision	Decreased pupillary dilatation and light sensitivity of retina	Poor night vision, affecting night driving and nocturnal ambulation
Hearing	Decreased high-frequency perception	Impaired understanding of certain sounds; some prefixes or suffixes drop out from perception
Immune	Decreased T-cell function	Propensity for infections
Nervous	Decreased neural connectivity	Slower recall even in the setting of preserved memory

A-a = alveolar-arterial; LV = left ventricular.

2. **How does change in body composition with aging affect drug treatment?**
A marked increase in fat mass and decrease in lean body mass associated with aging leads to an altered volume of distribution of some drugs. Patients who appear trim may still have these changes. As a result, water-soluble (hydrophilic) drugs such as digoxin or lithium have higher concentrations owing to a lower volume of distribution. Fat-soluble (lipophilic) drugs such as benzodiazepines or thiopental have a higher volume of distribution and will have longer times for steady-state concentration and elimination.

3. **How does sleep change with aging?**
Sleep latency (time to fall asleep) increases, and **sleep efficiency** (time asleep divided by time in bed) decreases. Elder patients tend to have an earlier bedtime, earlier morning awakening, more nocturnal arousals, and more daytime napping. Sleep structure changes include a notable decline in stage N3 (deep sleep) and an increase in stages N1 (transitional sleep) and N2 (intermediate sleep).

ASSESSMENT OF OLDER PATIENTS

4. **What are the essential elements of an evaluation for an elderly patient with recurrent falls?**
   - **History:** Focused on the circumstances of the fall and associated symptoms
   - **Gait:** Assessed with get-up-and-go test
   - **Balance:** Tested by observing side-by-side, semi-tandem, and tandem stance
   - **Muscle strength:** Including quadriceps, hip flexors, abductors and extensors, and foot dorsiflexion
   - **Vision**
   - **Feet and footwear:** Inspected for any deformities
   - **Orthostatic blood pressure measurement:** If history suggests postural weakness or lightheadedness
   - **Dix-Hallpike maneuver:** If positional vertigo suspected
   - **Home safety evaluation:** If appropriate

5. **What is the "get-up-and-go" test?**
A maneuver to assess the ease with which the patient can:
   - Rise from a chair without using arm supports
   - Stand still momentarily
   - Walk a short distance (~10 feet)
   - Turn around
   - Walk back to the chair
   - Turn around
   - Sit down in the chair without using the arm supports

   The test is scored both on qualitative observations of ability to perform the task and an age-adjusted time.

   Mathias S, Nayak USL, Isaacs B. Balance in elderly patients: The "get-up and go" test. *Arch Phys Med Rehabil.* 1986;67:387–389.

6. **What is the Dix-Hallpike maneuver?**
A procedure to reproduce positional vertigo. The physician supports the patient while the patient goes from a sitting to a supine position with head tilted back approximately 20 degrees below shoulder level and turned 45 degrees to one side. The eyes are observed for rotatory nystagmus, and the patient is asked about reproduction of symptoms. The patient then returns to the sitting position, and the maneuver is repeated on the opposite side.

7. **Describe the usefulness of an assessment of function and activities of daily living (ADLs).**
To provide insight into the symptomatic impact and current status of the patient's various health problems that allows the provider to monitor the trajectory of a patient's health and ensures attention is given to maximizing quality of life. Many older patients value quality of life over quantity of life. Also, a change in function is often the first sign of decompensation of a medical problem.

8. **How is such a functional assessment performed?**
By evaluating whether there are any recent changes in the patient's ability to perform ADLs (bathing, dressing, toileting, maintaining continence, grooming, feeding, and transferring) or whether the patient now needs assistance or has difficulty with some ADLs. Some of these observations are best made by others.

9. **What are the essential aspects of evaluating driving safety in an older adult?**
   - **Vision:** Including a formal eye examination (Snellen chart)
   - **Cognition:** Using the clock drawing test
   - **Neuromuscular status:** Including active range of motion of the feet, shoulders, hands, and neck
   - **Referral** to a driver rehabilitation specialist if indicated

10. **How can one assess driving safety in a patient with dementia?**
    The following may indicate higher risk of unsafe driving:
    - Clinical dementia rating score $\geq$ 2.0
    - Assessment by caregiver that patient's driving is unsafe
    - History of traffic citations
    - History of crashes
    - Voluntary reduction of driving mileage by patient
    - Voluntary avoidance of certain situations by patient
    - Mini-Mental State Examination (MMSE) score $\leq$ 24
    - Aggressive or impulsive personality characteristics

    Iverson DJ, Gronseth GS, Roger MA, et al. Practice parameter update: evaluation and management of driving risk in dementia. Report of the Quality Standards Subcommittee of the American Academy of Neurology. *Neurology.* 2010;74:1316–1324.

    Morris JC. The clinical dementia rating (CDR): current version and scoring rules. *Neurology.* 1993;43:2412–2414.

    Tombaugh TN, McIntyre NJ. The Mini-Mental State Examination: a comprehensive review. *J Am Geriatr Soc.* 1992;40:922–935.

NUTRITION

11. **A patient with severe dementia has recurrent admissions with pneumonia, likely due to aspiration. Will gastrostomy tube placement prevent further pneumonias?**
    No. Aspiration is considered an expected consequence of advanced dementia. Oral secretions are often aspirated even in patients not fed by mouth. There is currently no evidence that a gastrostomy tube prevents aspiration or pneumonias in advanced dementia. Caregivers should be instructed on techniques to help reduce the risk of aspiration such as sitting up at 90 degrees when eating and tipping the chin forward.

12. **Is megestrol useful and effective in increasing lean body mass in underweight older patients?**
    No, because of numerous side effects. Although megestrol often increases appetite, the weight gain is due to an increase in fat mass with decline of skeletal muscle mass in many patients. Megestrol can also blunt the beneficial effects of resistance exercise on strength. In addition, megestrol causes a decline in testosterone concentration in men to castrated levels and has catabolic effects from its glucocorticoid properties. Other side effects include Cushing syndrome, adrenal suppression, hyperglycemia, and thromboembolism.

13. **For most oral supplements and enteral feeding tube products, how many calories are there in each milliliter?**
    Around 1 kcal/mL. As a result, most cans of oral supplement, which are usually 8 ounces in volume, contain roughly 250 calories. Patients subsisting just on enteral feeds will typically require 1400–2000 mL of enteral feeding per day to meet their caloric needs. Calorically dense products containing 2 kcal/mL are available.

METABOLIC AND RENAL DISORDERS

14. **What are appropriate hemoglobin A_{1c} targets in older patients?**
    The American Geriatrics Society advises that reasonable targets would be 7.0–7.5% in healthy older adults with long life expectancy, 7.5–8.0% in those with moderate comorbidity and a life expectancy less than 10 years, and 8.0–9.0% in those with multiple comorbid conditions and shorter life expectancy. Tight control has been shown to produce higher rates of hypoglycemia in older adults, and there is no evidence that using medications to achieve tight glycemic control in most older adults is beneficial.

American Geriatrics Society. Choosing wisely. Available at: www.choosing wisely.org/societies/american-geriatrics-society/. Revised 4/23/15. Accessed October 1, 2016.

15. **What are the physiologic changes that predispose older people to dehydration?**
    - Diminution of thirst perception in response to volume depletion or hyperosmolality
    - Decline in basal and stimulated renin levels with reduction in aldosterone secretion
    - Reduced renal responsiveness to antidiuretic hormone (ADH)
    - Impaired sodium conservation by kidneys when salt intake is restricted

16. **What laboratory tests best determine dehydration?**
    Blood urea nitrogen (BUN), which is usually elevated. Other indicators include a BUN-to-creatinine ratio > 20 or a BUN greater than twice the baseline BUN.

17. **What is the significance of severe hypernatremia in frail elderly patients?**
    As a sign of severe dehydration. In mobile patients, hypernatremia induces the thirst response that leads to increased fluid intake. Frail elders may have inadequate intake of free water owing to immobility or cognitive impairment, leading to more severe hypernatremia. An elder with severe hypernatremia may be neglected, and the physician should look for other signs or symptoms of elder abuse or neglect.

18. **Does serum creatinine accurately reflect changes in glomerular filtration rate (GFR) in the elderly?**
    No. The aging process is accompanied by a significant deterioration of the renal function. On average the GFR declines by ~8 mL/min/1.73 m^2 per decade after the fourth decade of life. The age-related reduction in creatinine clearance is accompanied by a reduction in the daily urinary creatinine excretion owing to reduced muscle mass. Accordingly, the relationship between serum creatinine and creatinine clearance changes. The net effect is near-constancy of serum creatinine (S_{Cr}) while true GFR (and creatinine clearance) declines, and consequently, substantial reduction of GFR despite a relatively normal S_{Cr} level occurs.
    Pompei P. Preoperative assessment and perioperative care. In: Cassel C, Leipzig R, Cohen H, et al, eds. *Geriatric Medicine: An Evidence-Based Approach.* 4th ed. New York: Springer-Verlag; 2003. p 213–227.

MUSCULOSKELETAL DISORDERS

See also Chapter 2, General Medicine and Ambulatory Care; Chapter 10, Rheumatology; and Chapter 16, Endocrinology.

19. **What are "red flag" symptoms that raise suspicion for malignancy in an older patient with back pain?**
    - Unexplained weight loss
    - >1-month duration of symptoms
    - No relief of pain by lying down (suggesting cancer or infection)
    - History of cancer
    - Focal neurologic deficit

20. **How is an acute vertebral compression fracture managed?**
    With pain management and brief bed rest. Symptomatic acute vertebral fractures are a common problem for osteoporotic patients. Pain at the site of the fracture is often severe and requires initial bed rest and occasionally even hospitalization. Pain control is normally achieved with nonopioid analgesics, opioids, and nasal calcitonin spray. Imaging studies (including magnetic resonance imaging [MRI]) should be obtained if neurologic examination suggests radiculopathy or if malignancy is suspected. Older patients with uncontrolled focal back pain related to a nonmalignant vertebral compression fracture may benefit from balloon kyphoplasty or vertebroplasty; however, these procedures are invasive and should be reserved for older patients who did not respond well to conservative management. Clinical trials show only mild benefit compared to a sham procedure.

21. **If temporal arteritis is suspected, how soon must one perform a temporal artery biopsy?**
    The pathologic changes of temporal arteritis remain present for at least 2 weeks, even with corticosteroid treatment. Corticosteroid treatment should be initiated immediately when temporal arteritis is suspected, and the biopsy can be scheduled when convenient.

22. **How long do most temporal arteritis patients require drug treatment?**
One to 2 years. Patients receiving corticosteroids for this lengthy period benefit from early bisphosphonate therapy to prevent osteoporosis. Because prolonged corticosteroid therapy is associated with significant risks and side effects, the diagnosis of temporal arteritis should be confirmed to avoid unnecessary treatment.

23. **Does Medicare routinely cover screening bone mineral density (BMD) scans for older men and women?**
Yes, every 2 years for women 65 years and older. BMD scans are covered for older men only if there is an underlying suspicion for osteoporosis such as vertebral abnormalities on x-ray studies or treatment with corticosteroids for over 3 months.

24. **Should we screen older men for osteoporosis?**
Maybe. Health advisory organizations have issued recommendations regarding screening men. The U.S. Preventive Services Task Force (USPSTF) gives a grade I, meaning current evidence is insufficient to assess the balance of benefits and harms of screening older men. The National Osteoporosis Foundation recommends BMD testing for all men older than 70 years and men aged 50–69 years based on risk factors. The American College of Physicians recommends assessing older men for risk factors. Men who are considered at increased risk (and who are candidates for drug therapy) should be screened with a BMD scan.

25. **What are the risk factors for fractures for older men?**
    - Previous minimal trauma fracture
    - Glucocorticoid therapy
    - Low body weight
    - Current cigarette smoking
    - Excessive alcohol use
    - Rheumatoid arthritis
    - Hypogonadism
    - Malabsorption syndromes
    - Chronic liver disease
    - Parental history of hip fracture

26. **What is a T score?**
The number of standard deviations the patient's bone density is above or below the average value for a young adult of the same sex. Osteoporosis is defined by the World Health Organization as a T score < -2.5.

27. **What is sarcopenia? How can it be prevented?**
Loss of muscle mass related to aging and physiologic changes seen with muscle disuse. Sarcopenia significantly contributes to disability in the elderly and can be prevented with physical activity, especially moderate- to high-intensity resistance exercise.

28. **What laboratory test measures vitamin D levels in the body?**
25-Hydroxyvitamin D (25-OH-D). According to a 2011 Institute of Medicine report, levels > 20 ng/mL are adequate for bone health.
    IOM (Institute of Medicine). Dietary Reference Intakes for Calcium and Vitamin D. Washington, DC: The National Academies Press; 2011.

29. **Why is vitamin D deficiency important to diagnose in older adults?**
Because vitamin D deficiency is common in elders and can contribute to osteoporosis, fractures, muscle weakness, and falls. Active people get most of their vitamin D from sun exposure, because few foods contain or are fortified with vitamin D. Many older adults who get little skin exposure to the sun have insufficient vitamin D levels.

30. **What are the recommended daily dietary allowances for calcium and vitamin D in older adults?**
1200 mg of calcium/day in adults older than 50 years and 800 IU of vitamin D/day for adults older than 71 years. An 8-ounce glass of milk has 300 mg of calcium and 100 IU of vitamin D.

31. **Does calcium supplementation affect the absorption of other medications?**
Yes. Supplements such as calcium and iron (which are divalent cations) can reduce the absorption of commonly used medications such as levothyroxine and some quinolone antibiotics. Patients taking such medications should take the medications and supplements at least 2 hours apart.

32. **Why is lumbar spinal stenosis (LSS) sometimes misdiagnosed as claudication associated with peripheral vascular disease?**
Because spinal stenosis symptoms of leg pain increase with walking (neurogenic claudication), as do those of vascular claudication. LSS in older adults is most commonly caused by degenerative bone disease and is a common cause of disability. Treatment may involve spine surgery. Typical symptoms of LSS include pain in the buttocks or upper legs associated with sensory loss and weakness. Many patients also have associated low back pain. Symptoms tend to increase with walking, standing, and back extension and tend to improve with lying, sitting, and back flexion. Vascular claudication is usually described as calf tightness and cramps on exertion that typically resolve immediately after rest. Neurogenic claudication symptoms are relieved within minutes of sitting/lying but persist with standing erect.

CARDIOVASCULAR DISORDERS

33. **In an older patient with chronic atrial fibrillation (AF), is "rate control" or "rhythm control" preferable?**
Rate control. Randomized trials have shown that outcomes with a "rhythm control" strategy are no better than with a "rate control" strategy, and in some aspects, outcomes are inferior. For rhythm control, one attempts to convert the rhythm to sinus. For rate control, the rhythm remains AF, but the ventricular rate is controlled to a resting rate of less than 100 beats per minute (bpm) with beta blockers and calcium channel blockers. Unless a patient has significant symptoms, such as bothersome palpitations or exercise intolerance, treatment should focus on controlling ventricular rate both at rest and with exertion.

34. **Elderly people often fall every few months. Are oral anticoagulants for AF contraindicated in such patients?**
No. Advanced age is considered one of the major risk factors for thromboembolic events in patients with AF. Studies comparing the protective effect of warfarin versus antiplatelet therapy in elderly patients with AF have shown significantly higher risk reduction of cardioembolic events with warfarin. Advanced age is also considered a risk factor for bleeding with anticoagulation therapy, and therefore, older patients should have a risk of bleeding assessment before initiation of therapy. Elderly people tend to have multiple episodes of falls, but studies have shown only a small risk for intracranial hemorrhages with the use of anticoagulation. As a general rule, anticoagulant use is not contraindicated in elderly people who fall on occasion. Warfarin or novel oral anticoagulants (NOACs) are options for anticoagulation.

Mant J, Hobbs FD, Fletcher K, et al. Warfarin versus aspirin for stroke prevention in an elderly community population with atrial fibrillation (The Birmingham Atrial Fibrillation Treatment of the Aged Study, BAFTA): a randomized controlled trial. *Lancet.* 2007;370:493–503.

Hart RG, Pearce LA, Aguilar MI. Adjusted-dose warfarin versus aspirin for preventing stroke in patients with atrial fibrillation. *Ann Intern Med.* 2007;147:590–592.

Man-Son-Hing M, Laupacis A. Anticoagulant-related bleeding in older persons with atrial fibrillation: physicians' fears often unfounded. *Arch Intern Med.* 2003;163:1580–1586.

35. **What tests are and are not routinely indicated as part of a syncope work-up in an older adult?**
Routinely indicated tests:
- Orthostatic blood pressure measurements
- Electrocardiogram (ECG) and prolonged arrhythmia monitoring
- Echocardiogram (if unknown history of heart disease)
- Stress testing (if unknown history of heart disease)
- Tilt table testing (if cardiac work-up negative)

Tests not routinely indicated (unless dictated by clinical presentation):
- Electrophysiologic studies
- Computed tomography (CT) scan or magnetic resonance imaging (MRI) of head
- Electroencephalogram (EEG)
- Noninvasive carotid examination (NICE)

The most common causes of syncope in the elderly include neurally mediated syndromes, orthostatic hypotension, cardiac disease, and the presence of multiple abnormalities (including polypharmacy and acute or chronic medical problems in the setting of age-related physiologic impairments). A syncope work-up in an older adult should start with a complete history and physical examination, including an evaluation for orthostatic hypotension. A detailed history and physical examination and an ECG will generally suffice to identify the causes of syncope in the majority of patients. Older patients with known heart disease should be evaluated for arrhythmic syncope. Older patients without known heart disease who present with unexplained syncope should undergo further cardiac assessment to include echocardiogram and stress testing. Physicians should try to identify and treat all factors contributing to syncope before ordering more invasive tests, such as electrophysiologic studies. Patients with a normal cardiac work-up may benefit from an upright tilt table test to look for signs of neurocardiogenic syncope. Further diagnostic tests can be ordered as dictated by this initial assessment. Unless clinically indicated, imaging studies of the head, lumbar puncture, EEG, and NICE should not be part of the syncope work-up.

36. Because systolic blood pressure increases with age, what level of systolic hypertension should be treated in the elderly?
More than 160 mm Hg. According to randomized trials, patients older than 80 years with sustained systolic blood pressure > 160 mm Hg benefit from treatment. Evidence is less clear for treating elderly patients with systolic blood pressure between 140 and 160 mm Hg unless they have an additional indication such as chronic kidney disease or heart failure. In one study, patients over 75 years without diabetes benefited from treatment of systolic blood pressure to a target of 120 mm Hg versus a target of 140 mm Hg. Patients with coronary artery disease should maintain the diastolic blood pressure > 70 mm Hg.

Beckett NS, Peter R, Fletcher AE, et al. Treatment of hypertension in patients 80 years of age or older. *N Engl J Med.* 2008;358:1887–1898.

The SPRINT Research Group. A randomized trial of intensive versus standard blood-pressure control. *N Engl J Med.* 2015;373:2103–2116.

37. Does a normal ejection fraction (EF) on echocardiogram rule out congestive heart failure (CHF) as a cause of dyspnea on exertion?
No. In older patients with CHF almost 50% have diastolic heart failure (DHF) as the cause of CHF symptoms. DHF is also called "heart failure with preserved ejection fraction (HFpEF)." Diastolic dysfunction occurs with stiffened ventricular walls owing to hypertension and other aging-related changes that lead to elevated left ventricular end-diastolic pressure and the symptoms of CHF. Systolic CHF is typically considered a "pumping" abnormality, and DHF is considered a "filling" abnormality.

38. Is metolazone uniquely synergistic with furosemide in diuresis of older patients with refractory CHF?
No. Although metolazone is usually added to loop diuretic treatment in patients with refractory heart failure, other thiazide-type diuretics used in full dosage are also highly effective. Metolazone has an elimination half-life of 2 days, making dose titration difficult and leading to excessive diuresis in some patients.

39. What factors contribute to orthostatic hypotension in older patients?
Autonomic dysfunction frequently leads to orthostatic hypotension, even in patients with chronic hypertension. Hypertension can lead to reduced arterial wall compliance. Bed rest in frail elderly patients also contributes to orthostasis because of autonomic dysfunction and plasma volume loss. Nitrates, vasodilators, and tricyclic antidepressants accentuate orthostasis. Chronic antihypertensive therapy rarely leads to orthostatic hypotension.

40. How are orthostatic blood pressure changes measured properly?
- Patient reclines for 5 minutes.
- Measure blood pressure and pulse.
- Patient stands quietly for 3 minutes.
- Measure blood pressure and pulse.
- If there is no change and clinical suspicion of orthostasis remains high, patient remains standing for several more minutes with repeat blood pressure and pulse measurement.
- Repeat this process at different times during the day to fully document the presence or absence of orthostasis.

41. What nonpharmacologic approaches reduce orthostatic hypotension?
- Discontinue medications that cause orthostatic hypotension.
- Minimize bed rest.
- Elevate the head of the bed when sleeping.

- Liberalize dietary salt and water, if appropriate.
- Use compression gradient stockings, preferably waist high, with a pressure at least 20 mm Hg when out of bed.

42. **What are the side effects of medications used to treat orthostatic hypotension?**
    - **Fludrocortisone** (mineralocorticoid): Supine hypertension, fluid retention, hypokalemia
    - **Midodrine** (alpha$_1$-adrenergic agonist): Supine hypertension, piloerection, urinary retention, pruritus
    - **Pyridostigmine** (acetylcholinesterase inhibitor): Diarrhea, urinary urgency, bradycardia

NEUROLOGY

43. **What are potential pitfalls to avoid when performing a Mini-Mental State Examination (MMSE)?**
    The MMSE lacks sensitivity for diagnosing mild cognitive impairment, especially in the highly educated. The English version is valid only in patients who are fluent in English and has not been well validated for patients who have completed less than 8 years of education. In assessing serial 7s, tell the patient to "keep going" but do not repeat your directions after each answer.

44. **What symptoms and signs suggest a cause for dementia other than Alzheimer disease (AD)?**
    Variable progression (either stepwise or gradual) of symptoms and cortical findings such as prominent aphasia or motor weakness can suggest vascular dementia. Subcortical vascular dementias often disrupt frontal lobe function and present with mild memory deficits but prominent personality changes such as passivity, abulia, and psychomotor retardation. Subcortical vascular dementia is often undiagnosed and misperceived as depression or apathy. Patients lack internal drive and, therefore, require consistent external cueing. Lewy body dementia presents with parkinsonian signs, fluctuating mental status, and visual hallucinations and often can be misdiagnosed as Parkinson disease or primary psychosis. Patients typically respond poorly to antipsychotic medications and have prominent extrapyramidal symptoms.

45. **What are treatable or reversible causes of cognitive impairment in older people?**
    - **Metabolic disorders:** Vitamin B$_{12}$ deficiency; electrolyte disturbances (hypercalcemia, hyponatremia); thyroid, renal, or hepatic dysfunction
    - **Drug-induced:** Neuroleptics, sedative hypnotics, antidepressants, anticholinergics, analgesics, muscle relaxants, steroids
    - **Alcohol intoxication and withdrawal**
    - **Depression**
    - **Neurologic disorders:** Meningitis, subdural hematomas, normal-pressure hydrocephalus (NPH), tumors

46. **How prevalent is dementia in older people?**
    At age 65, the prevalence is approximately 1–2% but increases each year thereafter, approaching 20–25% by age 85.

47. **When a patient with dementia has behavioral problems, what nonpharmacologic approaches are helpful?**
    - Determine what immediately preceded the behavioral outburst and avoid such triggers.
    - Remove challenges from the environment.
    - Simplify required tasks.
    - Explain activities before asking the patient to perform them.
    - Provide a predictable routine.
    - Avoid corrections of behavior or language unless absolutely necessary.
    - Distract the patient from an undesirable activity and redirect when possible.
    - Encourage daily exercise.
    - Encourage restful sleep.
    - Consider pet therapy.

48. **What medications are potentially useful for treating dementia?**
    Cholinesterase inhibitors such as donepezil, rivastigmine, and galantamine in general have minimal benefit in reversing dementia but are often given with the hope of slowing progression. Memantine

is an *N*-methyl-D-aspartate (NMDA) receptor antagonist that has modest benefit in moderate to severe dementia and may be combined with a cholinesterase inhibitor. Patients with mild to moderate dementia should be assessed for depression and treated appropriately. Severe agitation with delusions or hallucinations warrants consideration of an antipsychotic, but adverse effects are common. Severe sleep disturbance that has not responded to nonpharmacologic measures warrants a trial of a nonbenzodiazepine hypnotic. Avoid use of anticholinergic medications because these drugs can worsen dementia.

49. **How does one differentiate pseudodementia and dementia?**
Initially by assessing the patient for symptoms of depression. Major depression is commonly associated with cognitive difficulties (pseudodementia), and many patients in the early stages of dementia become depressed. The differentiation of pseudodementia from true dementia can be a clinical challenge. Clues that depression is the cause of cognitive difficulties include decline over weeks to months rather than years and whether the patient has overt concern for the memory loss. Referral for complete neuropsychological testing can be helpful in elucidating the diagnosis in many cases. Treatment with antidepressants will significantly improve cognitive function in patients with pseudodementia, whereas truly demented patients may see improvements in overall function but will continue to have cognitive impairment.

50. **How can one prevent the development of AD?**
To date, modifiable risk factors for AD have not been identified, though vascular disease appears to contribute. There are no currently available pharmaceutical agents or dietary supplements that prevent cognitive impairment or AD. Current research, though, focuses on antihypertensive agents, omega-3 fatty acids, physical activity, and cognitive activities as possibly effective.

    Daviglus ML, Bell CC, Berrettini W, et al. NIH State-of-the-Science Conference Statement: Preventing Alzheimer's disease and cognitive decline. NIH Consens State Sci Statements 2010;27: 1–30. Available at: www.ncbi.nlm.nih.gov/pubmed/20445638. Accessed 01.10.16.

51. **How do you distinguish an essential tremor (ET) from the tremor associated with Parkinson disease?**
See Table 18.2.

Table 18.2. Tremor Characteristics of Essential Tremor and Parkinson Disease

CHARACTERISTIC	PARKINSON DISEASE	ESSENTIAL TREMOR
Symmetry	Usually asymmetrical	Usually symmetrical
Occurrence	At rest	Postural or kinetic
Frequency (Hz)	4–6	4–10
Parts of the body affected	Hands, legs, tongue, and chin	Hands, arms, trunk, head, and voice

52. **Why is Parkinson disease frequently under- or overdiagnosed?**
Because the diagnosis relies entirely on clinical impression. There are no blood tests or imaging studies for confirming the diagnosis, and other medical conditions present with similar features. For this reason, clinicians can easily underdiagnose or overdiagnose Parkinson disease, especially at the early stages.

53. **What presenting features can lead to underdiagnosis or overdiagnosis of Parkinson disease?**
Presenting features leading to **underdiagnosis** include:
- Absence of resting tremor on initial presentation that occurs in 25% of patients with early Parkinson disease
- Attribution of stooped posture, gait unsteadiness, and loss of facial expression to aging
- Attribution of postural instability and bradykinesia to cerebrovascular disease

Presenting features leading to **overdiagnosis** include:
- Tremor related to other causes (e.g., ET)
- Bradykinesia and loss of facial expression due to hypothyroidism or depression

54. How is ET treated?
Several drugs can be used for the treatment of ET. The most commonly used are nonselective beta blockers (such as propanolol) and primidone. Other useful drugs are phenobarbital and benzodiazepines. Surgical procedures may be tried in patients who had an unsatisfactory response to drug therapy and after carefully weighing the benefit-to-risk ratio. Available surgical procedures include thalamotomy or placement of electrodes for high-frequency stimulation of the thalamus.

55. Why is restless leg syndrome commonly undiagnosed? How is it treated?
Because many patients fail to mention restless legs, periodic limb movements, or nocturnal myoclonus unless specifically questioned and only describe "poor sleep." The bed partner frequently provides a more specific history of nocturnal movement disorders. Evening treatment with a dopaminergic medication such as ropinirole or pramipexole is highly effective in many patients.

56. An elderly hospital patient is acting oddly. What are the diagnostic criteria to determine whether it is delirium?
- Presence of disturbance of consciousness with reduced ability to focus, sustain, or shift attention.
- A change in cognition that is not better accounted for by an evolving dementia.
- Rapid development of the disturbance over hours to days with fluctuation during the course of the day.

American Psychiatric Association, eds. Diagnostic and Statistical Manual of Mental Disorders. 5th ed. Arlington, VA: American Psychiatric Publishing; 2013.

57. What are the most common risk factors and causes of delirium?

Risk Factors	Causes
Advanced age	Medications
Dementia	Infection
Male sex	Dehydration
Sensory impairment	Metabolic disturbance
Impaired function	Urinary retention
Comorbid conditions	Indwelling devices
Chronic alcoholism	Bed rest
Pain	Restraints
	Fecal impaction

58. In an elderly patient who is incapable of giving a medical history, how can one differentiate dementia and delirium?
See Table 18.3. Interviewing family members or friends is also helpful in obtaining an accurate history in a confused patient.

Table 18.3. Differentiation Between Delirium and Dementia

CHARACTERISTIC	DELIRIUM	DEMENTIA
Onset	Abrupt	Insidious
Duration	Hours to days	Months to years
Attention	Impaired	Normal unless severe
Speech	Incoherent, disorganized	Ordered, anomic/aphasic
Consciousness	Fluctuating, reduced	Clear

GENITOURINARY DISORDERS

59. **What percentage of older adults are sexually active?**
Among adults aged 57–64 years, 74% report sexual activity, declining to 26% among those aged 75–85 years.

60. **What sexual problems are most prevalent in older adults?**
See Table 18.4.

Table 18.4. Sexual Dysfunction Symptoms Among Older Men and Women

SYMPTOM	Frequency (%)	
	Men	Women
Low desire	—	43
Erectile dysfunction	37	
Inability to climax	—	34
Difficulty with vaginal lubrication	—	39
Climaxing too quickly	28	—
Finding sex not pleasurable	—	23
Pain	—	17
Performance anxiety	27	—

From Lindau ST, Schumm LP, Laumann EO, et al. A study of sexuality and health among older adults in the United States. *N Engl J Med*. 2007;357:762–777.

61. **What are the common types of urinary incontinence in older adults?**
   - **Stress:** Urinary leakage with increased abdominal pressure
   - **Urge or detrusor instability:** Involuntary bladder contraction at a modest volume
   - **Overflow:** Urinary leakage out of a distended bladder due to bladder outlet obstruction or a very weak detrusor muscle that does not empty the bladder
   - **Functional:** Failure to reach the toilet in a timely manner owing to physical or cognitive debility or both
   There may be overlap among the types of incontinence.

62. **What is the innervation of the urethral sphincter and detrusor muscle?**
Urethral sphincter: Alpha$_1$-adrenergic receptors in the sympathetic nervous system
Detrusor muscle: Sympathetic nervous system and activated by the parasympathetic system, largely through M2 and M3 muscarinic (cholinergic) receptors

63. **How does this innervation affect the choice of pharmacologic treatments for urinary incontinence?**
For men with prostatic hypertrophy and a tendency to urinary retention, resting urethral sphincter pressure is usually high so **alpha$_1$-receptor blockers** are used to reduce sphincter tone and facilitate emptying of the bladder. For patients with urge incontinence, **anticholinergic** medications with activity in blocking the M2 and M3 receptors are used to relax the bladder, as is mirabegron, a beta$_3$-adrenergic agonist.

KEY POINTS: CAUSES OF URINARY INCONTINENCE

1. **Delirium**
2. **Restricted mobility, retention**
3. **Infection, inflammation, impaction (fecal)**
4. **Polyuria, pharmaceuticals**

64. **What is a postvoid residual (PVR) measurement, and why is it so helpful in assessing the patient with urinary incontinence?**
The quantity of urine left in the bladder after an attempt at complete emptying. The PVR can be measured by in-and-out catheterization or noninvasively with a bladder ultrasound scanner. In most patients with incontinence, it is diagnostically useful to measure the residual urine to determine whether urinary retention is occurring. The residual volume should be measured before bladder relaxant drugs are given because they are contraindicated if the residual volume > 200 mL.

65. **What are the risks of and indications for an indwelling catheter?**
The most significant risk is urinary tract infection (UTI) if the catheter remains for a week or more. Within 30 days of catheterization, infection is almost universal. Besides infection risk, patients attached to an indwelling catheter remain in bed more than usual, which is highly detrimental in older patients. The indications for an indwelling catheter are urinary retention, severe pressure ulcers where healing is compromised by incontinence, or for hemodynamically unstable patients whose urinary output must be closely monitored.

66. **Is it true that clamping a Foley catheter before pulling it out helps "train the bladder"?**
No. When an indwelling catheter is no longer needed, it should be removed. There is no advantage to intermittently clamping the catheter for a day or two before removal.

67. **Can medications improve the symptoms of benign prostatic hypertrophy (BPH)?**
Yes. Several medicines are currently approved by the U.S. Food and Drug Administration (FDA) for the control of BPH symptoms. The alpha$_1$-adrenergic antagonists improve bladder outlet obstruction by acting in the prostatic urethra, bladder neck, and prostate. These drugs provide immediate therapeutic benefits and are considered first-line therapy for symptomatic BPH. The nonselective alpha$_1$-adrenergic antagonists (such as terazosin and doxazosin) also have antihypertensive effects and are useful agents for patients who suffer from BPH and hypertension. Tamsulosin and alfuzosin are selective alpha$_1$-adrenergic antagonists and have less effect on blood pressure. The 5-alpha-reductase inhibitors (finasteride and dutasteride) work by reducing the size of the prostate over time. They work better for larger prostates (>40 g) and provide symptomatic improvement only after 3–6 months of therapy. The alpha$_1$-adrenergic antagonists and 5-alpha-reductase inhibitors can be used together for optimal results in patients with larger prostates. Specialty referral is indicated when BPH symptoms are not relieved by the use of available medicines. Consultation with a urologist is recommended for men who develop complications such as hydronephrosis, renal dysfunction, recurrent UTIs, urinary incontinence, or bladder stones.
    Roehrborn CB, Siami P, Barkin J, et al. The effects of dutasteride, tamsulosin and combination therapy on lower urinary tract symptoms in men with benign prostatic hyperplasia and prostatic enlargement: 2-year results from the CombAT study. *J Urol.* 2008;179:616–621.

68. **Should asymptomatic UTIs > 100,000 colonies in older patients be treated with a brief course of antibiotics?**
No. Asymptomatic bacteriuria is common in older patients, especially women. Studies show that treating it does not improve clinical outcomes. In a large proportion of patients who receive treatment, the bacteriuria recurs within a few months.

69. **Why do men with symptomatic UTIs require longer antibiotic treatment than women?**
Because the prostate gland complicates UTI treatment. Quite often, the prostate gland harbors bacteria even if prostatitis is not overt. Because antibiotics penetrate the prostate poorly and because in older men the prostate often contains prostatic calculi, short-course (3-day) antibiotic treatment of UTI in men is associated with a high recurrence rate. In addition, many times older men with UTI have a high residual volume because of prostatic hypertrophy, and this urinary stasis is an additional risk factor for recurrence with short-course therapy. Usually, UTI in men is treated with 7–10 days of antibiotics.

70. **How is testosterone deficiency diagnosed in older adults?**
The Endocrine Society recommends checking morning total testosterone levels on more than one occasion in men with consistent signs and symptoms of androgen deficiency. Evaluation should not occur during acute or subacute illness. There is evidence that insulin release following food ingestion can transiently lower testosterone levels. Therefore, levels are preferably obtained when fasting in the morning.

71. **What are the clinical manifestations and prevalence of testosterone deficiency in older men?**
The most typical and specific symptoms are decreased libido, erectile dysfunction, and minimal trauma fracture or osteoporosis. The aging process in men is accompanied by a gradual decline in serum testosterone levels. Approximately 50% of men in their 80s have total testosterone levels in the hypogonadal range, though severe deficiency is much less common. Physical examination may reveal significant decreases in muscle mass and strength, loss of body hair, gynecomastia, and testicular atrophy.
   Harmann SM, Metter EJ, Tobin JD, et al. Longitudinal effects of aging on serum total and free testosterone levels in healthy men. Baltimore Longitudinal Study of Aging. *J Clin Endocrinol Metab.* 2001;86:724–731.

72. **What are the contraindications to testosterone replacement in older men?**
Testosterone-dependent diseases such as prostate cancer and severe BPH. There is no proven benefit of testosterone supplementation for mild age-related declines in testicular function at this time. However, testosterone supplementation is commonly prescribed for symptomatic elderly men with serum concentrations < 200 ng/dL. Special caution is recommended for patients who suffer from sleep apnea, hyperlipidemia, and erythrocytosis, because testosterone supplementation may worsen these conditions. Patients should be screened for the presence of prostate cancer and evaluated for signs of the other mentioned conditions at the time of treatment initiation and periodically thereafter.

73. **Why is nocturia so common in older people?**
Because of age-related physiologic changes. Nocturia is defined as either excessive nocturnal urine output or increased nocturnal frequency. Age-related physiologic changes can alter the regular circadian pattern of urine excretion and lead to increased nocturnal urine formation. In addition, aging is associated with changes of the urinary tract itself that predispose to urinary frequency. These changes include prostatic hypertrophy as well as reduced bladder capacity and lowered threshold for urination. Detrusor muscle contractions become less effective, and PVR volumes are larger with aging. Some medical problems that typically affect older people such as BPH, fecal impaction, and recurrent UTIs can also predispose to nocturia.
   Resnick NM. Voiding dysfunction in the elderly. In: Yalla SV, McGuire EJ, Elbadauwi A, et al, eds. *Neurology and Urodynamics: Principles and Practice.* New York: Macmillan; 1988. p 303–330.

INFECTIOUS DISEASES

74. **If pneumonia is suspected to be secondary to aspiration, should the antibiotics chosen provide full coverage for anaerobic bacteria?**
Not necessarily. Treatment with specific anaerobic coverage is required only if the aspiration was large in volume and contained food or if there is a cavitary infiltrate on chest radiograph. Virtually all pneumonia is secondary to some degree of aspiration of oral secretions. Many older patients with suspected aspiration pneumonia have gram-negative organisms, especially if the pneumonia was acquired in a hospital or nursing home.

75. **How does aging affect tuberculosis skin testing?**
Delayed hypersensitivity from latent tuberculosis may wane with age, causing a nonreactive tuberculin skin test in patients with latent tuberculosis. If a second skin test is placed days to months later, a booster phenomenon can occur with a resultant positive skin test. The second skin test can be falsely interpreted as a recent conversion. Patients who will undergo annual testing such as in nursing homes should undergo two-step testing on initial evaluation.

76. **What immunizations are recommended for older persons?**
   • Tetanus and diphtheria toxoid every 10 years (with at least one dose of tetanus toxoid, reduced diphtheria toxoid, and acellular pertussis [Tdap])
   • Herpes zoster vaccine after age 60
   • Pneumococcal vaccine (PCV13, then PCV23) at age 65
   • Influenza vaccine every fall. A high-dose inactivated influenza vaccine has been licensed specifically for persons aged ≥65 years to try to increase antibody titers after vaccination. At this time, the ACIP (Advisory Committee on Immunizations Practices) has not yet expressed a preference for this vaccine for older persons.

Centers for Disease Control and Prevention (CDC). Licensure of a high-dose inactivated influenza vaccine (Fluzone High-Dose) and Guidance for Use—United States, 2010. *MMWR Morb Mortal Wkly Rep.* 2010;59:485–486.

77. **When do older patients need revaccination with PCV23 pneumococcal vaccine?**
If they were vaccinated more than 5 years previously and were younger than 65 years at the time of primary vaccination.

78. **Why are so many of the excess deaths during influenza outbreaks from cardiovascular disease?**
Because influenza is a major physiologic stress on an older patient and frequently causes cardiovascular decompensation in patients with ischemic heart disease or CHF.

DERMATOLOGY

79. **Where are pressure ulcers most likely to develop?**
- Sacrum
- Posterior heels
- Trochanteric areas

80. **What are the principles to follow in treating pressure ulcers?**
- Avoid or minimize pressure on the wound.
- Provide adequate pain control.
- Correct nutritional deficiencies.
- Perform chemical or surgical débridement of necrotic tissues.
- Maintain a moist wound environment yet keep surrounding skin dry.
- Intensify preventive measures such as frequent body repositioning and use of pressure-reducing products and special mattresses.
- Stage and monitor pressure wounds very closely.

KEY POINTS: PRESSURE ULCER STAGING SYSTEM

1. Stage I: Area of persistent redness (or red, blue, or purple discoloration in darker skin tones) in intact skin.
2. Stage II: Partial-thickness skin loss involving epidermis or dermis or both, such as abrasion, blister, or shallow crater.
3. Stage III: Full-thickness skin loss that may extend to but not include the fascia such as deep crater.
4. Stage IV: Full-thickness skin loss with tissue necrosis and may involve muscle, bone, and adjacent structures.
5. Suspected deep tissue injury: Area of significant discoloration that may represent deeper tissue injury.
6. Unstageable: Ulcers covered with eschar cannot be staged.

81. **In the management of pressure ulcers on the trunk or pelvis in a patient with limited bed mobility, what type of mattress is necessary?**
There are two categories of mattresses: nonpowered and powered. Nonpowered pressure-reducing mattresses or overlays are filled with air, water, gel, foam, or a combination of these materials. They should meet the criteria for group 1 support surfaces in the recommendations of the Agency for Health Care Policy and Research Treatment of Pressure Ulcers Guidelines Panel. For patients with large or multiple deeper ulcers (stage III or IV) or multiple stage II ulcers without improvement after use of a group 1 support surface for 1 month, powered mattresses are recommended. These group 2 support surfaces are designed to mechanically vary the pressure beneath the patient and thereby reduce the duration of the applied pressure.
Bergstrom N, Bennett MA, Carlson CE, et al. Treatment of pressure ulcers. Clinical Practice Guideline No. 15. AHCPR Publication No. 95-0652. Rockville, MD: Agency for Health Care Policy and Research; December 1994.

82. Why do so many older people have pruritus?

Because the aging skin is associated with a decrease in eccrine and sebaceous gland function, as well as an increase in transepidermal water loss that predisposes to dryness. Xerosis (dry skin) is frequently seen in older people and is the most common cause of pruritus in the geriatric population. Xerosis can be treated or prevented by avoiding the use of strong soaps and by regular use of topical emollients containing urea such as lactic acid 12% lotion (Lac-Hydrin) or occlusive preparations such as Eucerin cream or petroleum jelly.

HEMATOLOGY

83. What are the common clinical manifestations of multiple myeloma?
    - Fatigue
    - Unexplained anemia
    - Hypercalcemia
    - Renal failure
    - Osteoporosis
    - Lytic bone lesions on skeletal films
    - Increased total serum protein concentration
    - Presence of urine or serum monoclonal protein

84. Does hemoglobin normally decrease with aging?

Only slightly. There is a modest increase in the prevalence of anemia, particularly in men older than 75 years. The mechanism probably relates at least partially to reduced sensitivity to erythropoietin because of decline in testosterone concentration. In mild anemia (hemoglobin > 12 g/dL) among elderly patients, a comprehensive work-up often fails to identify a cause. Anemia of chronic disease becomes increasingly common with aging and is typified by very low serum iron, low transferrin saturation, low total iron-binding capacity, and normal to increased ferritin.

85. Should the normal range for erythrocyte sedimentation rate (ESR) be adjusted for age and gender?

Yes. ESR is a common hematology test and is a nonspecific measure of inflammation that is useful for diagnosing diseases such as temporal arteritis, polymyalgia rheumatica, and various autoimmune diseases. The ESR can also be used to monitor therapeutic response. ESR values tend to rise with age and to be slightly higher in women. The formula to calculate normal maximum ESR values in adults is:

$$\text{ESR (mm/hr)} < \frac{[\text{Age (in years)} + 10 \text{ (if female)}]}{2}$$

Bottiger LE, Svedberg CA. Normal erythrocyte sedimentation rate and age. *Br Med J.* 1967;2:85–87.

Miller A, Green M, Robinson D. Simple rule for calculating normal erythrocyte sedimentation rate. *Br Med J (Clin Res Ed)*. 1983;286:266.

86. Why are patients with chronic lymphocytic leukemia (CLL) not always immediately treated?

Because survival with CLL does not improve with early treatment. CLL is the most common form of leukemia and occurs mainly in older patients. The diagnosis is often made incidentally when a blood count reveals a lymphocyte count > 5000/μL. In these asymptomatic patients, many years may go by without disease progression. There is little evidence that early treatment improves survival or that CLL can be cured with present standard treatment. Therapy is recommended for the following:
    - Disease-related symptoms such as fever, weight loss, or night sweats
    - Significant anemia (hemoglobin < 10 g/dL) or thrombocytopenia (platelet count < 100,000/μL)
    - Autoimmune hemolytic anemia or thrombocytopenia that is poorly responsive to corticosteroids
    - Rapidly progressive disease, as manifested by lymphocyte count doubling in < 6 months or rapidly enlarging lymph nodes, spleen, and liver

87. What are the common clinical manifestations of vitamin B_{12} deficiency?
    Hematologic:
    - Megaloblastic anemia
    - Hypersegmented neutrophils on peripheral blood smear

- Leukopenia (severe deficiency)
- Thrombocytopenia (severe deficiency)

Neurologic:
- Symmetrical peripheral neuropathy
- Cognitive impairment
- Ataxia

88. If a patient presents with pancytopenia, what other diagnoses should be considered in addition to vitamin B_{12} deficiency?
Aplastic anemia, myelodysplastic syndrome, and acute myeloid leukemia.

89. Why does subacute combined degeneration of the spinal cord occur with vitamin B_{12} deficiency?
Because of a defect in myelin formation due to cobalamin deficiency. This life-threatening neurologic complication may be reversed with an aggressive vitamin B_{12} supplementation over a period of several months.

90. How prevalent is vitamin B_{12} deficiency in older people, and what is the major cause?
10–20%. The major causes are food source cobalamin malabsorption related to gastric atrophy and achlorhydria and loss of intrinsic factor (pernicious anemia).

91. In a patient with vitamin B_{12} deficiency, does replacement have to be given by intramuscular injection?
No. Although, vitamin B_{12} deficiency is typically treated with frequent intramuscular injections for several weeks, followed by a monthly injection for maintenance, studies support the efficacy of alternative forms of administration such as oral and nasal. Oral and nasal treatments require high doses (1000 μg per day) owing to erratic absorption and the need for good patient compliance for optimal results.

Slot WB, Merkus FW, Van Deventer SJ, et al. Normalization of plasma vitamin B_{12} concentration by intranasal hydroxocobalamin in vitamin B_{12}–deficient patients. *Gastroenterology.* 1997;113:430–433.

Hathcock JN, Troendle GH. Oral cobalamin for the treatment of pernicious anemia. *JAMA.* 1991;265:96–97.

MEDICATION USE

92. Among the tricyclic antidepressants, is amitriptyline especially effective for neuropathic pain?
No. All the tricyclic antidepressants have similar efficacy for the treatment of neuropathic pain. Amitriptyline should be avoided in older patients because it has the most anticholinergic activity and frequently causes orthostatic hypotension.

93. What body systems are adversely affected by anticholinergic medications?
- **Genitourinary:** weakness of bladder muscle contractions
- **Gastrointestinal:** constipation, dry mouth
- **Central nervous system:** impaired cognition

94. What medications have highly significant anticholinergic properties?
- Antihistamines (diphenhydramine, chlorpheniramine, and hydroxyzine)
- Tricyclic antidepressants
- Cyclobenzaprine
- Scopolamine and meclizine
- Promethazine
- Anticholinergic bladder relaxants

95. Some of my older patients do not know why they are taking many of their pills. Do pharmacists routinely write the medication indication on the pill bottle label?
No, because there may be multiple indications for the same medications. For example, hydrochlorothiazide can be taken for edema or for hypertension. To improve patient understanding and compliance with medication regimens, providers should always write the indication on the prescription (e.g., "HCTZ, take 1 daily for HTN").

96. Patients often do not admit they are not taking their medications. How can one best inquire about medication compliance?

Try asking the question about compliance in several ways. When reviewing the patient's medication list, ask:
- Are you taking all your medications?
- Have you missed any pills in the past week?
- Are any of your pills causing you problems?

97. What over-the-counter medications greatly increase or decrease the international normalized ratio (INR) by affecting liver metabolism of warfarin?

Cimetidine (increased INR) and St. John's wort (decreased INR).

98. What common medications are renally excreted and require dose reduction in older patients, even those with serum creatinine in the "normal" range?
- Fluoroquinolones
- Colchicine
- Glyburide
- Low-molecular-weight heparin
- Ceftriaxone
- Digoxin
- Gabapentin
- Pregabalin
- Lithium
- Trimethoprim/sulfa
- Ranitidine

Because muscle mass is reduced in many older patients, reduced renal function is not reflected by a commensurate increase in serum creatinine.

PREVENTION

See also Chapter 2, General Medicine and Ambulatory Care.

99. Should certain older adults be screened for abdominal aortic aneurysms (AAAs)?

Yes. AAA rupture is a common cause of death in older adults. The most important risk factors for AAA are advanced age, male sex, and smoking. Several organizations recommend one-time screening for AAA in men between ages 65–75 who have ever smoked. Men in this age group who have a first-degree relative who required repair of an AAA are also considered for screening.

100. How is such screening performed?

With abdominal ultrasonography, a noninvasive test with a high sensitivity and specificity for diagnosing AAA. Medicare currently reimburses for AAA screening within the first 6 months of Medicare enrollment as part of the "Welcome to Medicare" physical for:
- Men aged 65–75 who have smoked at least 100 cigarettes during their lifetime
- Men and women who have a family history of AAA.

Fleming C, Whitlock EP, Beil TL, et al. Screening for abdominal aortic aneurysm: a best-evidence systematic review for the U.S. Preventive Services Task Force. *Ann Intern Med.* 2005;142:203–211.

Salo JA, Soisalon-Soininen S, Bondestam S, et al. Familial occurrence of abdominal aortic aneurysm. *Ann Intern Med.* 1999;130:637–642.

U.S. Preventive Services Task Force. Screening for abdominal aortic aneurysm: recommendation statement. *Ann Intern Med.* 2005;142:198.

HEALTH SYSTEMS

101. Which elderly patients qualify for home care services, and what services are covered by Medicare?

Those who need skilled services on an intermittent rather than a continuous basis **and** are homebound. **Skilled services** are defined as those provided by nursing (including teaching self-care skills, performing skilled procedures, and assessing changing or fluctuating medical conditions), physical therapy, speech therapy, and occupational therapy. **Homebound** is defined as leaving home infrequently but only with assistance and considerable effort; 24-hour care is not provided nor is personal care provided if such assistance is the only care needed.

102. Does Medicare part D provide at least partial coverage for all medications?

No. Part D plans are required to cover medications in all of the major therapeutic categories but are not required to cover every medication in each category. Each plan utilizes a unique formulary. In addition, coverage in many plans includes a "donut hole." This means payment for medications are covered up to a certain amount, but then coverage is reduced for further expenditures until the patient finally exceeds a certain yearly expenditure, at which point enhanced coverage resumes.

103. When is an occupational therapy referral appropriate? Physical therapy referral?

When the patient needs assistance in ADLs, adaptive equipment, splint or orthotic fabrication, or a home safety assessment. Most occupational therapy focuses on optimizing use of the upper extremities. Physical therapy referrals are appropriate if the patient has significant balance or gait disturbance, needs an ambulatory aid, has mobility or transfer difficulty, or has range of motion or strength impairment.

104. What percentage of American adults aged 65 and older lives in a nursing home?

Approximately 3.5%, though it is 11% for those over age 85. The number of older adults living in nursing homes has been declining over the past few years.

105. What is an older American's lifetime chance of spending at least some time residing in a nursing home?

Over 40% after age 65. Many of these nursing home admissions are for post acute care and patients who have short stays for rehabilitation after hospital discharge.

WEBSITE

1. www.americangeriatrics.org

BIBLIOGRAPHY

1. Cassel CK, Leipzig R, Cohen HJ, eds. *Geriatric Medicine: An Evidence-Based Approach.* 4th ed. New York: Springer; 2007.
2. Hatler J, Ouslander J, Tinetti M, eds. *Hazzard's Geriatric Medicine & Gerontology.* 6th ed. New York: McGraw Hill Medical; 2009.
3. Durso SC, Sullivan GM, eds. *Geriatrics Review Syllabus: A Core Curriculum in Geriatric Medicine.* New York: American Geriatrics Society; 2016.
4. Reuben DB, Herr KA, Pacala JT, et al. *Geriatrics at Your Fingertips 2016.* New York: American Geriatrics Society; 2016.

PALLIATIVE MEDICINE

Jason A. Webb, MD, FAPA, and Nathan A. Gray, MD

CHAPTER 19

1. **What is palliative care?**
   A specialized medical care approach for people with serious illness that focuses on providing relief from the symptoms and stress of serious illness. The goal is to improve quality of life for both the patient and the family. Palliative care is provided by a specially trained team of doctors, nurses, social workers, and other specialists who work together with a patient's doctors to provide an extra layer of support. It is appropriate at any age and at any stage in a serious illness and can be provided along with curative treatment.
   Center to Advance Palliative Care. Available at www.capc.org.

2. **What is hospice care?**
   A specific type of palliative care that provides multidisciplinary, noncurative care to patients with a life expectancy of ≤ 6 months if the disease follows its expected course. Hospice provides team-based multidisciplinary support services to patients and family in the home or an institution (e.g., skilled nursing facility [SNF]).

EARLY INTEGRATION

3. **When should patients be referred for palliative care?**
   At any point in a patient's life-limiting or serious illness process, regardless of prognosis (Fig. 19.1). Specifically, patients with complicated symptom needs, psychosocial distress, or anticipated complex medical decision-making needs may benefit from earlier referral. A study of patients with stage IV non–small cell lung cancer found that patients referred early to palliative care had better quality of life and survival.

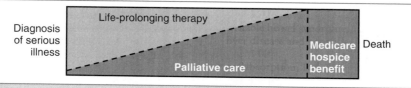

Fig. 19.1. Model for early integration of palliative care. *(Adapted from Ferris FD, Balfour HM, Bowen K, et al. A model to guide patient and family care,* J Pain Symptom Manage, *24:106-123, 2002.)*

Temel JS, Greer JA, Muzikansky A, et al. Early palliative care for patients with metastatic non-small-cell lung cancer. *N Engl J Med.* 2010;363:733–742.

4. **Which patients should be considered for a palliative care consultation in the hospital?**
   Any patient with a potentially life-limiting or life-threatening condition and:
   - Primary criteria:
     - The surprise question: "No" in answer to the question: "Would you be surprised if the patient died within 12 months or before adulthood?"
     - Frequent admissions: More than one admission for the same condition within several months
     - Sentinel admission: Prompted by difficult-to-control physical or psychological symptoms
     - Complex care requirements: Functional dependency or home support needed for ventilator, antibiotics, or enteral feedings
     - Failure to thrive: Decline in function, feeding intolerance, or unintended decline in weight

- Secondary criteria:
  - Admission to a long-term care facility or medical foster home
  - Elderly patient with cognitive impairment and new, complex injury or illness (e.g., hip fracture)
  - Metastatic or locally advanced incurable cancer
  - Chronic home oxygen use
  - Out-of-hospital cardiac arrest
  - Current or past hospice program enrollment
  - Limited social support (e.g., family caregiver stressors, chronic mental illness)
  - Lack of known advance care planning discussion or document

  Weissman DE, Meier DE. Identifying patients in need of a palliative care assessment in the hospital setting: a consensus report from the Center to Advance Palliative Care. *J Palliat Med.* 2011;14:17–23.

DEATH TRAJECTORIES

5. **How can one predict the course of an illness over time?**
   Although predicting exact prognosis and trajectory is challenging, illnesses generally follow one of several patterns. Recognizing these patterns can help clinicians and patients anticipate future needs and decisions (Fig. 19.2).
   - Short period of rapid decline: Cancer
   - Long-term limitations with intermittent serious episodes: Chronic heart and lung disease
   - Prolonged dwindling: Alzheimer disease, many neurodegenerative disorders

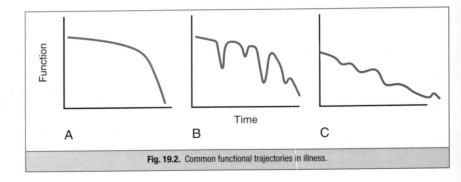

Fig. 19.2. Common functional trajectories in illness.

Murray SA, Kendall M, Boyd K, et al. Illness trajectories and palliative care. *BMJ.* 2005;330:1007–1011.

6. **Who is eligible for the Hospice Medicare Benefit?**
   Patients with Medicare Part A and a diagnosis of a terminal illness with a probable life expectancy of 6 months or less. The patient's doctor and the hospice medical director (two independent physicians) must certify the limited life expectancy.

7. **What does the Hospice Medicare Benefit cover?**
   - Physician services
   - Nursing care
   - Medical supplies: Bandages and catheters
   - Medications: For symptom control and pain relief
   - Medical equipment: Wheelchairs, walkers, and hospital beds
   - Short-term care in the hospital, including respite care
   - Home health aide and homemaker services

- Physical and occupational therapy
- Speech therapy
- Social work services
- Dietary counseling
- Family grief counseling

8. **Can hospice patients request cardiopulmonary resuscitation?**
Yes. Hospice programs cannot require that the patient or family request no resuscitation in order to receive services, but the majority of hospice patients do not want aggressive interventions of likely low benefit. Once enrolled in hospice, many patients who initially requested resuscitation later ask for no resuscitation after they are assured that pain relief and symptom management will continue.

9. **When does a patient with cancer meet criteria for hospice eligibility?**
When the patient has the following:
- Clinical findings of malignancy with widespread, aggressive, or progressive disease as evidenced by increasing symptoms, worsening laboratory values, or evidence of metastatic disease.
- Impaired performance status with a palliative performance score less than 70%.
- Continued decline despite definitive therapy.
  Decline is evidenced by:
  - Serum calcium greater than 12 mg/dL.
  - Cachexia or weight loss of 5% in the preceding 3 months.
  - Recurrent disease after surgery, radiation, or chemotherapy.
  - Refusal to pursue additional curative or prolonging cancer treatment.
  - Signs and symptoms of advanced disease (e.g., nausea, transfusions, malignant ascites, or pleural effusion).

  Finally, patients who refuse further curative therapy may be hospice eligible.
  Anderson F, Downing GM, Hill J, et al. Palliative performance scale (PPS): a new tool. *J Palliat Care.* 1996;12:5–11.

10. **When does a patient with heart failure meet criteria for hospice eligibility?**
When the patient has the following symptoms:
- Poor response to (or patient's choice not to pursue) optimal treatment with diuretics, vasodilators, and angiotensin-converting enzyme (ACE) inhibitors

OR
- Angina pectoris at rest resistant to standard nitrate therapy in a patient who is not a candidate for invasive procedures or has declined revascularization procedures

AND
- New York Heart Association (NYHA) class IV symptoms with one of the following:
  - The presence of significant symptoms of dyspnea or angina at rest
  - Inability to carry out even minimal physical activity without symptoms of dyspnea or angina
- Symptoms or features that support hospice eligibility:
  - Treatment-resistant symptomatic dysrhythmias
  - History of unexplained or cardiac-related syncope
  - Cerebrovascular accident (CVA) secondary to cardiac embolism
  - History of cardiac arrest or resuscitation
  - Hyponatremia

SPIRITUAL ASSESSMENT

11. **Do patients wish to discuss their spirituality with their medical providers?**
Yes. A majority of Americans feel that spirituality is important, and many wish for their medical providers to be aware of their spiritual beliefs.

12. **Where should I start in assessing someone's spiritual needs?**
By asking general questions, such as whether patients have religious or spiritual beliefs that help them cope with challenges, whether they are part of a faith community, or how they might like

their beliefs to influence their care. These questions can provide an opening for patients to share their spiritual needs or wishes. Although medical providers may not be equipped to address these concerns, acknowledging the patient's faith perspective can facilitate respectful care and allow providers to appropriately direct patients to spiritual resources within the health system or within the patient's own faith community.

Saguil A, Phelps K. The spiritual assessment. *Am Fam Physician.* 2012;86:546–550.

COMMUNICATION

13. **How do skilled communicators approach difficult conversation?**

    By beginning the conversation from the patient's perspective: what the patient already knows and what the patient wants to know. Always ask questions before giving information, and always follow up after giving information to assess what the patient heard. The phrase **"ASK-TELL-ASK"** can be a helpful reminder.

14. **What methods can be used to guide a bad news discussion?**

    The acronym **"SPIKES"** can provide a helpful structure for having a bad news meeting:

    S—Setup: Determine the best setting, participants, and timing for the discussion.

    P—Perception: Find out what the patient understands or is concerned about.

    I—Invitation: Ask permission to share news, especially if bad.

    K—Knowledge: Provide the relevant information in straightforward and direct language.

    E—Empathize: Acknowledge the patient's emotional response.

    S—Summarize and Strategize: Describe the situation and outline the plan for next steps. When appropriate, reassure the patient of ongoing support or your availability to answer further questions.

15. **How should one respond when patients express strong emotions, such as anger or grief?**

    The acronym **"NURSE"** can help to provide a compassionate response:

    N—Naming: Identify the emotion present: "I imagine you might feel disappointed right now."

    U—Understanding: Explore the patient's reaction: "What's most frustrating about this?"

    R—Respecting: Express respect for the patient's experience or coping: "I appreciate your being so honest with me. I know this can't be easy."

    S—Supporting: Avoid unrealistic promises, but respond with a statement of support: "I will continue to be here for you, even though these test results are not what we were hoping for."

    E—Exploring: Solicit additional concerns or needs: "Is there anything else I'm missing?"

    Back AL, Arnold RM, Baile WF, et al. Approaching difficult communication tasks in oncology. *CA Cancer J Clin.* 2005;55:164–177.

SYMPTOM MANAGEMENT: PAIN (OPIATES)

16. **How can pain be classified?**

    With the patient's description because it may direct the clinician to the underlying cause and to the most appropriate medication for that pain type.

    - **Nociceptive:** Mechanical or inflammatory activation of peripheral nerve fibers (nociceptors)
      - **Visceral:** *"Deep, crampy,"* poorly localized occurring in abdominal, pelvic, and thoracic regions.
      - **Somatic:** *"Dull, aching, throbbing"* occurring in bone, ligaments, and skin
    - **Neuropathic:** *"Pins-and-needles, stabbing, shooting"* due to direct damage to nerves

17. **How should escalating pain symptoms be managed?**

    The World Health Organization (WHO) provides a stepwise guide to managing escalating cancer-related pain and reminds clinicians to use adjuvant medications (discussed later) as well (Fig. 19.3). This guide can be helpful for cancer pain but should be regarded with caution in *non*cancer patients, in whom escalating opioid doses may not be effective as a long-term solution to pain and may worsen issues with substance dependence.

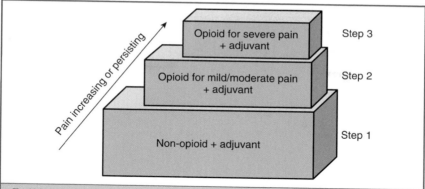

Fig. 19.3. World Health Organization pain relief ladder. *(Adapted from Cancer pain relief and palliative care. Report of a WHO Expert Committee, World Health Organ Tech Rep Ser, 804:1-75, 1990.)*

18. How does one pick an opiate?

Tables like the ones provided here are useful in choosing a starting dose or converting dosage from one opioid to another (Tables 19.1 and 19.2). However, decisions about selection and dosing of pain medications should always be individualized for each patient's situation and characteristics.

	Route of delivery	
Medication*	*PO (Onset 30–60 min)*	*SQ/IV/IM (Onset 15–30 min)*
Morphine	30 mg	10 mg
Oxycodone	20 mg	N/A
Hydromorphone	7.5 mg	1.5 mg
Fentanyl†	N/A	100 μg
Hydrocodone	30 mg	N/A
Codeine	200 mg	130 mg

*Methadone is not included in the table, as dosing conversion can be highly variable and methadone should be used with the assistance of an experienced clinician or pharmacist.
†Fentanyl transdermal should be dosed based on the manufacturer's guidelines.
IM, intramuscular; IV intravenous; N/A, not applicable; PO, by mouth (per os); SQ, subcutaneous.
Adapted from Foley KM. The treatment of cancer pain. *N Engl J Med.* 1985;313:84–95.

19. What is the first rule of opiate prescribing?

To provide a plan to address the constipation that these medications cause. Daily senna (a stimulant laxative) can be a useful starting regimen for patients new to opiates.

20. In addition to constipation, are there other side effects caused by opiates?

Yes. Opiates may also cause nausea, pruritus, urinary retention, myoclonus, and sedation. Many of these side effects lessen once patients become accustomed to the medication, but intolerable side effects may require rotation to a different opiate, dose modification, or an additional medication to address the side effect (such as antihistamines for itching).

21. How should patients who require frequent dosing of opiates be managed?

With the addition of a long-acting pain medication. The dose of long-acting medication is calculated as 50–75% of the patient's prior 24-hour short-acting opiate dosage. Breakthrough doses for acute pain should generally be 10–15% of the patient's total daily dose as a short-acting opiate.

22. Will opiates make patients stop breathing?

Rarely. Respiratory depression is a manifestation of overdose. When dosed appropriately and adjusted judiciously, clinically significant respiratory suppression is uncommon. Sedation almost universally precedes respiratory suppression and should be a clear indicator to modify dosage before patients reach the level of impaired respiratory drive.

Gallagher R. Killing the symptom without killing the patient. *Can Fam Physician.* 2010;56:544–546.

Table 19.1. Opioids for Mild-to-Moderate Pain

DRUG	ROUTE	EQUIANALGESIC DOSE (mg)*	PEAK EFFECT (hr)	DURATION OF EFFECT (hr)	COMMENTS
Codeine	PO	200	0.5	3–6	Ceiling for analgesia reached at doses >240 mg/day PO
	IV/IM	130	0.5	3–6	
Oxycodone	PO	20–30	0.5	3–6	No ceiling dose if given without fixed combinations; parenteral formulation not available
Hydrocodone	PO	30	0.5	4–6	Only available as fixed combination with acetaminophen or aspirin

*Approximate potency relative to 10 mg of parenteral morphine.
IM, intramuscular; IV, intravenous; NA, not available; PO, oral (per os).
From Grossman SA, Nesbit S: Cancer pain. In Abeloff MA, Armitage JO, Niederhuber JE, et al, editors. *Abeloff's Clinical Oncology*. 4th ed. Philadelphia: Churchill Livingstone; 2008.

Table 19.2. Strong Opiates for Moderate-to-Severe Cancer Pain

DRUG	ROUTE	EQUIANALGESIC DOSE (mg)*	DURATION OF EFFECT (hr)	COMMENTS
Oxycodone	PO	20–30	3–6	No ceiling dose if given without fixed combinations; parenteral formulations not available
	PO (SR)		12	
Morphine	PO	30	4–6	Many PO formulations for individual patient needs
	PO (SR)		8–12	
	IV/IM	10	3–5	
Hydromorphone	PO	7.5	3–4	Good choice for SC due to potency
	PR	(?)	Unknown	
	IV/IM	1.5	3–4	
Meperidine	PO	300	3–6	Not preferred due to CNS toxic metabolite that accumulates in renal failure
	IV/IM	75	2–3	
Levorphanol	PO	4.0	6–8	Long $t_{1/2}$ (11 hr) necessitates slow dose titration; drug accumulation may occur

Table 19.2. Strong Opiates for Moderate-to-Severe Cancer Pain *(Continued)*

DRUG	ROUTE	EQUIANALGESIC DOSE (mg)*	DURATION OF EFFECT (hr)	COMMENTS
	IV/IM	2.0	6–8	
Fentanyl	TD	(?)	≥12	Short $t_{1/2}$ (<1 hr); TD dose titration difficult with depot in SC adipose tissue; TD fentanyl 25 µg/hr ~45 mg/day PO morphine
	IV/IM	0.1	0.5–1.0	
Methadone[†]	PO	10	6–8	Despite long $t_{1/2}$ (15– >150 hr), duration of analgesia is not prolonged; however, drug accumulation can result in toxicities Caution is warranted when converting to methadone in patients with high opioid tolerance
Oxymorphone	PO	10	7–9	Now available as immediate-release formulations
	PO (SR)		12	
	IV	1	7–9	

*Approximate potency relative to 10 mg of parenteral morphine.
[†]Ripamonti C, Groff L, Brunelli C, et al. Switching from morphine to oral methadone in treating cancer pain: what is the equianalgesic dose ratio? *J Clin Oncol.* 1998;16:3216–3221; Moryl N, Santiago-Palma J, Kornick C, et al. Pitfalls of opioid rotation: substituting another opioid for methadone in patients with cancer pain. *Pain.* 2002;96:325–328; Bruera E, Neumann CM. Role of methadone in the management of pain in cancer patients. *Oncology.* 1999;13:1275–1282; Pereira J, Lawlor P, Vigano E, et al. Equianalgesic dose ratios for opioids: a critical review of proposals for long term dosing. *J Pain Symptom Manage.* 2001;22:672–687; Bruera E, Sweeny C. Methadone use in cancer patients with pain: a review. *J Palliat Med.* 2002;5:127–138.
CNS, central nervous system; IM, intramuscular; IV, intravenous; PO, oral; SC, subcutaneous; SR, slow-release formulation; $t_{1/2}$, half-life; TD, transdermal; (?), unknown.
From Grossman SA, Nesbit S: Cancer pain. In Abeloff MA, Armitage JO, Niederhuber JE, et al, editors. *Abeloff's Clinical Oncology.* 4th ed. Philadelphia: Churchill Livingstone; 2008.

23. **What can be done if a patient really does suffer an opiate overdose that causes respiratory suppression?**
   In cases of true overdose, naloxone (an opioid antagonist), given intravenously, can be used to temporarily reverse opioid effects. Patients should be monitored closely afterward, because naloxone is short acting and symptoms of overdose may recur. In palliative care patients, it may be prudent to reduce the dose of naloxone to avoid causing complete opiate withdrawal, which can be painful and distressing to patients.

KEY POINTS: SYMPTOM MANAGEMENT: PAIN

- Always provide treatments for constipation when starting opiate medications.
- Use acetaminophen and NSAIDs in addition to opiates for pain control.

NSAIDs, nonsteroidal anti-inflammatory drugs.

SYMPTOM MANAGEMENT: PAIN (NONOPIATE ADJUVANTS)

24. **In addition to opioids, what other first-line treatment modalities can be used for pain management for patients with a serious illness?**
    All patients with acute or chronic pain should be treated with acetaminophen and adjuvant pain medications. The WHO pain ladder recommends a stepped management strategy with combination therapy with adjuvants to decrease the total daily dosage of opiates to reduce the risks of opiate-induced side effects and toxicity.

25. **Is acetaminophen really effective for pain relief, or is it just a placebo?**
    In placebo-controlled trials acetaminophen has been shown to be effective for pain relief, and it is the recommended first-line agent by the WHO, given the excellent overall safety profile. Patients, however, should never exceed 3000 mg/day because of the risk of toxicity and liver failure.

26. **How helpful are NSAIDs for pain management?**
    Oral nonsteroidal anti-inflammatory drugs (NSAIDs) are more effective compared to acetaminophen for pain reduction, stiffness, and physical functioning. NSAIDs can also be very effective for bone pain due to metastatic cancer, as well as other types of inflammation-mediated nociceptive pain. However, NSAIDs should be used with caution and for the shortest duration possible given the established gastrointestinal, renal, and cardiovascular toxicities. Oral NSAIDs such as naproxen, ibuprofen, diclofenac, and celecoxib are the preferred agents, especially in older adults. Topical NSAIDs such as diclofenac gel are generally well tolerated, have lower systemic absorption, and are more effective than placebo in reducing pain and improving physical function.
    Makris UE, Abrams RC, Gurland B, et al. Management of persistent pain in the older patient: a clinical review. *JAMA*. 2014;312:825–836.

27. **What are the most effective medications for painful peripheral neuropathy?**
    Duloxetine, venlafaxine, amitriptyline, gabapentin, and pregabalin have shown evidence of pain reduction in diabetic neuropathy and neuropathic pain syndromes associated with cancer. Gabapentin has been shown to be the most favorable in terms of balance between efficacy and safety.
    Rudroju N, Bansal D, Talakokkula ST, et al. Comparative efficacy and safety of six antidepressants and anticonvulsants in painful diabetic neuropathy: a network meta-analysis. *Pain Physician*. 2013;16:E705–E714.

28. **What medications are effective for chemotherapy-induced peripheral neuropathy?**
    No medications or treatments are currently available to prevent chemotherapy-induced peripheral neuropathy; however, duloxetine has the best clinical trial evidence for its effectiveness and receives a moderate recommendation from the American Society of Clinical Oncology.
    Hershman DL, Lacchetti C, Dworkin RH, et al. Prevention and management of chemotherapy induced peripheral neuropathy in survivors of adult cancers: American Society of Clinical Oncology Clinical Practice Guideline. *J Clin Oncol*. 2014;32:1964–1967.

SYMPTOM MANAGEMENT: NAUSEA, VOMITING, AND CONSTIPATION

29. **What are common treatment strategies for constipation?**
    Good hydration, ambulation or exercise, and added dietary fiber can be useful nonpharmacologic strategies. Patients with ongoing chronic constipation will benefit from stimulant laxatives such as senna (1–2 tablets by mouth twice a day) or bisacodyl (10 mg by mouth daily). Nonabsorbable osmotic laxatives such as polyethylene glycol or lactulose have strong evidence for effectiveness.

30. **What are the management options for a patient with severe opiate-induced constipation (OIC)?**
    Newer medications, including lubiprostone and linaclotide, have good clinical trial evidence of effectiveness. These drugs are intestinal secretagogues. Some data suggest the opioid receptor antagonist methylnatrexone is also effective for patients with opiate-induced constipation, though this medication is an injectable, which makes it less favorable for outpatient use.
    Wald A. Constipation: advances in diagnosis and treatment. *JAMA*. 2016;315:185–191.

31. **What are the common causes of nausea and vomiting?**
Remember the acronym "**VOMIT**":
   - **V**estibular
   - **O**bstruction of bowel
   - **D**ys**m**otility of upper gastrointestinal tract
   - **I**nfection, **i**nflammation
   - **T**oxins stimulating the chemoreceptor trigger zone
   Hallenbeck J. The causes of nausea and vomiting (V.O.M.I.T.): fast facts concept #5, Palliative Care Network of Wisconsin. Published July 2005, Updated May 2015. Available at: http://www.mypcnow.org [accessed 05.09.16].

32. **What medications are used for the treatment of nausea and vomiting in patients with serious illnesses?**
   - **Dopamine antagonists (D_2):** Metoclopromide, prochlorperazine, haloperidol, olanzapine
   - **Antihistamines (H_1):** Promethazine, diphenhydramine
   - **Serotonin antagonists (5-HT_3):** Ondansetron, granisetron, olanzapine, mirtazapine
   - **Cannabinoids (CB1):** Dronabinol
   - **Muscarinic acetylcholine:** Scopolamine, promethazine
   - **Neurokinin 1/substance P antagonists:** Aprepitant, fosaprepitant
   - **Corticosteroids:** Dexamethasone, prednisone
   Wood GJ, Shega JW, Lynch B, et al. Management of intractable nausea and vomiting in patients at the end of life: "I was feeling nauseous all of the time . . . nothing was working." *JAMA.* 2007;298:1196–1207.

33. **What therapies can be used to manage a malignant bowel obstruction?**
   - **Decompression:** Placement of a nasogastric tube or venting gastrostomy tube
   - **Hydration:** Intravenous fluids for dehydration
   - **Symptom management:** Intravenous corticosteroids (dexamethasone) and antiemetics (haloperidol, ondansetron)
   - **Antacids:** Intravenous proton pump inhibitor or H_2 blockers
   - **Antisecretory agents:** Octreotide, anticholinergic agents
   - **Analgesics:** Opiates and consideration for a patient-controlled analgesia (PCA) pump
   Laval G, Marcelin-Benazech B, Guirimand F, et al. Recommendations for bowel obstruction with peritoneal carcinomatosis. *J Pain Symptom Manage.* 2014;48:75–91.

34. **What are some of the causes of hiccups in terminally ill patients?**
Liver disease, gastroesophageal reflux disease (GERD), diaphragmatic irritation, central nervous system (CNS) tumor, and medication side effects (e.g., steroids).

35. **What medications are helpful for treatment of hiccups?**
The antipsychotic chlorpromazine is U.S. Food and Drug Administration (FDA) approved for hiccup treatment. Baclofen and gabapentin have also been found to be effective in trials, although at times hiccups can be nearly intractable.
   Hernandez JL, Pajaron M, Garcia-Regata O, et al. Gabapentin for intractable hiccup. *Am J Med.* 2004;117:279–281.
   Ramirez FC, Graham DY. Treatment of intractable hiccup with baclofen: results of a double-blind randomized, controlled, cross-over study. *Am J Gastroenterol.* 1992;87:1789–1791.

SYMPTOM MANAGEMENT: SHORTNESS OF BREATH/ DYSPNEA

36. **How can medications be used to alleviate shortness of breath?**
In addition to medications for the primary cause of a patient's shortness of breath (such as diuretics for heart failure or bronchodilators for COPD), the following interventions can be helpful:
   - **Opioids:** first-line drugs for severe shortness of breath. As mentioned previously, when dosed appropriately, opioids can ease shortness of breath without suppressing respirations.
   - **Benzodiazepines:** second-line drugs for shortness of breath and can ease the anxiety associated with severe dyspnea.

37. **Is there anything in addition to medicine to help patients who have dyspnea?**
Paying attention to proper body positioning, airway, and management of oral/nasal secretions can help. Breathing and relaxation techniques may be useful for certain situations. Room cooling and bedside fans may benefit some patients.

    Thomas JR, von Gunten CF. Management of dyspnea. *J Support Oncol.* 2003;1:23–32;discussion 32–24.

38. **Should everyone who is short of breath receive oxygen therapy?**
No. Supplemental O_2 is helpful for patients with hypoxia but is generally not better than room air for patients with normal O_2 levels.

    Kamal AH, Maguire JM, Wheeler JL, et al. Dyspnea review for the palliative care professional: treatment goals and therapeutic options. *J Palliat Med.* 2012;15:106–114.

39. **What medications can be given to help a patient with persistent cough?**
After removing any obvious triggers (including noxious environmental stimuli, infection, aspiration, or medications [such as ACE inhibitors]), symptom-directed medications, including centrally acting cough suppressants (opioids, dextromethorphan, gabapentin) or peripherally acting suppressants (benzonatate) can be used. Patients with reactive or inflammatory processes may benefit from bronchodilators or steroids.

    Wee B, Browning J, Adams A, et al. Management of chronic cough in patients receiving palliative care: review of evidence and recommendations by a task group of the Association for Palliative Medicine of Great Britain and Ireland. *Palliat Med.* 2012;26:780–787.

SYMPTOM MANAGEMENT: DEPRESSION

40. **How should depression be assessed in patients with advanced illnesses?**
Patients with advanced illness often suffer from distress or grief, which may be normal and adaptive in the context of a new diagnosis and change in life planning. Maladaptive symptoms may progress to frank depression with increasing mood symptoms such as hopelessness/helplessness, anhedonia, sleep and appetite disturbances, cognitive changes, low energy/fatigue, and suicidal ideation. All patients with cancer should be screened for depression using the Patient Health Questionnaire 9 (PHQ9).

    See also Chapter 2, General Medicine and Ambulatory Care.
    Widera EW, Block SD. Managing grief and depression at the end of life. *Am Fam Physician.* 2012;86:259–264.
    Kroenke K, Spitzer RL, Williams JB, et al. The Patient Health Questionnaire Somatic, Anxiety, and Depressive Symptom Scales: a systematic review. *Gen Hosp Psychiatry.* 2010;32:345–359.

41. **What medications are recommended for depression treatment in advanced illnesses?**
    - **Selective serotonin reuptake inhibitors (SSRIs):** Sertraline, citalopram, escitalopram, fluoxetine, and paroxetine
    - **Serotonin norepinephrine reuptake inhibitors (SNRIs):** Venlafaxine, duloxetine, desvenlafaxine
    - **Dopamine reuptake inhibitor:** Buproprion (avoid with brain tumors/metastasis due to seizure risk)
    - **Serotonin norepinephrine receptor antagonist:** Mirtazapine
    - **Psychostimulants:** Dextroamphetamine, methylphenidate, modafinil, and armodafinil
    - **Tricyclic antidepressants (TCAs):** Nortriptyline, desipramine, amitriptyline

    Cipriani A, Furukawa TA, Salanti G, et al. Comparative efficacy and acceptability of 12 new-generation antidepressants: a multiple-treatments meta-analysis. *Lancet.* 2009;373:746–758.

42. **Does psychotherapy have a role in managing depression in serious illnesses?**
Yes. Psychotherapy can be delivered to patients with serious illnesses, and specific therapies such as cognitive behavior therapy, acceptance and commitment therapy, and dignity therapy have specific roles in patients with terminal illnesses.

Table 19.3. Symptoms at the End of Life: Cancer Versus Other Causes of Death

SYMPTOM	Cause of Death	
	Cancer (%)	Other (%)
Pain	84	67
Trouble breathing	47	49
Nausea and vomiting	51	27
Sleeplessness	51	36
Confusion	33	38
Depression	38	36
Loss of appetite	71	38
Constipation	47	32
Bedsores	28	14
Incontinence	37	33

Adapted from Seale C, Cartwright A. *The Year Before Death*. Aldershot, UK: Avebury; 1994.

SYMPTOM MANAGEMENT: ANXIETY

43. **How can the physician manage anxiety in patients with serious illness?**
With both nonpharmacologic and pharmacologic approaches.
    - **Nonpharmacologic approaches:** Psychotherapy, behavioral therapies, and complementary therapies such as guided imagery may be useful in certain patients.
    - **Pharmacologic approaches:**
        - **Benzodiazepines** (for acute anxiety): Clonazepam, alprazolam, lorazepam, midazolam
        - **SSRI** (for chronic or persistent anxiety): Sertraline, fluoxetine, citalopram, and others
    In addition, providers should always look for ways to ease the underlying triggers for anxiety (such as uncertainty about treatments or expectations).
    Roth AJ, Massie MJ. Anxiety and its management in advanced cancer. *Curr Opin Support Palliat Care.* 2007;150–156.

SYMPTOM MANAGEMENT: DELIRIUM

44. **How common is delirium in patients with advanced illnesses?**
Delirium is the most common neuropsychiatric complication experienced by patients with advanced illnesses (Table 19.3). Delirium either can be attributed to a reversible cause or can be irreversible or terminal. Both require assessment and management for symptom control.

45. **How should delirium be managed without medications?**
    - Minimize immobilization with catheters, IV lines, and physical restraints.
    - Avoid immobility and institute early mobilization.
    - Provide visual and hearing aids.
    - Monitor dehydration and nutrition.
    - Control pain.
    - Monitor bowel and bladder function.
    - Avoid deliriogenic medications.
    - Place an orientation board, clock, and familiar objects in the room.
    - Minimize noise and interventions at night.

46. **Can delirium be treated with medications if nonpharmacologic strategies fail?**
Yes. Despite no medication having FDA approval for the treatment or management of delirium, many dopamine antagonist medications can improve the psychomotor and cognitive effects of delirium.
    - **Typical antipsychotics** (highest level of evidence): Haloperidol, chlorpromazine
    - **Atypical antipsychotics:** Olanzapine, risperidone, aripiprazaole, quetiapine

- **Benzodiazepines** (avoid unless agitation/aggression cannot be managed with an antipsychotic medication as there can be a paradoxical worsening of agitation): lorazepam, diazepam
  Breitbart W, Alici Y. Agitation and delirium at the end of life: "We couldn't manage him." *JAMA.* 2008;300:2898–2910.

WEBSITE

Center to Advance Palliative Care: www.capc.org

INDEX

Page numbers followed by "*f*" indicate figures, "*t*" indicate tables, and "*b*" indicate boxes.

Atrioventricular (AV) block, types of, 62
Atrophic vaginitis, 27
Atypical hemolytic uremic syndrome
  (aHUS), with complement proteins/
  factors, 273
Atypical lymphocytosis, differential
  diagnosis of, 318, 318t–319t
Atypical squamous cells of uncertain
  insignificance, 27
Autoantibodies, in systemic sclerosis, 241
Autoimmune hemolytic anemia, 364
  Coombs test for, 365
Autoimmune lymphoproliferative
  syndrome (ALPS), 274
  with hepatosplenomegaly, 275
Autoimmune regulatory (AIRE) protein,
  in thymus, 260–261
Autoinflammatory disorders, 281–282
Autonomy, 5
Auto-positive end-expiratory pressure
  (PEEP), 135
Autosomal dominant hyper-IgE
  syndrome, 274
Autosomal dominant polycystic kidney
  disease, 194t
Autosomal recessive polycystic kidney
  disease, 194t
Avascular necrosis, of bone, 256
"Average" blood cholesterol levels, MI
  survivors with, 80–81
Azathioprine, allopurinol and, 192
Azoles, 305
Azotemia, 180

B

B lymphocytes (B cells), 262
  biology, 262
  deficiencies, 262
  immunodeficiencies, 275–278
Babesia microti, 330
Bacteria overgrowth, small bowel, 166
Bacterial conjunctivitis, 38t
Bacterial infection, nephrotic syndrome
  and, 174
Bacterial meningitis, acute, 201
Balloon angioplasty, 78
Barrett esophagus, 163
Bartholin cyst, 329
Bartonella species, 308
Bartter syndrome, 206
Baseline functional status, preoperative
  interview and, 45

Basophils, 258, 259t
Bayes theorem, 67
Behçet disease (BD), 100, 247
Bell palsy, 483
Beneficence, 5
Benign (paroxysmal) positional vertigo
  (BPV/BPPV), 481
Benign primary hepatic lesions, 161
Benign prostatic hypertrophy
  (BPH), 508
Berger disease, 177
Best interest, 9
Beta blockers
  in anaphylaxis, 297
  angina pectoris and, 81
  "cardioselectivity" of, 96
  congestive heart failure and, 84–85
  with heart failure, 85
  hypertension and, 71
  intrinsic sympathomimetic activity
    and, 96
  perioperative period and, 50
Beta-D-glucan assay, 311–313
Beta-lactam antibiotic, 303
Betamethasone, potencies and effects of,
  287t
Bethesda titer, 396
Bezoars, 167
Bicipital tendinitis, detecting, 221
Biguanides, for type 2 diabetes mellitus,
  436t
Bile acid resin sequestrants, 95
Biliary tract disease, 168–169
  air in biliary system, 168–169
  Charcot triad, 168
  computed tomography and, 168
  endoscopic ultrasound and, 168
  in ethnic groups, 168–169
  gallstones, 168–169
  liver scans in, 168
  magnetic retrograde
    cholangiopancreatography
    (MRCP) in, 168
  obstructive jaundice, 168
  Reynold pentad, 168
Binet staging system, 382t
Binocular diplopia
  differential diagnosis of, 480
  localization of, 480
Biologic disease-modifying
  antirheumatic drugs, 232, 232t
Biologic warfare agents, 314t–315t

Sleep study, 476
SLICC. *see* Systemic Lupus International
    Collaboration Clinics
SLR. *see* Straight leg raising
Small airways, 109
Small bowel bacteria overgrowth, 166
Small bowel ileus, 167
Small bowel obstruction, 167–168
Small cell carcinoma, 133
Small cell lung cancer (SCLC)
    stages of, 421
        IV, 422
    treatment of, 421–422
Small intestine neoplasms, 150
Smell, acute loss/impairment of, 34
Sodium bicarbonate, 205
Soft tissue calcification, diseases
    associated with, 226
Soft tissue rheumatism, 253–254
    de Quervain tenosynovitis
      and, 254
    fibromyalgia and, 253–254
    patellofemoral syndrome and, 254
Solitary pulmonary nodule (SPN), 114
Somatostatinomas, 150
SPACE organisms, 308–309
Specificity of tests, 12, 12f
Speech, slurred, 479
Speed test, for bicipital tendinitis, 221
Spherocytosis, 365
SPICE organisms, 308–309
SPIKES acronym, 518
Spinal anesthesia, 43
Spinal cord compression
    diagnosis of, 407
    malignancies causing, 407
    signs and symptoms of, 407
    treatment of, 407
Spinal stenosis syndrome, 249
Spirituality, 517–518
Splenectomy, 33, 365
SPN. *see* Solitary pulmonary nodule
Spondyloarthropathies, 243–245
    ankylosing spondylitis and, 244
    definition of, 243–245
    HLA-B27 with, 243
    osteophyte in, 244
    psoriasis and, 244
    psoriatic arthritis and, 244
    reactive arthritis and, 244
    Schober test in, 221
    syndesmophyte in, 244

Spontaneous bacterial peritonitis (SBP),
    327
Spurious hyponatremia, 200
Sputum sample, pneumonia and, 325
Squamous cell carcinoma, of esophagus
    incidence of, 409–414
    risk factors for, 409
Squeeze test, 220
SSRIs. *see* Selective serotonin reuptake
    inhibitors
St. Vitus dance, 249
ST elevation myocardial infarction
    (STEMI), 72
    ACE inhibitor, ARB, and aldosterone
      antagonist from, 80
    treatment of, 74–75
Stalk effect, 446
Stanford classification system, 101
Staphylococcus aureus, 307
Staphylococcus haemolyticus, 307
Staphylococcus lugdunensis, 307
Staphylococcus saprophyticus, 307
Statins, 81, 95–96
    stroke prevention, 488
Status approach, decisional capacity and,
    8
Status epilepticus, 491
    management of, 491
Stavudine, for human immunodeficiency
    virus infection, 340t
Steatorrhea, 166
STEMI. *see* ST elevation myocardial
    infarction
Stevens-Johnson syndrome, 299
Still disease, 255
Straight leg raising (SLR), in low back
    pain, 221
Streptokinase, 76
"Stress tests", 49
Stroke, 486–489, 489b
    antiplatelet therapy in, 488
    behavioral risk factors assessed in, 488
    hemorrhagic, causes and locations of,
      489, 489t
    ischemic
      blood pressure controlled in, 488
      mechanisms of, 486
      treatment of, 486
    severity of, standard rating scale for,
      487
    tests for, 486
Stroke-in-evolution, 106